Oncologic Imaging: Urology

Seung Hyup Kim • Jeong Yeon Cho
Editors

Oncologic Imaging: Urology

Springer

Editors
Seung Hyup Kim
Department of Radiology
Seoul National University Hospital
Seoul
Korea

Jeong Yeon Cho
Department of Radiology
Seoul National University Hospital
Seoul
Korea

ISBN 978-3-662-45217-2 ISBN 978-3-662-45218-9 (eBook)
DOI 10.1007/978-3-662-45218-9

Library of Congress Control Number: 2016953772

Printed on acid-free paper

This Springer imprint is published by Springer Nature
The registered company is Springer-Verlag GmbH Berlin Heidelberg

Preface

Today's medicine is directing patient-centered multidisciplinary approach, and imaging is an integral part of it. In line with this direction, "Oncologic Imaging: Urology" is a book presenting oncological diseases of the urinary tract including renal tumors, urothelial tumors, prostatic tumors, tumors of the male genitalia, adrenal tumors, and retroperitoneal tumors.

This book was edited and written by specialists of urologic oncology in radiology, urology, pathology, nuclear medicine, and radiation oncology of the Seoul National University Hospital and the members of the Korean Society of Urogenital Radiology. We deeply appreciate all contributors named and unnamed for their works for this book. We hope this book is read by physicians of a variety of specialties who are interested in oncological diseases of the urinary tract.

Seoul, Korea — Seung Hyup Kim, MD
Seoul, Korea — Jeong Yeon Cho, MD

Contents

Contributors

Gi Jeong Cheon Department of Nuclear Medicine, Seoul National University Hospital, Seoul National University College of Medicine, Seoul, Republic of Korea

Jeong Yeon Cho Department of Radiology, Seoul National University Hospital, Seoul National University College of Medicine, Seoul, Korea

Hyuck Jae Choi Department of Radiology, Kangwon National University Hospital, Seoul National University College of Medicine, Gangwon-do, Seoul, Republic of Korea

Seung Beom Ha Seoul Urology Group, Seoul, Republic of Korea

Keon Wook Kang Department of Nuclear Medicine, Seoul National University Hospital, Seoul National University College of Medicine, Seoul, Republic of Korea

Minyong Kang Department of Urology, Seoul National University Hospital, Seoul, Republic of Korea

Bohyun Kim Department of Radiology, Mayo Clinic, Rochester, MN, USA

Hyung Suk Kim Department of Urology, Seoul National University Hospital, Seoul, Republic of Korea

Jin Ho Kim Department of Radiation Oncology, Seoul National University Hospital, Seoul National University College of Medicine, Seoul, Republic of Korea

Myong Kim Department of Urology, Asan Medical Center, University of Ulsan College of Medicine, Seoul, Republic of Korea

Seung Hyup Kim Department of Radiology, Seoul National University, Seoul, Korea

Sun Ho Kim Department of Radiology, National Cancer Center, Gyeonggi-do, Seoul, Republic of Korea

Ja Hyeon Ku Department of Urology, Seoul National University Hospital, Seoul National University College of Medicine, Seoul, Republic of Korea

Cheol Kwak Department of Urology, Seoul National University Hospital, Seoul National University College of Medicine, Seoul, Republic of Korea

Hak Jong Lee Department of Radiology, Bundang Seoul National University Hospital, Seoul National University College of Medicine, Gyeonggi-do, Seoul, Republic of Korea

Young Ju Lee Department of Urology, Incheon St. Mary's Hospital, The Catholic University of Korea, Incheon, Republic of Korea

Kyung Chul Moon Department of Pathology, Seoul National University Hospital, Seoul National University College of Medicine, Seoul, Republic of Korea

Min Hoan Moon Department of Radiology, SMG-SNU Boramae Medical Center, Seoul National University College of Medicine, Seoul, Republic of Korea

Byung Kwan Park Department of Radiology, Samsung Medical Center, Sungkyunkwan University School of Medicine, Seoul, Republic of Korea

Chang Kyu Sung Department of Radiology, SMG-SNU Boramae Medical Center, Seoul National University College of Medicine, Seoul, Republic of Korea

Renal Tumors

1

Sun Ho Kim, Seung Hyup Kim, Byung Kwan Park, Keon Wook Kang, Kyung Chul Moon, Cheol Kwak, Young Ju Lee, and Jin Ho Kim

1.1 Introduction

Malignant renal cell tumor (renal cell carcinoma: RCC) is the most common malignant renal tumor, and the most common benign renal tumor is angiomyolipoma (AML). Malignant renal mesenchymal tumor (sarcoma) is rare. Other renal tumors include oncocytoma, metanephric adenoma, mixed epithelial and stromal tumor, rare mesenchymal tumors such as leiomyoma or hemangioma, nephroblastoma, and neuroendocrine tumors. Lymphoma and metastasis should be differentiated from these primary renal tumors.

Most renal masses are detected by ultrasonography (US), but computed tomography (CT) is considered as the dominant imaging modality for evaluating renal masses, especially for RCC in its staging and treatment planning. Some subtypes of RCC show typical CT finding and can be differentiated from other subtypes, which is important in planning treatment and expecting prognosis. Magnetic resonance imaging (MRI) is usually used in limited cases, in which US and CT fail to give sufficient information.

1.2 Detection

Although most renal masses are discovered incidentally, some tumors are detected during the work-up of patients' symptoms such as hematuria or flank pain. Most symptomatic tumors are large,

S.H. Kim (✉)
Department of Radiology, National Cancer Center, Goyang, Gyeonggi-do, Republic of Korea
e-mail: 11888@ncc.re.kr

S.H. Kim (✉)
Department of Radiology, Seoul National University, Seoul, Korea
e-mail: kimshrad@snu.ac.kr

B.K. Park
Department of Radiology, Samsung Medical Center, Sungkyunkwan University School of Medicine, Seoul, Republic of Korea

K.W. Kang
Department of Nuclear Medicine, Seoul National University Hospital, Seoul National University College of Medicine, Seoul, Republic of Korea

K.C. Moon
Department of Pathology, Seoul National University Hospital, Seoul National University College of Medicine, Seoul, Republic of Korea

C. Kwak
Department of Urology, Seoul National University Hospital, Seoul National University College of Medicine, Seoul, Republic of Korea

Y.J. Lee
Department of Urology, Seoul National University Hospital, Seoul, Republic of Korea

J.H. Kim
Department of Radiation Oncology, Seoul National University Hospital, Seoul National University College of Medicine, Seoul, Republic of Korea

S.H. Kim, J.Y. Cho (eds.), *Oncologic Imaging: Urology*, DOI 10.1007/978-3-662-45218-9_1

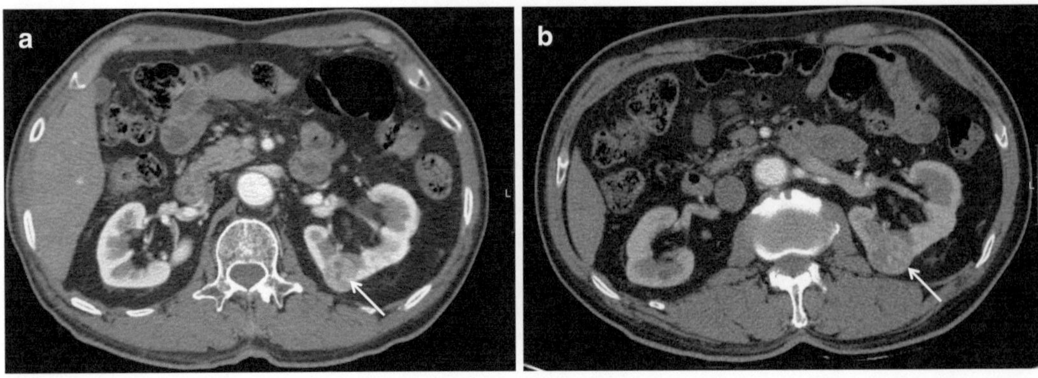

Fig. 1.1 Small RCC discovered incidentally on CT. (**a**) Contrast-enhanced CT shows a 2.4 cm-sized, hypervascular mass (*arrow*) in the left kidney. (**b**) The diameter of the mass increased as much as 2 mm during 2-year follow-up without metastasis. Clear cell RCC was confirmed after partial nephrectomy

but even small renal masses can cause significant symptom, and renin-producing juxtaglomerular cell tumor (reninoma) is an example. RCC with renal vein thrombus may be an underlying cause of scrotal varicocele, especially on the right side where the incidence is relatively rare.

Most renal masses are detected on imaging performed for no or unrelated symptom. These masses are usually small, mostly smaller than 3 cm in diameter (Fig. 1.1). Some lesions are too small to characterize on imaging. Because most incidentally discovered renal mass (incidentaloma) is detected by US, the first step is the differentiation of these lesions from pseudotumor, a mass-like finding that mimics a neoplasm. The most common renal pseudotumor is congenital variations or anomalies such as a prominent column of Bertin and dromedary hump. Doppler US can be helpful in the differential diagnosis to show normal vascular pattern in these pseudotumors [1, 2]. Echogenic mass such as AMLs or small RCCs can be easily detected on US. 50 % of small RCC (<3 cm) can be detected by US. However, isoechoic masses, masses embedded totally in renal parenchyma, or masses located in polar regions are apt to be missed.

1.3 Characterization

1.3.1 US

Renal masses can be divided into solid and cystic lesions. Although it is well known that US is accurate in differentiating between cystic and solid renal masses, it is also known that often this differentiation is difficult. Sometimes a homogeneous solid renal mass may be difficult to differentiate from a simple renal cyst if it accompanies posterior sonic enhancement and edge shadowing. The diagnosis of a simple renal cyst can be made if a renal mass is round, well demarcated, and anechoic and accompanies posterior acoustic enhancement. If a renal mass does not meet these criteria but also does not appear as an overt RCC, it can be defined as an indeterminate renal mass and should be evaluated further. Indeterminate renal masses can be categorized into mainly cystic, mixed cystic and solid, and mainly solid renal masses, and the amount of solid portions is important in the suspicion of malignancy [1, 2].

Although the main role of US in renal masses is detection and CT or MRI is usually used for further characterization, US may be required to provide additional information of renal masses detected on CT or MRI. Technical advances in US including tissue harmonic imaging, Doppler US, and contrast-enhanced US (CEUS) increase the ability of US in characterizing renal masses (Fig. 1.2).

1.3.1.1 Solid Renal Mass

The most common solid renal tumor is RCC. Solid renal mass on US in adult should be considered as RCC unless strong evidence of other tumors is present. Differential diagnosis includes AML, oncocytoma, adenoma, lymphomas, metastases, and various benign mesenchymal tumors and sarcomas. A study showed that oncocytomas and

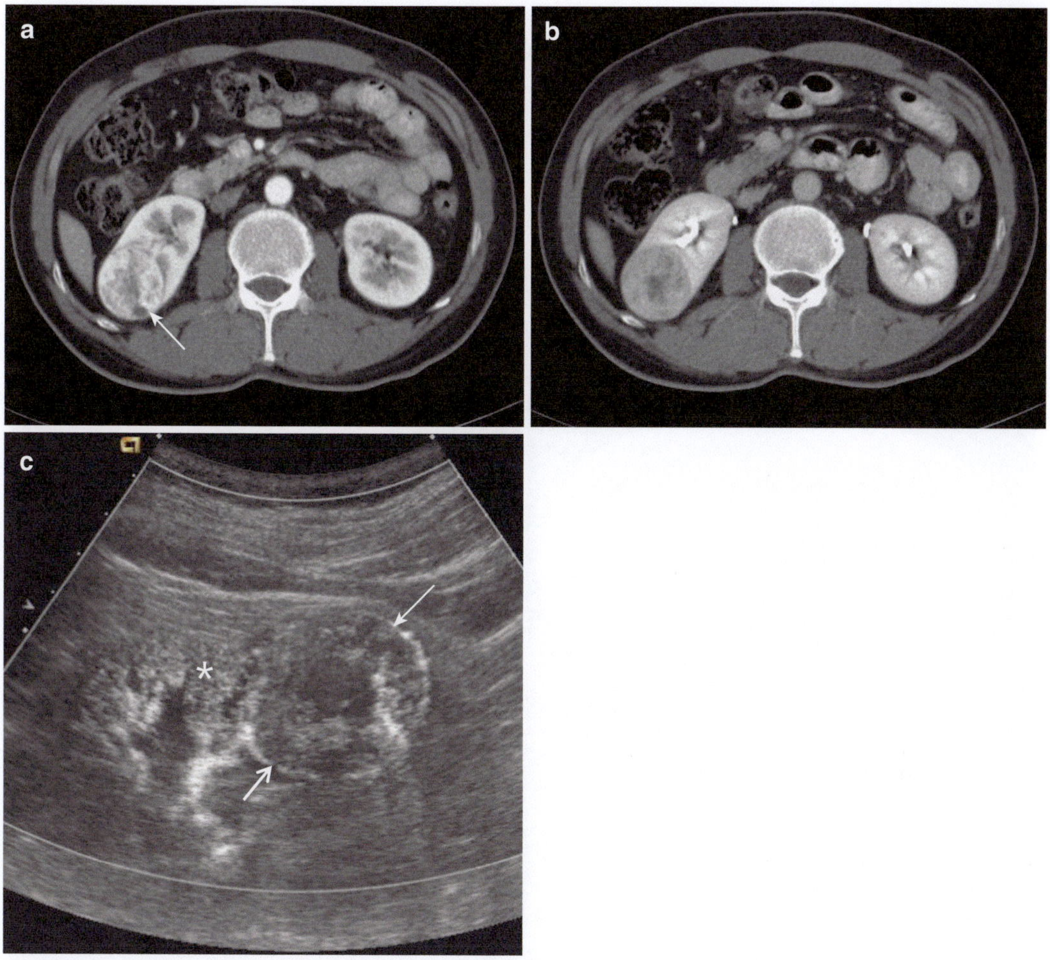

Fig. 1.2 Clear cell RCC. (**a**) Contrast-enhanced CT in corticomedullary phase shows a hypervascular mass (*arrow*) in the right kidney. The degree of the enhancement is similar to that of the renal cortex. (**b**) In nephrographic phase, the mass enhances less than the renal parenchyma. (**c**) Contrast-enhanced US shows early enhancement of the mass (*arrows*), similar to the renal cortex (*)

AMLs were almost all of benign masses (12.8 %) among 2770 solid renal masses that were surgically removed [3]. AML can show typical US findings such as bright high echo comparable to renal sinus fat (Fig. 1.3). Small RCCs are also usually hyperechoic but may show characteristic findings such as intratumoral cysts and hypoechoic rim (Fig. 1.4). Lymphomas and metastases may be differentiated by clinical settings, but other tumors usually show nonspecific US finding, and other imaging modalities such as CT or MRI are required for further characterization.

1.3.1.2 Cystic Renal Mass

Simple cyst is the most common renal mass detected incidentally. If a cystic mass does not show typical findings of a simple cyst on US, it should be considered a complicated cyst. In evaluating cystic masses based on US findings, internal echoes, septa, wall thickness, calcification, and mural nodularity are important in assessing the risk of malignancy.

Bosniak proposed a four-category classification system of cystic renal masses. Although it is based on CT findings, this classification is widely used also in US or MRI [4].

Bosniak I: Clearly simple cysts that have hairline-thin wall without septa, calcifications, or solid components. Hounsfield units (HU) of CT in the content is usually smaller than 20 (0–20), and does not enhance.

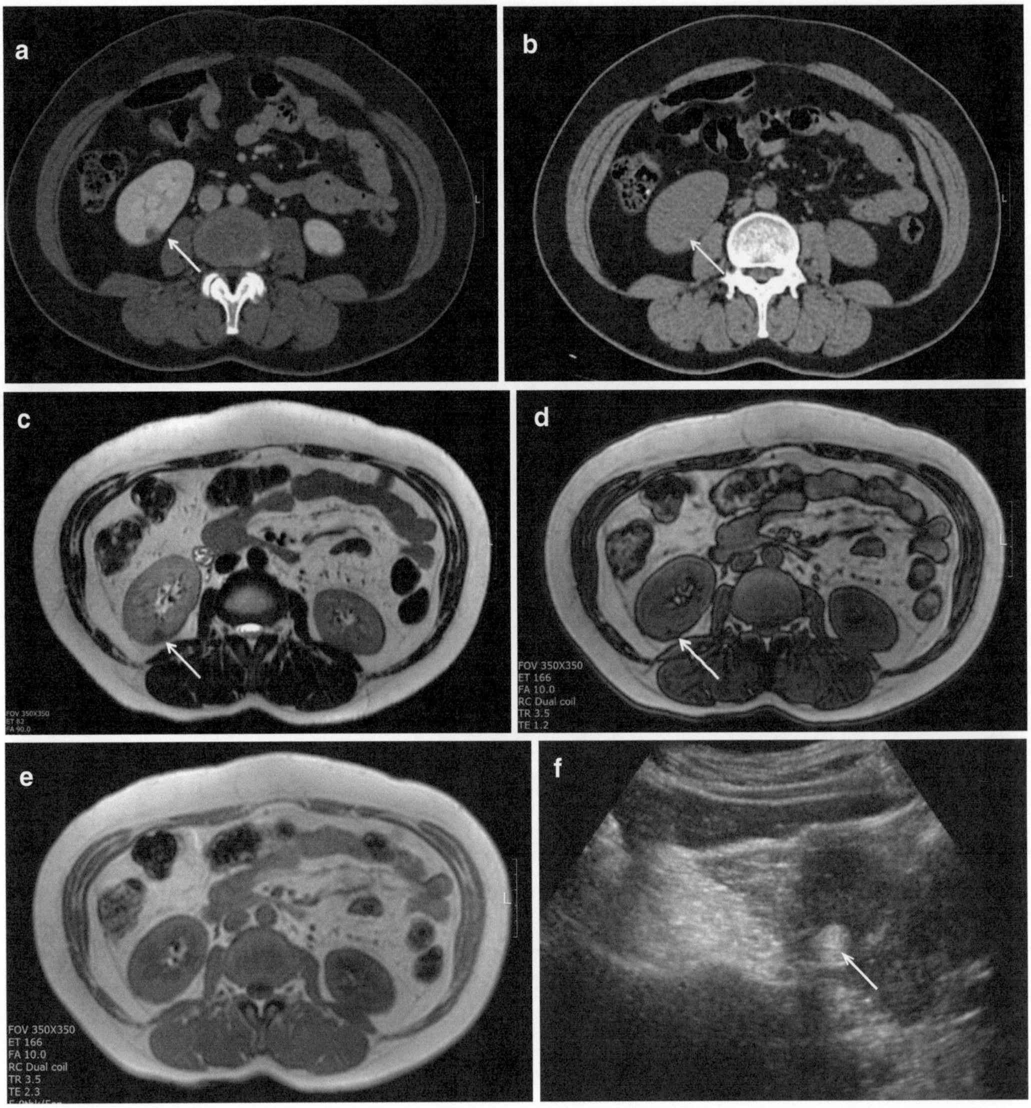

Fig. 1.3 AML. (**a**) Contrast-enhanced CT shows a small, poorly enhancing mass (*arrow*) in the right kidney. (**b**) Noncontrast CT shows subtle low attenuation in the mass (*arrow*). (**c**) The mass (*arrow*) shows low SI on T2-weighted MR image. (**d, e**) Small area of signal drop (*arrow*) is detected in the mass on out-of-phase T1-weighted MR image (**d**) compared with in-phase image (**e**). (**f**) The mass appears as a brightly high-echoic mass (*arrow*) on US

Bosniak II: Minimally complicated cysts with few, thin septa, or thin, fine calcification. The septa may be minimally thickened (Fig. 1.5).

Bosniak III: More complicated cystic masses that contain thick or irregular walls or septa in which enhancement can be measured (Fig. 1.6).

Bosniak IV: Clearly malignant cystic masses that not only contain all the characteristics of Bosniak III lesions but also contain enhancing soft tissue components adjacent to, but independently of, the wall of septa. Most malignant complex renal cysts are cystic renal cell carcinomas (Fig. 1.7).

In Bosniak classification, the probability of malignancy is virtually 0 % for I and almost 100 % for IV. The problem in this classification is almost always the differentiation between II and III, because the criteria are apt to be subjective. In 1993, Bosniak added class IIF, which is a little bit more complicated than class II, but less than class III, and so needs close follow-up (Fig. 1.8).

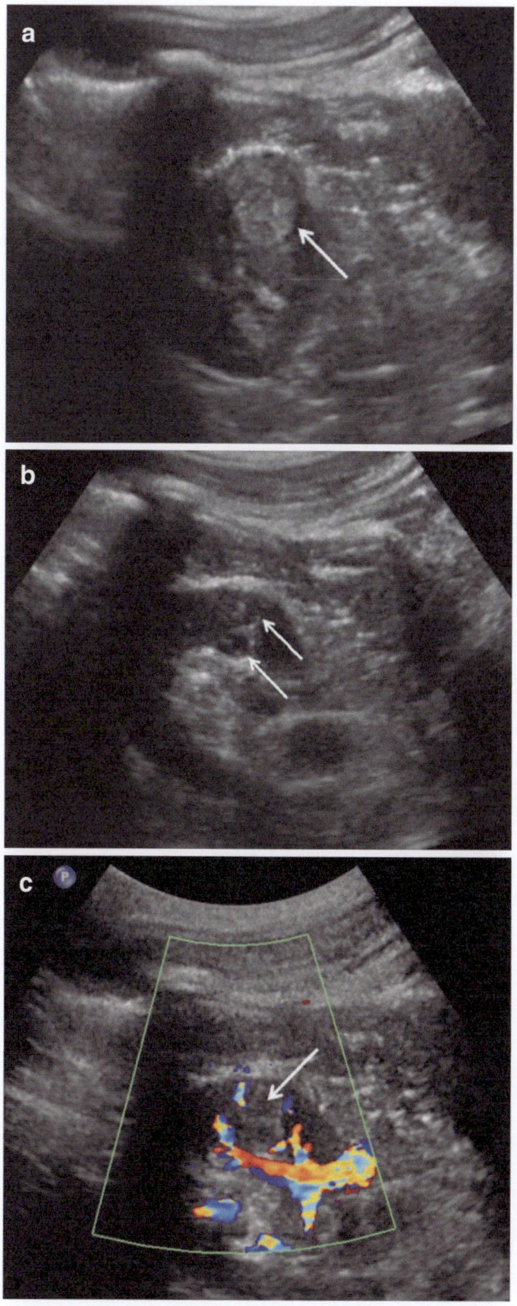

Fig. 1.4 US of small RCC. (**a**) About 2 cm-sized, high-echoic mass shows low-echoic rim (*arrow*). (**b**) Small cysts (*arrows*) are visible in the mass on another plane. (**c**) Increased vascularity is noted around the mass (*arrows*) on color Doppler US

Malignant risk of Bosniak IIF and III lesions is known as 5–10 % and 40–60 %, respectively [5]. A recent study retrospectively evaluated the outcome of Bosniak IIF and III cysts and reported higher malignancy rate (25 %) in IIF

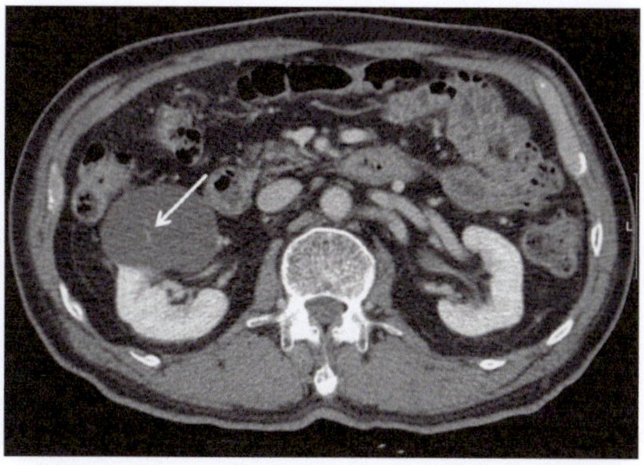

Fig. 1.5 Bosniak II cyst. Thin septal calcification (*arrow*) is noted on contrast-enhanced CT

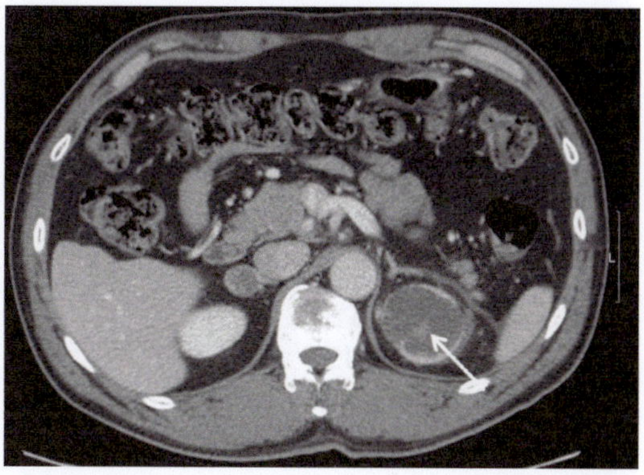

Fig. 1.6 Bosniak III cyst. Irregular wall and nodular thickening of a septum (*arrow*) is visible on contrast-enhanced CT. This cyst turned out to be cystic nephroma after surgery

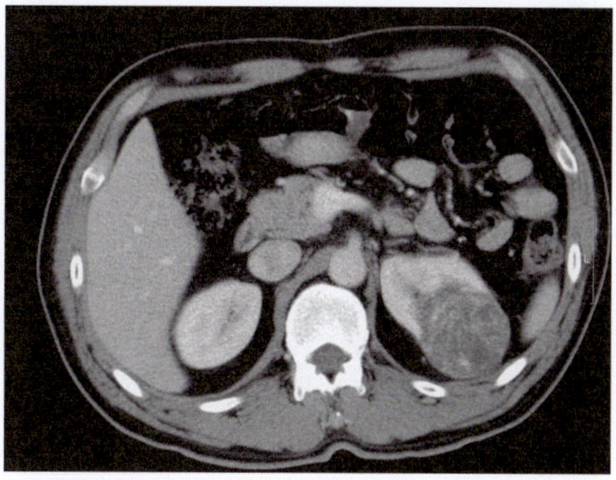

Fig. 1.7 Bosniak IV cyst. A complex cystic lesion in the left kidney shows multiple irregular septa with enhancement on contrast-enhanced CT. Multilocular cystic RCC was the pathologic diagnosis

lesions and similar rate (54 %) in III lesions. However, in this study, resected Bosniak IIF

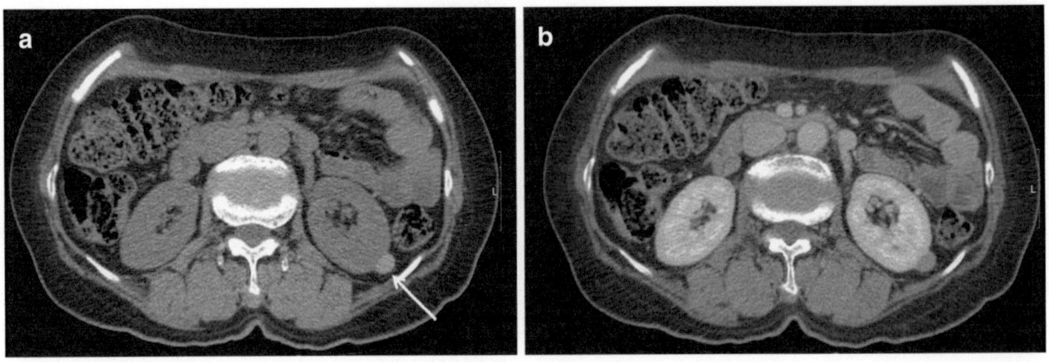

Fig. 1.8 Bosniak IIF cyst. (**a**). Noncontrast CT shows a hyperattenuating nodule (*arrow*) in the left kidney. (**b**). This nodule shows no definite enhancement on contrast-enhanced CT, suggesting hemorrhagic cyst

lesions were highly selected in patients with a high number of risk factors associated with malignancy: a history of primary renal malignancy, coexisting Bosniak IV lesion, and/or solid renal neoplasm [6].

1.3.1.3 Doppler US and Contrast-Enhanced US

Color Doppler US (CDUS) or power Doppler US (PDUS) can be helpful in evaluating indeterminate renal masses by depicting vascularity in the mass (Fig. 1.4). Increased vascularity in a renal mass can suggest malignancy, whereas the absence of flow signals may suggest high likelihood of benign lesion. However, the presence of flow signals in the septa of a cystic mass does not always indicate malignancy, because benign neoplasms such as cystic nephroma or even nonneoplastic cysts may show flow signals in the septa. Flow signals on CDUS or PDUS should be confirmed by using spectral Doppler US, because artifacts may mimic flow signals.

Contrast-enhanced Doppler US can increase the detection of intratumoral vascularity compared to CDUS and PDUS. Recent development of contrast-enhanced harmonic US imaging has provided for a better assessment of the vascular morphology and the enhancing patterns of renal tumors, such as early enhancement and washout of RCC, in contrast to delayed and prolonged enhancement of AML (Fig. 1.2). Ultrasound contrast agents are strictly intravascular and not excreted by or retained in kidneys, so that they can be used in patients with renal failure or urinary obstruction, unlike CT or MRI. Because CEUS is very sensitive for vascularity, it is especially useful in the differential diagnosis of hypovascular renal tumors or the detection of blood flow in the septa of complex renal cysts, even if enhancement on CT is equivocal [7]. A study showed higher sensitivity of CEUS in the diagnosis of hypovascular renal tumors compared with contrast CT (94.4% vs 88.9%) [8]. In a prospective study comparing CEUS with CT in the assessment of complex renal cysts, CEUS was proved to be appropriate for renal cyst classification with the Bosniak system, and complete concordance between CT and CEUS was observed regarding the need for surgery [9]. Another study demonstrated the superiority of CEUS as compared to grayscale US and to CT for the diagnosis of complex renal cysts [10].

1.3.2 CT

1.3.2.1 Unenhanced CT

Renal cysts show low attenuation (0–20 HU) on CT images regardless of contrast enhancement, but hemorrhagic cysts may show higher attenuation on unenhanced CT. These high-attenuation cysts should be categorized as Bosniak IIF, and follow-up is required (Fig. 1.8). Complicated cysts may show septal or wall calcifications, and close comparison with contrast-enhanced images should be made to differentiate from enhancing part. Solid RCCs usually show attenuation similar to surrounding renal parenchyma. However,

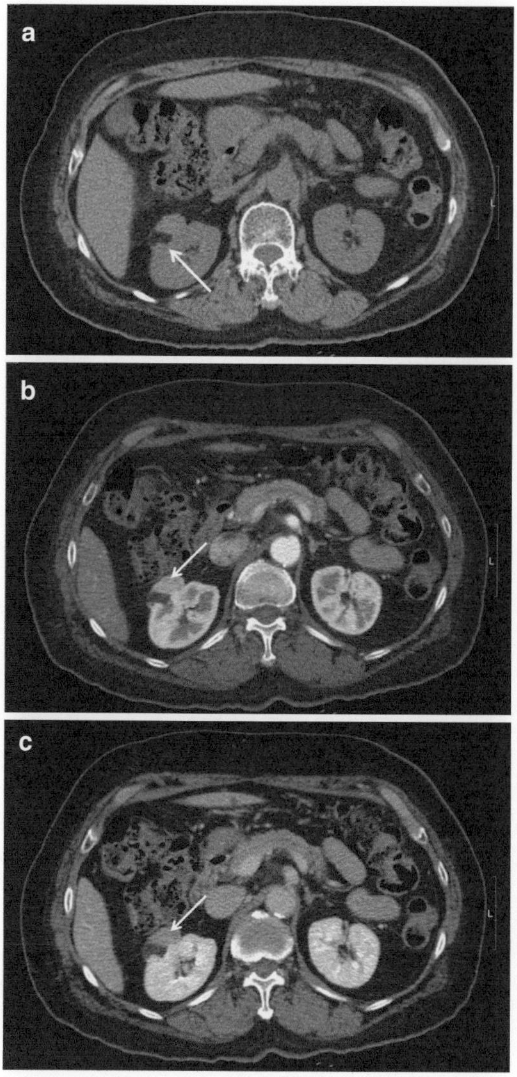

Fig. 1.9 AML. (**a**) Noncontrast CT shows fatty component (*arrow*) of a mass in the right kidney. (**b**, **c**) Nonfatty component of the mass (*arrow*) enhances well in corticomedullary phase (**b**) and shows persistent enhancement in nephrographic phase (**c**)

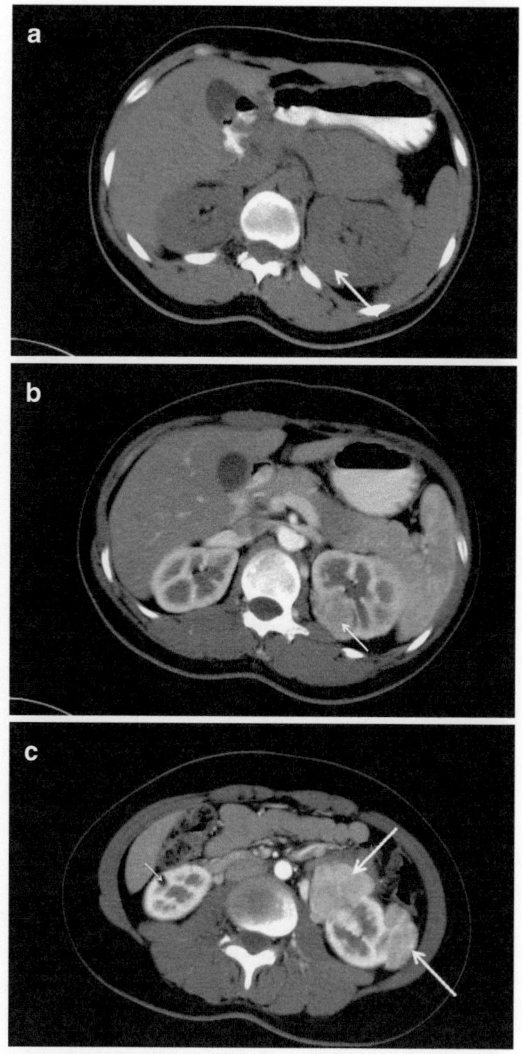

Fig. 1.10 Multiple AMLs in tuberous sclerosis. (**a**) Noncontrast CT shows a hyperattenuating mass (*arrow*) without detectable fatty component in the left kidney. (**b**) This mass (*arrow*) shows heterogeneous enhancement on contrast-enhanced CT. (**c**) Other AMLs (*arrows*) are also found in bilateral kidneys. Note fatty component of an AML (*small arrow*) in the right kidney

the attenuation becomes heterogeneous in large tumors due to hemorrhage or necrosis. Calcifications in a renal mass may suggest malignancy, because RCCs can contain calcifications but AMLs do not. AMLs usually show higher attenuation than RCCs on unenhanced CT and contain low-attenuation part comparable to fat (Fig. 1.9). However, 5 % of AMLs do not contain enough fat to be detected on CT (Fig. 1.10). In these fat-free or fat-deficient AMLs, the analysis of the shape and the enhancement pattern of the mass may be clues for the differentiation.

A recent study with 193 pathologically proven RCCs reported that all RCCs contained substantial noncalcified regions that measured 20–70 HU in ROI attenuation on unenhanced CT. Therefore, indeterminate renal lesions on unenhanced CT measuring within this range warrant further workup, whereas lesions that fall entirely outside this range may be considered benign [11].

1.3.2.2 Contrast Enhancement

Renal masses that do not enhance after the injection of contrast material are almost always benign, such as Bosniak I and II cysts. Enhancement in the septa and the wall of a cyst raises the probability of malignancy, and the enhancing solid part strongly suggests the malignancy. However, in small renal masses, enhancement itself is not definite evidence of malignancy because several investigators have reported that about 20 % of the enhancing renal masses smaller than 4 cm turned out to be benign tumors after surgery [12]. On the other hand, severely necrotic masses may fail to demonstrate contrast enhancement in rare instances. Hemorrhage in the mass may mask subtle or small enhancing part, and close comparison with unenhanced CT or follow-up is required. In mildly enhancing lesions, true enhancement should be differentiated from pseudoenhancement due to strongly enhancing renal parenchyma. Although there is no strict cutoff value, a threshold of 20 HU is commonly used to indicate definitive enhancement and values of less than 10 HU as indicating no enhancement [13].

Dynamic contrast enhancement is essential for the differential diagnosis of solid renal masses. RCCs usually show strong enhancement on early or corticomedullary phase, and lower attenuation than renal parenchyma on delayed or nephrographic/excretory phase (Fig. 1.2). This is true in most clear cell-type RCCs, but may be not in other types, such as papillary or chromophobe type. AMLs show variable degree of enhancement according to the ratio of components in the mass. Strong and early enhancement may be visible in AMLs with dominant angiomatous component, and the differentiation from RCC may be difficult. However, most AMLs show less and delayed enhancement compared with clear cell-type RCCs [14, 15].

1.3.3 MRI

MRI can be useful in some circumstances to further evaluate a renal mass. It is usually used as a problem-solving modality in suspicious or undetermined renal masses. MRI can replace CT if patients cannot receive iodinated contrast agent. Furthermore, if the lesion has features such as endophytic property, small size (<1 cm), equivocal enhancement, or confluent areas of dense calcification, MRI may give more sensitive or specific information than CT.

1.3.3.1 Signal Intensity

Cyst or cystic masses show low signal intensity (SI) on T1-weighted image (T1WI) and high SI on T2-weighted image (T2WI), identical to water. Hemorrhagic cysts show various signal, and recent hemorrhage tends to show high SI on T1WI and low SI on T2WI. The septa and wall of complicated cysts usually show low SI on T2WI. Most solid renal lesions appear isointense to the surrounding normal renal parenchyma on T1WI and variable in SI on T2WI. Therefore, SI itself cannot provide many clues to the diagnosis. Chemical shift imaging is helpful to detect small amount of fat in AMLs, which may show signal drop on out-of-phase images (Fig. 1.3). However, this should be interpreted with caution because a similar signal drop can be visible in clear cell RCC due to intracytoplasmic lipid [16]. Renal mass signal on T2WI may be helpful in differentiating fat-deficient AML from clear cell RCC. Fat-deficient AML shows low SI due to its smooth muscle content, whereas clear cell RCC usually shows iso- or high SI on T2WI. Papillary RCC, however, also shows low SI on T2WI. Therefore, T2WI cannot be used to differentiate papillary RCC from AML (Figs. 1.3 and 1.11).

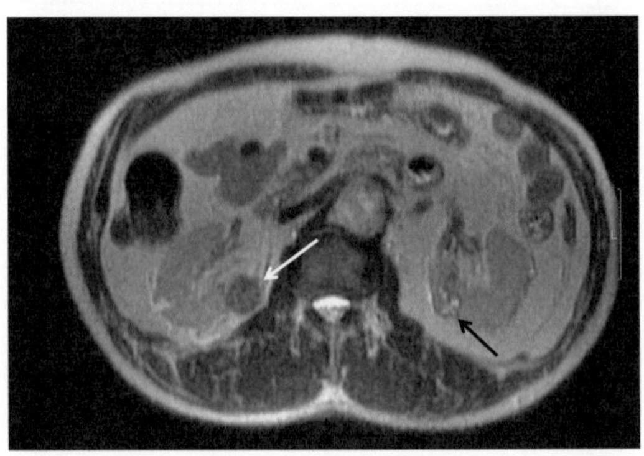

Fig. 1.11 Clear cell RCC in the left kidney and papillary RCC in the right kidney in the same patient. T2-weighted MR image shows bilateral renal masses (*arrows*). The right renal mass shows low SI but the left mass appears as a heterogeneous mass with high SI

1.3.3.2 Contrast Enhancement

Gadolinium-enhanced dynamic images can increase the diagnostic accuracy of renal masses. However, in MRI, there is no widely accepted method in determining enhancement objectively in renal masses. Subjective comparison of unenhanced and contrast-enhanced images is usually used and may be useful in hypervascular tumors, but the detection of enhancement may be difficult in hypovascular tumors. Hyperintense masses on unenhanced T1WI, such as hemorrhagic masses, are another problem in evaluating enhancement.. In such cases, subtraction technique can be helpful to detect enhancement (Fig. 1.12), and calculation of percent enhancement using arbitrary SI units can be also applied [17, 18].

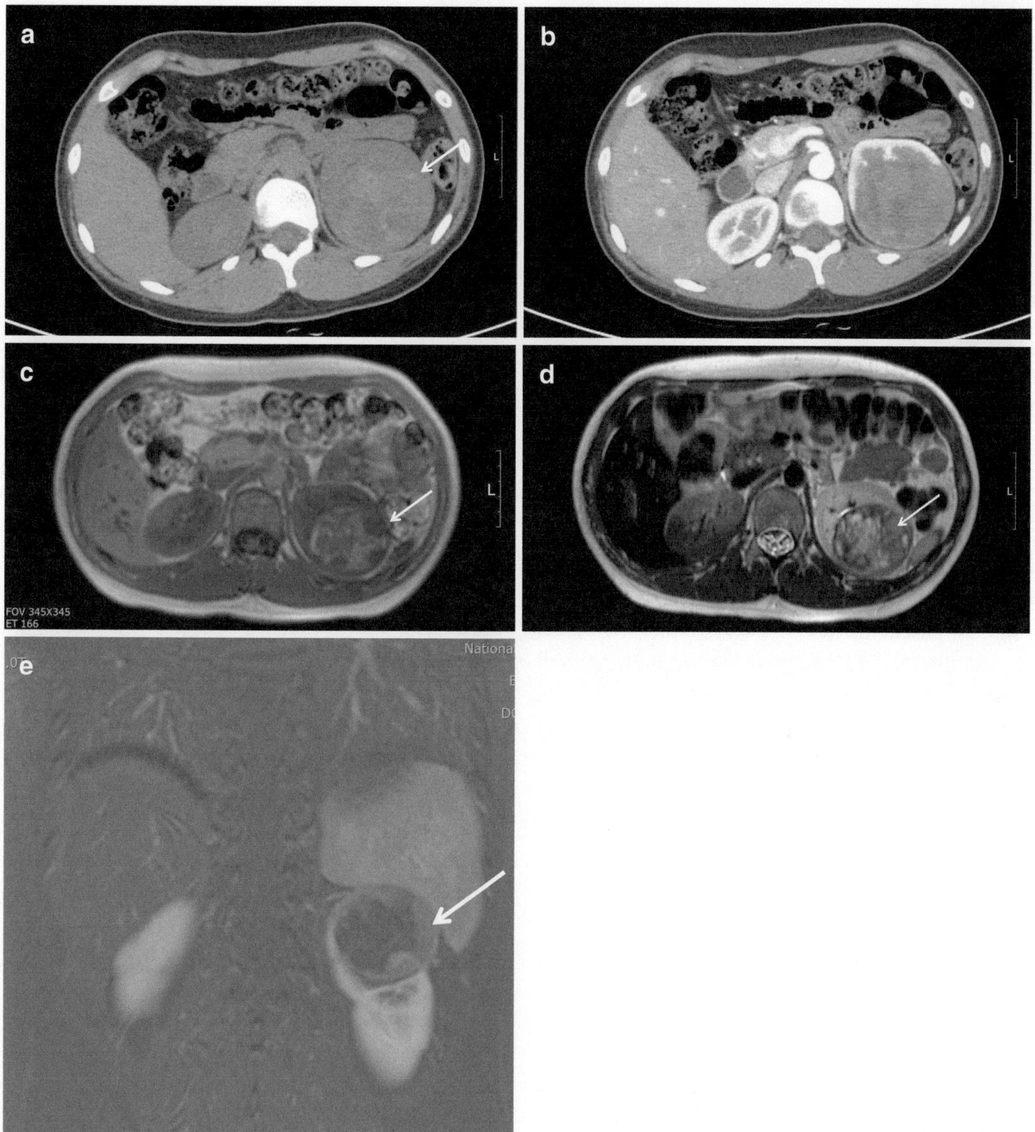

Fig. 1.12 Xp11.2 translocation–TFE3 gene fusion carcinoma. (**a**) Noncontrast CT shows a heterogeneous, highly attenuating mass (*arrow*) in the left kidney, suggesting hemorrhage inside. (**b**) The enhancement in the mass is difficult to assess due to hemorrhage. (**c**, **d**) The mass (*arrow*) shows high SI on T1WI of MRI (**c**) and heterogeneous SI on T2WI (**d**). (**e**). Subtraction image obtained from dynamic contrast-enhanced MRI shows mildly enhancing component (*arrow*) in the mass

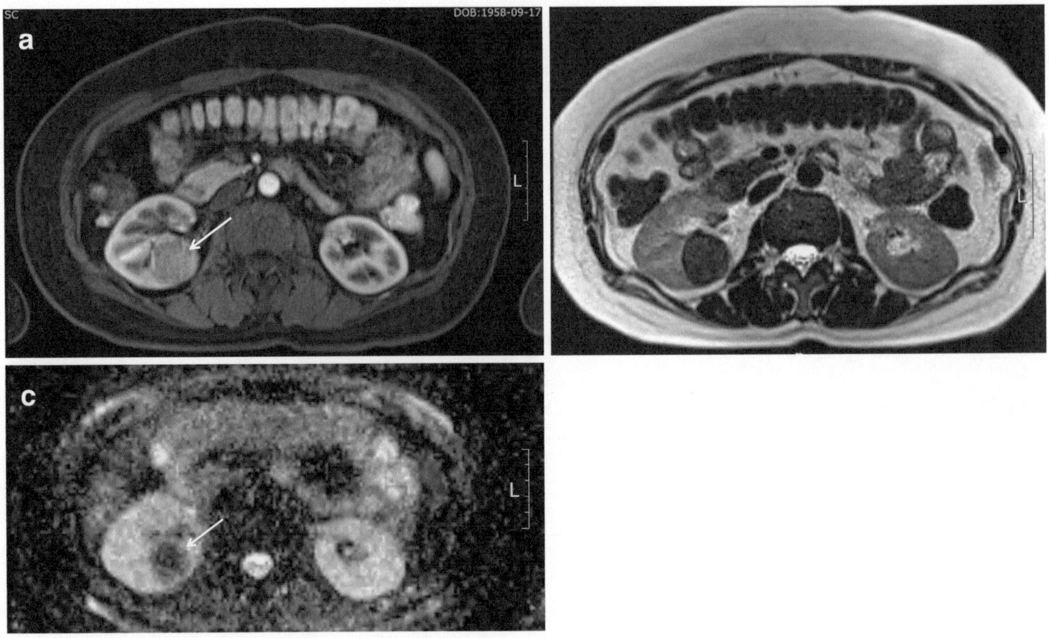

Fig. 1.13 Diffusion-weighted MR imaging of RCC. (**a**) Contrast-enhanced T1WI of MR shows a round, mildly enhancing mass (*arrow*). (**b**) The mass shows low SI on T2WI. Note low-SI rim (*arrow*) in the periphery of the mass. (**c**) The mass (*arrow*) shows decreased diffusion on ADC image

1.3.3.3 Diffusion-Weighted Imaging (DWI)

DWI is a functional MR imaging based on the diffusion of water molecules in biological tissues. Apparent diffusion coefficient (ADC) can be calculated and mapped on imaging, which reflects the random thermal motion of protons. DWI in renal masses can be useful in identifying solid renal masses and evaluating the possibility of malignancy (Fig. 1.13). Previous studies suggested that DWI could provide comparable accuracy to contrast-enhanced MRI in identifying renal lesions, and combined DWI and contrast-enhanced MRI had more specificity when compared to using those two methods alone [19]. ADC values of malignant solid masses are known to be lower than those of benign masses. Furthermore, the mean ADC value of clear cell RCC was reported to be significantly higher than other subtypes [20]. In a recent study with 3.0Tesla DWI MRI, the mean ADC value was significantly lower in RCC than in normal renal parenchyma, and the ADC value was also statistically different between clear cell RCC and other subtypes of RCCs [21]. However, objective evaluation of DWI is not easy because there is substantial inter- and intra-scanner variability in ADC measurement. ADC values also depend on selected b values that vary across institutions and protocols.

1.3.4 Positron Emission Tomography

FDG PET is capable of visualizing malignant tumors and associated lymph nodes and distal metastatic sites in a single test. In renal cell carcinoma, FDG PET can detect the renal cell carcinoma with various uptake patterns according to the histologic grades. Despite higher specificity, the sensitivity for the detection of malignant renal tumors is quite low of 47–60 % because of the urinary excretion of FDG and incapability of discrimination of tumor uptake and excreted urine activity [22] (Fig. 1.14). However, FDG PET can detect the regional node or distant metastasis for the staging. About 30 % of patients

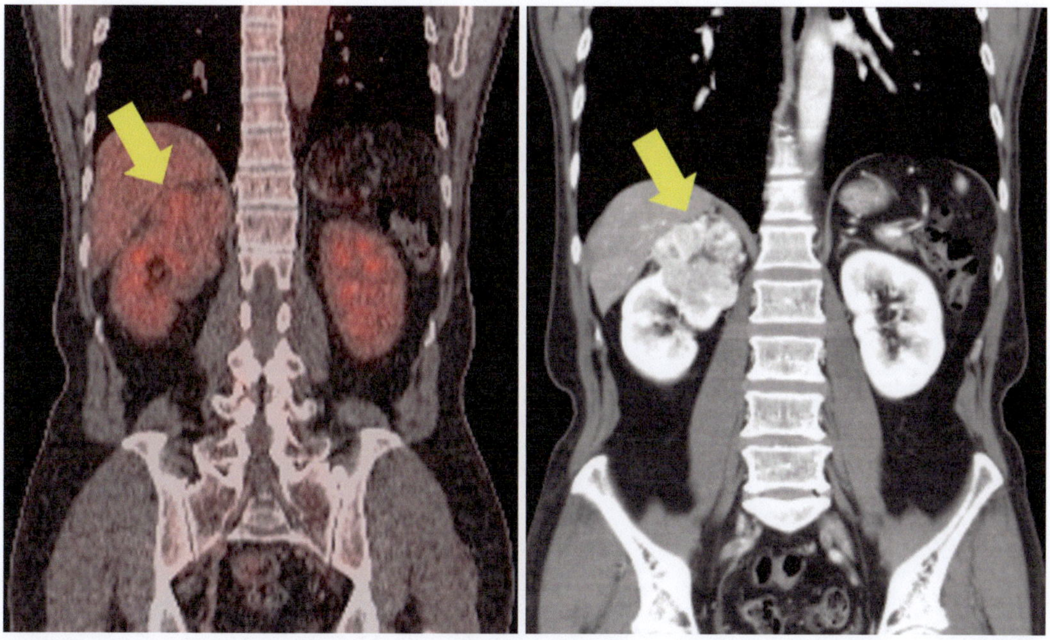

Fig. 1.14 A 63-year-old man presented with incidentally detected mass in the right kidney. FDG PET shows mild hypermetabolism (3.2 of SUVmax) in the corresponding mass (*arrow*) on enhanced CT scan. The hypermetabolic mass lesion is discriminated from the adjacent urine activity with an aid of CT localization. Renal cell carcinoma is confirmed on histopathology after radical nephrectomy

with renal cell carcinoma have metastatic diseases at the initial diagnosis [23] (Fig. 1.15). The lung, bone, and brain are the most common sites of distant metastasis. The sensitivity for detecting metastases is higher than the detection of primary tumors in renal cell carcinoma [24] (Fig. 1.16). Moreover, FDG PET has better diagnostic performance in restaging and recurrence. Nakatani et al. [25] studied the value of FDG PET to detect recurrence disease in 23 postsurgical RCC patients with the sensitivity, specificity, and diagnostic accuracy of FDG PET for detecting recurrent malignancy of 81%, 71%, and 79%, respectively. The higher detection rate of recurrence in renal cell carcinoma enables FDG PET with positive findings as a prognostic marker in patients with recurrent renal cell carcinoma [26]. FDG PET seems to be useful in characterizing anatomic lesions of unknown significance in patients with renal cell carcinoma [27] (Fig. 1.17). However, we need the clinical results in larger-scale patient numbers to establish the clinical utility of FDG PET in staging and restaging renal cell carcinoma.

Recently, targeted drugs have been developed and approved for use in metastatic renal cell carcinoma. Multikinase inhibitors inhibit the receptor tyrosine kinase VEGF receptor or the platelet-derived growth factor receptor in the endothelial cells and pericytes, respectively [28]. These drugs can be administered in patients with metastatic renal cell carcinoma as single agent, which makes PET imaging with a specific radiotracer that visualizes steps in the metabolic pathway of the targeted drug an attractive biomarker for predicting and monitoring the effect of the drug [29]. The expression of glucose transporter (GLUT) is a downstream product of HIF transcriptional activity. Thus, the intensity of FDG uptake on PET may be reflective of the entire pathway of hypoxia [25]. FDG PET with its variable intensity in renal cell carcinoma may reflect the variable expression of the HIF signaling pathways in tumor hypoxia and expression of its downstream products, which may be predictive marker of the effect of the inhibitors of this pathway [30, 31]. Kayani et al. reported that tumors of renal cell carcinoma

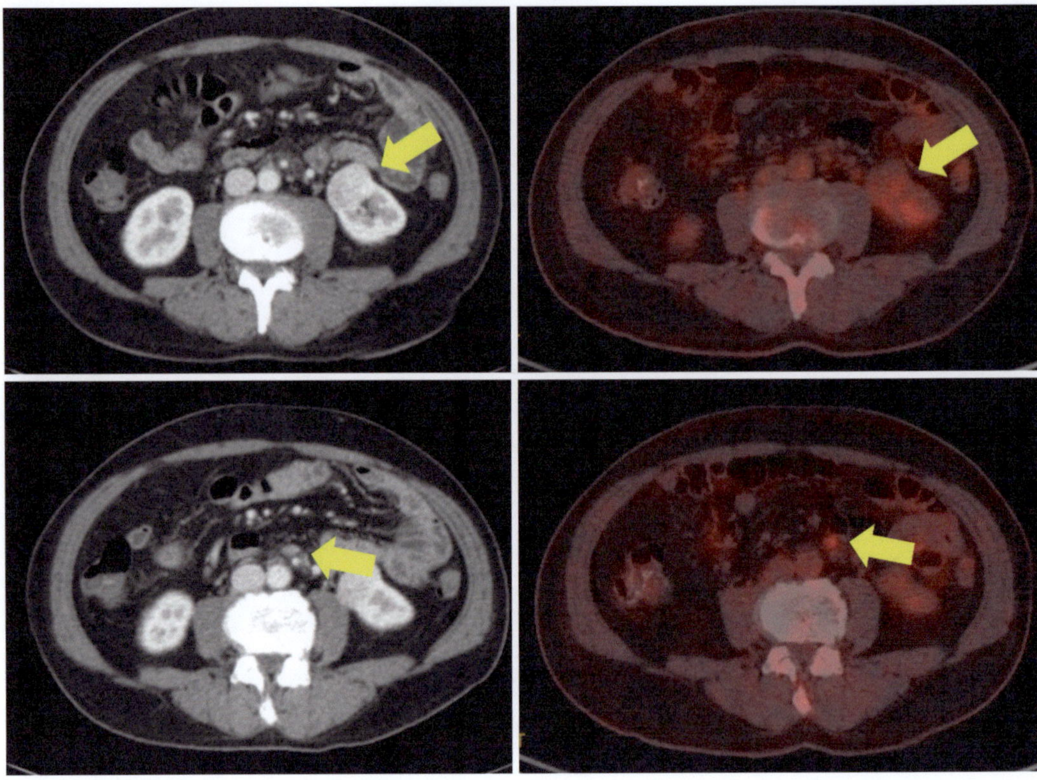

Fig. 1.15 A 60-year-old man underwent FDG PET for staging of renal cell carcinoma. Para-aortic lymph node as well as left renal mass shows hypermetabolism (*arrows*), which were confirmed as renal cell carcinoma with node metastasis after radial nephrectomy

with a lower pretherapy uptake on FDG PET demonstrate a larger size decrease on CT after treatment with tyrosine kinase inhibitors [29, 31]. They proposed that the reduction of metabolic activity of more than 20 % in SUV on FDG PET can be used as a predictive marker for targeted therapeutics.

Other kinds of molecular imaging targets have been proposed in order for more specific to renal cell carcinoma. The PET with 11C-acetate can also detect renal cell cancer. 11C-acetate, as a metabolic substrate of beta-oxidation, that is, precursors of amino acid, fatty acid, and sterol, has been proved useful in detecting various malignancies [32]. In addition, it is an advantage for the 11C-acetate that the urinary excretion is negligible compared with FDG on PET imaging. Liu et al. [33] proposed another radiotracer of FLT on PET to characterize and quantify changes in tumor proliferation during sunitinib exposure and its temporary withdrawal and to explore pharmacodynamics changes that may yield insight into predicting treatment response. In another view point of metabolic alteration by hypoxia, tumor hypoxia can be evaluated by 18F-FMISO (Fig. 1.18). However, Hugonne et al. [34] reported that hypoxia in metastatic RCC as assessed by FMISO PET was less frequent and less pronounced than initially suspected.

In summary, FDG is the most commonly used PET radiopharmaceutical in assessing malignant tumors. However, urinary tract tumor assessment is hampered by the renal elimination of FDG. On the contrary, PET scan using C-11 labeled acetate or other molecular tracers enables us to obtain pelvic images with molecular target specific information in order for staging, restaging, prognosis assessment, response evaluation, and/or prediction as well as without radioactivity of eliminated tracers in the urinary tract [32]. Larger studies are required before it can be advocated for clinical use in the field of urology.

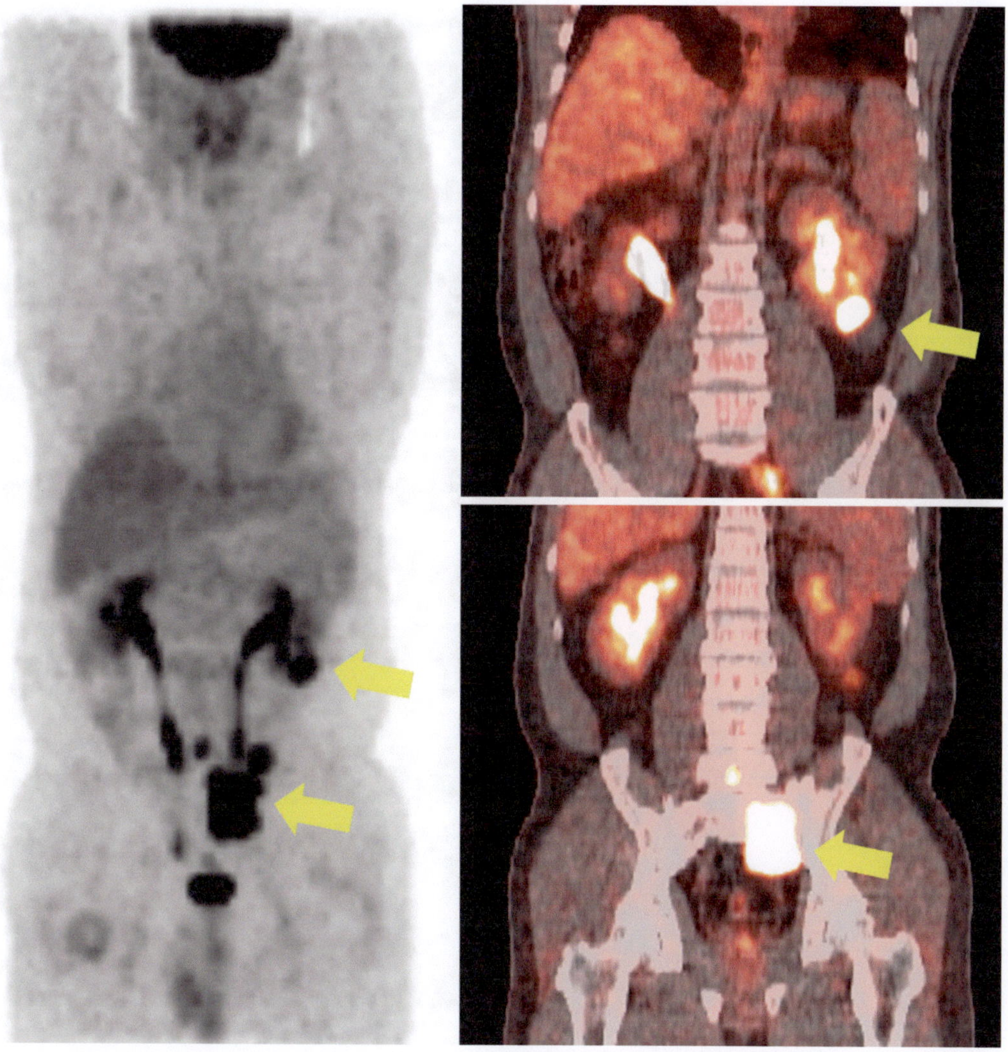

Fig. 1.16 A 57-year-old man presented with incidentally detected renal mass. FDG PET shows an exophytic hypermetabolic mass in the inferior pole of the left kidney with hypermetabolic bone lesion in the sacrum (*arrows*). FDG PET is a useful method to detect unexpected metastasis in a single test

1.3.5 Biopsy

Percutaneous biopsy of renal masses has been usually performed in the suspicion of metastatic renal tumor, for the pathologic diagnosis of unresectable renal mass including multiple, bilateral masses, or suspicion of renal involvement of inflammatory or autoimmune diseases. However, biopsy is also frequently performed in other renal masses nowadays, because nephron-saving surgery becomes popular. Core biopsy can provide an accurate and safe diagnostic tool in small renal masses, which turn out to be benign in 13–16 % after surgery. In a study of 268 small renal masses (≤4 cm) biopsied, diagnostic yield was obtained in 80 % and 26 % of them were benign. The accuracy of biopsy in determining benign or malignant lesions was 100 % in cases where nephrectomy was done [35]. Therefore, biopsy should be offered before surgical intervention in indeterminate small renal masses. US is usually used for guiding biopsy, and CT-guided biopsy is being also used for small masses.

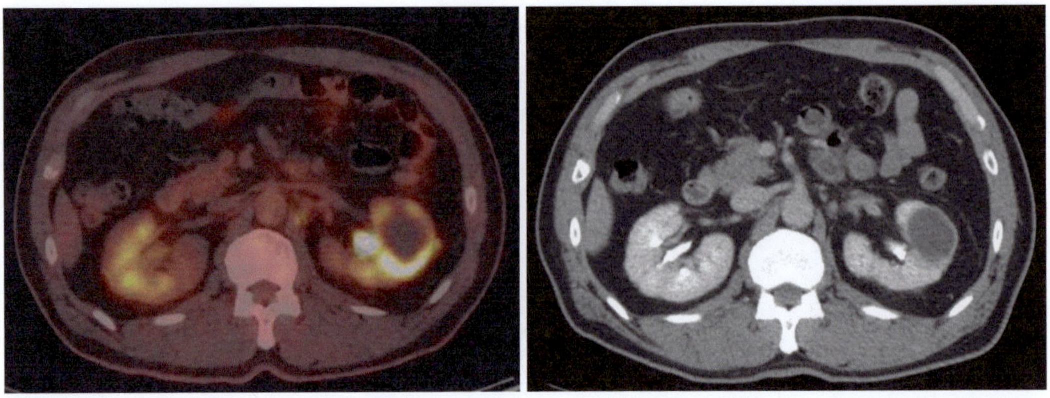

Fig. 1.17 A 58-year-old man underwent diagnostic work-up for the evaluation of incidentally detected lymph node enlargement in the left aortic lymph node, which was metastatic adenocarcinoma on biopsy. FDG PET shows hypermetabolism in the solid area of the cystic mass which is corresponding with cystic mass in the left kidney on contrast-enhance CT. Clear cell RCC was confirmed on histopathology after resection

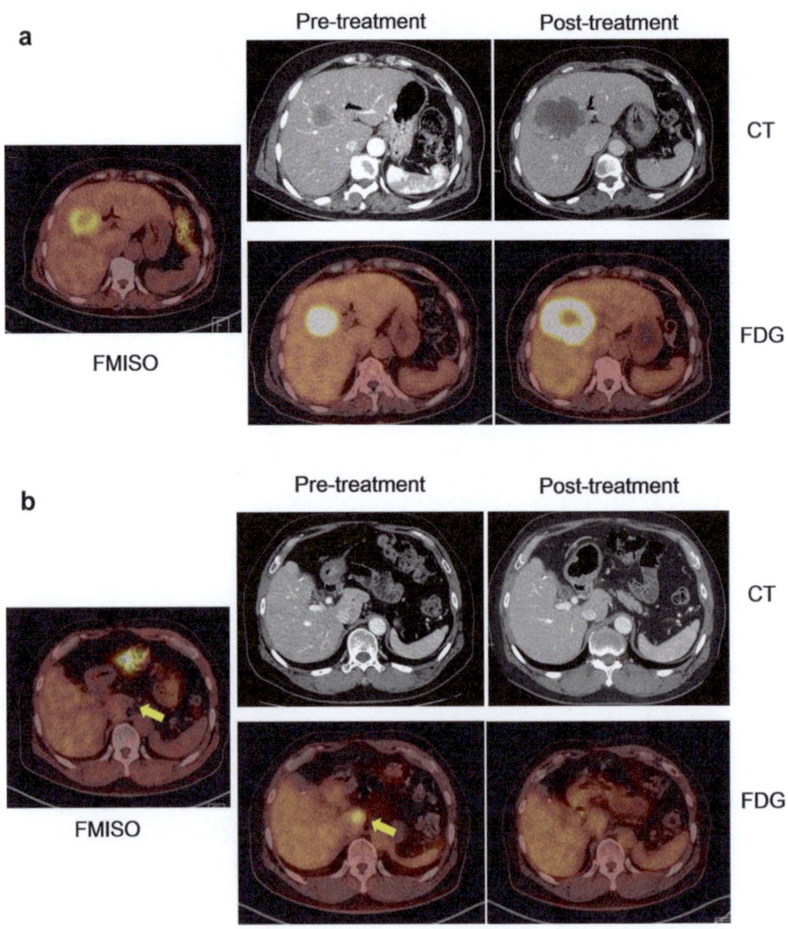

Fig. 1.18 Tumor hypoxia can be evaluated by 18F-FMISO PET. Two patients with liver metastasis underwent palliative chemotherapy. (**a**) One patient with a metastatic lesion of high FMISO uptake shows progression and (**b**) the other patient with a metastasis of low FMISO uptake shows response after palliative chemotherapy (*arrow*)

1.4 Malignant Renal Cell Tumors: Renal Cell Carcinoma

The most common renal cell tumor is RCC in adults. It is also the most common renal malignant tumor, comprising more than 90 % of them. Owing to early detection, the incidence of RCC is rising, as 30–40 % of RCCs are detected incidentally by imaging. It is more common in males than females and the most common in 40–60-year-old patients.

In the WHO classification proposed in 2004, several distinct histologic subtypes of RCC include clear cell RCC, papillary RCC, chromophobe RCC, hereditary cancer syndromes, multilocular cystic RCC, collecting duct carcinoma, medullary carcinoma, mucinous tubular and spindle cell carcinoma, neuroblastoma-associated RCC, Xp11.2 translocation–TFE3 carcinoma, and unclassified lesions. Sarcomatoid RCC is considered as the result of sarcomatoid dedifferentiation of other RCCs and no longer a subtype [36].

1.4.1 Pathologic Consideration

1.4.1.1 Clear Cell Renal Cell Carcinoma

Grossly, clear cell renal cell carcinoma is relatively well demarcated and frequently uncapsulated but occasionally has fibrous pseudocapsule. On cut surface, clear cell renal cell carcinoma typically reveals golden yellow color, and high-grade area shows white to gray cut surface (Fig. 1.19).

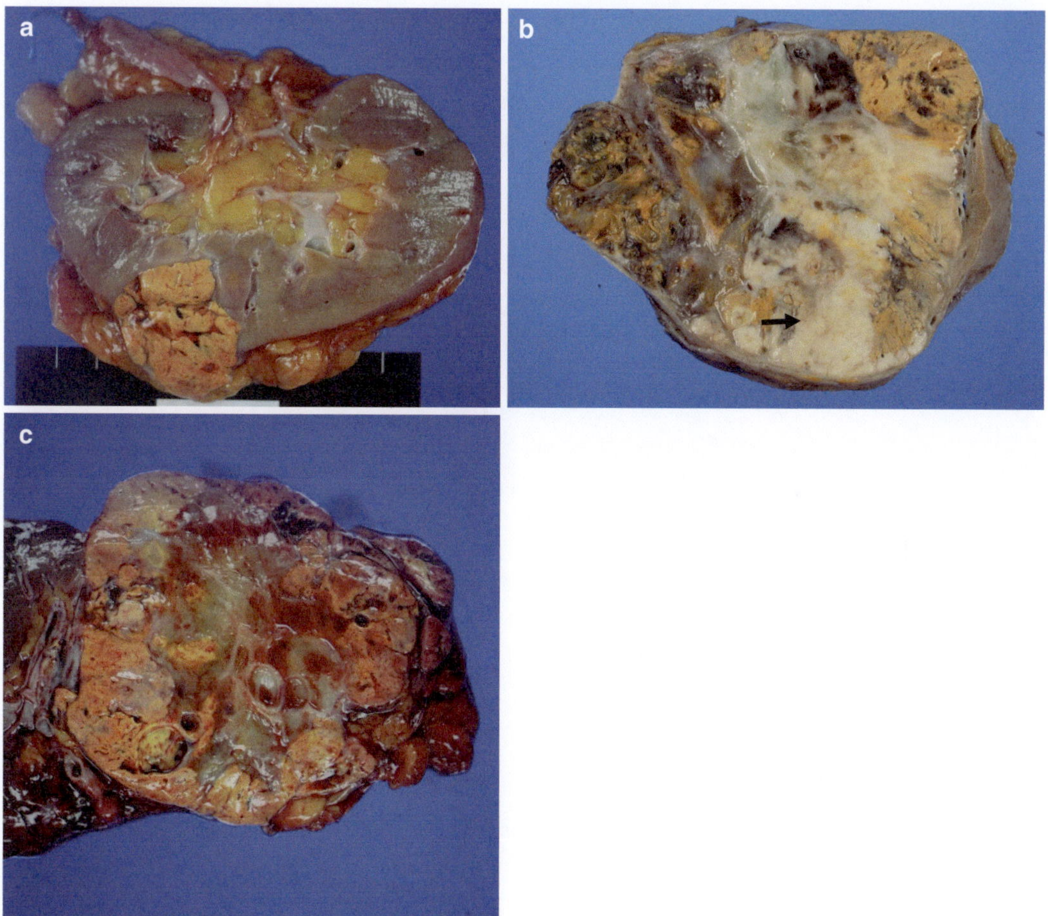

Fig. 1.19 Macroscopic findings of clear cell renal cell carcinoma. (**a**) Grossly, clear cell renal cell carcinoma typically shows *golden-yellow-colored* cut surface. (**b**) Occasionally *whitish- to grayish-colored* area (*arrow*) can be found in high-grade clear cell renal cell carcinoma. (**c**). Hyaline changes, cystic changes, or hemorrhages are frequently found

They frequently have variable cystic change, hyaline change, necrosis, and hemorrhage (Fig. 1.19c). Calcification or ossification is rarely found.

Histologically clear cell renal cell carcinoma shows various architectural patterns such as solid sheet, nest, alveolar, tubular, or microcyst formations. Tumor cells typically have clear cytoplasm with distinct cell border (Fig. 1.20a), but eosinophilic granular cytoplasm can be found especially in high-grade area. Rhabdoid feature of tumor cells is rarely found (Fig. 1.20b) [37, 38] and is associated with aggressive behavior and metastasis [39, 40]. Tumor cell nuclei of low-grade clear cell renal cell carcinoma are small, round, and uniform with fine chromatin. High-grade clear cell renal cell carcinomas generally have larger nuclei with prominent nucleoli. Highly pleomorphic nuclei can be found in high-grade tumor. Sarcomatoid change is also found in about 4–5 % of clear cell renal cell carcinomas [41, 42] (Fig. 1.20c).

1.4.1.2 Multilocular Cystic Renal Cell Carcinoma (Multilocular Cystic Neoplasm of Low Malignant Potential)

Multilocular cystic renal cell carcinoma is a well-demarcated multicystic mass without solid or expansile tumor nodules. Generally, this tumor is entirely cystic with fibrous capsule, thin septa, and multiple cysts containing clear or bloody fluid (Fig. 1.21).

Microscopically, multilocular cystic renal cell carcinoma is composed of multiple cysts lined by mainly single layer of clear tumor cells, but lining cells are often absent. Small clear cell clusters

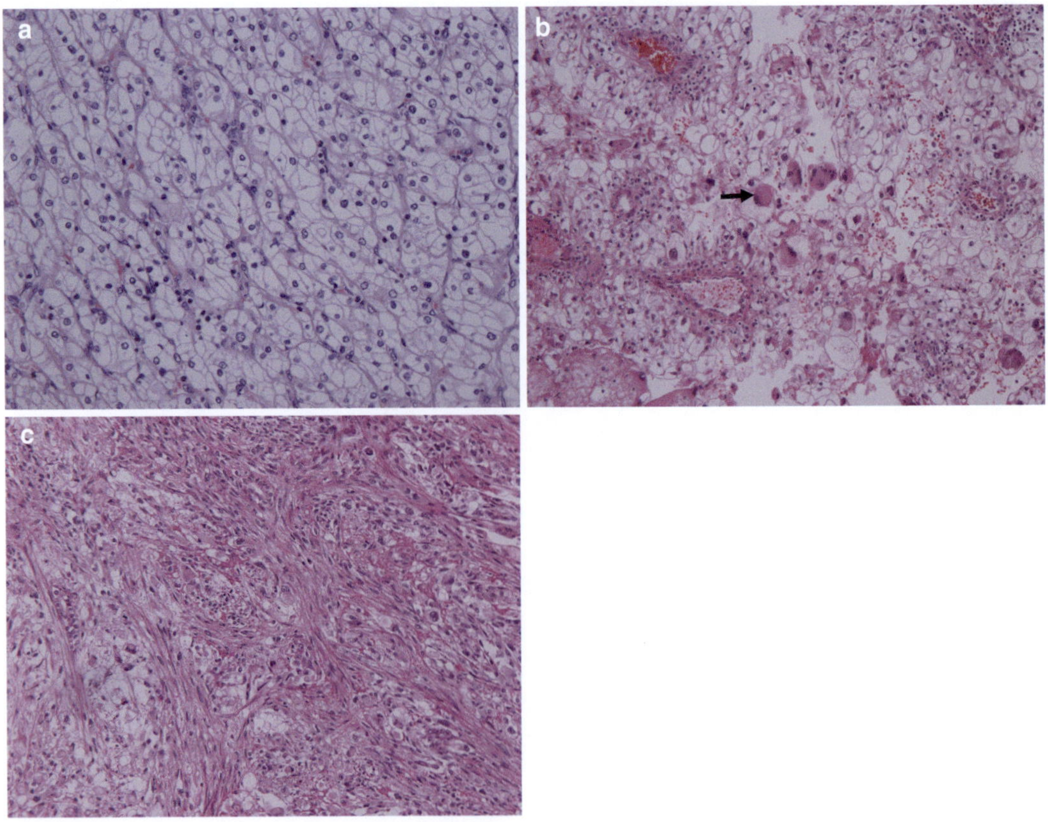

Fig. 1.20 Microscopic findings of clear cell renal cell carcinoma. (**a**) Tumor cells of clear cell renal cell carcinoma typically have clear cytoplasm and distinct cell border. (**b**) Some tumor cells of this clear cell renal cell carcinoma reveal rhabdoid changes (*arrow*). (**c**) Sarcomatoid change of clear cell renal cell carcinoma shows malignant spindle cells between clear tumor cell nests

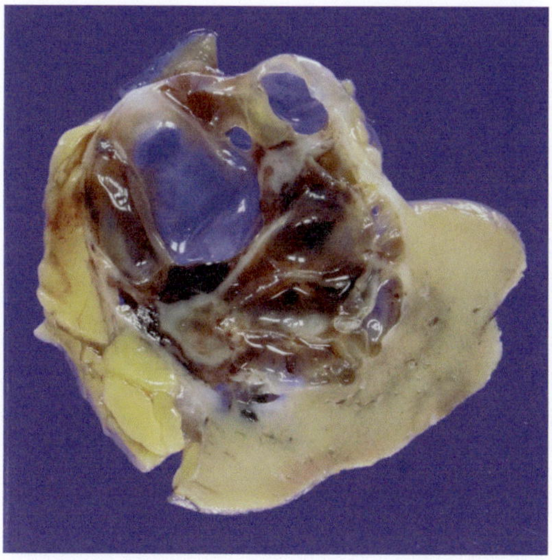

Fig. 1.21 Multilocular cystic renal cell carcinoma shows well-circumscribed multiple cysts without solid tumor nodules

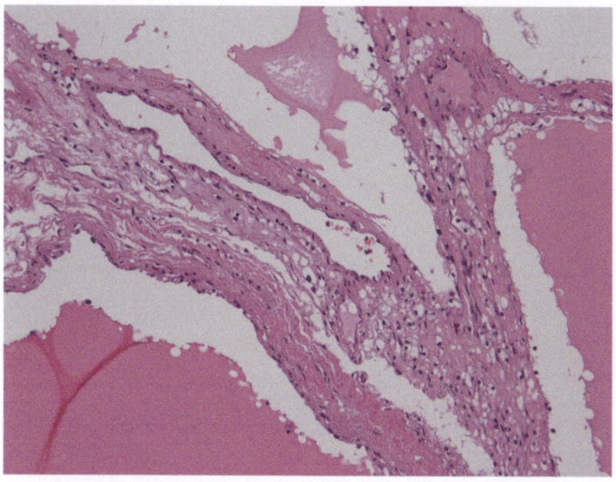

Fig. 1.22 Microscopically, cyst wall is lined by tumor cells with clear cytoplasm and low-grade nuclei

can be present in fibrous septa. Tumor cells have small low-grade nuclei with clear cytoplasm (Fig. 1.22).

1.4.1.3 Papillary RCC

Papillary renal cell carcinoma is a well-demarcated mass with frequent fibrous pseudocapsule. Cut surface of papillary renal cell carcinoma reveals gray to red brown to golden yellow color with frequent hemorrhage and necrosis (Fig. 1.23).

Microscopically, the main architectural pattern of papillary renal cell carcinoma is papillary arrangement with fibrovascular core and occasionally shows tubular arrangement. The papillae are covered by single layer of tumor cells or occasionally pseudostratified tumor cells. Varying degrees of aggregates of lipid-laden macrophages are frequently found in fibrovascular core. Psammomatous calcifications are occasionally present. Papillary renal cell carcinoma is classified into two subtypes, type 1 and type 2 [43, 44]. Type 1 papillary renal cell carcinoma shows small tumor cells with scanty basophilic cytoplasm, small nuclei, and inconspicuous nucleoli. Covered tumor cells mainly form single layer (Fig. 1.24a). Type 2 papillary renal cell carcinoma is characterized by tumor cells with voluminous eosinophilic cytoplasm, large nuclei, and prominent nucleoli. Tumor cells are frequently pseudostratified (Fig. 1.24b). Type 2 papillary renal cell carcinomas show more aggressive behavior [43].

1.4.1.4 Chromophobe RCC

Grossly, chromophobe renal cell carcinoma is a well-circumscribed mass with yellow-tan- to brown-colored, homogeneous cut surface (Fig. 1.25). Hemorrhage or necrosis is rarely found. Central fibrous scar can be present.

Microscopically, tumor cells of chromophobe renal cell carcinoma are mainly arranged in solid sheet or trabecular pattern. Tumor cells have distinctive thick cell border and abundant pale eosinophilic to clear cytoplasm (Fig. 1.26a). Perinuclear halo is frequently found (Fig. 1.26b). Nuclei of chromophobe renal cell carcinoma are small and uniform and occasionally have irregular nuclear membrane. Binucleated nuclei are also present. Sarcomatoid change is rarely found in chromophobe renal cell carcinoma (Fig. 1.26c).

1.4.1.5 Carcinoma of Collecting Duct of Bellini (Collecting Duct Carcinoma)

Collecting duct carcinoma is mainly located in renal medulla and often involves renal cortex. Generally, this tumor shows white- to gray-colored, firm cut surface with infiltrative border (Fig. 1.27). Hemorrhage and necrosis are frequent.

Microscopically, collecting duct carcinoma is mainly composed of irregular-shaped tubules and

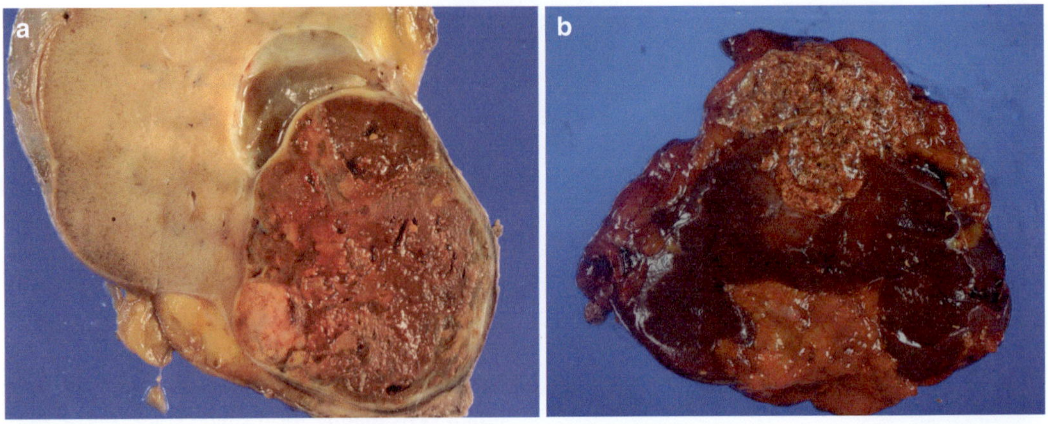

Fig. 1.23 Macroscopic findings of papillary renal cell carcinoma. (**a**) A papillary renal cell carcinoma shows a well-circumscribed mass with encapsulation. On cut surface, massive hemorrhage and necrosis are found. (**b**) This papillary renal cell carcinoma reveals *prominent yellow color*, indicating lipid-laden macrophage collections

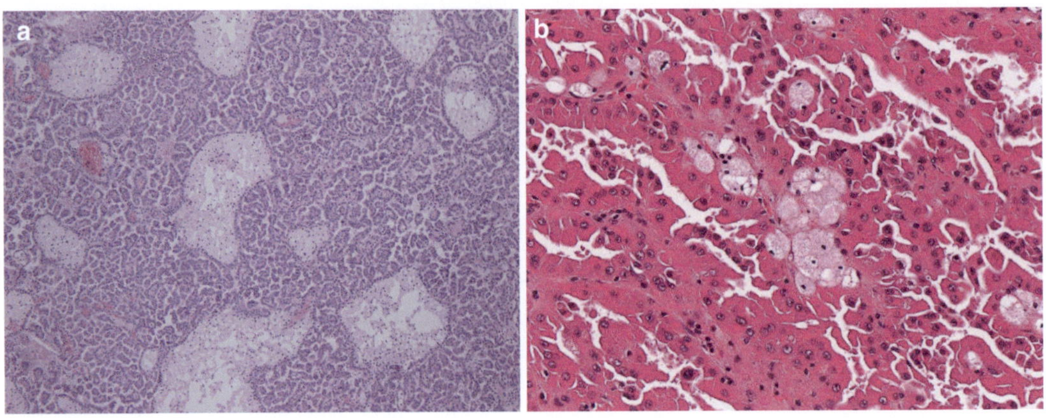

Fig. 1.24 Microscopic findings of papillary renal cell carcinoma. (**a**) Type 1 papillary renal cell carcinoma shows well-formed papillary configurations lined by small tumor cells with scanty cytoplasm and small nuclei. Foamy macrophage collections are found. (**b**) Type 2 papillary renal cell carcinoma reveals papillary architectures lined by eosinophilic tumor cells with abundant cytoplasm and prominent nucleoli. Tumor cells show pseudostratification. Foam cell collections are also found

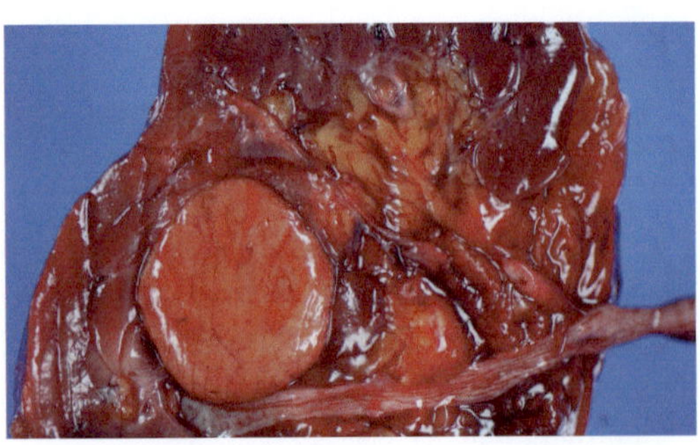

Fig. 1.25 Grossly, chromophobe renal cell carcinoma is a well-defined mass with *yellowish* cut surface

papillae. Tumor cells have high-grade morphology with eosinophilic cytoplasm and pleomorphic nuclei (Fig. 1.28). Frequent mitosis, desmoplastic stroma, and infiltration into surrounding renal parenchyme are typical features of collecting duct carcinoma.

1.4.1.6 MiTF/TFE Family Translocation-Associated Carcinoma

This specific renal cell carcinoma subtype is defined by gene translocations between MiTF/TFE family gene (TFE3 (Xp11.2), TFEB (6p21)), and

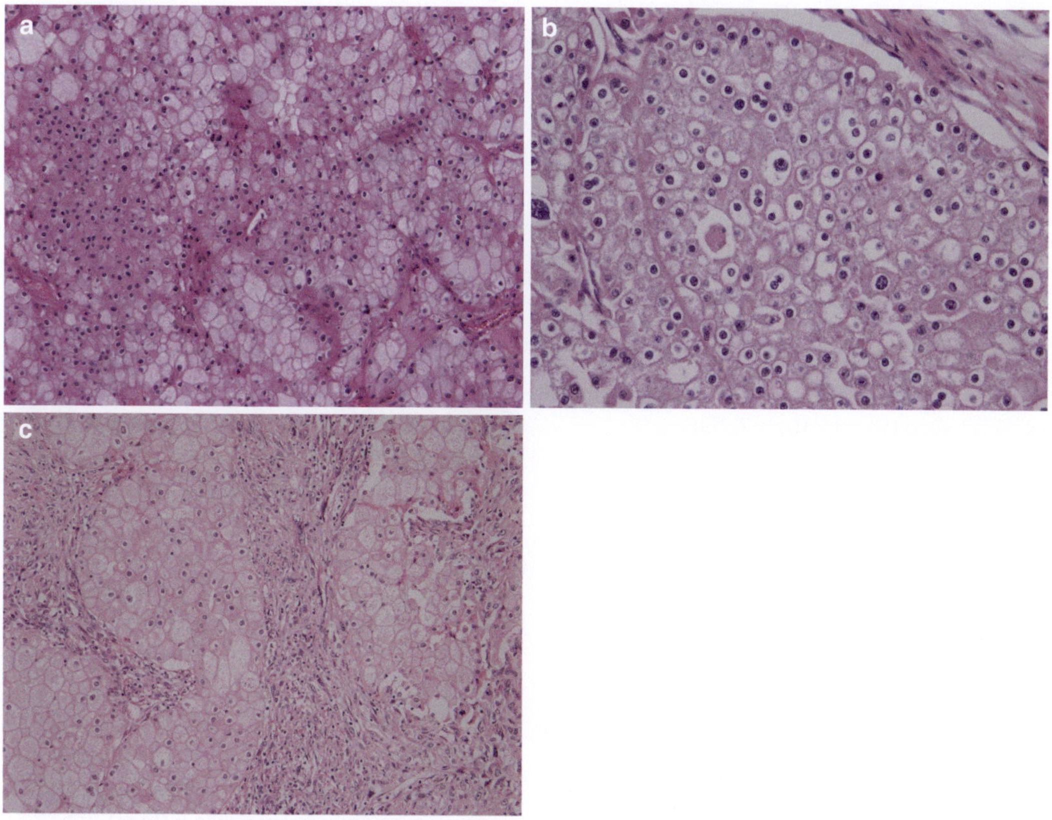

Fig. 1.26 Microscopic findings of chromophobe renal cell carcinoma. (**a**) Tumor cells are arranged in solid pattern. Cytoplasms are clear or eosinophilic with thick cell border. (**b**) Perinuclear halo is frequently found. (**c**) Sarcomatoid change of chromophobe renal cell carcinoma shows malignant spindle cells between typical tumor cell nests

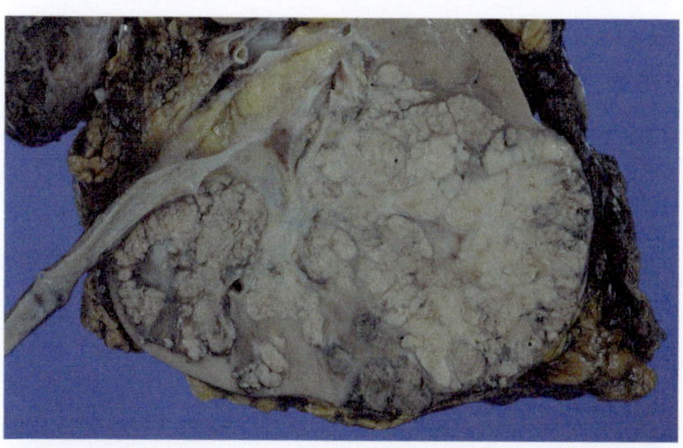

Fig. 1.27 Collecting duct carcinoma is a *whitish firm* mass with infiltration into the renal parenchyma

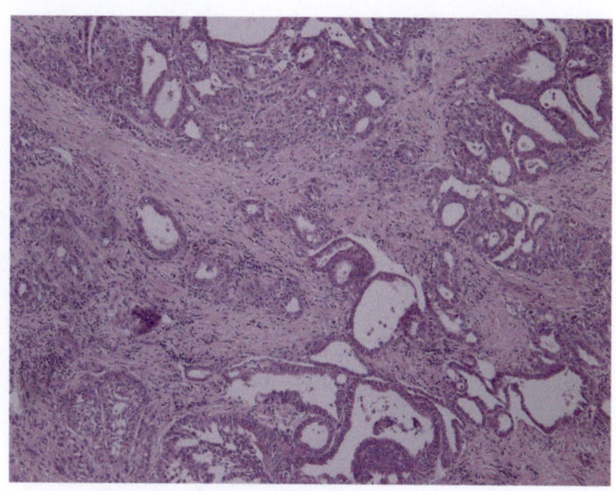

Fig. 1.28 Microscopic findings of collecting duct carcinoma. Tumor shows tubulopapillary architecture with fibrotic stroma. Nucleoli are prominent

variable partner genes including PRCC (1q21) and ASPL (17q25) [45–50]. TFE3 translocation renal cell carcinomas and TFEB translocation renal cell carcinomas are included in this category.

Grossly, TFE3 translocation renal cell carcinoma has variable gross appearance. Sometimes this tumor has infiltrative border. Cut surface shows white, tan, or yellow color with occasional necrosis and hemorrhage (Fig. 1.29) [46, 47].

Microscopic features can be variable according to translocation type. Many reported cases show tubulopapillary architecture with voluminous clear to eosinophilic cytoplasm and often psammomatous calcification in TFE3 traslocation renal cell carcinomas (Fig. 1.30) [46, 47].

Immunohistochemistry and FISH study help in the correct diagnosis of these translocation carcinomas [51]. Immunohistochemical staining for TFE3 shows strong and diffuse nuclear positivity in TFE3 translocation carcinoma (Fig. 1.31a). TFE3 break-apart FISH study reveals split signals of TFE3 gene (Fig. 1.31b) [52, 53].

1.4.1.7 Mucinous Tubular and Spindle Cell Carcinoma

Grossly, mucinous tubular and spindle cell carcinoma is a well-demarcated solid homogeneous mass with pale yellow- to gray-colored cut surface (Fig. 1.32).

Microscopically, mucinous tubular and spindle cell carcinoma is composed of small tightly packed tubules and spindle cells with mucinous stroma (Fig. 1.33). Tumor cells generally have low-grade nuclei and scanty cytoplasm.

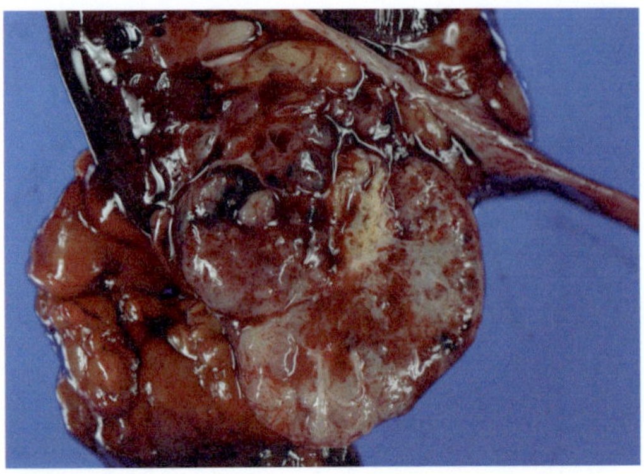

Fig. 1.29 This TFE3 translocation renal cell carcinoma is a *whitish* mass with focal hemorrhage

1.4.1.8 Renal Cell Carcinoma Associated with End-Stage Renal Disease (ESRD)

Two specific renal cell carcinoma types are frequently related to end-stage renal disease [54].

Acquired Cystic Disease-Associated Renal Cell Carcinoma

Acquired cystic disease-associated renal cell carcinoma is generally found in acquired cystic disease patients on dialysis. Grossly, acquired cystic disease-associated renal cell carcinoma is a well-circumscribed small tumor and is often found within cysts (Fig. 1.34a). Microscopically, this tumor shows acinar, alveolar, solid, and cystic pattern. The tumor cells have abundant eosinophilic cytoplasm and prominent nucleoli (Fig. 1.34b) [55].

Clear Cell Papillary Renal Cell Carcinoma

Clear cell papillary renal cell carcinoma is found in ESRD or non-ESRD patients. Grossly, this tumor is a well-circumscribed yellowish or whitish mass with fibrous capsule and occasional cystic change (Fig. 1.35a). Microscopically, clear cell papillary renal cell carcinoma is composed

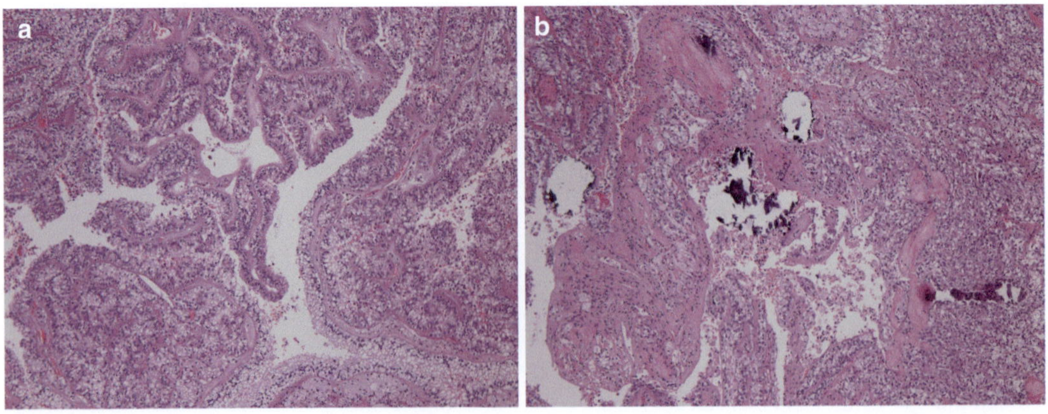

Fig. 1.30 Microscopic findings of TFE3 translocation renal cell carcinoma. (**a**) TFE3 translocation renal cell carcinoma frequently shows papillary configurations. (**b**) Clear tumor cells and calcifications are found in this tumor

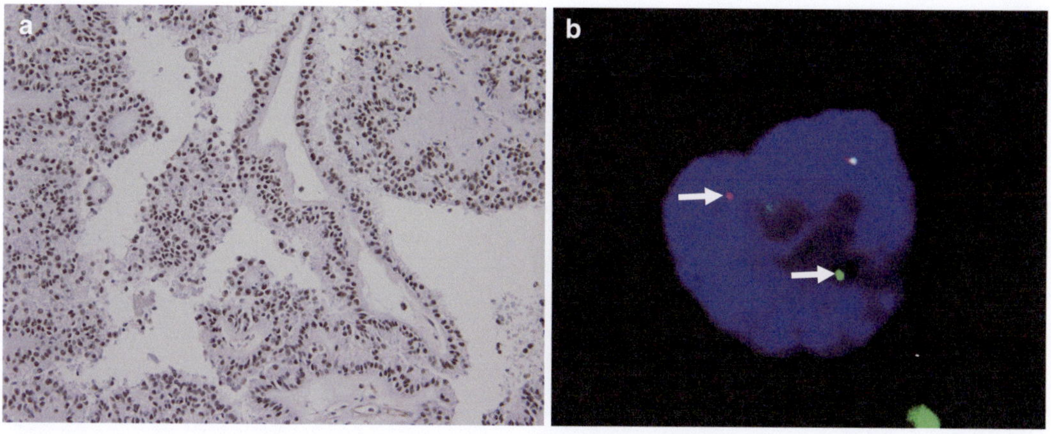

Fig. 1.31 Ancillary tests for TFE3 translocation renal cell carcinoma. (**a**) Immunohistochemical staining for TFE3 shows diffuse strong nuclear staining in TFE3 translocation carcinoma. (**b**) TFE3 break-apart FISH study shows one set of fused signal and one set of *red and green* split signals (*arrows*) in TFE3 translocation renal cell carcinoma

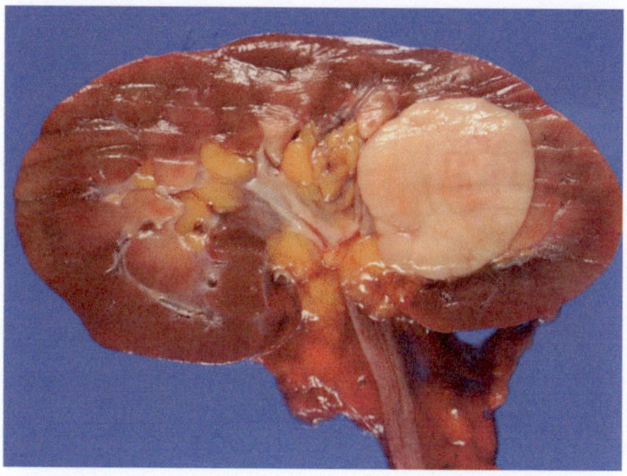

Fig. 1.32 Gross photograph of mucinous tubular and spindle cell carcinoma shows a well-demarcated solid *whitish* mass with homogeneous cut surface

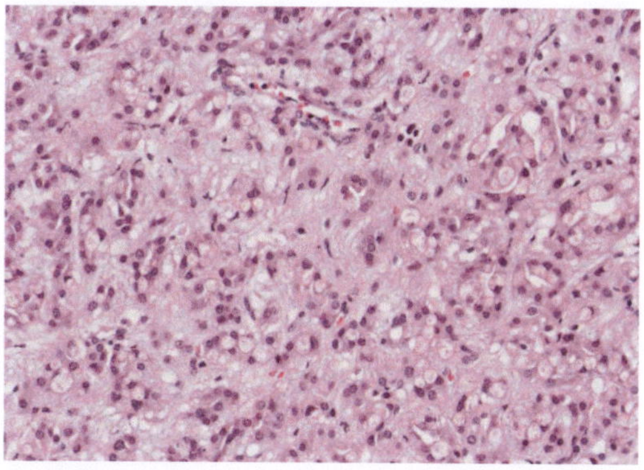

Fig. 1.33 Microscopically, this mucinous tubular and spindle cell carcinoma reveals vague tubule formation and spindle-shaped cells with mucinous background. Tumor cells have low-grade nuclei

of exclusively clear cells with tubule–papillary architecture (Fig. 1.35b). Nuclei are generally low grade. Unlike papillary renal cell carcinoma, foamy macrophages are not present. Cystic change is frequently found [56].

1.4.1.9 Unclassified Renal Cell Carcinoma

Unclassified renal cell carcinoma is defined as renal cell carcinomas that cannot fit into one renal cell carcinoma category. Some cases have morphologic features of two or more renal cell carcinoma types. Other cases are high-grade undifferentiated cases or pure sarcomatoid renal cell carcinoma [57].

1.4.1.10 Nuclear Grading of RCC

Fuhrman nuclear grading is a very important prognostic factor of renal cell carcinoma [58]. This grading system is mainly defined by nuclear size and nucleolar prominence. Tumors of Fuhrman grade 1 have small dense nuclei with no visible nucleoli in × 10 objective lens. Grade 2 tumors have fine granular open chromatin with inconspicuous nucleoli. Nucleoli are identifiable at higher magnification (×40 objective lens). Grade 3 tumors reveal prominent nucleoli that can be easily identifiable at × 10 objective lens. Grade 4 nuclei show nuclear pleomorphism with large nucleoli (Fig. 1.36).

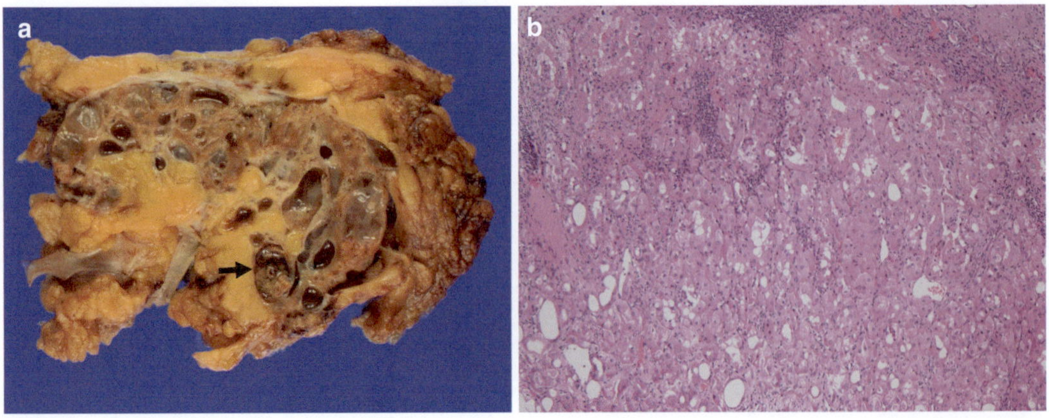

Fig. 1.34 Pathologic features of acquired cystic disease-associated renal cell carcinoma. (**a**) Grossly, acquired cystic disease-associated renal cell carcinoma is a well-circumscribed mass with cystic change. (**b**) Microscopically, tumor cells have abundant eosinophilic cytoplasm

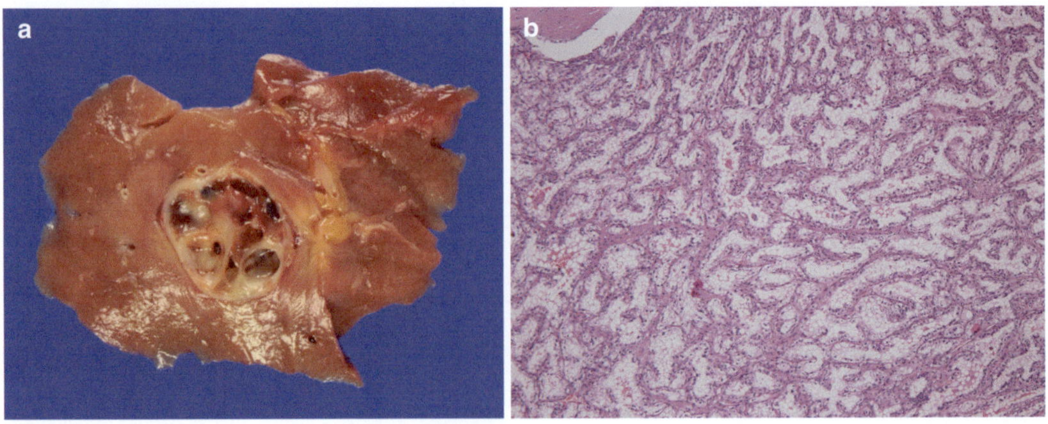

Fig. 1.35 Pathologic features of clear cell papillary renal cell carcinoma. (**a**) Grossly, clear cell papillary renal cell carcinoma is a well-circumscribed whitish mass with encapsulation and frequent cystic change. (**b**) Microscopically, clear cell papillary renal cell carcinoma is composed of clear cells with tubule–papillary architecture. Tumor cell nuclei are low grade

1.4.2 Imaging

1.4.2.1 Staging

The TNM staging system of RCC is summarized in Table 1.1. T1 and T2 tumor without nodal or distant metastasis belongs to Stage I and II, respectively. Stage III means T3 or N1 disease without distant metastasis, and T4 or M1 disease are in stage IV [59]. The staging is important not only in predicting the prognosis but also planning the treatment, because tumorectomy or partial nephrectomy is preferred in locally noninvasive tumors nowadays.

In staging of RCC, invasion into renal fascia or adjacent organs, renal vein thrombosis, regional lymph node enlargement, or distant metastasis are important CT findings (Fig. 1.37). Multidetector-row CT (MDCT) is now the imaging modality of choice for staging and preoperative planning of RCCs. MDCT increases the accuracy of CT in staging RCC compared with MRI. In a prospective study to compare the diagnostic accuracy of MRI and MDCT, similar accuracy (0.78–0.87 vs 0.80–0.83) was shown. MDCT also yields similar staging results in evaluating the extent of venous thrombosis as MRI [60].

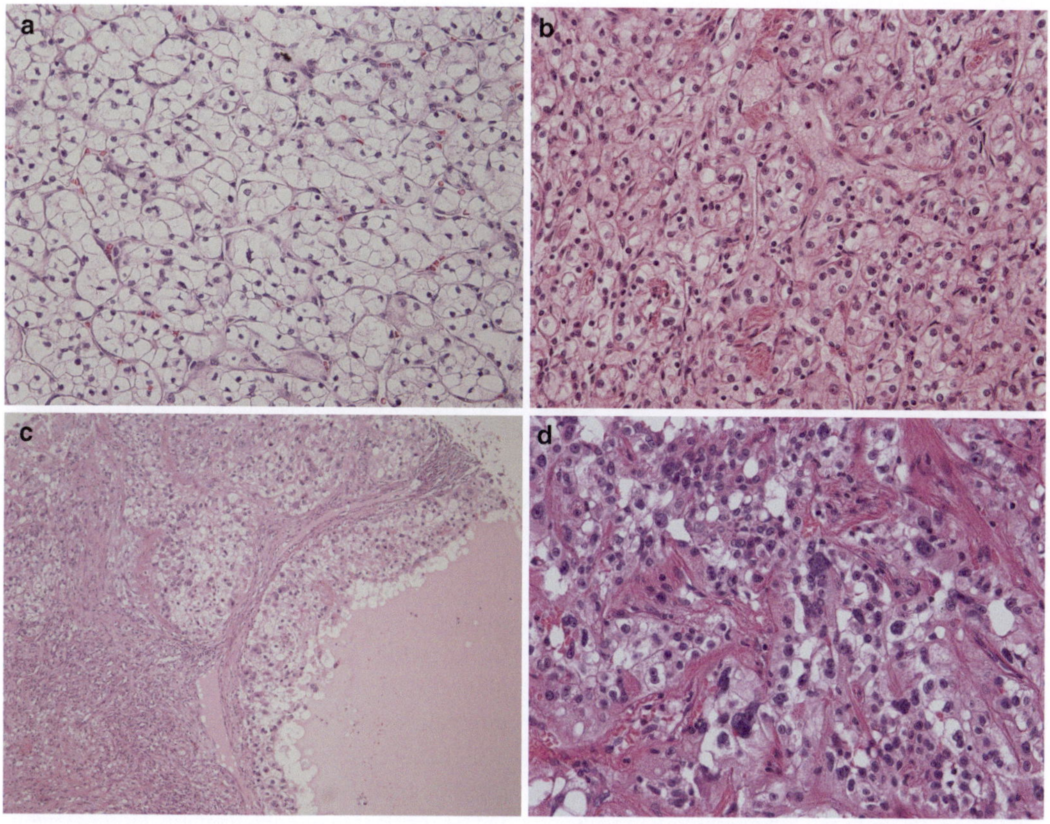

Fig. 1.36 Fuhrman nuclear grading of renal cell carcinoma. (**a**) Fuhrman nuclear grade I. Tumor cells have small nuclei and inconspicuous or invisible nucleoli (×400). (**b**) Fuhrman nuclear grade II. Tumor cells show distinct nucleoli at high magnification (×400) but not conspicuous at × 10 objective lens. (**c**) Fuhrman nuclear grade III. Tumor cells reveal distinct nucleoli at this magnification (×100). (**d**). Fuhrman nuclear grade IV. Tumor cells have large and pleomorphic nuclei

Table 1.1 TNM Staging system of RCC (7th edition)

T1	Tumor confined to renal capsule
T1a	≤4 cm
T1b	4–7 cm
T2	Tumor confined to kidney
T2a	7–10 cm
T2b	>10 cm
T3a	Spreading into perinephric tissue, renal sinus, or renal vein
T3b	Spreading into inferior vena cava (IVC) below diaphragm
T3c	Spreading into IVC above diaphragm or invasion into wall of IVC at any level
T4	Beyond Gerota's fascia or direct invasion into ipsilateral adrenal gland
N0	No nodal involvement
N1	Regional lymph node(s) metastasis
M0	No distant metastasis
M1	Distant metastasis

When considering nephron-sparing surgery, the detection of intrarenal infiltrations of RCC is important. MDCT shows good sensitivity in predicting arterial infiltration but the lowest specificity in excluding infiltration of the renal pelvis [61]. In the detection of perirenal fat invasion, stranding, collateral vessels, fat obliteration, discrete soft tissue mass, and fascial thickening are suggestive CT findings. Among them, mass over than 1 cm is the only strong evidence of perirenal invasion. The interruption of the pseudocapsule, which is formed by compressed renal parenchyma around RCC, is an important sign of locally invasive tumor within perirenal fat. On MRI, the pseudocapsule appears as low SI rim in the periphery of tumor on T2WI (Fig. 1.13). Multiplanar images are required to prove an intact pseudocapsule, which implies a lack of perinephric fat

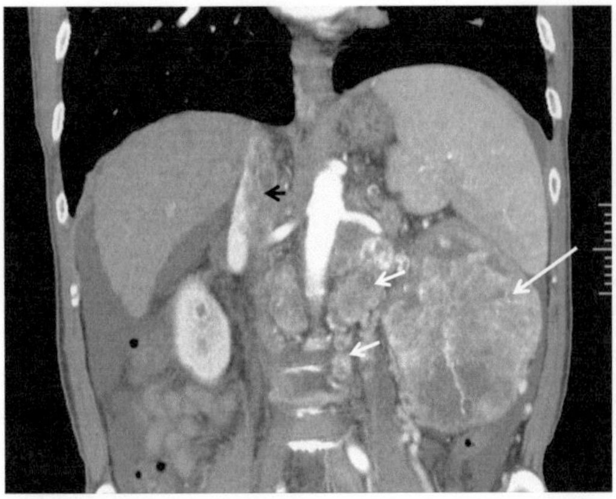

Fig. 1.37 RCC staging on CT. Contrast-enhanced CT in coronal plane shows a large RCC (*large arrow*) in the left kidney. Multiple lymph node metastases (*white small arrows*) and thrombus in the inferior vena cava (*black small arrow*) are important findings for staging

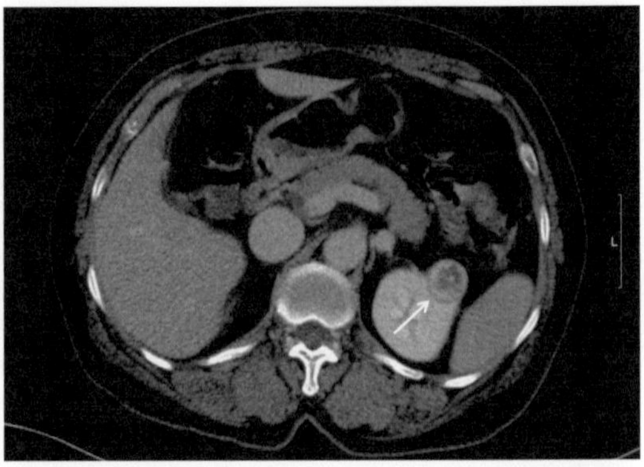

Fig. 1.38 Pseudocapsule of RCC on CT. Contrast-enhanced CT shows a hypervascular mass in the left kidney. Note thin, low-attenuation rim (*arrow*) between the mass and renal parenchyma

invasion and that the tumor can be removed by partial surgery. The pseudocapsule also appears as low-attenuation rim on contrast-enhanced CT (Fig. 1.38), and a recent study reported that the accuracy of MDCT in the detection of pseudocapsule was 83 % with the histopathologic results as the standard of reference. Imaging in the portal and nephrographic phases with coronal and sagittal reformations proved more accurate in the detection of pseudocapsule [62].

MDCT is also important in providing renal vascular information before surgery. Multiplanar reformation (MPR) and 3D volume-rendering (VR) images can provide the accurate information of the renal vasculature including the number, early branching and late confluence of renal vessels, the relations with the collecting system, and the depiction of anatomic variants. In a series of 47 cases with two-phase MDCT angiography, the accuracy for the only-arterial anatomy was 97.9 % and only-venous anatomy was 100 %. This result can suggest the MDCT angiography can fully replace catheter-based angiography for assessing vascular supply of the kidney before surgery [63].

1.4.2.2 Subtypes of RCC

Because prognosis is significantly different among subtypes of RCCs, preoperative knowledge of the subtype is important in planning treatment. CT may differentiate these subtypes based on the degree of enhancement, enhancement pattern, calcification, and tumor-spreading patterns. 91–100 % specificity was reported in differentiating clear cell RCCs from other subtypes on biphasic contrast-enhanced CT, depending on the degree of enhancement. Homogeneous enhancement is the most common in chromophobe type, and calcification is more common in papillary and chromophobe types. Perinephric change and venous invasion are common in collecting duct carcinoma [64].

Clear Cell RCC

Clear cell RCCs are the most common subtype of RCC (70–75 %). Multicentric (5 %) or bilateral (1–2 %) tumors are rarely encountered. They are usually spherical and the margin is smooth and well demarcated. They are located in the renal cortex with expansile growth. The tumors are often surrounded by the pseudocapsule formed by the compressed surrounding renal parenchyma (Fig. 1.38) [65].

On imaging, they commonly appear heterogeneous due to hemorrhage, necrosis, and cysts. Calcification can be found in 10–15 % and gross fat is seldom detected on CT. Clear cell RCCs are typically hypervascular on contrast-enhanced CT and show earlier and stronger enhancement than other subtypes. Characteristically, they enhance similarly to or stronger than renal cortex at early arterial or corticomedullary phase of contrast-enhanced CT (Fig. 1.2). A recent study reported that multiphasic MDCT could discriminate clear cell RCC from oncocytoma, papillary RCC, and chromophobe RCC with the accuracies of 77 %, 85 %, and 84 %, respectively, because clear cell RCCs exhibit significantly greater enhancement at the corticomedullary phase [66].

On MRI, clear cell RCCs usually show high SI on T2WI and iso SI on T1WI to that of the renal parenchyma (Fig. 1.11). Hemorrhage and necrosis make the tumor appear heterogeneous on T2WI. Pseudocapsule of the mass appears as low-signal rim at the periphery of the mass. Considerable signal drop within the solid portions of a clear cell RCC on opposed phase MR images can be detected in up to 60 %, due to the presence of intracytoplasmic fat. Dynamic contrast-enhanced MRI can provide important information in differentiating from other subtypes. A study reported that tumor-to-cortex enhancement indexes at the corticomedullary and nephrographic phases of dynamic contrast-enhanced MRI were the largest for clear cell RCCs and the smallest for papillary RCCs. SI changes on corticomedullary phase images was the most effective parameter for the differentiation [67].

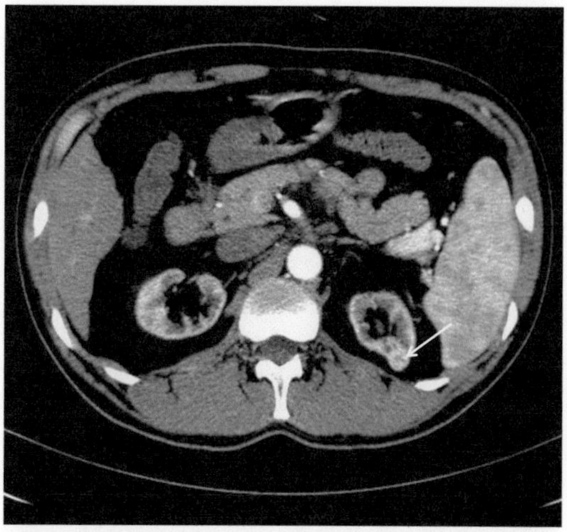

Fig. 1.39 Papillary RCC in ESRD. Contrast-enhanced CT shows a small hypervascular mass (*arrow*) in the left kidney, suggesting RCC. Note atrophic kidneys

Papillary RCC

It accounts for 10–15 % of all RCC and the second most common subtype. There are two histomorphologic subtypes (type 1 and 2), and type 1 tumors are typically of a lower stage and grade than type 2 tumors and associated with a better prognosis. Bilateral or multifocal tumors are more common in papillary RCC than in other subtypes, which is especially common in hereditary syndromes. Papillary type is the most common in RCCs arising in patients with ESRD. Long duration of dialysis may be a predisposing factor (Fig. 1.39). It is usually solid, slow growing, and in intrarenal location in 70 % at presentation [65]. On US, it usually appears as a homogeneous mass of variable echogenicity and hypovascular on Doppler US. On CT, high attenuation within tumor on unenhanced images may be visible due to hemorrhage, even in small tumors. Fat is rarely detected. Papillary RCCs show weak, homogeneous, and persistent enhancement on dynamic contrast-enhanced images (Fig. 1.40). These findings are not different between type 1 and 2 tumors [68]. On MRI, they show homogeneous low SI compared with the cortex on T2WI. This low SI on T2WI, which may be due to hemosiderin deposition, hemorrhage, or necrosis, is an important MR characteristic in differentiating from clear cell RCCs [69] (Fig. 1.11). Clear cell RCCs usually show heterogeneously high SI on T2WI and strongly enhance on corticomedullary phase, but papillary RCCs enhance minimally on early phase and less than renal parenchyma on nephrographic phase.

Chromophobe RCC

It is the third most common subtype and accounts for approximately 4–11 % of RCCs. There is no gender preponderance, and it is most common in the sixth decade of life. It has the best prognosis among RCCs, although large tumors may be accompanied by hepatic metastases. On US, chromophobe RCCs tend to be homogeneously echogenic. On CT, and MRI, they enhance homogeneously and mildly. This homogeneous enhancement is also visible in even large tumors (Fig. 1.41). On dynamic contrast-enhanced images, they enhance intermediately on corticomedullary phase and show variable enhancement (early washout or constant

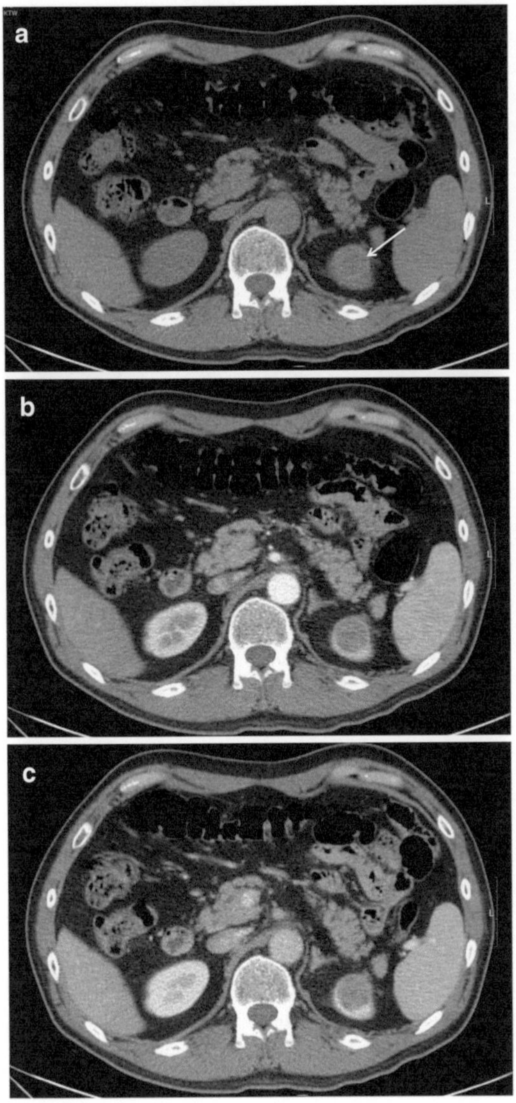

Fig. 1.40 Papillary RCC. (**a**–**c**) In three-phased contrast-enhanced CT, a mass (*arrow*) in the left kidney is slightly hyperattenuating on noncontrast CT (**a**) and mildly enhancing both in corticomedullary (**b**) and in nephrographic (**c**) phase

enhancement) on delayed phases. Fine reticular enhancement has been reported on corticomedullary phase in 70 % of cases, which may be helpful for the differentiation from other subtypes [65]. Spoke-wheel pattern of enhancement has been also described, similar to the enhancement pattern of oncocytoma. Oncocytomas share similar histologic features with chromophobe RCCs and may show similar imaging findings [70]. On MRI, chromophobe RCCs may show signal intensity similar to that of clear cell RCCs or might appear low SI on T2WI compared with renal parenchyma [71].

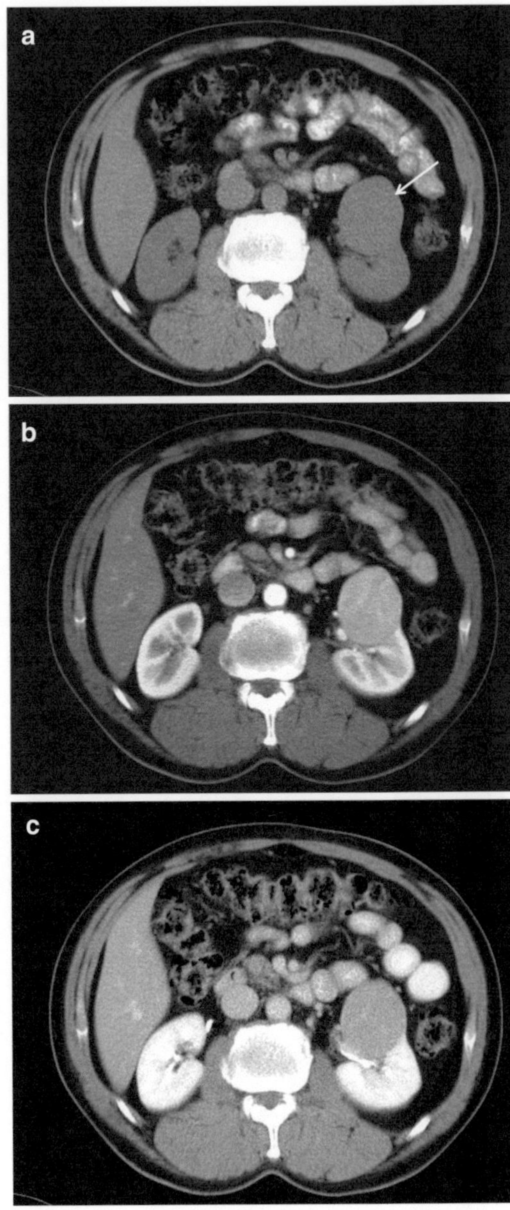

Fig. 1.41 Chromophobe RCC. (**a**–**c**) Three-phased contrast-enhanced CT show a mass (*arrow*) in the left kidney, which is homogenous and mildly enhancing ((**a**) noncontrast scan, (**b**) corticomedullary phase, (**c**) nephrographic phase)

Multilocular Cystic RCC

Multilocular cystic RCC is a rare subtype and constitutes 1–4 % of all RCCs. The incidence is more common in males than females and higher in middle-aged patients (around 50 years old). Its prognosis is usually favorable, and the cure can be almost achieved by nephrectomy. It appears as a multilocular cystic mass on imaging with septa of variable thickness. It is separated from renal parenchyma by a fibrous capsule, and the septa and the capsule enhances mildly or minimally on CT and MRI (Fig. 1.7). They may show enhancing nodular thickening and can contain calcifications in 20 %. They appear as cystic masses of variable Bosniak category from IIF to IV, and the higher the category, the larger the volume of malignant cells and/or vascularized fibrous tissue [72].

Collecting Duct Carcinoma

It is a rare and highly aggressive subtype, accounting for less than 1 % of all RCCs. Metastasis is present at the time of diagnosis in one-third of the patients. The prognosis is very poor, and two-thirds of patients cannot live for more than 2 years after the diagnosis. It is more common in males (male to female ratio: 2:1) and the mean age is 55 years. Its typical imaging appearance is an infiltrative tumor with the epicenter in the medullary portion of the kidneys near the renal pelvis. US appearance is nonspecific and usually shows heterogeneous echogenicity due to necrosis and hemorrhage. CT and MRI findings are also nonspecific, especially in larger tumors, and the differentiation from other subtypes is often difficult. On CT, it is poorly enhancing and may have calcifications. The enhancement pattern is heterogeneous or predominantly peripheral. Its infiltrative pattern of growth preserves renal contour (Fig. 1.42). On MRI, it shows variable SI on T1WI and usually low SI on T2WI. Heterogeneous SI is common due to necrosis, hemorrhage, and calcification, and a cystic portion may be visible in 50 % [65, 73].

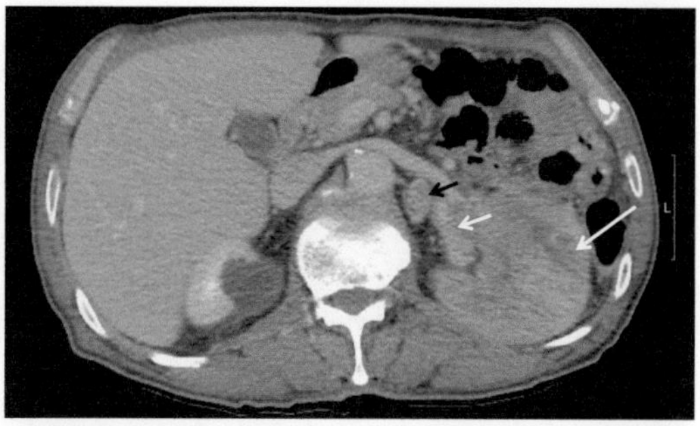

Fig. 1.42 Collecting duct carcinoma. Contrast-enhanced CT shows a large, ill-defined mass (*large arrow*) in the left kidney. Renal contour is preserved, and enlarged regional lymph node (*black small arrow*) and renal vein thrombus (*white small arrow*) are visible

Renal Medullary Carcinoma

It is also rare, accounting for less than 1 % of all RCCs. It occurs exclusively in patients with sickle cell trait. The patients are almost always young, aged between 11 and 40 years. The male-to-female ratio is 2:1. Medullary carcinomas are aggressive tumors with early local invasion and distant metastasis and the prognosis is unfavorable. On imaging, they appear as ill-defined and infiltrative masses centered on the renal medulla. The renal contour is usually persevered, and caliectasis is commonly associated. On CT and MRI, they are hypovascular and heterogeneously enhancing. They show heterogeneous SI on T2WI due to necrosis and hemorrhage [65, 74].

Mucinous Tubular and Spindle Cell Carcinoma

It has been often diagnosed as a sarcomatoid RCC or a renal sarcoma but newly classified as a distinctive subtype. Its clinical course is indolent and the prognosis is favorable. Imaging findings are nonspecific.

Xp11.2 Translocation–TFE3 Gene Fusion Carcinoma

It is also a newly classified subtype and accounts for 20 % of RCCs in the first and second decades of life. The prognosis is favorable, although it is discovered in the advanced stage. Its imaging findings are rarely described in the literature, and reported CT and MRI findings include hyperdense and hypovascular mass on CT and hypointense on T2-weighted MR images (Fig. 1.12). The imaging finding may be similar to papillary RCC due to histopathological resemblance [75].

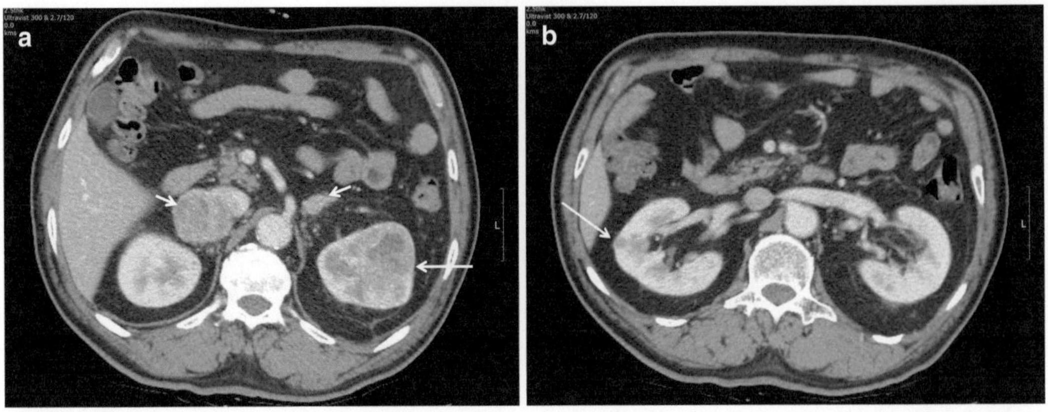

Fig. 1.43 Von Hippel–Lindau syndrome. (**a**) Contrast-enhanced CT shows a large mass (*large arrow*) in the left kidney. Note bilateral adrenal masses (*small arrows*). (**b**) Another small mass (*arrow*) suggesting RCC is also found in the right kidney

Hereditary RCC Syndromes

Von Hippel–Lindau syndrome is the most famous hereditary RCC syndromes, in which multiple RCCs are developed in bilateral kidneys associated systemic syndromes including retinal angiomas, central nervous system hemangioblastomas, and pheochromocytomas (Fig. 1.43). In Birt–Hogg–Dube' syndrome, renal tumors including chromophobe RCC, oncocytoma, or hybrid tumors are associated with skin lesions or lung cysts. Hereditary syndromes associated with papillary type include hereditary papillary RCC (type 1) and hereditary leiomyoma RCC (type 2). Recently, PTEN hamartoma tumor syndrome (PHTS) is newly reported as a hereditary syndrome associated with papillary RCC [65, 76].

1.5 Benign Renal Cell Tumors

Of renal epithelial tumors, 5–10 % are benign and represented mostly by oncocytoma, papillary adenoma, and metanephric adenoma.

1.5.1 Oncocytoma

1.5.1.1 Pathologic Consideration

Grossly, oncocytoma is a well-circumscribed solid homogeneous mass with typically mahogany brown color (Fig. 1.44a). Oncocytoma often has central fibrous scar.

Microscopically, oncocytoma is composed of round- to oval-shaped tumor cells having deeply eosinophilic cytoplasm (Fig. 1.44b). Nuclei are round and uniform without prominent nucleoli (Fig. 1.44c). The main architectural pattern is variable-sized tumor cell nests in loose hypocellular fibrous or hyalinized stroma. Occasionally, tubular or cystic architectures are found.

1.5.1.2 Imaging

Oncocytoma is the second most common benign renal tumor after AML, accounting for 3–7 % of all renal tumors. It is more common in males than females, and the peak age is in the seventh decade. Most patients are asymptomatic, and the tumors are discovered incidentally. Most of them occur sporadically, but multiple, bilateral tumors in a patient can occur (Fig. 1.45). Some oncocytomas may be associated with RCCs either as hybrid tumors or as collision tumors.

On imaging, they usually appear as well-demarcated but unencapsulated masses with homogeneous enhancement, located in renal cortex. Hemorrhage may be found in up to 20 %. Several imaging characteristics has been described, including a central stellate fibrotic scar, which is more common in larger tumors, and an arterial spoke-wheel pattern of enhancement. The central scar has been reported to be seen in up to 33 % (Fig. 1.46) [77]. However, these findings are neither sensitive nor specific enough to affect the treatment option. Recently, it has been described

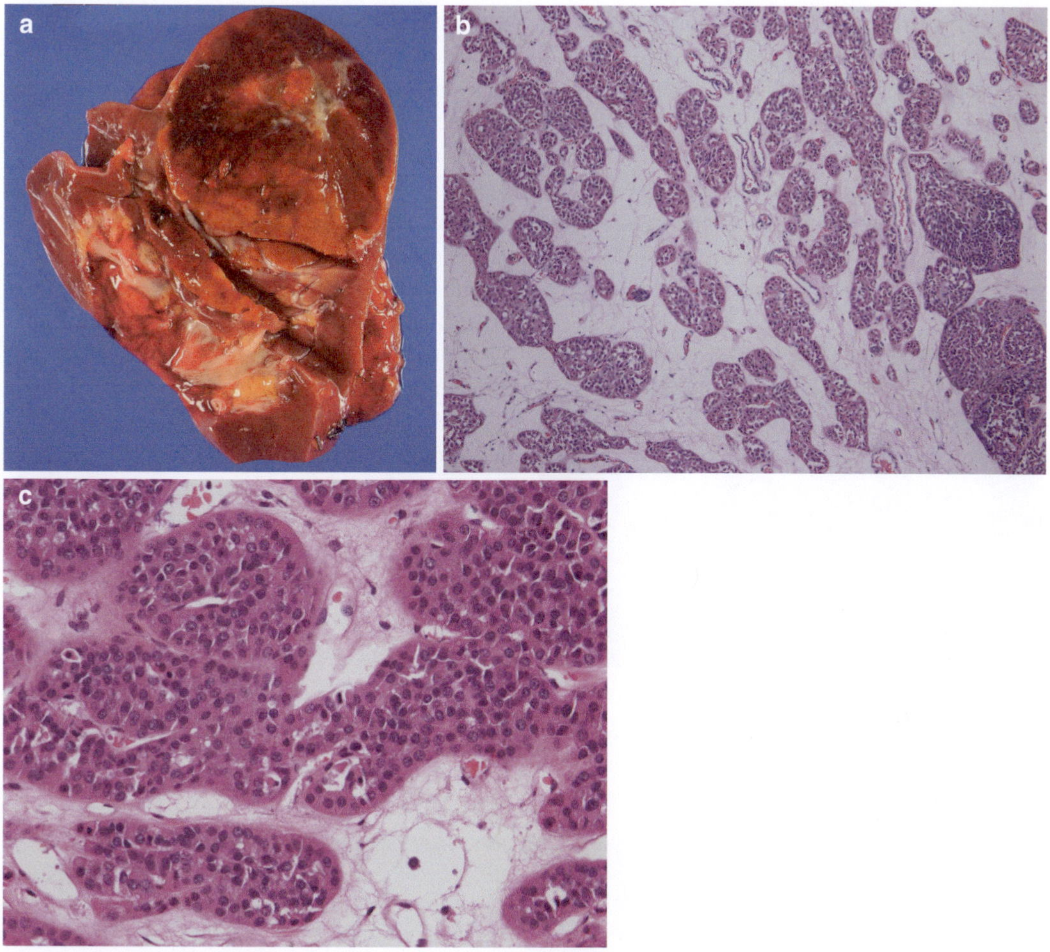

Fig. 1.44 Pathologic features of oncocytoma. (**a**) Grossly, oncocytoma is a well-demarcated mass with typically mahogany *brown color*. This tumor shows central scar. (**b**) Variable-sized tumor cell nests are present in loose hypocellular stroma. (**c**) Tumor cells have deeply eosinophilic cytoplasm and low-grade nuclei

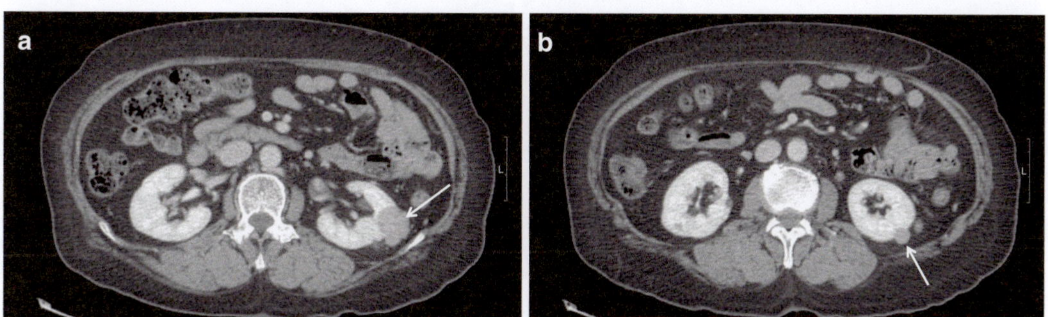

Fig. 1.45 Multiple oncocytomas in the kidney. (**a**) Contrast-enhanced CT shows a lobulating, homogeneously enhancing mass (*arrow*) in the left kidney. (**b**) Another similar mass (*arrow*) is also found in the lower pole of the kidney

that many small (<4 cm) oncocytomas exhibit "segmental inversion enhancement" on CT (Fig. 1.47). This sign is segmental differences of enhancement in a mass, and the highly enhanced area on the corticomedullary phase converts into the relatively less enhanced area on the excretory phase image, while the less enhanced area converts into relatively highly enhanced area [78]. This finding was initially thought to be highly sensitive and specific, but there has been much debate in later studies, especially in large tumors which tend to have fibrous septa, cystic change, hemorrhage, or necrosis [79, 80]. Segmental enhancement inversion is more common in tumors measuring 1.5–2.9 cm, in which these pathologic changes are not frequently visible [81]. Chromophobe RCCs are known to be especially difficult to differentiate from oncocytoma, because both of them share the similar histologic origin and features. A recent study reported that the segmental enhancement inversion on biphasic MDCT might be useful in differentiating small renal oncocytomas from chromophobe RCCs [82].

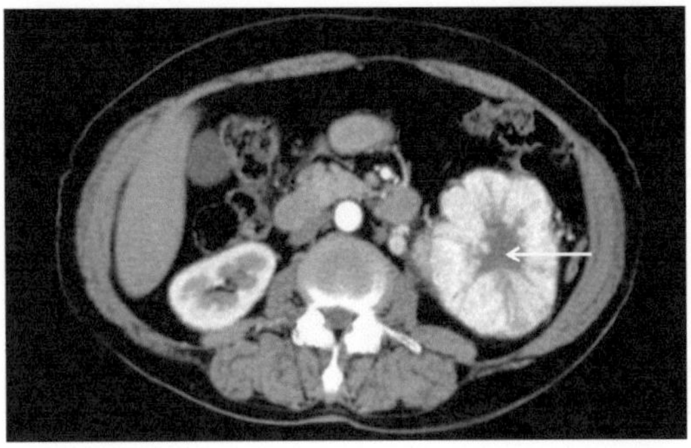

Fig. 1.46 Oncocytoma. Contrast-enhanced CT shows a large, well-enhancing mass in the left kidney. Note low-attenuation central scar (*arrow*) in the mass

1.5.2 Papillary Adenoma

It is the most common neoplasm of the epithelium of renal tubules. An autopsy study reported that 40% of prevalence in patients older than 70 years. Papillary adenoma is a small (0.5 cm or less) tubulopapillary lesion having low-grade nuclei (Fig. 1.48).

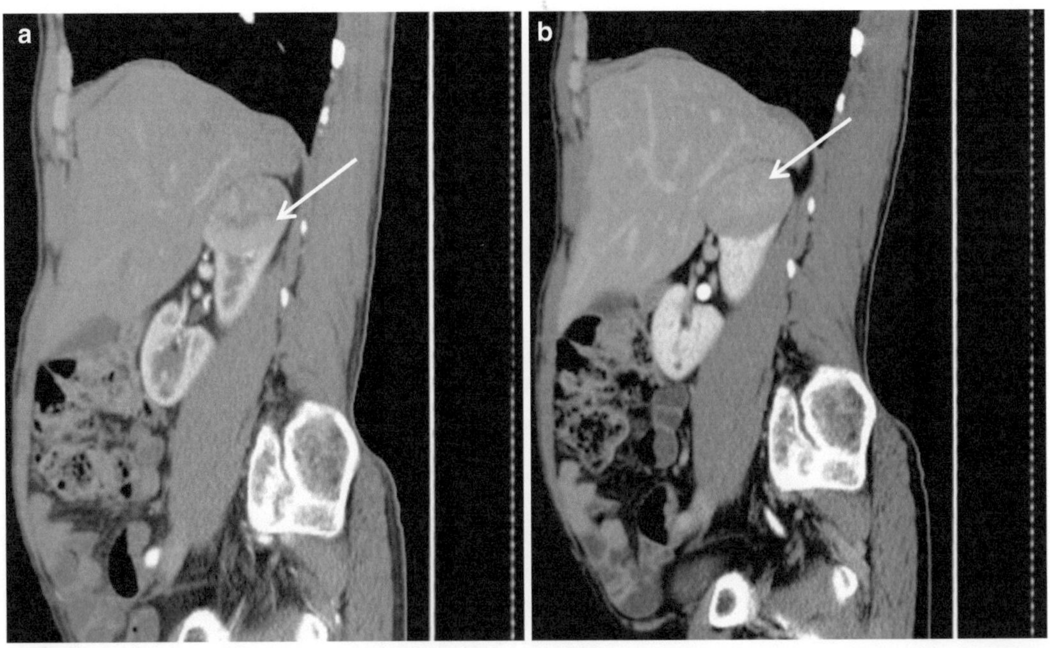

Fig. 1.47 Segmental inversion in an oncocytoma. (**a**) Corticomedullary phase CT in sagittal plane shows a heterogeneously enhancing mass in the right kidney. Note the posteroinferior part of the mass (*arrow*) enhances more than the anterosuperior part. (**b**) In nephrographic phase, the enhancement of the anterosuperior part becomes more prominent than the posteroinferior part (segmental inversion)

1.6 Metanephric Tumors

1.6.1 Metanephric Adenoma

Metanephric adenoma is a rare benign tumor and mostly occurs in young and middle-aged women. Female-to-male ratio is 2.6, with a mean age of 41 years. It is detected incidentally in 40 %, and 12 % of cases are associated with polycythemia [83].

1.6.1.1 Pathologic Consideration

Grossly, metanephric adenoma is a well-demarcated mass with gray, yellow, or white cut surface (Fig. 1.49a).

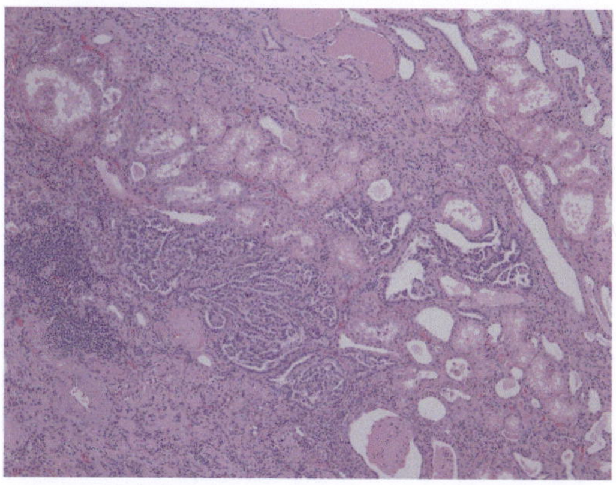

Fig. 1.48 Papillary adenoma is small tubulopapillary lesion composed of tumor cells with scanty cytoplasm and low-grade nuclei

Microscopically, metanephric adenoma is composed of small uniform tubules. Papillary architectures are commonly found. Tumor cells have scanty cytoplasm and small round nuclei (Fig. 1.49b).

1.6.1.2 Imaging

The tumor is well circumscribed and shows variable echogenicity on US. Hyperechogenicity is more commonly encountered due to calcifications or intratumoral interphases. It is hypovascular on Doppler US. On unenhanced CT, the attenuation may be high due to microscopic calcifications. Calcifications are common and were reported to present in two-thirds of the patients. On contrast-enhanced CT, the tumor appears as a well-defined, homogeneous hypovascular mass (Fig. 1.50). On MRI, metanephric adenomas appear as hypo- or isointense masses on both T1WI and T2WI [83, 84].

1.7 Mesenchymal Tumors

Mesenchymal tumors of the kidney are uncommon except angiomyolipoma. They can occur in various tissues of the kidney: differentiated stromal tissue (leiomyoma/leiomyosarcoma, lipoma/liposarcoma, schwannoma, rhabdomyosarcoma),

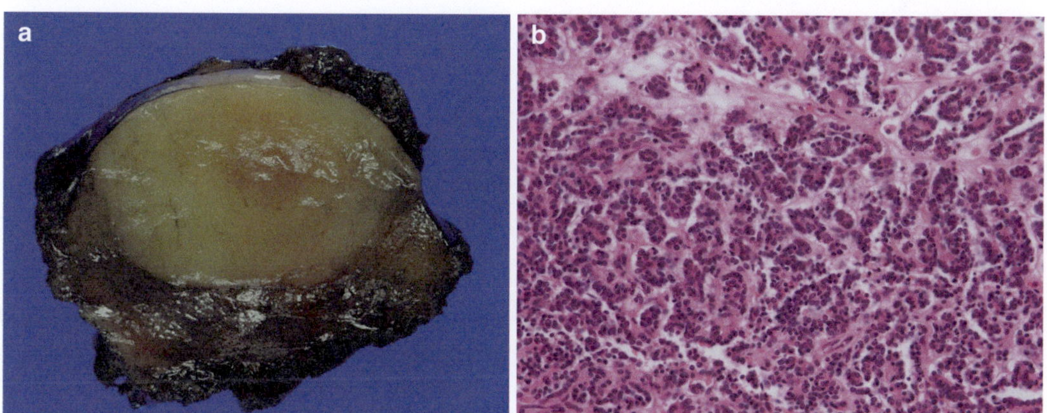

Fig. 1.49 Pathologic findings of metanephric adenoma. (**a**) Metanephric adenoma is a well-demarcated mass with *gray or yellow* color. (**b**). Microscopically, tumor cells are small and uniform having scanty cytoplasm and low-grade nuclei. This tumor is mainly composed of small uniform tubules

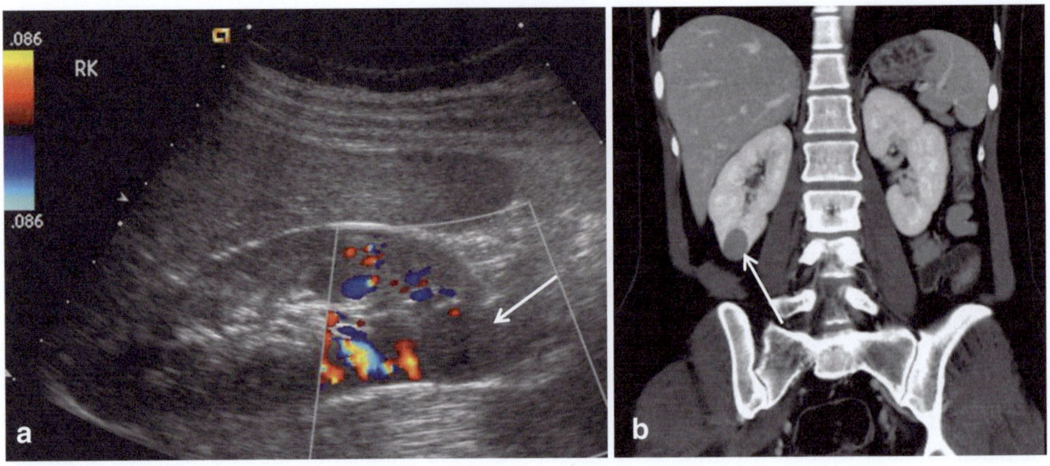

Fig. 1.50 Metanephric adenoma. (**a**) Color Doppler US shows an isoechoic and hypovascular mass (*arrow*) in the right kidney. (**b**) On contrast-enhanced CT in coronal plane, the mass (*arrow*) is homogeneous and poorly enhancing

vascular origin (hemangioma, glomus tumor, myopericytoma, hemangioblastoma, lymphangioma, angiosarcoma), and other miscellaneous origin (myxoma, renomedullary interstitial cell tumor, juxtaglomerular cell tumor, solitary fibrous tumor, desmoplastic small round-cell tumor, synovial sarcoma). In some cases, the criteria to differentiate between benign and malignant tumors is not definitely defined currently [85].

1.7.1 Sarcoma

In children, clear cell sarcoma and rhabdoid tumor are common renal sarcomas. In adult, leiomyosarcoma is the most common and accounts more than 50 % of renal sarcomas.

1.7.1.1 Pathologic Consideration

Clear Cell Sarcoma of Kidney

This pediatric malignant renal tumor has aggressive clinical behavior. Grossly, this tumor is a large well-demarcated mass with solid tan- to gray-colored cut surface (Fig. 1.51a). Microscopically, this tumor is composed of ovoid to spindle tumor cells with pale, often clear cytoplasm (Fig. 1.51b). And this tumor frequently shows "chicken-wire" vascular pattern.

Malignant Rhabdoid Tumor

Malignant rhabdoid tumor is a highly malignant pediatric renal tumor. Grossly, it is a large tumor with ill-defined border and tan to gray cut surface (Fig. 1.52a). Occasionally, hemorrhage and necrosis are found. Microscopically, malignant rhabdoid tumor is composed of sheets of large ovoid tumor cells with rhabdoid morphology. Tumor cells have large eosinophilic cytoplasm with eccentrically located high-grade nucleus (Fig. 1.52b) [86]. Typically, INI1 immunohistochemistry shows loss of nuclear expression in tumor cells (Fig. 1.52c) [87].

Other Malignant Mesenchymal Tumors

Pathological features of these sarcomas are identical to those of soft tissue counterparts.

1.7.1.2 Imaging

Renal sarcomas usually appear as very large and heterogeneous masses on imaging. Necrosis and cystic change are common, and lobulated contour, irregular and indistinct edges, heterogeneous enhancement are frequently observed. They may present with or without metastases and generally show no renal vein or inferior vena cava invasion. Leiomyosarcoma often arises from renal capsule and is commonly centered at the periphery of the kidney with exophytic growth. However, in most cases, renal sarcomas are indistinguishable from RCCs (Fig. 1.53) [88].

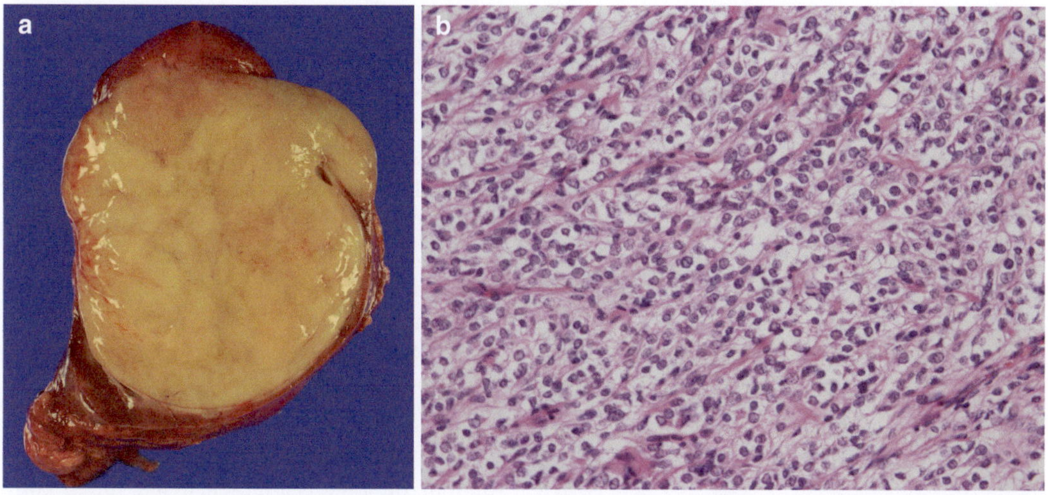

Fig. 1.51 Pathologic findings of clear cell sarcoma of the kidney. (**a**) Grossly, clear cell sarcoma of the kidney is a large well-demarcated mass with homogeneous *whitish to yellowish* cut surface. (**b**) Microscopically, clear cell sarcoma of the kidney is composed of oval-shaped cells with clear cytoplasm

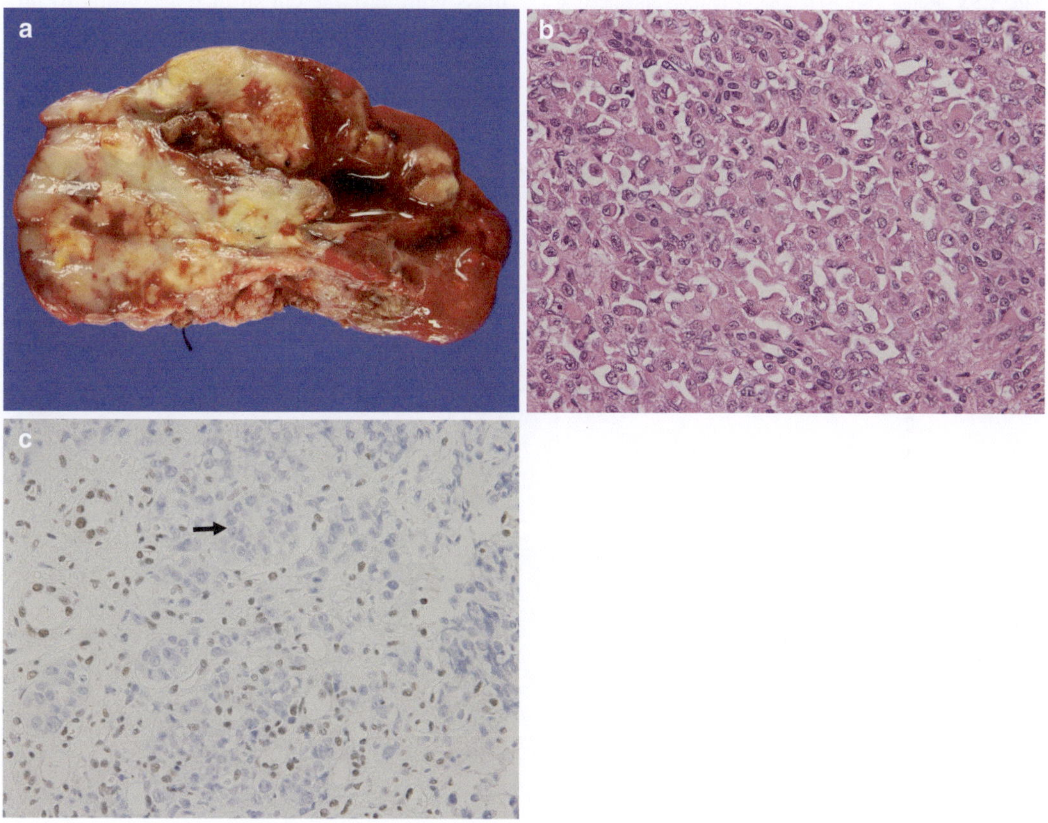

Fig. 1.52 Pathologic findings of malignant rhabdoid tumor. (**a**) Grossly, malignant rhabdoid tumor of kidney is a large tumor with ill-defined border. Focal hemorrhage and necrosis are found in this tumor. (**b**) Microscopically, malignant rhabdoid tumor is composed of rhabdoid cells with eccentrically located nuclei and abundant eosinophilic cytoplasm. (**c**) INI-1 immunohistochemistry shows loss of nuclear expression in tumor cell nuclei (*arrow*). Normal tubular epithelial cells and endothelial cells show INI-1 nuclear positivity in this tumor

1.7.2 Angiomyolipoma

AML is the most common benign renal tumor. Actually, it is a hamartoma of the kidney, containing blood vessels, smooth muscle, and fat in variable proportions. It is common in middle-aged women. Eighty percent of AMLs are sporadic, whereas 20 % are associated with tuberous sclerosis. AMLs with tuberous sclerosis tend to be bilateral and multifocal and grow faster (Fig. 1.10). The growth of AMLs is mainly due to increased fatty component or intratumoral hemorrhage. Risk of bleeding in AML increases when the size of the mass increases to greater than 4 cm or the intratumoral aneurysm is larger than 5 mm (Fig. 1.54). Rarely, AMLs may have necrosis and calcification within them.

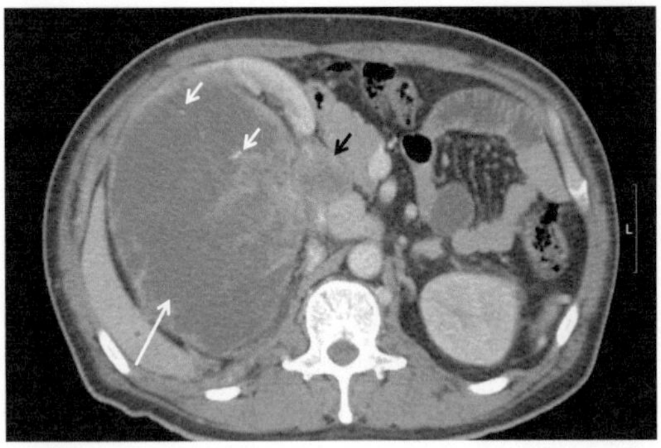

Fig. 1.53 Renal osteosarcoma. Contrast-enhanced CT shows a large necrotic mass (*arrow*) with small calcifications (*white small arrow*) and renal vein thrombus (*black small arrow*) in the right kidney. The appearance cannot be differentiated from that of RCC

1.7.2.1 Pathologic Consideration

Angiomyolipoma is a mesenchymal tumor composed of adipose tissue, smooth muscle, and blood vessels.

Grossly, angiomyolipoma is a well-demarcated mass with variable cut surface according to proportion of adipose tissue, smooth muscle component, and vessels (Fig. 1.55a). It often extends into perinephric fat.

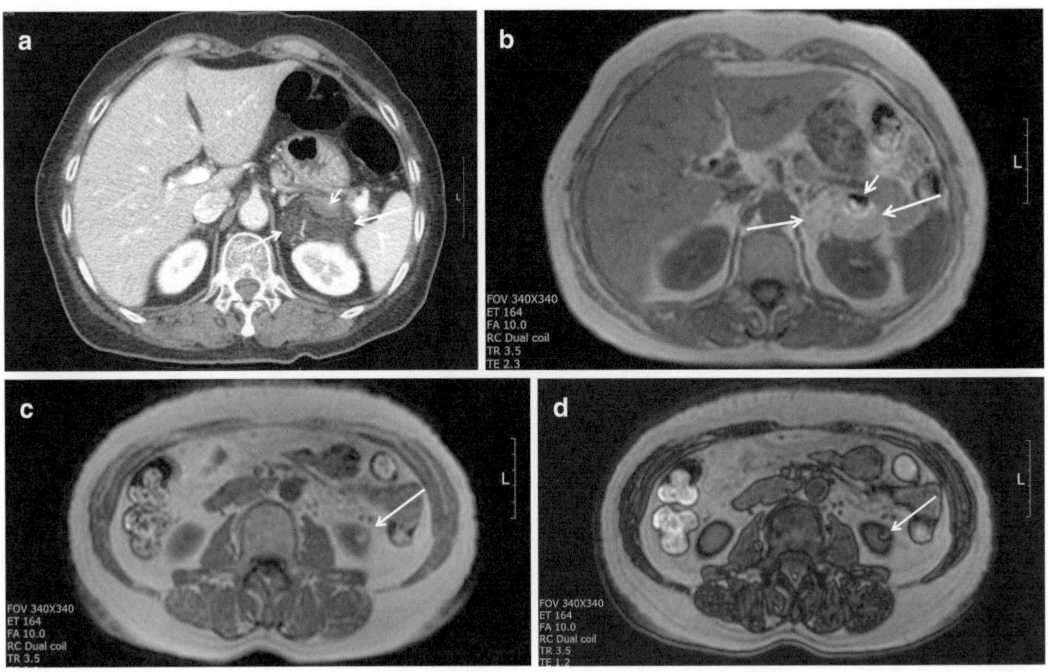

Fig. 1.54 Angiomyolipoma with intratumoral hemorrhage. (**a**) Contrast-enhanced CT shows a fatty mass (*large arrows*) in the left kidney. The mass contains a high-attenuation part (*small arrow*). (**b**) The mass (*large arrows*) shows high SI on T1WI of MR and contains a nodule (*small arrow*) composed of dark and high SI, suggesting hemorrhage. (**c**) Another small mass (*arrow*) with high SI is found in the lower pole on T1WI. (**d**) The lower pole mass (*arrow*) shows signal drop in opposed phase, suggesting another AML

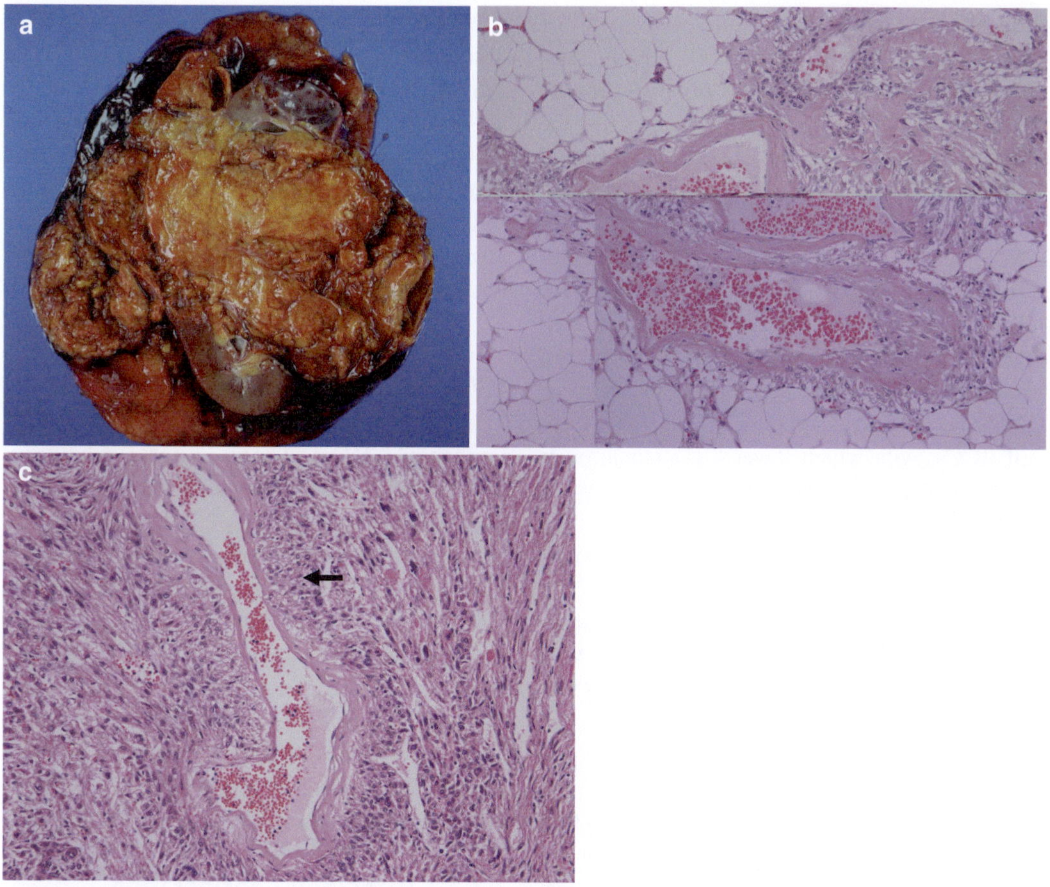

Fig. 1.55 Pathologic findings of angiomyolipoma. (**a**) Gross photograph of angiomyolipoma shows large mass with fat and hemorrhage. This tumor extends to perinephric tissue. (**b**) Microscopically, angiomyolipoma is composed of fat, blood vessels, and smooth muscle cells. Vascular wall is hyalinized. (**c**) Radiating smooth muscle cells from vascular wall (*arrow*) are typical finding of angiomyolipoma

Microscopically, angiomyolipoma contains variable amount of fat, smooth muscle cells, and vessels (Fig. 1.55b). Around the vessels, smooth muscle cells radiate from the vascular wall (Fig. 1.55c). Vessels often have thick and hyalinized vascular wall.

1.7.2.2 Imaging

US

AMLs are usually hyperechoic on US due to fat or hemorrhage. The echogenicity is often similar or even higher than that of renal sinus fat. However, small RCCs can also appear hyperechoic and have similar imaging features to AML. In such cases, intratumoral cysts and hypoechoic rim, which are characteristic US findings of small RCCs, may help the differentiation (Fig. 1.3).

CT

Macroscopic fat demonstrates negative Hounsfield units on CT. Fat is identified with a region-of-interest (ROI) circle on unenhanced CT images, and in routine practice, this method is sufficient to confirm an AML. Using ROI circles ≤−10 HU as a criteria for the diagnosis of AML, the specificity is very high (100 %), but the sensitivity is about 73 %. An attenuation threshold of −10 HU or lower with an ROI of at least 19–24 mm^2 is optimal for the diagnosis of AML. The use of smaller ROIs leads to unacceptably high false-positive rates, increasing the risk of misdiagnosing an RCC as an AML [89]. A more precise method for the analysis of small clusters of fat is pixel mapping, which analyzes the Hounsfield units of individual pixels. This method is especially useful in AMLs with no or minimal fat [90]. These fat-poor AMLs account for 5 % of AML and do not contain enough fat to be diagnosed with confidence on unenhanced CT (Figs. 1.3 and 1.10). However, a study reported that once lesions with macroscopic fat have been excluded, pixel attenuation histogram analysis cannot be used to distinguish AMLs from clear cell RCCs, with which lower CT attenuation is more strongly associated due to intracytoplasmic fat [91].

AML tends to show angular interface with normal renal parenchyma, which can be seen in 79 % of benign renal masses. AMLs are nonencapsulated and never show a pseudocapsule. AMLs with dominant smooth muscle component show higher attenuation than renal parenchyma on unenhanced CT (Fig. 1.10). However, this hyperattenuation is nonspecific, and 22 % of clear cell RCCs share this feature on CT images [92, 93].

On contrast-enhanced CT, uniform, prolonged contrast enhancement can be observed in contrast to clear cell RCCs, but the enhancement pattern can be variable according to vascular components of AMLs (Fig. 1.9). Therefore, CT cannot differentiate fat-poor AML from RCC conclusively.

MRI

Fat in AMLs shows high SI on T1WI and dark SI with fat saturation. Double-echo gradient chemical shift MR imaging can be used to differentiate AML with minimal fat from other renal neoplasms (Fig. 1.3). In AMLs, a higher signal intensity index and tumor-to-spleen ratio can be observed between in- and out-of-phase images. A prospective study reported the sensitivity of 96 % and the specificity of 93 %, using a signal intensity index of 25 % as a threshold [94]. However, this signal drop on out-of-phase MR images should be interpreted with caution because a similar signal drop can be identified in the clear cell subtype of RCC secondary to intracytoplasmic lipid.

Renal mass signal on T2WI may be helpful in differentiating AML with minimal fat from clear cell RCC. AML with minimal fat is low SI due to its smooth muscle content, whereas clear cell RCC usually shows iso- or high SI on T2WI. Papillary RCC, however, also shows typically low SI on T2WI. Therefore, T2WI image cannot be used to differentiate papillary RCC from a fat-poor AML.

1.7.3 Epithelioid Angiomyolipoma

Epithelioid AML is a variant of AML with little or no fat, which was previously reported as RCC. One-third of epithelioid AML have been found to present with malignant biological behaviors, including local invasion, recurrence, and metastasis. Large masses with infiltrative growth are common, hemorrhage and necrosis may be present, and extrarenal extension or venous invasion may occur. It is classified as a potentially malignant mesenchymal neoplasm in 2004 WHO classification of renal tumors. More than half of patients are associated with tuberous sclerosis [95].

1.7.3.1 Pathologic Consideration

Epithelioid angiomyolipoma is defined as angiomyolipoma with predominant epithelioid features [96]. Grossly, epithelioid angiomyolipoma is a solid well-demarcated mass with occasional extrarenal extension and occasionally shows hemorrhagic or necrotic cut surface (Fig. 1.56a). Epithelioid angiomyolipoma is composed of sheets of large epithelioid cells and spindle cells. Epithelioid cells have clear to eosinophilic cytoplasm, and some tumor cells show considerable nuclear pleomorphism (Fig. 1.56b). Epithelioid angiomyolipoma can have frequent mitotic figures, multinucleated giant cells, and necrosis. There are less prominent vasculature and adipose tissue than classic angiomyolipoma.

1.7.3.2 Imaging

Imaging findings of most epithelioid AMLs are nonspecific and difficult to differentiate from RCC (Fig. 1.57). They could be a heterogeneously

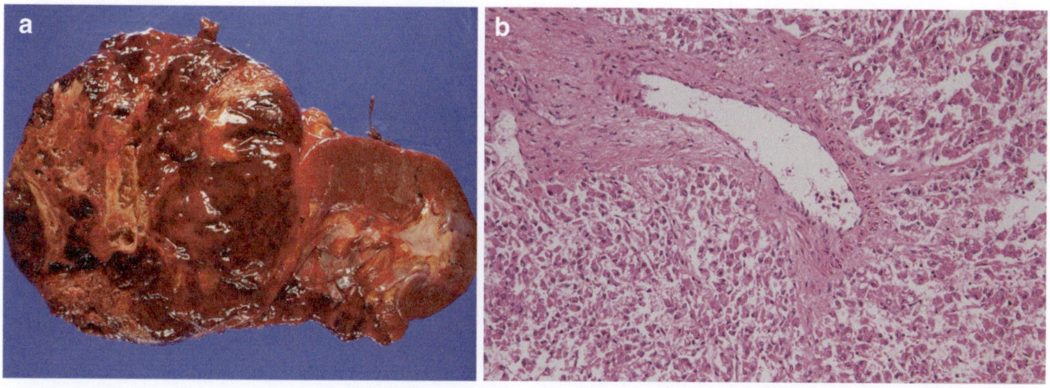

Fig. 1.56 Pathologic findings of epithelioid angiomyolipoma. (**a**) Epithelioid angiomyolipoma shows hemorrhage and necrosis. Fatty tissue was not identifiable at this gross photograph. (**b**) Tumor cells of epithelioid angiomyolipoma are epithelioid and have abundant eosinophilic cytoplasm with prominent nucleoli

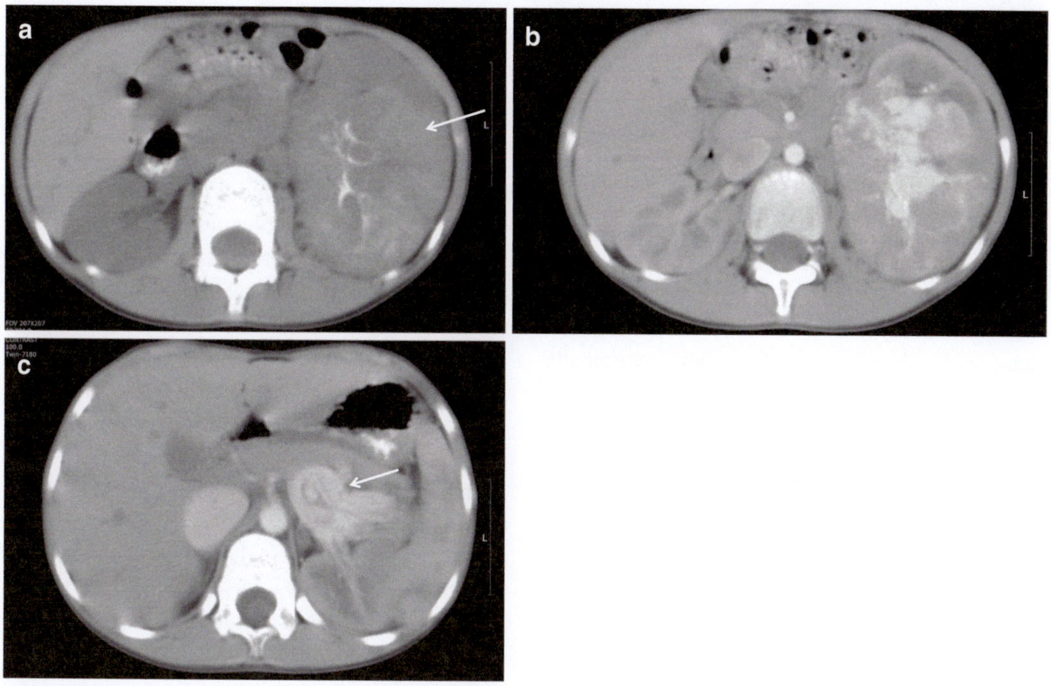

Fig. 1.57 Epithelioid AML. (**a**) Noncontrast CT shows a large mass (*arrow*) with calcifications in the left kidney. No fatty component is detected. (**b**, **c**) The mass is hypervascular and shows a large amount of tumor thrombus (*arrow*) in the renal vein

solid, homogeneously solid, or multilocular cystic lesion with massive hemorrhage. They tend to be hyperattenuating on unenhanced CT images and low SI on T2-weighted MR images due to muscle component, which is a characteristic finding of AMLs. Macroscopic fat may or may not be demonstrated [97, 98].

1.7.4 Rare Benign Renal Mesenchymal Tumors

1.7.4.1 Pathologic Consideration

Leiomyoma is a benign mesenchymal tumor composed of smooth muscle cells, and pathologic features are identical to soft tissue leiomyoma.

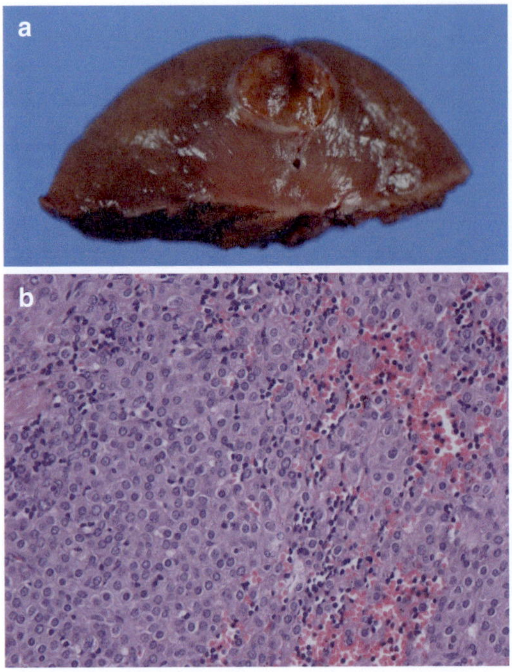

Fig. 1.58 (**a**) Juxtaglomerular cell tumor is a small well-circumscribed tumor with *tan to yellow color*. (**b**) Microscopically, tumor cells are uniformly small and round with distinct cell border

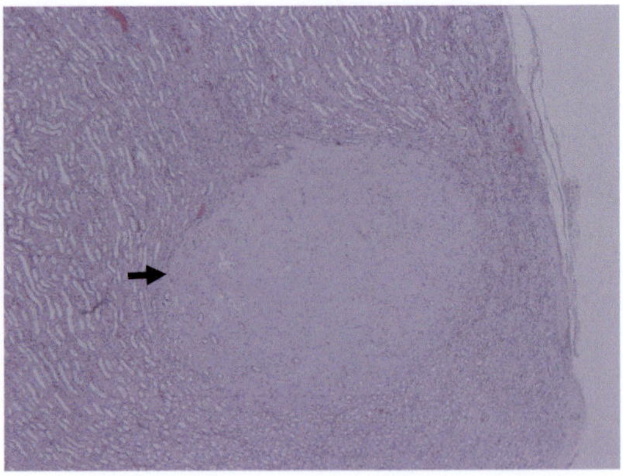

Fig. 1.59 Renomedullary interstitial cell tumor (*arrow*) is composed of hypocellular benign spindle cells in loose or collagenous stroma

Grossly, leiomyoma is a firm, well-demarcated mass with whitish cut surface. Microscopically, tumor cells have spindle nuclei without pleomorphism and show fascicular arrangement.

Grossly, juxtaglomerular cell tumor is 2–3 cm-sized well-demarcated tumor with tan to yellow cut surface (Fig. 1.58a). Microscopically, this tumor is composed of sheets of small uniform round cells with clear to eosinophilic cytoplasm and distinct cell border (Fig. 1.58b). Occasionally, it contains sheets of spindle cells. This tumor generally has abundant vasculature.

Renomedullary interstitial cell tumor is a small benign mesenchymal tumor located at the renal medulla, and it is composed of benign-looking spindle or stellate cells with loose or collagenous stroma (Fig. 1.59).

1.7.4.2 Imaging

Renal leiomyomas occur in the renal capsule most commonly, but it can also arise from the smooth muscle of the renal pelvis or vessels. On CT, well-demarcated, homogeneously enhancing solid mass is a common finding (Fig. 1.60). However, degenerative changes such as cyst and hemorrhage may be visible in larger tumors. The mass shows low SI on T2WI of MR.

Hemangioma can occur in the urinary tract, and the kidney is the most commonly affected organ. Males and females are equally affected. Renal pyramids and the renal pelvis are the most common sites of occurrence. The size of renal hemangiomas is usually small but may be larger than 10 cm, especially in a cavernous form. Symptoms may be none or recurrent episodes of hematuria with colicky pain. On US, renal hemangiomas may be hypoechoic with normal power Doppler signals. On CT, calcifications may be visible, and prolonged enhancement on delayed phase contrast-enhanced images can be characteristic (Fig. 1.61). On MRI, it usually shows high SI with some flow voids on T2WI [99].

Juxtraglomerular cell tumor or reninoma is a benign renin-secreting tumor. It is usually detected in young hypertensive patients with high plasma renin activity and hypokalemia. It is usually small, solid, and peripherally located. On US, it commonly shows isoechogenicity to renal parenchyma. On CT and MRI, the mass shows similar attenuation or signal intensity to renal parenchyma, and mild, delayed enhancement (Fig. 1.62) [100].

Renomedullary interstitial cell tumors, formerly called renal medullary fibromas, are found

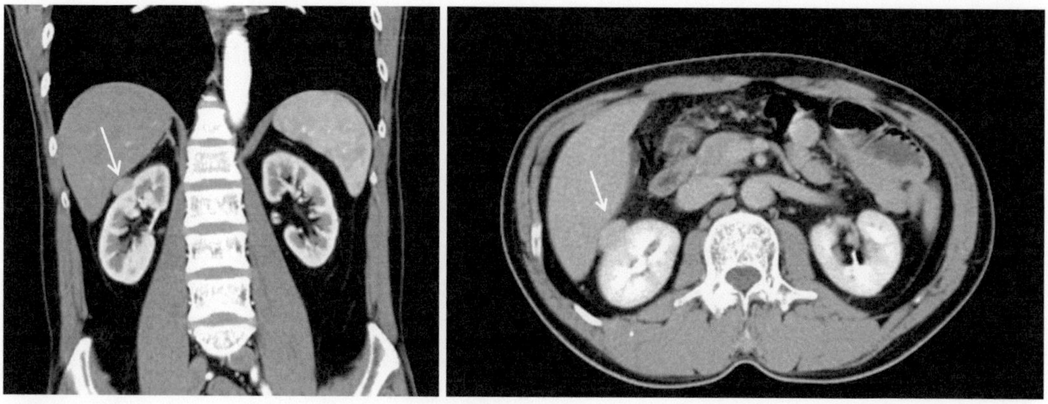

Fig. 1.60 Renal capsular leiomyoma. (**a**) Corticomedullary phase CT in coronal plane shows a small, mildly enhancing mass (*arrow*) in the right kidney, which is almost entirely exophytic. (**b**) The mass shows homogeneous and prolonged enhancement in nephrographic phase

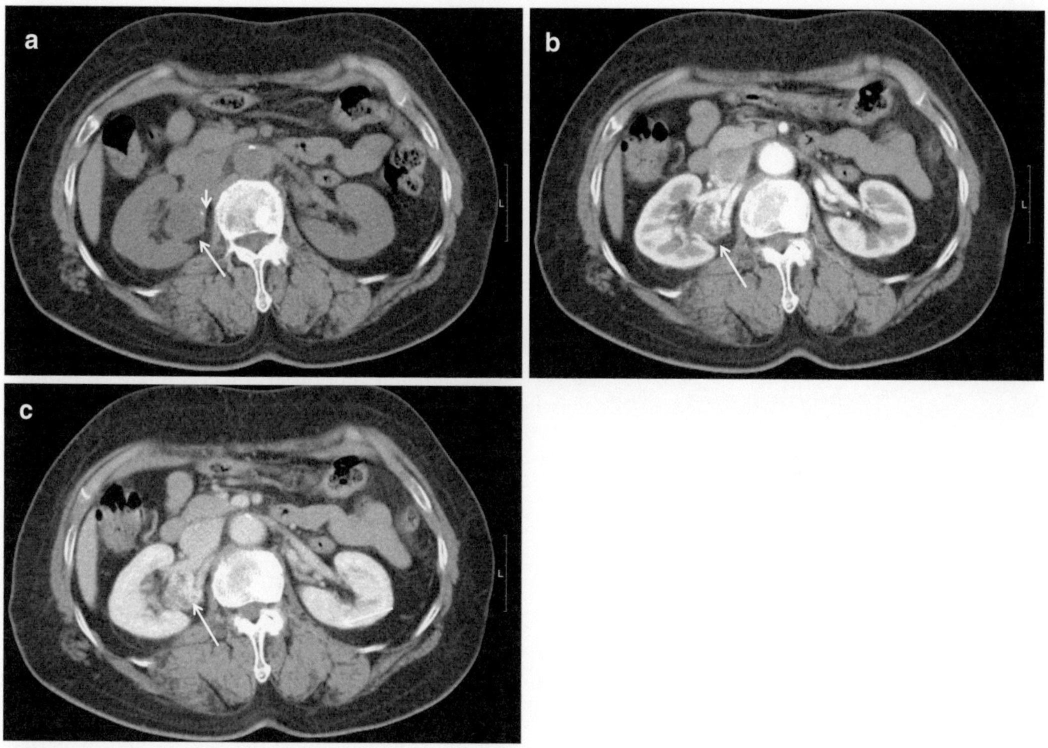

Fig. 1.61 Renal hemangioma. (**a**) Noncontrast CT shows a lobulating mass (*large arrow*) with small calcification (*small arrow*) in the sinus of the right kidney. (**b**, **c**) The mass (*arrow*) enhances from the periphery to the center in dynamic contrast-enhanced CT (**b** corticomedullary phase, **c** nephrographic phase)

in nearly 50% of adult at autopsy. They are located at renal medullary pyramid and mostly smaller than 5 mm. Larger mass may occur in rare instances and appears as a nonenhancing solid mass in the renal medulla [101].

Solitary fibrous tumors are fibrous tumors arising from serosal surfaces of organs. They are most common in pleura, but it also arises in the kidney. Renal capsule or peripelvic connective tissue is thought as sites of origin. Most solitary

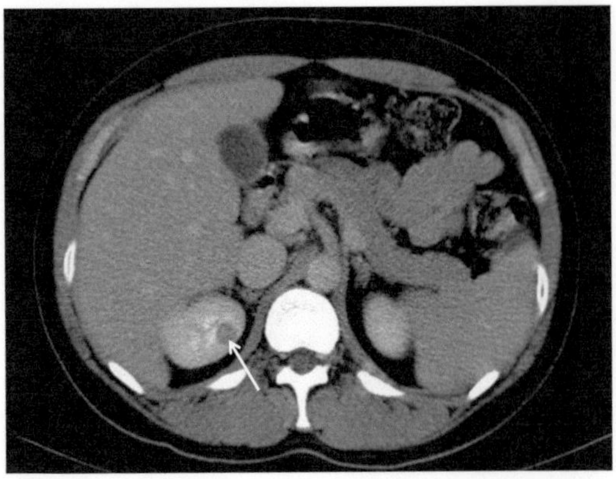

Fig. 1.62 Juxtraglomerular cell tumor in a hypertensive patient. Contrast-enhanced CT shows a small, poorly enhancing mass (*arrow*) in the right kidney

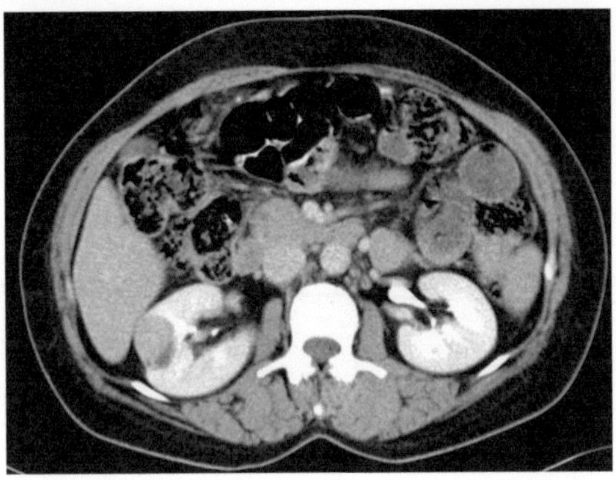

Fig. 1.63 Solitary fibrous tumor. Contrast-enhanced CT shows a well-defined mass (*arrow*) in the right kidney. The enhancing part of the mass appears homogeneous

fibrous tumors are benign, but 10–15 % of extra-pleural solitary fibrous tumors show malignant behavior such as recurrence or metastasis. Mean age is 52 years, and there is no sex predilection. The patients are usually asymptomatic. On CT, a well-defined, lobulated mass in the renal sinus or capsule shows homogeneous enhancement despite the large size (Fig. 1.63). Necrosis, hemorrhage, and calcifications are rarely found. On T2WI MR, alternate areas of low SI and moderately high SI are reported to be found in solitary fibrous tumor with a radial configuration. Spoke-wheel pattern of enhancement has been also reported [102, 103].

1.8 Cystic Nephroma and Mixed Mesenchymal and Epithelial Tumors

1.8.1 Pathologic Consideration

Cystic nephroma is a benign neoplasm composed entirely of cysts. Grossly, cystic nephroma is a well-demarcated mass with multiple cysts without solid component, and cysts contain serous fluid (Fig. 1.64a). Microscopically, cysts are lined by epithelial cells with variable features including flat, cuboidal, or columnar appearance (Fig. 1.64b). Stroma between cysts have fibrous component with variable amount of spindle cells. Sometimes, ovarian stroma-like feature is found.

Mixed epithelial and stromal tumor is composed of variable amount of epithelial and stromal components. Mixed epithelial and stromal tumor and cystic nephroma are considered as morphologic spectrum of same entity. Grossly, mixed epithelial and stromal tumor is a well-demarcated mass with variable amounts of cysts (Fig. 1.65a). Microscopically, this tumor is composed of variable-sized cysts and stroma. Stromal and epithelial components of this tumor are similar to those of cystic nephroma. Cyst lining cells are flat, cuboidal, or columnar epithelium (Fig. 1.65b).

1.8.2 Imaging

Mixed epithelial and stromal tumor (MEST) and adult cystic nephroma (ACN) are included in this category of renal tumors. MEST of the kidney is a rare, benign cystic neoplasm, characterized by a biphasic proliferation of epithelium and stroma. Recent studies suggest that MEST and ACN may be in a morphologic spectrum of the same disease, although 2004 WHO classification of renal tumors considered MEST and ACN as separate entities. MEST and ACN also share clinical features: 6:1 female predominance, predominantly perimenopausal, and common history of estrogen therapy. ACN is a multilocular cystic mass with no solid portion and thin septa (< 5 mm in thickness) (Fig. 1.66), whereas MEST shows solid portions

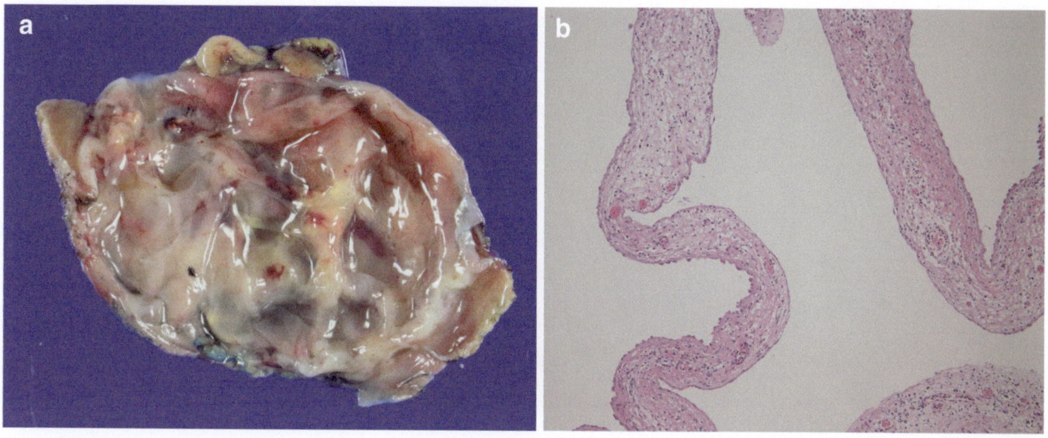

Fig. 1.64 (**a**) Gross morphology of cystic nephroma shows multiloculated cyst. (**b**) Microscopic findings of cystic nephroma shows thin cyst wall with flat or cuboidal lining epithelial cells

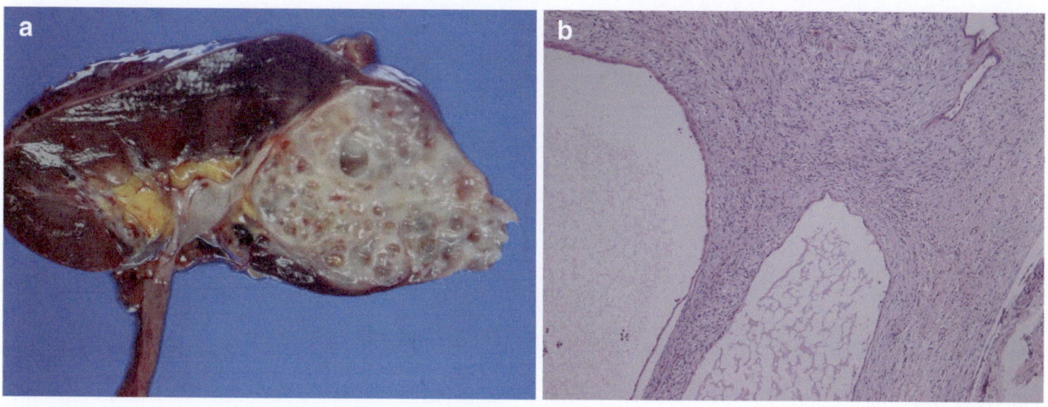

Fig. 1.65 (**a**) Grossly, mixed epithelial and stromal tumor is a well-demarcated, partly solid and partly cystic mass. (**b**) Mixed epithelial and stromal tumor shows benign-looking spindle cells in solid area with multiple cysts lined by flat to cuboidal epithelial cells

grossly with thicker septa (Fig. 1.67). However, the differentiation is difficult on imaging and not important clinically because both of them are benign cystic renal lesions. Because most MESTs appear as Bosniak category III or IV lesions, a cystic RCC should be differentiated first. Other differential diagnosis includes complex cyst, multicystic dysplastic kidney, obstructed duplicated renal collecting system, and renal abscess.

On CT, MEST appear as a mixed cystic and solid or a solid mass according to the proportion of epithelial and stromal components. The septa

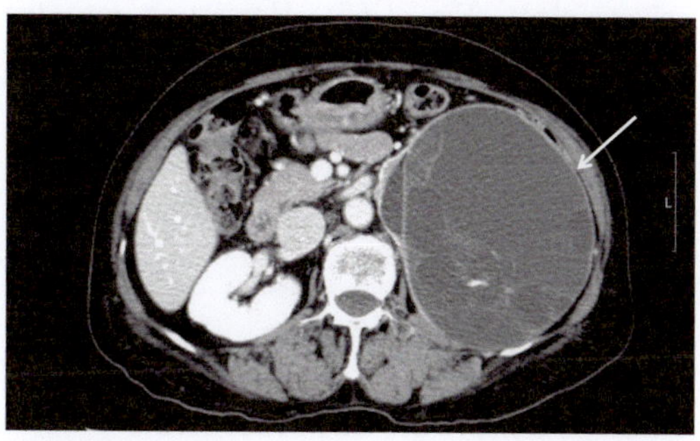

Fig. 1.66 Adult cystic nephroma. Contrast-enhanced CT shows a large cystic mass (*arrow*) with multiple septa and calcifications in the left kidney

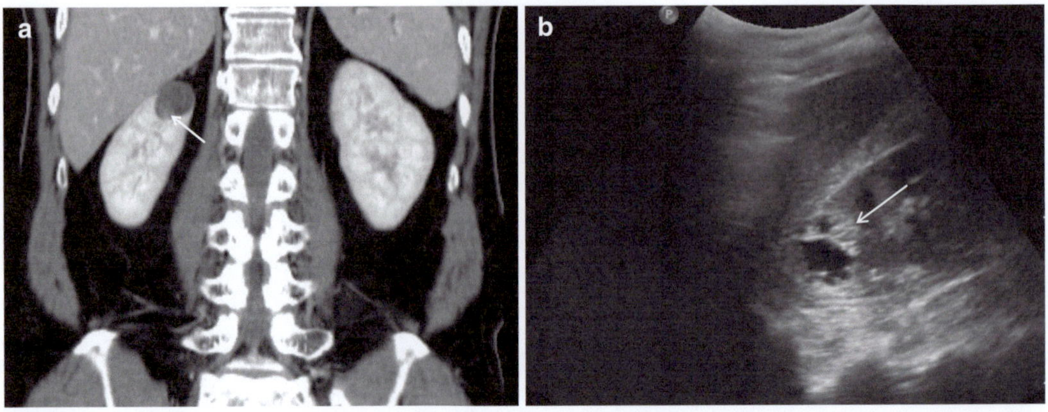

Fig. 1.67 MEST. (**a**) Contrast-enhanced CT in coronal plane shows a cystic mass containing small enhancing solid part (*arrow*) in the right kidney. (**b**) On US, the mass (*arrow*) shows mixed echogenicity

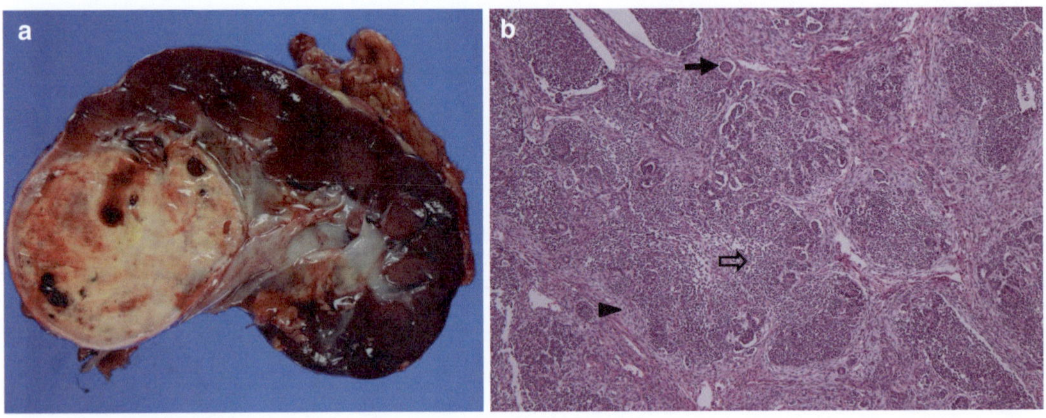

Fig. 1.68 (**a**) This nephroblastoma is a large well-demarcated tumor with focal hemorrhage. (**b**) Microscopically, nephroblastoma shows triphasic pattern including blastemal, epithelial, and stromal component. This photograph shows these three components: epithelial components reveal immature glomerular structures (*arrow*); blastemal components are small tightly packed immature cells (*open arrow*); stromal components are spindle cells between epithelial and blastemal components (*arrowhead*)

are usually thin and show mild and delayed enhancement (Fig. 1.67). Herniation into the renal pelvis is sometimes observed, which may be a cause of hemorrhage or urinary obstruction. On MRI, the stromal component of MEST shows low SI on T2WI and enhances mildly [104].

1.9 Nephroblastoma

1.9.1 Pathologic Consideration

Nephroblastoma is a malignant embryonal tumor composed of blastemal, epithelial, and stromal components. Grossly, nephroblastoma is a well-demarcated mass with uniform tan to gray cut surface (Fig. 1.68a). After chemotherapy, necrosis and hemorrhage are common. Typically, this tumor shows triphasic pattern having blastemal, epithelial, and stromal component (Fig. 1.68b). Blastemal cells are small, closely packed immature cells with scanty cytoplasm. Epithelial components show primitive or mature tubules, immature-looking glomerular structure or papillary structure. Stromal components consist of spindle cells of smooth muscle or skeletal muscle differentiation or undifferentiated spindle cells. Sometimes other mesenchymal components such as fat, bone, or cartilage also can be found.

1.9.2 Imaging

Nephroblastoma, also known as Wilms' tumor, is mainly a tumor of childhood. It can occur in adult but its incidence is rare. Its imaging findings in adult do not differ from those of RCC, and preoperative diagnosis is very difficult or impossible.

1.10 Neuroendocrine Tumors

1.10.1 Pathologic Consideration

Renal carcinoid is very rare. Grossly, carcinoid is a well-demarcated mass with homogeneous yellow to tan cut surface (Fig. 1.69a). Microscopic features of renal carcinoid are similar to those of carcinoid tumors at other sites. Architectural patterns of renal carcinoid are cord, trabeculae, solid sheets, or glandular structures (Fig. 1.69b). Tumor cells have small uniform round nuclei with finely granular chromatin.

Primitive neuroectodermal tumor (PNET) is a malignant small blue round-cell tumor showing gene fusion between EWS gene and ETS gene family. Renal PNET is very rare. Grossly, PNET is large tan to yellow mass with often hemorrhage and necrosis. Microscopic features of renal PNET are same as soft tissue PNET. It is mainly composed of large sheets of small round cells with scanty cytoplasm [105, 106].

1.10.2 Imaging

Carcinoid, neuroendocrine carcinoma, PNET, neuroblastoma, and pheochromocytoma belong to this group. Primary renal carcinoid tumors are extremely uncommon. They usually show indolent behavior compared with RCCs. However, metastasis to lymph nodes, liver, or bone has been reported.

PNET is an uncommon, highly aggressive tumor with a poor prognosis. Outside the central nervous system, they can involve the chest wall, paraspinal areas, and rarely organs. Its incidence in the abdomen and pelvis, including the retroperitoneum, is 14 %. The peak age incidence is in the second and third decades of life and male-to-female ratio is 2:1. On imaging, it usually appears as a minimally enhancing, large mass with multiple septum-like structures, peripheral hemorrhage, venous thrombosis, and is accompanied by distant metastasis (Fig. 1.70) [107].

1.11 Lymphoma

1.11.1 Pathologic Consideration

Primary malignant lymphoma of kidney is very rare. Diffuse large B cell lymphoma is the most common lymphoma subtype of kidney [108].

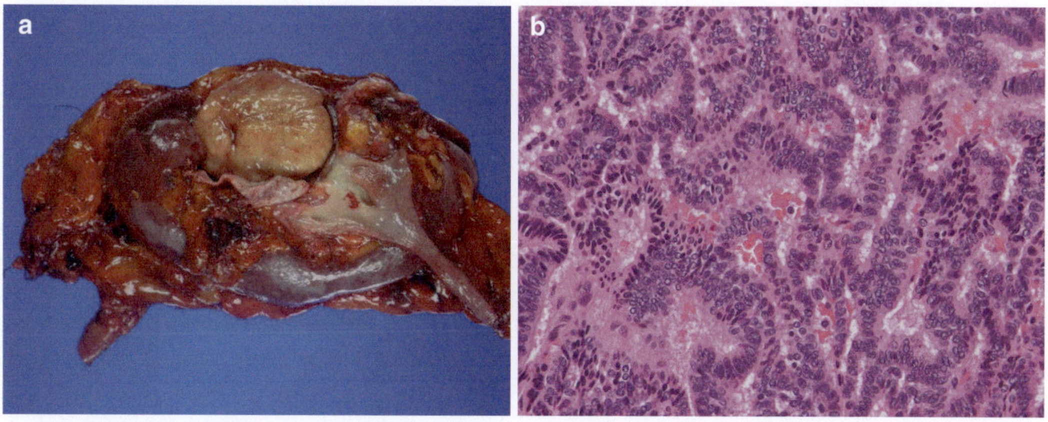

Fig. 1.69 Pathologic findings of renal carcinoid. (**a**) Grossly, renal carcinoid is a well-demarcated mass with *yellowish* homogeneous cut surface. (**b**) Microscopically, this carcinoid shows trabecular or glandular structure

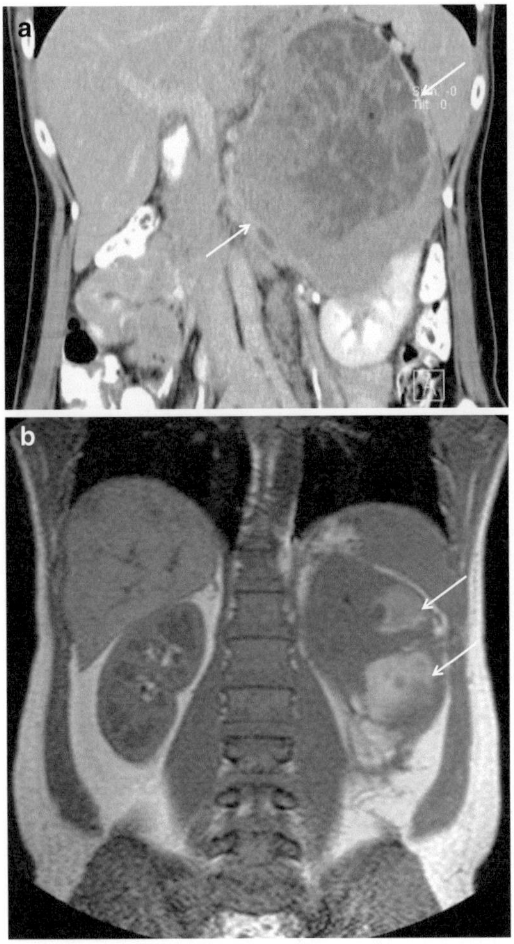

Fig. 1.70 Renal PNET. (**a**) Contrast-enhanced CT in coronal plane shows a large solid and cystic mass (*arrow*) in the left kidney. (**b**) The mass shows large hemorrhagic components (*arrows*) on coronal T1WI of MR

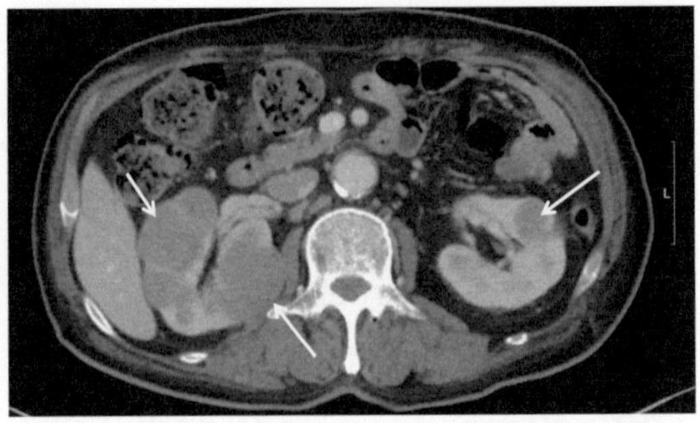

Fig. 1.71 Renal lymphoma. Contrast-enhanced CT shows multiple, homogeneous masses (*arrows*) with mild enhancement in bilateral kidneys

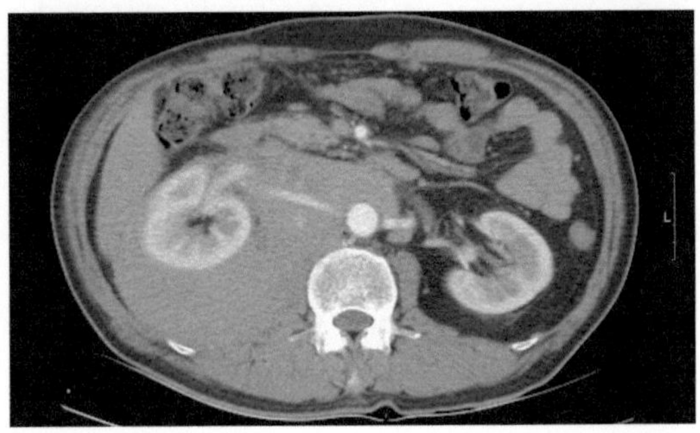

Fig. 1.72 Right renal involvement of lymphoma by retroperitoneal spread on contrast-enhanced CT

1.11.2 Imaging

Primary renal lymphoma is very rare because kidney has no intrinsic lymphoid tissue. However, kidney is frequently involved by lymphoma in the setting of widespread disease and usually with non-Hodgkin's lymphoma. Lymphoma may enter the kidney hematogenously or through the sinus, perinephric, or capsular lymphatics, and the radiological findings depend upon these mechanisms of involvement. The most common finding is multiple, bilateral, or unilateral renal masses of variable size (Fig. 1.71). This pattern is seen in 50–60 % of cases, and retroperitoneal lymphadenopathy is mostly associated. Contiguous, infiltrative spread from adjacent retroperitoneal lymphadenopathy is the second most common pattern, seen on 25–30 % of cases (Fig. 1.72). Smooth, generalized, bilateral renal enlargement occurs in approximately 20 %, due to diffuse lymphomatous infiltration in kidneys. A solitary renal mass is seen in 10–25 %. Other findings include perirenal mass, and preferential renal sinus involvement [109, 110].

On US, lymphoma mass is mostly homogeneous and hypoechoic. Sometimes it is markedly hypoechoic and even shows posterior sonic enhancement, mimicking a renal cyst (Fig. 1.73).

Renal lymphoma is a soft tissue mass with slightly higher attenuation than that of the surrounding parenchyma on unenhanced CT. Calcifications are rarely visible. It enhances homogeneously but less intensely than normal renal parenchyma. Large lesions tend to be more heterogeneous. Nephrographic phase contrast-enhanced CT is essential in the detection of lymphomatous deposits

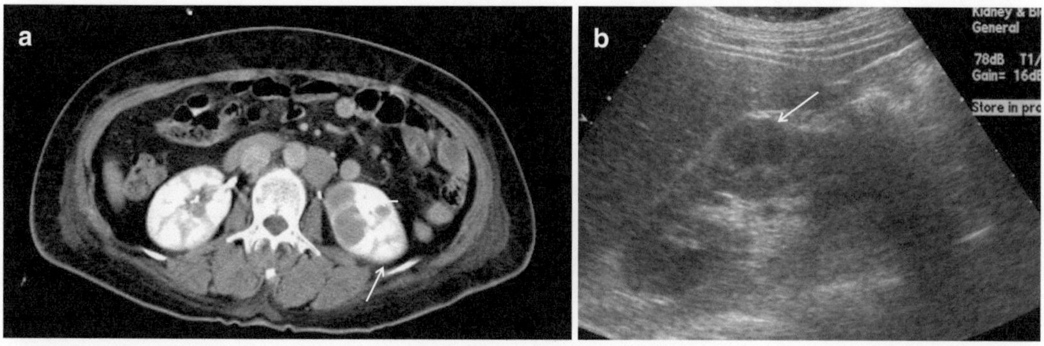

Fig. 1.73 US of renal lymphoma. (**a**) Contrast-enhanced CT shows multiple low-attenuation masses (*large arrow*) in the left kidney. Note enlarged para-aortic lymph node (*small arrow*). (**b**) On US, a renal mass (*arrow*) shows low echo, almost looks like a cyst

in the kidney, because they may be small and medullary in location with relatively little cortical deformity. The presence of retroperitoneal lymphadenopathy may be a clue to the diagnosis.

On MR, renal lymphomas show high SI on T1WI and are slightly hypointense or isointense relative to normal renal cortex on T2WI. They enhance less than the renal parenchyma, and some lesions may enhance progressively on delayed images [109, 110].

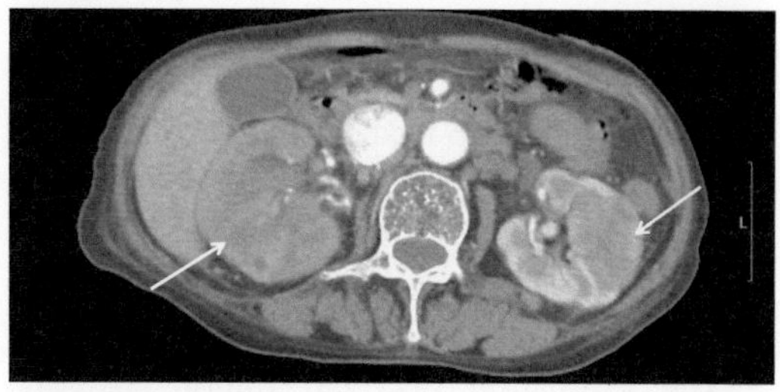

Fig. 1.74 Renal metastasis from lung cancer. Contrast-enhanced CT shows ill-defined masses (*arrows*) preserving renal contour in bilateral kidneys

1.12 Metastatic Tumors

1.12.1 Pathologic Consideration

Metastatic tumors from various primary sites can be encountered in the kidney. Common primary sites are the lung, breast, skin (melanoma), gastrointestinal tract, and genitourinary tracts [111].

1.12.2 Imaging

Renal metastases are usually multiple, small, and ill marginated. They are frequently less exophytic or more infiltrative than RCCs on CT (Fig. 1.74). On US, they are usually isoechoic and often difficult to detect (Fig. 1.75). Tissue biopsy is needed when the differentiation between primary and metastatic tumor is uncertain to make a therapeutic plan [88, 112].

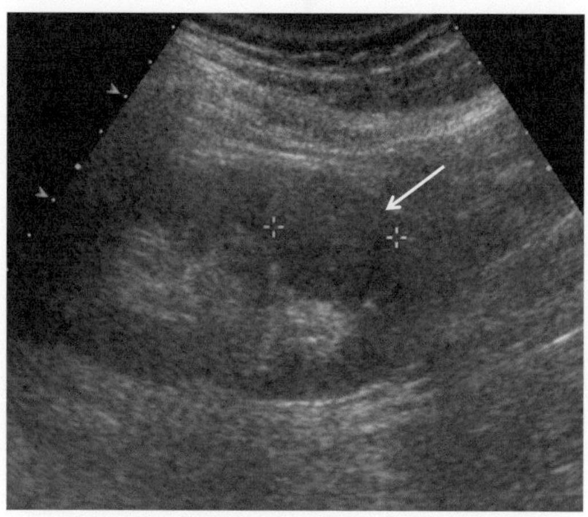

Fig. 1.75 US of renal metastasis. US shows an isoechoic mass (*arrow*) preserving renal contour in the kidney. The mass was confirmed as metastasis from lung cancer by biopsy

1.13 Therapeutic Considerations

1.13.1 Active Surveillance of Renal Tumor

Small RCCs grow slowly and metastasis is very rare, and the metastatic risk grows when tumor diameter is larger than 3 cm (Fig. 1.1). In one meta-analysis, 30 % of small (<3 cm) solid renal masses did not grow during a 23–39-month observation interval [113].

Therefore, active surveillance can be an option in small renal masses to avoid the morbidity of surgical or ablative treatment in elderly and/or infirm patients. In a multicenter, prospective study, active surveillance was done in 209 small renal masses in 178 patients by serial imaging with CT, MRI, or US in an average of 28 months. Local progression occurred in 12 % and metastases in 1.1 %. Tumor growth rate was an average of 0.13 cm/year, which was not affected significantly by the presence of RCC on biopsy [114].

The estimation of renal tumor size and growth rate is essential to active surveillance protocols. A prospective study reported that US, which has advantages in terms of radiation and accessibility, was not inferior in the assessment of renal mass size compared with MRI or CT [115].

1.13.2 Ablation of Renal Tumor

1.13.2.1 Introduction

Increasing utilization of cross-sectional imaging contributes to the increasing detection of RCC. Radical or partial nephrectomy is a treatment of choice for RCC. However, renal tumor ablation is an alternative treatment for RCC in patients who are not able to undergo surgery. Percutaneous ablation has been accepted as a minimally invasive surgery for treating a small RCC (<4 cm) [116].

1.13.2.2 Patient Selection and Preparation

For treating an RCC, patients should be meticulously selected because ablation is an alternative treatment for patients with serious comorbidity. Still, this treatment does not have evidence for replacing surgery in treatment of RCC in healthy patients. Patients should be fasting for at least 8 hours prior to ablation. Renal mass biopsy is a mandatory procedure because a smaller tumor increases a higher probability for benign diagnosis [117]. Patients are asked not to have medication increasing a risk for bleeding or coagulopathy at least 1 or 2 week before ablation. The use of antibiotics is not mandatory pretreatment. Serum creatinine, blood cell count, and a coagulation profile are all checked. Platelet count of less than 50,000 or an International normalized ratio of greater than 1.5 may increase a risk for bleeding or coagulaopathy and thus should be corrected before ablation. Pre-ablation CT or MR images should be reviewed to evaluate how to access or treat a tumor and avoid complication [118].

1.13.2.3 Procedures

Conscious sedation for cryoablation or general anesthesia for radiofrequency ablation is recommended to control pain. Most of the patients are placed prone on the CT table, and a baseline unenhanced CT is obtained. The appropriate entry site is prepared and draped sterilely. Ablation margin should range from 5 to 10 mm to reduce local tumor progression [119]. Generally, cryoablation protocol consists of a 10-min freeze, an 8-minutes active thaw, and a 10-minutes freeze under CT or MRI guidance. RFA protocol lasts 10–12 minutes under CT guidance.

1.13.2.4 Complications

Major complication rate is reported to be 2–3 % and requires specific treatment. This complication includes bowel perforation, ureter stricture, uncontrolled bleeding, and tension pneumothorax [118]. Hematuria is the most common complication but spontaneously disappears. Prevention methods such as patient position change, levering applicator, and hydrodissection are necessary to avoid injury to adjacent organs.

1.13.2.5 Follow-Up

Pre- and post-contrast CT scan is recommended at 1–3 months after ablation. Thereafter, pre- and post-contrast CT should be performed every 6 months or annually. Patients with reduced renal function can undergo unenhanced MRI protocols consisting of T1-weighted, T2-weighted, and diffusion-weighted images. Contrast-enhanced US is one of the options in these patients.

1.13.2.6 Outcomes

Reportedly, intermediate- or long-term survival rates of percutaneous ablation for T1a RCC (<4 cm) range between 88 and 99 % [116, 120–122]. These outcomes are very similar to those of partial nephrectomy [120]. Therefore, percutaneous ablation is a safe and effective treatment for RCC in poor surgical candidate.

1.13.3 Surgery

1.13.3.1 Radical Nephrectomy

The objective of oncologic surgery is to excise all tumors with adequate surgical margin. In 1969, Robson established the basic principle and the concept of radical nephrectomy, an early ligation of renal vessels to prevent vascular tumor emboli, and an en bloc resection of the kidney with Gerota's fascia and the ipsilateral adrenal gland as well as complete regional lymphadenectomy from the crus of the diaphragm to the aortic bifurcation [123]. Historically, it has been known that ipsilateral adrenal metastasis was present in 1–10 % of patients. However, ipsilateral adrenal involvement of renal cell carcinoma is rare (1–2 %), and many patients with ipsilateral adrenal involvement present with hematogenous metastasis. No survival gain has been demonstrated by concurrent ipsilateral adrenalectomy. Therefore, ipsilateral adrenalectomy is indicated if there is an evidence of ipsilateral adrenal involvement in CT/MRI, tumors located in upper pole, or large tumors [124, 125]. Otherwise, the risk of future adrenal insufficiency should be weighed against the benefit. Nodal involvement status is important in the prognosis of RCC. However, level 1 evidence showed that no therapeutic benefit of lymphadenectomy was demonstrated over nephrectomy alone [126]. Radical nephrectomy is the standard of care for tumors ≥T2.

1.13.3.2 Open Radical Nephrectomy

Traditionally, radical nephrectomy is considered to be the standard treatment for localized renal cell carcinoma. Although surgery remains to be the main treatment of RCC, open radical nephrectomy (ORN) is no longer the gold standard. ORN has inevitable morbidity associated with the incision through muscle and fascia, and postoperative recovery is longer than that of minimally invasive surgery (Fig. 1.76). Procedure-related morbidity and resultant renal insufficiency and risk of dialysis are the major drawbacks of it [127, 128].

1.13.3.3 Laparoscopic Radical Nephrectomy

Laparoscopic radical nephrectomy (LRN) was first described by Clayman et al. in 1990s [129]. The strength of laparoscopic approach lies in its minimally invasive nature with better perioperative outcomes, such as shorter length of hospital stay, decreased blood loss, less pain, and better cosmesis [130]. The oncologic outcome of LRN is comparable and equivalent to that of ORN [131]. Three laparoscopic approaches exist for radical nephrectomy: transperitoneal, retroperitoneal, and hand assisted. The original description of LRN was in a transperitoneal approach.

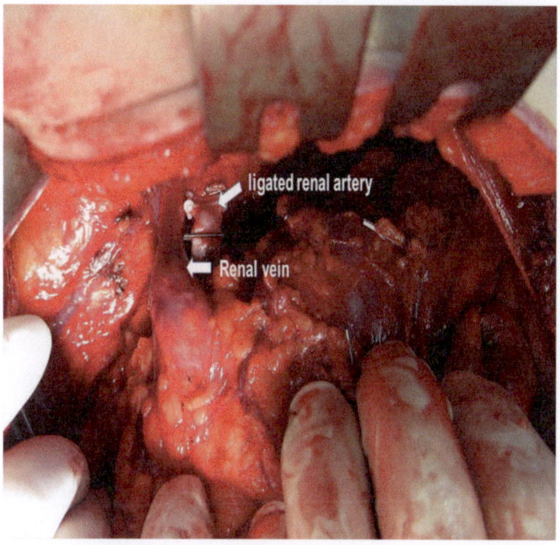

Fig. 1.76 Open radical nephrectomy of 55-year-old male with tumor thrombus in the renal vein. After identifying the vasculature, renal artery is ligated first, and then renal vein can be ligated

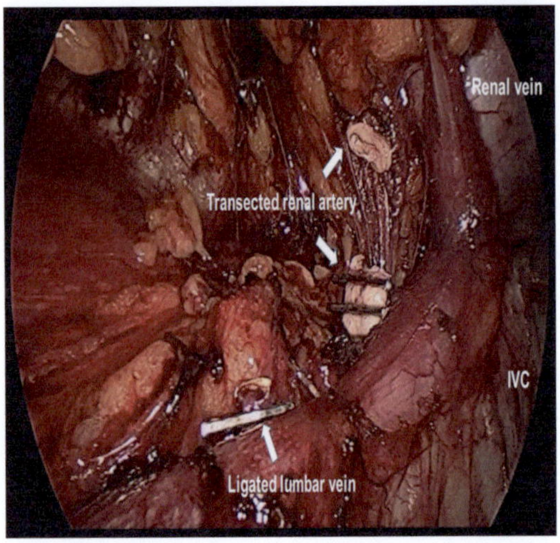

Fig. 1.77 Right laparoscopic radical nephrectomy was performed for a 58-year-old male. Renal artery is first ligated using multiple metal clips

Hand-assisted nephrectomy can be an alternative to open conversion for novice surgeons. Retroperitoneal approach mimics the open retroperitoneal surgery and facilitates the access of hilar vessels without violating the peritoneal cavity. The choice of surgical method depends on the surgeon's preferences.

For transperitoneal laparoscopic radical nephrectomy, four ports (12 mm × 2, 5 mm × 2) are placed. Additional 5 mm port can be placed for right nephrectomy. The procedures are as follows: (1) Take down the bowels and incise along the line of Toldt to expose the Gerota's fascia. (2) Identify the retroperitoneal organs and major vessels illuminating behind the whitish tissue. (3) Dissect the tissues between the gonadal vein and IVC in the right, aorta in the left to encounter the back muscles. (4) Lift up the ureter and gonadal vein and proceed the dissection proximally to the renal hilum. (5) Control the renal artery first and the renal vein. If the lumbar vein is encountered, it can be sacrificed (Fig. 1.77). (6) Dissect and ligate the ureter and gonadal vein. (7) Lateral dissection of the kidney is usually the last step because if it is done from the first time, the kidney can descend due to the gravity obscuring the hilar dissection. (8) If there is no bleeding from the surgical bed, the specimen can be retrieved in a bag through the caudal extension of the incision in camera port. 12 mm ports are usually closed under direct vision using angiocath and Carter–Thomason needle.

For right-side surgery, attention to duodenum and IVC is necessary. For left-side surgery, if the depth of resection is in the wrong plane, mesenteric vessels can be compromised, which can result in significant bleeding or otherwise, small bowel injury can happen.

Hand-assisted laparoscopic nephrectomy is good for inexperienced surgeons to get used to laparoscopic surgeries. The key steps are the same in principle. But the tractions and tactile sensation using the hand can be useful.

Single-port surgery is an option for nephrectomy. The incision can be made around the umbilicus or above the umbilicus. Home-made port, Octoport, or GelPort can be used. Unique devices are developed to prevent crush of both arm and camera. Although articulated instruments are not as strong as the conventional, non-articulated ones, better cosmesis is a strong point of this method.

1.13.3.4 Partial Nephrectomy, Nephron-Sparing Surgery

Partial nephrectomy is performed with the absolute indication in patients with bilateral RCC or tumor in a functionally or anatomically solitary kidney. Relative indications included unilateral tumor with future renal failure, such as baseline renal insufficiency or concurrent comorbid conditions such as renal artery stenosis, hypertension, or diabetes. With the modern imaging techniques and increased incidence of incidentally detected tumors, the trend of renal oncologic surgery has been shifted toward maximal renal functional preservation without compromising oncologic outcomes. Renal function after partial nephrectomy is determined by ischemic time, amount of preserved renal parenchyma, and baseline renal function [132]. Radical nephrectomy can lead to an increased risk of chronic kidney disease [133], which is associated with more cardiovascular events and mortality [134, 135].

Partial nephrectomy is a standard of care for tumors 4 cm or less (pT1a). Patients having T1b tumors or selected patients with unilateral T2a tumors can be treated with partial nephrectomy whenever feasible. Nephron-sparing surgery (NSS) is a treatment of choice whenever technically possible.

1.13.3.5 Open Partial Nephrectomy

Open partial nephrectomy (OPN) has been the primary approach for NSS. Postoperative complications such as urine leak and hemorrhage can occur after OPN.

OPN can be performed in flank position, not entering the peritoneal space. Flank incision with or without cutting the rib can be used. In general, the 11th rib can be used as an index, and it can be cut for 5 cm to have a better exposure. Alternatively, the 10th or 12th rib can be used as an index according to the location of tumors. After incision of flank muscles, the kidney and Gerota's fascia can be separated from the back muscles, and the peritoneum can be peeled off to expose the renal hilum. The renal artery can be dissected and tagged with vessel loop. Location of the ureter has to be identified to prevent potential ureteral injury. Intraoperative ultrasonography can be used before or after removal of the peritumoral fat to have an accurate margin if the tumor is not exophytic. Before clamping the renal artery with Bulldog clamp or Satinsky clamp, expected resection margin can be marked by electrocauterization at the renal capsule. After inducing the renal ischemia, the tumor can be removed by cold scissor or cutting current. Depending on situations, enucleation method or extracorporeal tumorectomy and autotransplantation or "zero ischemia" with unclamping can be used. After removal of the tumor with a certain safety margin, the collecting system or large vessels can be closed with 4–0 Prolene, if opened. Small vessels can be coagulated with bipolar electrocauterization. If the anticipated ischemic time is over 25–30 minutes due to difficult location or large size, cold ischemia can be induced with NaCl ice-slush. V-loc sutures are helpful in reducing the ischemic time. After applying Floseal in the resected bed and suturing the parenchyma with 1–0 Vicryl, the renal parenchyma can be approximated. If there is no bleeding after reperfusion of the kidney, Floseal and Surgicel are applied. Some surgeons use Tisseel to seal the needle hole in the parenchyma according to their preferences.

1.13.3.6 Minimally Invasive Partial Nephrectomy

With the advance of minimally invasive surgery, laparoscopic and robotic surgery is introduced in this field. Minimally invasive surgeries have better convalescence and better cosmesis compared to those of open surgeries because this method can prevent large, muscle-dissecting flank incision.

1.13.3.7 Laparoscopic Partial Nephrectomy

Laparoscopic partial nephrectomy (LPN) had been performed in a limited number of centers by experienced surgeons to small, exophytic peripheral tumors with two normal functioning kidneys, because it is technically difficult to perform. Complication rates of LPN were higher than that of OPN or LRN in early series, as high as 30 % [136, 137]. In experienced hands, the complication rates were decreased [138]. The survival of LPN was equivalent to that of OPN [131].

In laparoscopic partial nephrectomy, the location of ports is slightly different from those of radical nephrectomy. The surgeon's both hand ports should be designed to perform the suturing without difficulty. Tumor location is an important factor that should be considered. Key steps are similar to OPN in principle but using the laparoscopic instruments instead of the hand (Figs. 1.78 and 1.79). The kidney should be positioned to facilitate an easy resection and suturing. It can be done by an assistant using a grasper or tagging the pararenal tissue to the abdominal wall using sutures.

1.13.3.8 Robot-Assisted Laparoscopic Partial Nephrectomy

Da Vinci robot system enabled enhanced dexterity and stereoscopic 3-D vision. While LPN was a technically demanding procedure to be adopted for every surgeon due to the difficulty of suturing,

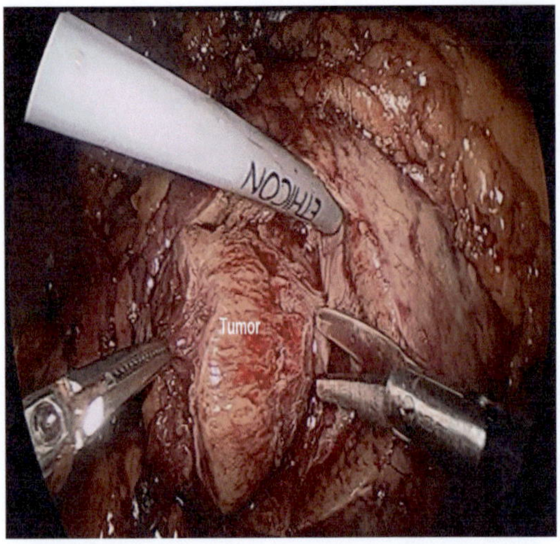

Fig. 1.78 Tumor with adequate resection margin, including peritumoral normal parenchyma is resected using endo-scissors

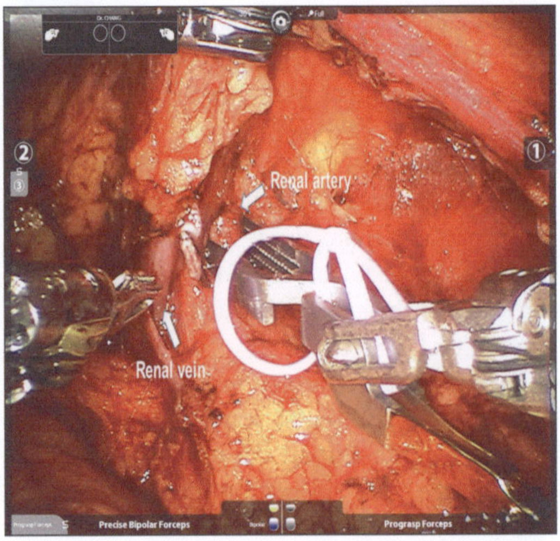

Fig. 1.80 Renal artery is clamped with Bulldog clamp in a robot-assisted laparoscopic partial nephrectomy

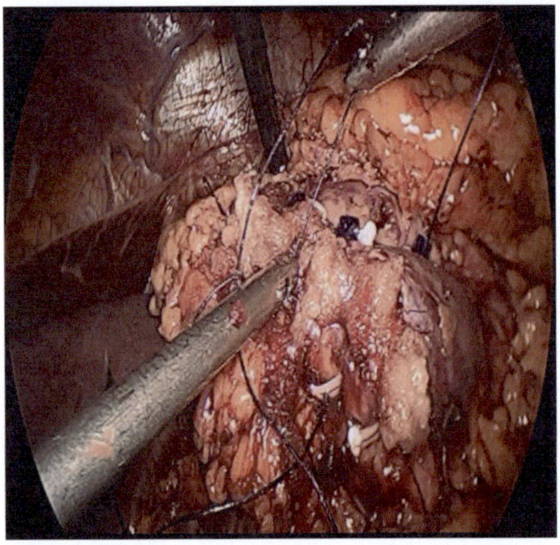

Fig. 1.79 After tumor resection and bed suture, the renorrhaphy using 1–0 Vicryl is done

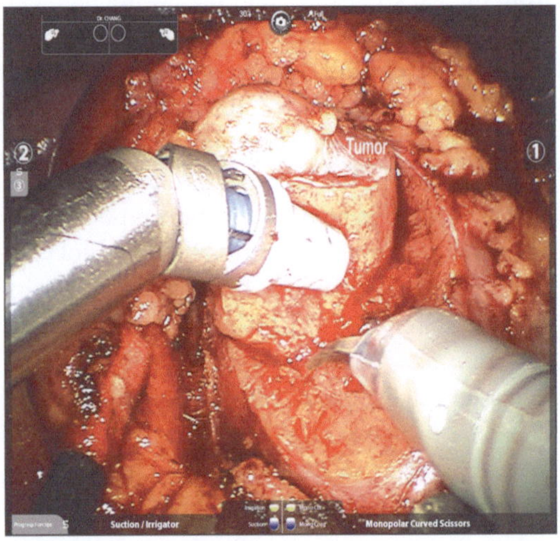

Fig. 1.81 Having a suction-irrigator at the *left hand*, the tumor is resected with decreased dependence on assistant

suturing using robotic system is easier to perform because this system has 7° of freedom and mimics the open surgery. This can relieve the surgeon's pressure to complete the resection and renorrhaphy within 25–30 minutes of warm ischemic time. This can be a viable alternative to OPN or LPN in small renal tumors [139], and also having the advantage of minimally invasive surgeries (Figs. 1.80 and 1.81).

1.14 Targeted Therapy in Metastatic Renal Cell Carcinoma: Advancing Paradigms

1.14.1 Introduction

The 5-year survival for renal cell carcinoma (RCC) improved from 52% in 1975 to 74% in

2014 [140]. Sixteen percent of individuals, however, will present with distant metastases. The contemporary 5-year survival for metastatic RCC is reported as only 12 % [140]. Consistent with the short survival associated with metastatic RCC, this malignancy is relatively unresponsive to traditional chemotherapeutic agents [141]. Until recently, patients were left with few options including the biologic response modifiers IL-2 and IFN-a.

1.14.2 Novel Agents in Metastatic RCC

Current clinical trials have been conducted focusing on clear cell RCC, because of their well-established molecular genetic mechanisms. Most patients with clear cell RCC have mutations of the von Hippel–Lindau (VHL) tumor suppressor gene resulting in cell signaling abnormalities [118]. Under normal conditions, VHL proteins complex with hypoxia-inducible factor (HIF) 1-a and 2-b, leading to degradation. However, in its absence, HIF 1-a and 2-b complex together leading to production of growth factors such as vascular endothelial growth factor (VEGF), platelet-derived growth factor (PDGF), and transforming growth factor-a (TGF-a). These growth factors activate cell surface growth factor receptors setting off intracellular signaling pathways, ultimately ending in angiogenesis and proliferation of malignant cells [142].

1.14.2.1 Tyrosine Kinase Inhibitors

Sorafenib

Sorafenib (BAY 43–9006, Nexavar), approved in 2005, is a multi-kinase inhibitor which was designed as a c-Raf and b-Raf inhibitor. The Ras/Raf signaling pathway is a mediator of tumor cell proliferation and angiogenesis [143]. Sorafenib also inhibits several tyrosine kinases on the intracellular domain of VEGFR and PDGFR. FDA approval of sorafenib was largely based on a multicenter, randomized, double-blind phase III trial (TARGET trial), comparing sorafenib 400 mg twice daily to placebo in 903 patients with previously treated metastatic clear cell RCC [144]. Overall, sorafenib was shown to be more efficacious than placebo with a 10 % RR and a 56 % reduction in risk of PFS (5.5 months vs 2.8 months) in second-line treatment of RCC.

Sunitinib

Sunitinib (SU11248, Sutent), approved in 2006, is the second TKI marketed in the United States for the treatment of RCC. It inhibits the same tyrosine kinases as sorafenib plus the colony-stimulating factor receptor type I, but it does not inhibit Raf [145]. A phase III trial conducted comparing sunitinib with IFN-a in 750 patients with untreated metastatic clear cell RCC [146]. Patients assigned to receive sunitinib achieved a median PFS of 11 months, which was more than double the 5-month PFS observed in the IFN-a group (HR: 0.42). OS difference between the groups was borderline for statistical significance possibly due to crossover to sunitinib after progression on IFN-a alone (26.4 months vs 21.8 months, $p=0.051$) [147].

Pazopanib

Pazopanib (Votrient) is a potent and selective multi-targeted receptor TKI. A phase III trial (COMPARZ trial) showed comparable efficacy (pazopanib ORR 31 %, PFS 8.4 months, OS 28.4 months vs sunitinib ORR 25 %, PFS 9.5 months, OS 29.3 months) with better safety compared to sunitinib [148].

Axitinib

Axitinib (AG013736, Inlyta) is a small-molecule TKI. A phase III trial (AXIS trial) for previously treated metastatic RCC showed significantly longer PFS compared to sorafenib (6.7 months vs 4.7 months, $p<0.001$) [149, 150].

TKI Adverse Effects

Adverse effects commonly associated with TKIs include diarrhea, nausea, vomiting, fatigue, rash, hand–foot syndrome, and leukopenia. Sunitinib can cause QT prolongation with torsades de pointe as well as thyroid and adrenal dysfunction, and patients should be monitored for such throughout therapy.

1.14.2.2 mTOR Inhibitor

Temsirolimus

Temsirolimus (CCI-779, Torisel) most recently received FDA approval for the treatment of advanced RCC. It inhibits the mammalian target of rapamycin (mTOR), which is regulated by upstream kinases, including phosphatidylinositol 3-kinase/Akt [151]. Interruption of mTOR signaling decreases levels of HIF, VEGF, and other intracellular factors involved in the progression of the cell through its cycle. In the only phase III trial reported to date, temsirolimus was compared with IFN-a2a and the combination of temsirolimus and IFN-a2a as first-line treatment in 626 patients with metastatic RCC [152]. Compared to IFN-a, temsirolimus monotherapy was associated with an increase in OS (10.9 months vs 7.3 months, $p=0.008$), PFS (5.5 months vs 3.1 months, $p<0.001$), and RR (8.6 % vs 4.8 %) and was better tolerated than IFN-a2a alone (grades 3–4 adverse effects, 69 % vs 85 %). The addition of temsirolimus to IFN-a did not add benefit in OS and was associated with an increase in adverse events (grades 3–4 adverse effects: 87 %).

Everolimus

Everolimus is the second-line treatment agent for patients who have already failed VEGF inhibitor therapy. Everolimus has been demonstrated to prolong PFS (4 months, 3.25–6.32 month) in these patients [153].

mTOR Inhibitor Adverse Effects

The most common adverse reactions are asthenia, rash, nausea, and anorexia. Temsirolimus inhibits the production of VEGF and is associated with adverse effects commonly observed in patients who receive anti-angiogenic therapy, including hypertension (7 %), bowel perforation (1 %), and abnormal wound healing (1 %). Surgery should be avoided during treatment, and adequate time for wound healing should be allowed before instituting temsirolimus.

1.14.2.3 Monoclonal Antibody

Bevacizumab (VEGF Monoclonal Antibody, Avastin)

Two phase III trials (AVOREN, CALGB90206) reported that bevacizumab plus IFN-a showed longer median PFS (10.2 months vs 5.4 months, $p=0.0001$ and 8.5 months vs 5.2 months, $p<0.0001$, respectively) compared to IFN-a monotherapy in patients with clear cell metastatic RCC [154, 155].

Bevacizumab Adverse Effects

Similar to other agents targeting VEGF and angiogenesis, bevacizumab has been associated with hemorrhage (4.7–5.2 %), arterial thromboembolism (4.4 %), venous thromboembolism (13.6–15.1 %), hypertension (8–18 %), left ventricular dysfunction (grades 2–4: 1.7 %), proteinuria (grades 3/4: 3 %), gastrointestinal perforation (0–3.7 %), and wound-healing complications (0.8 %) [156].

1.14.3 Combination and Sequencing Therapy of Targeted Agents

Given the differences in mechanisms of action, and the apparent lack of cross-resistance, combination therapy has been proposed to maximize VEGF inhibition and increase activity of these drugs in patients with metastatic RCC. As described above, bevacizumab plus IFN-a was efficacious. However, both RECORD-2 and INTORACT studies, recently reported phase II and phase III trials, did not ultimately prove superior to single agents [157, 158]. Despite increased toxicity, such combinations have not demonstrated improvements in RR or PFS. With this regard, there has been a need to sequence available agents.

Sequencing therapy is currently the best approach to treat resistance, because of limited cross-resistance between VEGF TKI-targeted agents. However, optimal order of sequencing targeted agents remains to be determined with prospective trials.

1.14.4 Conclusions

Targeted therapies represent a significant advance in the treatment of metastatic RCC and have been shown to be superior to IFN-a or placebo. Future treatment strategies for metastatic RCC will likely incorporate a combination of molecular approaches, using multidrug regimens consisting of small-molecule kinase inhibitors with biologic therapies, immune-modulatory therapies, or both.

1.15 Radiation Therapy

As complete surgical extirpation is the mainstay curative treatment of most renal tumors, primary irradiation is rarely used. Although radiotherapy may be given preoperatively or postoperatively, its role remains controversial. Addition of radiotherapy either preoperatively or postoperatively tends to improve local control in locally advanced renal tumors [159–161]. However, it is not clear whether radiotherapy confers survival benefit. Accurate evaluation of tumor extent and regional spread is important to determine target volumes of radiotherapy. Contrast-enhanced computed tomography is useful for target volume definition. Some preliminary results have been reported on the efficacy of stereotactic body radiotherapy (SBRT) of renal cell carcinomas. With the technological advance in image guidance and radiation delivery, SBRT can be an option to ablate small renal mass with excellent local control and acceptable toxicity profile [162–164]. In delivering SBRT of renal tumors, optimal imaging studies are of upmost importance to provide demarcation of lesions form normal renal parenchyma and spatial relations regarding adjacent critical structures. Contrast-enhance CT is mandatory to define target volumes for SBRT of small renal tumors.

References

1. Kim SH, Cho JY, Kim SY, et al. Ultrasound evaluation of renal masses: gray-scale, Doppler, and More. Ultrasound Clin. 2013;8:565–79.
2. Israel GM, Silverman SG. The incidental renal mass. Radiol Clin North Am. 2011;49:369–83.
3. Frank I, Blute ML, Cheville JC, et al. Solid renal tumors: an analysis of pathological features related to tumor size. J Urol. 2003;170:2217–20.
4. Israel GM, Hindman N, Bosniak MA. Evaluation of cystic renal masses: comparison of CT and MR imaging by using the Bosniak classification system. Radiology. 2004;231:365–71.
5. Whelan TF. Guidelines on the management of renal cyst disease. Can Urol Assoc J. 2010;4:98–9.
6. Smith AD, Remer EM, Cox KL, et al. Bosniak category IIF and III cystic renal lesions: outcomes and associations. Radiology. 2012;262:152–60.
7. Sirli R, Sporea I, Popescu A, et al. Contrast enhanced ultrasound evaluation of the kidney. Med Ultrason. 2009;11:47–54.
8. Tama H, Takiguchi Y, Oka M, et al. Contrast-enhanced ultrasonography in the diagnosis of solid renal tumors. J Ultrasound Med. 2005;24:1635–40.
9. Ascenti G, Mazziotti S, Zimbaro G, et al. Complex cystic renal masses: characterization with contrast-enhanced US. Radiology. 2007;243:158–65.
10. Quai E, Bertolotto M, Cioff V, et al. Comparison of contrast-enhanced sonography with unenhanced sonography and contrast-enhanced CT in the diagnosis of malignancy in complex cystic renal masses. AJR Am J Roentgenol. 2008;191:1239–49.
11. Pooler BD, Pickhardt PJ, O'Connor SD, et al. Renal cell carcinoma: attenuation values on unenhanced CT. AJR Am J Roentgenol. 2012;198:1115–20.
12. Duchene DA, Lotan Y, Cadeddu JA, et al. Histopathology of surgically managed renal tumors: analysis of a contemporary series. Urology. 2003;62: 827–30.
13. Bae KT, Heiken JP, Siegel CL, et al. Renal cysts: is attenuation artifactually increased on contrast-enhanced CT images? Radiology. 2000;216:792–6.
14. Zhang J, Lefkowitz RA, Ishill NM, et al. Solid renal cortical tumors: differentiation with CT. Radiology. 2007;244:494–504.
15. Alshumrani G, O'Malley M, Ghai S, et al. Small (< or=4 cm) cortical renal tumors: characterization with multidetector CT. Abdom Imaging. 2010;35:488–93.
16. Israel GM, Hindman N, Hecht E, et al. The use of opposed-phase chemical shift MRI in the diagnosis of renal angiomyolipomas. AJR Am J Roentgenol. 2005;184:1868–72.
17. Hecht EM, Israel GM, Krinsky GA, et al. MR imaging of renal masses: comparison of quantitative enhancement using signal intensity measurements versus qualitative enhancement with image subtraction. Radiology. 2004;232:373–8.
18. Ho VB, Allen SF, Hood MN, et al. Renal masses: quantitative assessment of enhancement with dynamic MR imaging. Radiology. 2002;224:695–700.
19. Taouli B, Thakur RK, Mannelli L, et al. Renal lesions: characterization with diffusion-weighted

imaging versus contrast-enhanced MR imaging. Radiology. 2009;251:398–407.

20. Wang H, Cheng L, Zhang X, et al. Renal cell carcinoma: diffusion-weighted MR imaging for subtype differentiation at 3.0 T. Radiology. 2010;257:135–43.
21. Yu X, Lin M, Ouyang H, et al. Application of ADC measurement in characterization of renal cell carcinomas with different pathological types and grades by 3.0T diffusion-weighted MRI. Eur J Radiol. 2012;81:3061–6.
22. Kim GH, Jo MK, Cheon GJ, Lee HM. Clinical role of F-18 fluorodeoxyglucose positron emission tomography for follow-up patients with renal cell carcinoma. Korean J Urol. 2007;48:765–70.
23. Figlin RA. Renal cell carcinoma: management of advanced disease. J Urol. 1999;161:381–6.
24. Kang DE, White RL, Zuger JH, et al. Clinical use of fluorodeoxyglucose F 18 positron emission tomography for detection of renal cell carcinoma. J Urol. 2004;171:1806–9.
25. Nakatani K, Nakamoto Y, Saga T, et al. The potential clinical value of FDG-PET for recurrent renal cell carcinoma. Eur J Radiol. 2011;79:29–35.
26. Volpe A, Patard JJ. Prognostic factors in renal cell carcinoma. World J Urol. 2010;28:319–27.
27. Ozülker T, Ozülker F, Ozbek E, et al. A prospective diagnostic accuracy study of F-18 fluorodeoxyglucose-positron emission tomography/computed tomography in the evaluation of indeterminate renal masses. Nucl Med Commun. 2011;32:265–72.
28. Hiles JJ, Kolesar JM. Role of sunitinib and sorafenib in the treatment of metastatic renal cell carcinoma. Am J Health Syst Pharm. 2008;65:123–31.
29. Khandani AH, Rathmell WK. Positron emission tomography in renal cell carcinoma: an imaging biomarker in development. Semin Nucl Med. 2012;42:221–30.
30. Revheim ME, Winge-Main AK, Hagen G, et al. Combined positron emission tomography/computed tomography in sunitinib therapy assessment of patients with metastatic renal cell carcinoma. Clin Oncol. 2011;23:339–43.
31. Kayani I, Avril N, Bomanji J, et al. Sequential FDG-PET/CT as a biomarker of response to sunitinib in metastatic clear cell renal cancer. Clin Cancer Res. 2011;17:6021–8.
32. Kim EE, Lee MC, Inoue T, Wong WH, editors. Clinical PET and PET/CT: principles and applications. New York: Springer; 2013.
33. Liu G, Jeraj R, Vanderhoek M, et al. Pharmacodynamic study using FLT PET/CT in patients with renal cell cancer and other solid malignancies treated with sunitinib malate. Clin Cancer Res. 2011;17:7634–44.
34. Hugonne F, Fournier L, Medioni J, et al; Hypoxia in Renal Cancer Multicenter Group. Metastatic renal cell carcinoma: relationship between initial metastasis hypoxia, change after 1 month's sunitinib, and therapeutic response: an 18F-fluoromisonidazole PET/CT study. J Nucl Med. 2011;52:1048–55.
35. Menogue SR, O'Brien BA, Brown AL, et al. Percutaneous core biopsy of small renal mass lesions: a diagnostic tool to better stratify patients for surgical intervention. BJU Int. 2013;111:E146–51.
36. Eble JN, Sauter G, Epstein JI, et al., editors. World Health Organization classification of tumours: tumours of the urinary system and male genital organs. Lyon: IARC Press; 2004.
37. Gokden N, Nappi O, Swanson PE, et al. Renal cell carcinoma with rhabdoid features. Am J Surg Pathol. 2000;24(10):1329–38.
38. Kuroiwa K, Kinoshita Y, Shiratsuchi H, et al. Renal cell carcinoma with rhabdoid features: an aggressive neoplasm. Histopathology. 2002;41(6):538–48.
39. Lee C, Park JW, Suh JH, et al. Histologic variations and immunohistochemical features of metastatic clear cell renal cell carcinoma. Korean J Pathol. 2013;47(5):426–32.
40. Przybycin CG, McKenney JK, Reynolds JP, et al. Rhabdoid differentiation is associated with aggressive behavior in renal cell carcinoma: a clinicopathologic analysis of 76 cases with clinical follow-up. Am J Surg Pathol. 2014;38(9):1260–5.
41. Kim H, Cho NH, Kim DS, et al. Renal cell carcinoma in South Korea: a multicenter study. Hum Pathol. 2004;35(12):1556–63.
42. Delahunt B. Sarcomatoid renal carcinoma: the final common dedifferentiation pathway of renal epithelial malignancies. Pathology. 1999;31(3):185–90.
43. Delahunt B, Eble JN, McCredie MR, et al. Morphologic typing of papillary renal cell carcinoma: comparison of growth kinetics and patient survival in 66 cases. Hum Pathol. 2001;32(6):590–5.
44. Delahunt B, Eble JN. Papillary renal cell carcinoma: a clinicopathologic and immunohistochemical study of 105 tumors. Mod Pathol Off J U S Can Acad Pathol Inc. 1997;10(6):537–44.
45. Altinok G, Kattar MM, Mohamed A, et al. Pediatric renal carcinoma associated with Xp11.2 translocations/TFE3 gene fusions and clinicopathologic associations. Pediatr Dev Pathol Off J Soc Pediatr Pathol Paediatric Pathol Soc. 2005;8(2):168–80.
46. Argani P, Antonescu CR, Couturier J, et al. PRCC-TFE3 renal carcinomas: morphologic, immunohistochemical, ultrastructural, and molecular analysis of an entity associated with the t(X;1)(p11.2;q21). Am J Surg Pathol. 2002;26(12):1553–66.
47. Argani P, Antonescu CR, Illei PB, et al. Primary renal neoplasms with the ASPL-TFE3 gene fusion of alveolar soft part sarcoma: a distinctive tumor entity previously included among renal cell carcinomas of children and adolescents. Am J Pathol. 2001;159(1):179–92.
48. Argani P, Yonescu R, Morsberger L, et al. Molecular confirmation of t(6;11)(p21;q12) renal cell carcinoma in archival paraffin-embedded material using a break-apart TFEB FISH assay expands its clinicopathologic spectrum. Am J Surg Pathol. 2012;36(10):1516–26.

49. Rao Q, Liu B, Cheng L, et al. Renal cell carcinomas with t(6;11)(p21;q12): a clinicopathologic study emphasizing unusual morphology, novel alpha-TFEB gene fusion point, immunobiomarkers, and ultrastructural features, as well as detection of the gene fusion by fluorescence in situ hybridization. Am J Surg Pathol. 2012;36(9):1327–38.
50. Smith NE, Illei PB, Allaf M, et al. t(6;11) renal cell carcinoma (RCC): expanded immunohistochemical profile emphasizing novel RCC markers and report of 10 new genetically confirmed cases. Am J Surg Pathol. 2014;38(5):604–14.
51. Argani P, Lal P, Hutchinson B, et al. Aberrant nuclear immunoreactivity for TFE3 in neoplasms with TFE3 gene fusions: a sensitive and specific immunohistochemical assay. Am J Surg Pathol. 2003;27(6): 750–61.
52. Kim SH, Choi Y, Jeong HY, et al. Usefulness of a break-apart FISH assay in the diagnosis of Xp11.2 translocation renal cell carcinoma. Virchows Arch Int J Pathol. 2011;459(3):299–306.
53. Rao Q, Williamson SR, Zhang S, et al. TFE3 break-apart FISH has a higher sensitivity for Xp11.2 translocation-associated renal cell carcinoma compared with TFE3 or cathepsin K immunohistochemical staining alone: expanding the morphologic spectrum. Am J Surg Pathol. 2013;37(6):804–15.
54. Lopez-Beltran A, Carrasco JC, Cheng L, et al. 2009 update on the classification of renal epithelial tumors in adults. Int J Urol Off J Jpn Urol Assoc. 2009;16(5):432–43.
55. Srigley JR, Delahunt B, Eble JN, et al. The International Society of Urological Pathology (ISUP) Vancouver classification of renal neoplasia. Am J Surg Pathol. 2013;37(10):1469–89.
56. Park JH, Lee C, Suh JH, et al. Clear cell papillary renal cell carcinoma: a report of 15 cases including three cases of concurrent other-type renal cell carcinomas. Korean J Pathol. 2012;46(6):541–7.
57. Eble JN, Sauter G, Epstein JI, et al. Pathology and genetics of tumours of the urinary system and male genital organs. Oxford: International Agency for Research on Cancer (IARC); 2004.
58. Fuhrman SA, Lasky LC, Limas C. Prognostic significance of morphologic parameters in renal cell carcinoma. Am J Surg Pathol. 1982;6(7):655–63.
59. Kidney. In: Edge SB, Byrd DR, Compton CC, et al., eds.: AJCC Cancer Staging Manual. 7th ed. New York, NY: Springer, 2010, pp 479–89.
60. Hallscheidt PJ, Bock M, Riedasch G, et al. Diagnostic accuracy of staging renal cell carcinomas using multidetector-row computed tomography and magnetic resonance imaging: a prospective study with histopathologic correlation. J Comput Assist Tomogr. 2004;28:333–9.
61. Hallscheidt P, Wagener N, Gholipour F, et al. Multislice computed tomography in planning nephron-sparing surgery in a prospective study with 76 patients: comparison of radiological and histopathological findings in the infiltration of renal structures. J Comput Assist Tomogr. 2006;30:869–74.
62. Tsili AC, Argyropoulou MI, Gousia A, et al. Renal cell carcinoma: value of multiphase MDCT with multiplanar reformations in the detection of pseudocapsule. AJR Am J Roentgenol. 2012;199:379–86.
63. Ferda J, Hora M, Hes O, et al. Assessment of the kidney tumor vascular supply by two-phase MDCT-angiography. Eur J Radiol. 2007;62:295–301.
64. Kim JK, Kim TK, Ahn HJ, et al. Differentiation of subtypes of renal cell carcinoma on helical CT scans. AJR Am J Roentgenol. 2002;178:1499–506.
65. Prasad SR, Humphrey PA, Catena JR, et al. Common and uncommon histologic subtypes of renal cell carcinoma: imaging spectrum with pathologic correlation. Radiographics. 2006;26:1795–806.
66. Young JR, Margolis D, Sauk S, et al. Clear cell renal cell carcinoma: discrimination from other renal cell carcinoma subtypes and oncocytoma at multiphasic multidetector CT. Radiology. 2013;267:444–53.
67. Sun MR, Ngo L, Genega EM, et al. Renal cell carcinoma: dynamic contrast-enhanced MR imaging for differentiation of tumor subtypes-correlation with pathologic findings. Radiology. 2009;250:793–802.
68. Herts BR, Coll DM, Novick AC, et al. Enhancement characteristics of papillary renal neoplasms revealed on triphasic helical CT of the kidneys. AJR Am J Roentgenol. 2002;178:367–72.
69. Oliva MR, Glickman JN, Zou KH, et al. Renal cell carcinoma: T1 and T2 signal intensity characteristics of papillary and clear cell types correlated with pathology. AJR Am J Roentgenol. 2009;192:1524–30.
70. Cochand-Priollet B, Molinie V, Bougaran J, et al. Renal chromophobe cell carcinoma and oncocytoma: a comparative morphologic, histochemical, and immunohistochemical study of 124 cases. Arch Pathol Lab Med. 1997;121:1081–6.
71. Rosenkrantz AB, Hindman N, Fitzgerald EF, et al. MRI features of renal oncocytoma and chromophobe renal cell carcinoma. AJR Am J Roentgenol. 2010;195:421–7.
72. Hindman NM, Bosniak MA, Rosenkrantz AB, et al. Multilocular cystic renal cell carcinoma: comparison of imaging and pathologic findings. AJR Am J Roentgenol. 2012;198:20–6.
73. Pickhardt PJ, Siegel CL, McLarney JK. Collecting duct carcinoma of the kidney: are imaging findings suggestive of the diagnosis? AJR Am J Roentgenol. 2001;176:627–33.
74. Taneja R, Bhargava P, Cuevas C, et al. Common and less-common renal masses and masslike conditions. Radiol Clin North Am. 2012;50:245–57.
75. Kato H, Kanematsu M, Yokoi S, et al. Renal cell carcinoma associated with Xp11.2 translocation/TFE3 gene fusion: radiological findings mimicking papillary subtype. J Magn Reson Imaging. 2011;33:217–20.
76. Mester JL, Zhou M, Prescott N, et al. Papillary renal cell carcinoma is associated with PTEN hamartoma tumor syndrome. Urology. 2012;79:1187.e1–7.

77. Abrahams NA, Tamboli P. Oncocytic renal neoplasms: diagnostic considerations. Clin Lab Med. 2005;25:317–39.
78. Kim JI, Cho JY, Moon KC, et al. Segmental enhancement inversion at biphasic Multidetector CT: characteristic finding of small renal oncocytoma. Radiology. 2009;252:441–8.
79. McGahan JP, Lamba R, Fisher J, et al. Is segmental enhancement inversion on enhanced biphasic MDCT a reliable sign for the noninvasive diagnosis of renal oncocytomas? AJR Am J Roentgenol. 2011;197: W674–9.
80. O'Malley ME, Tran P, Hanbidge A, et al. Small renal oncocytomas: is segmental enhancement inversion a characteristic finding at biphasic MDCT? AJR Am J Roentgenol. 2012;199:1312–5.
81. Woo S, Cho JY, Kim SH, et al. Segmental enhancement inversion of small renal oncocytoma: differences in prevalence according to tumor size. AJR Am J Roentgenol. 2013;200:1054–9.
82. Woo S, Cho JY, Kim SH, et al. Comparison of segmental enhancement inversion on biphasic MDCT between small renal oncocytomas and chromophobe renal cell carcinomas. AJR Am J Roentgenol. 2013;201:598–604.
83. Bastide C, Rambeaud JJ, Bach AM, et al. Metanephric adenoma of the kidney: clinical and radiological study of nine cases. BJU Int. 2009;103:1544–8.
84. Torricelli FC, Marchini GS, Campos RS, et al. Metanephric adenoma: clinical, imaging, and histological findings. Clinics (Sao Paulo). 2011;66:359–61.
85. Samaratunga H, Delahunt B. Mesenchymal tumors of adult kidney. Semin Diagn Pathol. 2015;32:160–71.
86. Weeks DA, Beckwith JB, Mierau GW, et al. Rhabdoid tumor of kidney. A report of 111 cases from the National Wilms' Tumor Study Pathology Center. Am J Surg Pathol. 1989;13(6):439–58.
87. Hollmann TJ, Hornick JL. INI1-deficient tumors: diagnostic features and molecular genetics. Am J Surg Pathol. 2011;35(10):e47–63.
88. Kim SH, Sim JS. Malignant renal parenchymal tumors. In Kim SH (ed): Radiology illustrated: uroradiology. 2nd ed. Heidelberg New York Dordrecht London: Springer; 2012. p. 145–251.
89. Davenport MS, Neville AM, Ellis JH, et al. Diagnosis of renal angiomyolipoma with hounsfield unit thresholds: effect of size of region of interest and nephrographic phase imaging. Radiology. 2011;260:158–65.
90. Simpson E, Patel U. Diagnosis of angiomyolipoma using computed tomography-region of interest<or=−10 HU or 4 adjacent pixels<or=−10 HU are recommended as the diagnostic thresholds. Clin Radiol. 2006;61:410–6.
91. Catalano OA, Samir AE, Sahani DV, et al. Pixel distribution analysis: can it be used to distinguish clear cell carcinomas from angiomyolipomas with minimal fat? Radiology. 2008;247:738–46.
92. Hafron J, Fogarty JD, Hoenig DM, et al. Imaging characteristics of minimal fat renal angiomyolipoma with histologic correlations. Urology. 2005;66:1155–9.
93. Kim JK, Park SY, Shon JH, et al. Angiomyolipoma with minimal fat: differentiation from renal cell carcinoma at biphasic helical CT. Radiology. 2004;230: 677–84.
94. Kim JK, Kim SH, Jang YJ, et al. Renal angiomyolipoma with minimal fat: differentiation from other neoplasms at double-echo chemical shift FLASH MR imaging. Radiology. 2006;239:174–80.
95. Cui L, Hu XY, Gong SC, et al. A massive renal epithelioid angiomyolipoma with multiple metastatic lymph nodes. Clin Imaging. 2011;35:320–3.
96. Eble JN, Amin MB, Young RH. Epithelioid angiomyolipoma of the kidney: a report of five cases with a prominent and diagnostically confusing epithelioid smooth muscle component. Am J Surg Pathol. 1997;21(10):1123–30.
97. Tsukada J, Jinzaki M, Yao M, et al. Epithelioid angiomyolipoma of the kidney: radiological imaging. Int J Urol. 2013;20:1105–11.
98. Froemming AT, Boland J, Cheville J, Kawashima A, et al. Renal epithelioid angiomyolipoma: imaging characteristics in nine cases with radiologic-pathologic correlation and review of the literature. AJR Am J Roentgenol. 2013;200:W178–86.
99. Geenen RW, Den Bakker MA, et al. Sonography, CT, and MRI of giant cavernous hemangioma of the kidney: correlation with pathologic findings. AJR Am J Roentgenol. 2004;182:411–4.
100. Wang JH, Sheu MH, Lee RC. MR findings of renin-secreting tumor: a case report. Abdom Imaging. 1998;23:533–5.
101. Hwang SI, Sim JS. Benign renal tumors. In: Kim SH, editor. Radiology illustrated: uroradiology. 2nd ed. Heidelberg/New York/Dordrecht/London: Springer; 2012. p. 103–44.
102. Znati K, Chbani L, El Fatemi H, et al. Solitary fibrous tumor of the kidney: a case report and review of the literature. Rev Urol. 2007;9:36–40.
103. Johnson TR, Pedrosa I, Goldsmith J, et al. Magnetic resonance imaging findings in solitary fibrous tumor of the kidney. J Comput Assist Tomogr. 2005;29:481–3.
104. Chu LC, Hruban RH, Horton KM, et al. Mixed epithelial and stromal tumor of the kidney: radiologic-pathologic correlation. Radiographics. 2010;30: 1541–51.
105. Jimenez RE, Folpe AL, Lapham RL, et al. Primary Ewing's sarcoma/primitive neuroectodermal tumor of the kidney: a clinicopathologic and immunohistochemical analysis of 11 cases. Am J Surg Pathol. 2002;26(3):320–7.
106. Thyavihally YB, Tongaonkar HB, Gupta S, et al. Primitive neuroectodermal tumor of the kidney: a single institute series of 16 patients. Urology. 2008;71(2):292–6.
107. Lee H, Cho JY, Kim SH, et al. Imaging findings of primitive neuroectodermal tumors of the kidney. J Comput Assist Tomogr. 2009;33:882–6.
108. Ferry JA, Harris NL, Papanicolaou N, et al. Lymphoma of the kidney. A report of 11 cases. Am J Surg Pathol. 1995;19(2):134–44.

109. Urban BA, Fishman EK. Renal lymphoma: CT patterns with emphasis on helical CT. Radiographics. 2000;20:197–212.
110. Sheth S, Ali S, Fishman E. Imaging of renal lymphoma: patterns of disease with pathologic correlation. Radiographics. 2006;26:1151–68.
111. Bracken RB, Chica G, Johnson DE, et al. Secondary renal neoplasms: an autopsy study. South Med J. 1979;72(7):806–7.
112. Choyke PL, White EM, Zeman RK, et al. Renal metastases: clinicopathologic and radiologic correlation. Radiology. 1987;162:359–63.
113. Chawla SN, Crispen PL, Hanlon AL, et al. The natural history of observed enhancing renal masses: meta-analysis and review of the world literature. J Urol. 2006;175:425–31.
114. Jewett MA, Mattar K, Basiuk J, et al. Active surveillance of small renal masses: progression patterns of early stage kidney cancer. Eur Urol. 2011;60:39–44.
115. Mucksavage P, Ramchandani P, Malkowicz SB, et al. Is ultrasound imaging inferior to computed tomography or magnetic resonance imaging in evaluating renal mass size? Urology. 2012;79:28–31.
116. Psutka SP, Feldman AS, McDougal WS, McGovern FJ, Mueller P, Gervais DA. Long-term oncologic outcomes after radiofrequency ablation for T1 renal cell carcinoma. Eur Urol. 2013;63(3):486–92.
117. Silverman SG, Israel GM, Herts BR, Richie JP. Management of the incidental renal mass. Radiology. 2008;249(1):16–31.
118. Park BK, Kim CK. Complications of image-guided radiofrequency ablation of renal cell carcinoma: causes, imaging features and prevention methods. Eur Radiol. 2009;19(9):2180–90.
119. Park SY, Park BK, Kim CK. Thermal ablation in renal cell carcinoma: what affects renal function? Int J Hyperthermia. 2012;28(8):729–34.
120. Sung HH, Park BK, Kim CK, Choi HY, Lee HM. Comparison of percutaneous radiofrequency ablation and open partial nephrectomy for the treatment of size- and location-matched renal masses. Int J Hyperthermia. 2012;28(3):227–34.
121. Zagoria RJ, Pettus JA, Rogers M, Werle DM, Childs D, Leyendecker JR. Long-term outcomes after percutaneous radiofrequency ablation for renal cell carcinoma. Urology. 2011;77(6):1393–7.
122. Schmit GD, Thompson RH, Kurup AN, et al. Percutaneous cryoablation of solitary sporadic renal cell carcinomas. BJU Int. 2012;110(11 Pt B):E526–31.
123. Robson CJ. Radical nephrectomy for renal cell carcinoma. J Urol. 1963;89:37–42.
124. O'Malley RL, Godoy G, Kanofsky JA, Taneja SS. The necessity of adrenalectomy at the time of radical nephrectomy: a systematic review. J Urol. 2009;181:2009–17.
125. Tsui KH, Shvarts O, Barbaric Z, Figlin R, De Kernion JB, Belldegrun A. Is adrenalectomy a necessary component of radical nephrectomy? UCLA experience with 511 radical nephrectomies. J Urol. 2000;163:437–41.
126. Blom JH, Van Poppel H, Marechal JM, Jacqmin JA, Schroder FH, De Prijck L, Sylvester R, Group EGTC. Radical nephrectomy with and without lymph-node dissection: final results of European Organization for Research and Treatment of Cancer (EORTC) randomized phase 3 trial 30881. Eur Urol. 2009;55:28–34.
127. Shuford MD, McDougall EM, Chang SS, Lafleur BJ, Smith Jr JA, Cookson MS. Complications of contemporary radical nephrectomy: comparison of open vs. laparoscopic approach. Urol Oncol. 2004;22:121–6.
128. Dunn MD, Portis AJ, Shalhav AL, Elbahnasy AM, Heidorn C, McDougall EM, Clayman RV. Laparoscopic versus open radical nephrectomy: a 9-year experience. J Urol. 2000;164:1153–9.
129. Clayman RV, Kavoussi LR, Soper NJ, Dierks SM, Meretyk S, Darcy MD, Roemer FD, Pingleton ED, Thomson PG, Long SR. Laparoscopic nephrectomy: initial case report. J Urol. 1991;146:278–82.
130. Maclennan S, Imamura M, Lapitan MC, Omar MI, Lam TB, Hilvano-Cabungcal AM, Royle P, Stewart F, Maclennan G, Maclennan SJ, Dahm P, Canfield SE, Mcclinton S, Griffiths TR, Ljungberg B, N'Dow J, Group USRR, Panel EAURCG. Systematic review of perioperative and quality-of-life outcomes following surgical management of localised renal cancer. Eur Urol. 2012;62:1097–117.
131. Maclennan S, Imamura M, Lapitan MC, Omar MI, Lam TB, Hilvano-Cabungcal AM, Royle P, Stewart F, Maclennan G, Maclennan SJ, Canfield SE, Mcclinton S, Griffiths TR, Ljungberg B, N'Dow J, Group USRR, Panel EAURCG. Systematic review of oncological outcomes following surgical management of localised renal cancer. Eur Urol. 2012;61:972–93.
132. Fergany A. Chronic renal insufficiency after partial nephrectomy for T1b tumors. Curr Opin Urol. 2013;23:394–8.
133. Huang WC, Levey AS, Serio AM, Snyder M, Vickers AJ, Raj GV. Scardin ions of contemporary laparoscopic partial nephrectomy: use of a standardized reporting system. J Urol. 2007;177:2067–73.
134. Go AS, Chertow GM, Fan D, Mcculloch CE, Hsu CY. Chronic kidney disease and the risks of death, cardiovascular events, and hospitalization. N Engl J Med. 2004;351:1296–305.
135. Thompson RH, Boorjian SA, Lohse CM, Leibovich BC, Kwon ED, Cheville JC, Blute ML. Radical nephrectomy for pT1a renal masses may be associated with decreased overall survival compared with partial nephrectomy. J Urol. 2008;179:468–73.
136. Ramani AP, Desai MM, Steinberg AP, Ng CS, Abreu SC, Kaouk JH, Finelli A, Novick AC, Gill IS. Complications of laparoscopic partial nephrectomy in 200 cases. J Urol. 2005;173:42–7.
137. Becker A, Ravi P, Roghmann F, Trinh QD, Tian Z, Larouche A, Kim S, Shariat SF, Kluth L, Dahlem R, Fisch M, Graefen M, Eichelberg C, Karakiewicz PI, Sun M. Laparoscopic radical nephrectomy vs laparoscopic or open partial nephrectomy for T1 renal

cell carcinoma: comparison of complication rates in elderly patients during the initial phase of adoption. Urology. 2014;83:1285–91.
138. Simmons MN, Gill IS, Hafron J, Fogarty JD, Hoenig DM, et al. Decreased complicat92. Imaging characteristics of minimal fat renal angiomyolipoma with histologic correlations. Urology. 2005;66:1155–9.
139. Lee S, Oh J, Hong SK, Lee SE, Byun SS. Open versus robot-assisted partial nephrectomy: effect on clinical outcome. J Endourol. 2011;25:1181–5.
140. Howlader N, Noone A, Krapcho M, et al. SEER Cancer statistics review, 1975–2010. Bethesda: National Cancer Institute; 2013.
141. Yagoda A, Abi-Rached B, Petrylak D, et al. Chemotherapy for advanced renal-cell carcinoma: 1983–1993. Semin Oncol. 1995;22:42–60.
142. Cohen HT, McGovern FJ. Renal-cell carcinoma. N Engl J Med. 2005;353:2477–90.
143. Mancuso A, Sternberg CN. New treatment approaches in metastatic renal cell carcinoma. Curr Opin Urol. 2006;16:337–41.
144. Escudier B, Eisen T, Stadler WM, Szczylik C, et al. TARGET Study Group. Sorafenib in advanced clear-cell renal-cell carcinoma. N Engl J Med. 2007;356:125–34.
145. Product information. Sutent (sunitinib). New York: Pfizer, Inc; 2008.
146. Motzer RJ, Hutson TE, Tomczak P, et al. Sunitinib versus interferon alfa in metastatic renal-cell carcinoma. N Engl J Med. 2007;356:115–24.
147. Figlin R, Hutson TE, Tomczak P, et al. Overall survival with sunitinib versus interferon (IFN)-alfa as first-line treatment of metastatic renal cell carcinoma (mRCC). J Clin Oncol. 2008;26(Suppl 18)(abstract 5024).
148. Motzer RJ, Hutson TE, Cella D, et al. Pazopanib versus sunitinib in metastatic renal-cell carcinoma. N Engl J Med. 2013;369:722–31.
149. Rini BI. SU11248 and AG013736: current data and future trials in renal cell carcinoma. Clin Genitourin Cancer. 2005;4:175–80.
150. Rini BI, Escudier B, Tomczak P, et al. Comparative effectiveness of axitinib versus sorafenib in advanced renal cell carcinoma (AXIS): a randomized phase 3 trial. Lancet. 2011;380:1818.
151. Product information. Torisel (temsirolimus). Philadelphia: Wyeth Pharmaceuticals Inc; 2007.
152. Hudes G, Carducci M, Tomczak P, et al. Temsirolimus, interferon alfa, or both for advanced renal-cell carcinoma. N Engl J Med. 2007;356:2271–81.
153. Fisher R, Gore M, Larkin J. Current and future systemic treatments for renal cell carcinoma. Semin Cancer Biol. 2013;23:38–45.
154. Escudier B, Pluzanska A, Koralewski P, et al. Bevacizumab plus interferon alfa-2a for treatment of metastatic renal cell carcinoma: a randomised, double-blind phase III trial. Lancet. 2007;370:2103–11.
155. Rini BI, Halabi S, Rosenberg JE, et al. Bevacizumab plus interferon alfa compared with interferon alfa monotherapy in patients with metastatic renal cell carcinoma: CALGB 90206. J Clin Oncol. 2008;26:5422–8.
156. Reeves DJ, Liu CY. Treatment of metastatic renal cell carcinoma. Cancer Chemother Pharmacol. 2009;64:11–25.
157. Ravaud A, Barrios CH, Alekseev B, et al. RECORD-2: phase II randomized study of everolimus and bevacizumab versus interferon α-2a and bevacizumab as first-line therapy in patients with metastatic renal cell carcinoma. Ann Oncol. 2015;26:1378–84.
158. Rini BI, Bellmunt J, Clancy J, et al. Randomized phase III trial of temsirolimus and bevacizumab versus interferon alfa and bevacizumab in metastatic renal cell carcinoma: INTORACT trial. J Clin Oncol. 2014;32:752–9.
159. Juusela H, Malmio K, Alfthan O, Oravisto KJ. Preoperative irradiation in the treatment of renal adenocarcinoma. Scand J Urol Nephrol. 1977;11(3):277–81.
160. Kjaer M, Frederiksen PL, Engelholm S. Postoperative radiotherapy in stage II and III renal adenocarcinoma. A randomized trial by the Copenhagen Renal Cancer Study Group. Int J Radiat Oncol Biol Phys. 1987;13(5):665–72.
161. Svedman C, Karlsson K, Rutkowska E, et al. Stereotactic body radiotherapy of primary and metastatic renal lesions for patients with only one functioning kidney. Acta Oncol. 2008;47(8):1578–83.
162. Svedman C, Sandström P, Pisa P, et al. A prospective phase II trial of using extracranial stereotactic radiotherapy in primary and metastatic renal cell carcinoma. Acta Oncol. 2006;45(7):870–5.
163. Van der Werf-Messing B. Carcinoma of the kidney. Cancer. 1973;32(5):1056–61.
164. Wersäll PJ, Blomgren H, Lax I, et al. Extracranial stereotactic radiotherapy for primary and metastatic renal cell carcinoma. Radiother Oncol. 2005;77(1):88–95.

2 Urothelial Tumors

Hyuck Jae Choi, Kyung Chul Moon, Jin Ho Kim, and Ja Hyeon Ku

2.1 Introduction

Primary bladder neoplasms consist 2–6 % of all tumors, and bladder cancer is the fourth common malignancy [1]. Tumors can arise from the urothelium or other layers of the bladder wall. The bladder wall consists of four layers. The first layer is the uroepithelium. This consists of 3–7 layers of stratified flat cells. More superficial cells are flexible and change shape from cuboidal to flat with distension of the bladder. This is why we call it "transitional epithelium." The second layer is the lamina propria. The third layer is the muscularis propria (detrusor muscle). The fourth layer is the adventitia. Bladder neoplasms arise from any of the four layers. They are classified into epithelial and nonepithelial tumors [1]. Epithelial tumors consist 95 % of bladder tumors. When epithelial tumor differentiates to normal urothelium, we call it urothelial. Other epithelial tumors include squamous cell carcinoma, adenocarcinoma, small cell/neuroendocrine carcinoma, carcinoid, and melanoma. These epithelial tumors occur at the surface of bladder lumen and usually show irregular, intraluminal mass.

Muscle, nerve, cartilage, and fat, fibrous tissues are derived from the mesenchymal tissue. Benign mesenchymal tumors include leiomyoma, paraganglioma, fibroma, plasmacytoma, neurofibroma, and lipoma. Malignant tumors include rhabdomyosarcoma, leiomyosarcoma, lymphoma, and osteosarcoma. They usually occur at the submucosal layer of the bladder wall and have a smooth intramural appearance.

Imaging findings of these tumors are sometimes nonspecific and tissue confirmation is needed for diagnosis. However, some tumors have specific imaging findings, and this preoperative diagnosis is helpful in the clinical setting.

2.2 Urothelial Tumors

2.2.1 Transitional Cell Carcinoma: Bladder

The urothelium is exposed to carcinogens, and both synchronous and metachronous transitional

H.J. Choi (✉)
Department of Radiology, Kanwon National University Hospital, Seoul National University College of Medicine,
Gangwon-do, Seoul, Republic of Korea
e-mail: choihj@amc.seoul.kr

K.C. Moon
Department of Pathology, Seoul National University Hospital, Seoul National University College of Medicine, Seoul, Republic of Korea

J.H. Kim
Department of Radiation Oncology, Seoul National University Hospital, Seoul National University College of Medicine, Seoul, Republic of Korea

J.H. Ku
Department of Urology, Seoul National University Hospital, Seoul National University College of Medicine, Seoul, Republic of Korea

S.H. Kim, J.Y. Cho (eds.), *Oncologic Imaging: Urology*, DOI 10.1007/978-3-662-45218-9_2

cell carcinomas (TCCs) can occur from urothelium. There are typical findings of TCCs occurring in the bladder, ureter, and renal pelvis although they have same pathologic findings. Carcinoma of the bladder is the most common neoplasm of the urinary tract, and more than 90 % of the primary bladder cancers are transitional cell carcinomas (TCCs). Tumors in the urothelium of the renal pelvis and ureter are rare compared with those in the bladder; tumors in the renal pelvis are more common compared with those in the ureter. Typical findings of TCCs are irregular mass from urothelium. TCCs in the urinary bladder are usually confined to the bladder lumen; however, they extend to outside of the bladder when they become larger. Focal wall thickening is a manifestation of TCCs of the ureter. Usually, they are confined to the lumen of the urinary tract; however, they can show infiltrative growth to the renal parenchyma when they become larger.

Bladder cancer is the most common malignancy of the urinary tract consisting about 90 % [2]. About 25 % of urothelial cancers have mixed histology such as small cell neuroendocrine, micropapillary, sarcomatoid, and plasmacytoid component. The most common etiologic factor for TCC is cigarette smoking [3]. Exposure to other carcinogens such as dyes, rubber, cable, and plastics and abuse of analgesics are also risk factors for transitional cell carcinomas. About 80–85 % of TCCs do not invade muscle and they occur from a hyperplastic epithelium. They have low histologic grade and are multifocal. They can recur in about 50 % after treatment; however, they have good prognosis [4, 5]. About 20–25 % of bladder TCCs invade muscle and have higher histologic grade [6].

2.2.1.1 CT

CT is the modality of choice for workup of bladder TCC patients. With CT urography, not only urinary system but also perirenal, periureteral, and extravesical tumor spread, lymph node metastases, and distant metastases can be evaluated simultaneously [7].

When CT urography is performed in MDCD, fast multiplanar and high-resolution images can be acquired. CT urography has 79 % sensitivity and 94 % specificity for diagnosis of bladder malignancies [5]. However, CT urography has limited utility in staging bladder TCCs and is more useful in advanced diseases [8]. Muscle-invasive and non-muscle-invasive bladder TCCs and microscopic perivesical tumor infiltration cannot be detected with CT urography [9]. CT cannot confidently detect flat lesions and lesions at the bladder base near prostate gland. For these reasons, CT urography cannot be used as a replacement for cystoscopy in patients with suspected bladder cancer. Another problem is that CT cannot differentiate inflammatory wall thickening from tumor after transurethral resection of bladder tumor (TURBT).

Virtual cystoscopy of the bladder can be performed with CT. This utilizes three different techniques: intravenous contrast injection to enhance tumor, bladder lumen filling with contrast with bladder catheter or opacification through intravenous contrast, and negative intraluminal contrast using air or CO_2 through bladder catheter [10, 11]. Bernhardt et al. reported that CT virtual endoscopy had 97.2 % sensitivity and 100 % specificity for bladder lumen pathologic lesions [12]. In spite of this relatively high diagnostic accuracy, this high performance should be carefully interpreted. Things to consider are first, virtual cystoscopy is more invasive compared with CT urography; second, cystoscopy is still needed for detection of flat lesion; and third, reduced sensitivity for dependant lesion is due to pool of urine obscuring the mucosa [13].

Bladder TCCs have various appearances (carcinoma in situ (CIS), papillary, infiltrative, and mixed papillary and infiltrative). Tumor with papillary growth has tendency to be less invasive to muscle and has better prognosis compared to that of infiltrative growth. Median survivals of tumors with papillary growth and infiltrative growth are 85 months and 29 months respectively [14].

Bladder wall thickening, focal nodular or irregular, is finding of bladder TCCS (Fig. 2.1). However in underdistended bladder, this finding should cautiously be interpreted [15]. In addition, diffuse wall thickening is rare presentation of bladder TCCs, except in case of irregular or nodular wall thickening [16]. In many cases, focal

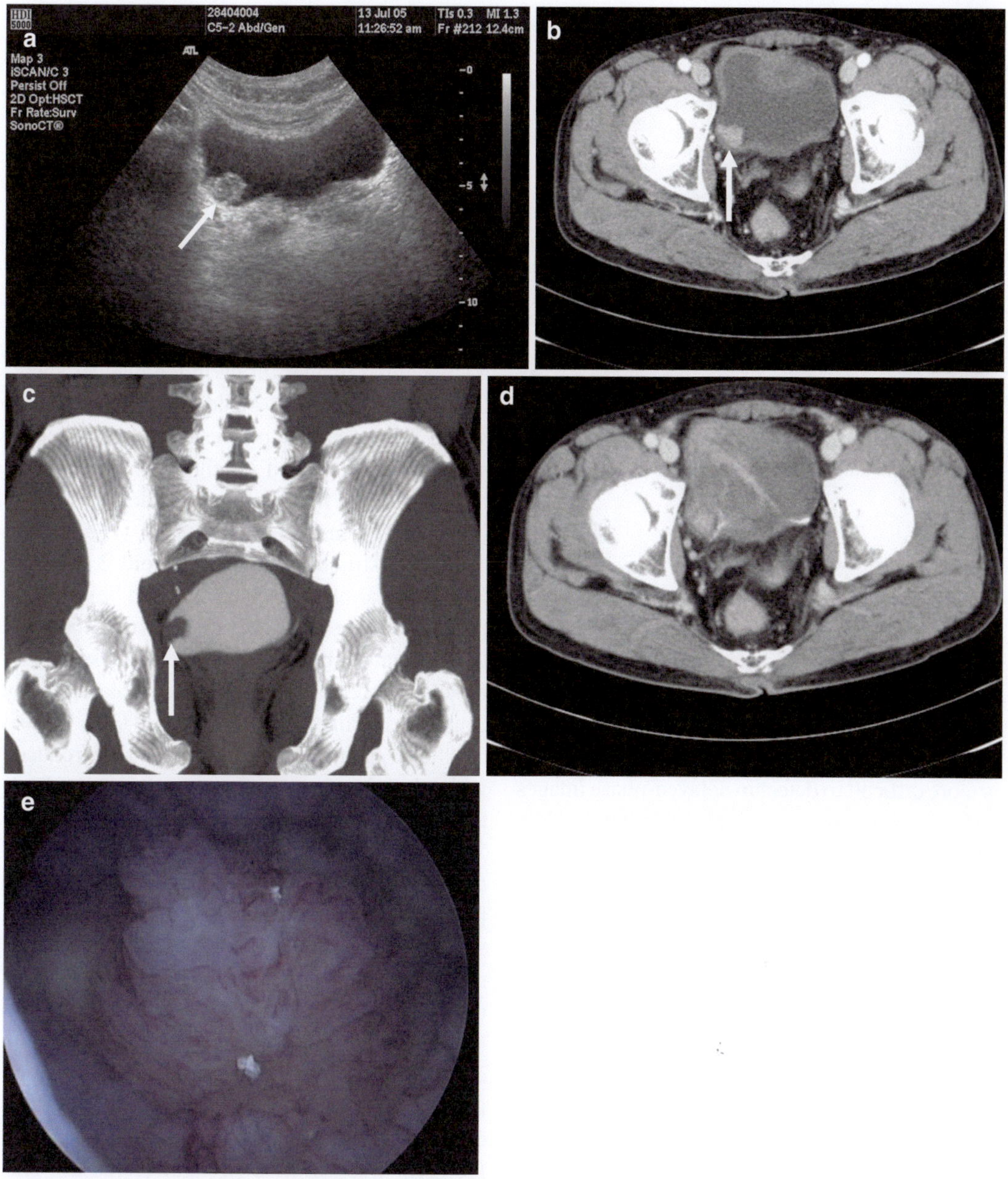

Fig. 2.1 A 69-year-old man with bladder cancer. (**a**) Axial US image of the bladder shows a lumen protruding mass (*arrows*) in the right lateral wall of the bladder. (**b**) Early-phase contrast-enhanced CT image demonstrates strong enhancing, nodular lesion (*arrow*) within the bladder. Note low attenuation of urine in the bladder with excreted contrast in the bladder lumen. (**c**) Maximum-intensity-projection image of bladder mass (*arrow*) with contrast material filled in the bladder lumen. (**d**) Nephrogenic phase contrast-enhanced CT image demonstrates obscured tumor contour due to excreted contrast to the bladder lumen. (**e**) Cystoscopic photograph shows papillary mass fungating into the bladder

wall thickening in dependent wall is hard to detect in delayed-phase images because of contrast material in the bladder lumen and associated beam-hardening artifact (Fig.2.1d).

Discrete bladder mass and nodule are findings of bladder TCCs. This lesion shows early enhancement after contrast injection (within 60 s) when the lesion is surrounded by low-attenuated urine.

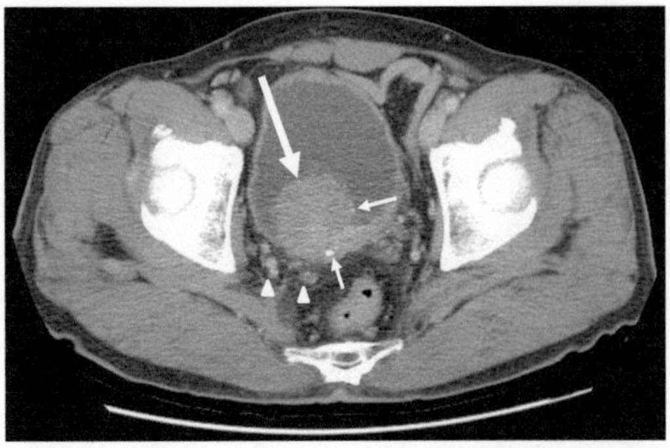

Fig. 2.2 A 74-year-old man with bladder cancer. Contrast-enhanced axial CT image of the bladder shows iso-attenuated mass (*large arrow*) in the posterior wall of the bladder. Note calcification in the mass (*small arrows*) and perivesical infiltration (*arrowheads*)

However, filling defect in delayed-phase image is also helpful in the detection of tumor when the nodule is large (Fig.2.1c). For this reason, focal hyperenhancement of the bladder urothelium should be considered as bladder TCCs. In other words, early-phase images are more important for detection of bladder TCCs because subtle lesion is more difficult to detect in delayed-phase images due to contrast material excreted to the bladder lumen. As a result, when patients suspected with bladder malignancy undergo contrast-enhanced CT, early-phase image should be obtained before contrast excretes to the bladder.

Presence of ureteral obstruction is observed when tumor invades the bladder muscle. Perivesical fat infiltration is seen when tumor extends to perivesical fat (Fig. 2.2) [17]. Calcification of bladder wall associated with bladder wall thickening should be suspected as malignancy, and further evaluation should be done. But, calcification can also be seen as sequelae of previous infections, bacilli Calmette Guérin (BCG) therapy.

2.2.1.2 MRI

MR imaging is known to allow more accurate staging of bladder TCCs than CT due to high soft tissue contrast [18]. MR imaging is better in assessing both muscle invasion and extravesical invasion in bladder TCCs. In addition, MR imaging has no radiation. In the evaluation of bladder TCCs, high spatial resolution is needed. For this purpose, phased-array external surface coil, thin section, and large matrix are needed. Twenty-eight to 32 cm axial field of view (FOV) is sufficient to evaluate bladder and adjacent structures. Optimal echo time (60–80 ms) is crucial for high contrast-to-noise ratio, which is important in evaluating bladder wall invasion depth with tumor [19].

Axial T1-weighted images are useful in detecting perivesical tumor infiltration. On T1-weighted images, urine in the bladder shows low signal intensity, bladder wall shows iso-signal intensity, and perivesical fat shows high signal intensity. On T2-weighted images, urine has high signal intensity and bladder wall shows low signal intensity.

With instructing patients to void 2 h before MR, optimal bladder distension can be achieved [20]. When the bladder is underdistended, small tumors cannot be detected due to thickening of bladder muscle. An overdistended bladder may cause obscuring of flat bladder TCCs. Bowel peristalsis causes artifact; this can be reduced with administering an intramuscular antiperistaltic agent and using anterior saturation bands. With swapping phase and frequency-encoding direction, motion artifact can also be reduced [13]. Chemical shift artifact is misregistration of spatial information caused by the difference of resonant frequencies of fat and water. This occurs in the interface of water and fat [21]. This artifact is seen in frequency-encoding direction and appears as low- and high-signal bands along the water-fat interface perpendicular to face-encoding direction. The pixel width of this artifact gets wide as field strength increases. This bandlike artifact can hinder detection of bladder wall tumor. To reduce this artifact, the increase of bandwidth and changing direction of frequency-encoding direction are needed [22]. T2-weighted images are obtained in three orthogonal planes. High-resolution images with plane perpendicular to the bladder mass are most crucial in the evaluation of muscle invasion depth and perivesical extension [18]. When the tumor does not invade bladder muscle, low signal intensity of muscle is not interrupted on

T2-weighted image. When the tumor invades bladder muscle, low signal intensity of muscle is interrupted by the tumor. When tumor extends to extravesical fat or organ, this can also be seen MR imaging (Fig. 2.3).

With multiplanar imaging, MR imaging can minimize partial volume averaging and allow accurate evaluation of bladder muscle invasion with tumor. Coronal images are useful in evaluating bladder lateral wall and dome. Sagittal images are useful in detecting lesions in the anterior and posterior wall [13].

Recently, 3D sequence MR imaging is feasible. Compared to 2D sequence, 3D sequence offers shorter acquisition time, volumetric coverage without interslice gaps, and higher signal-to-noise ratio [19]. With this technique, single-breath-hold imaging acquisition is possible.

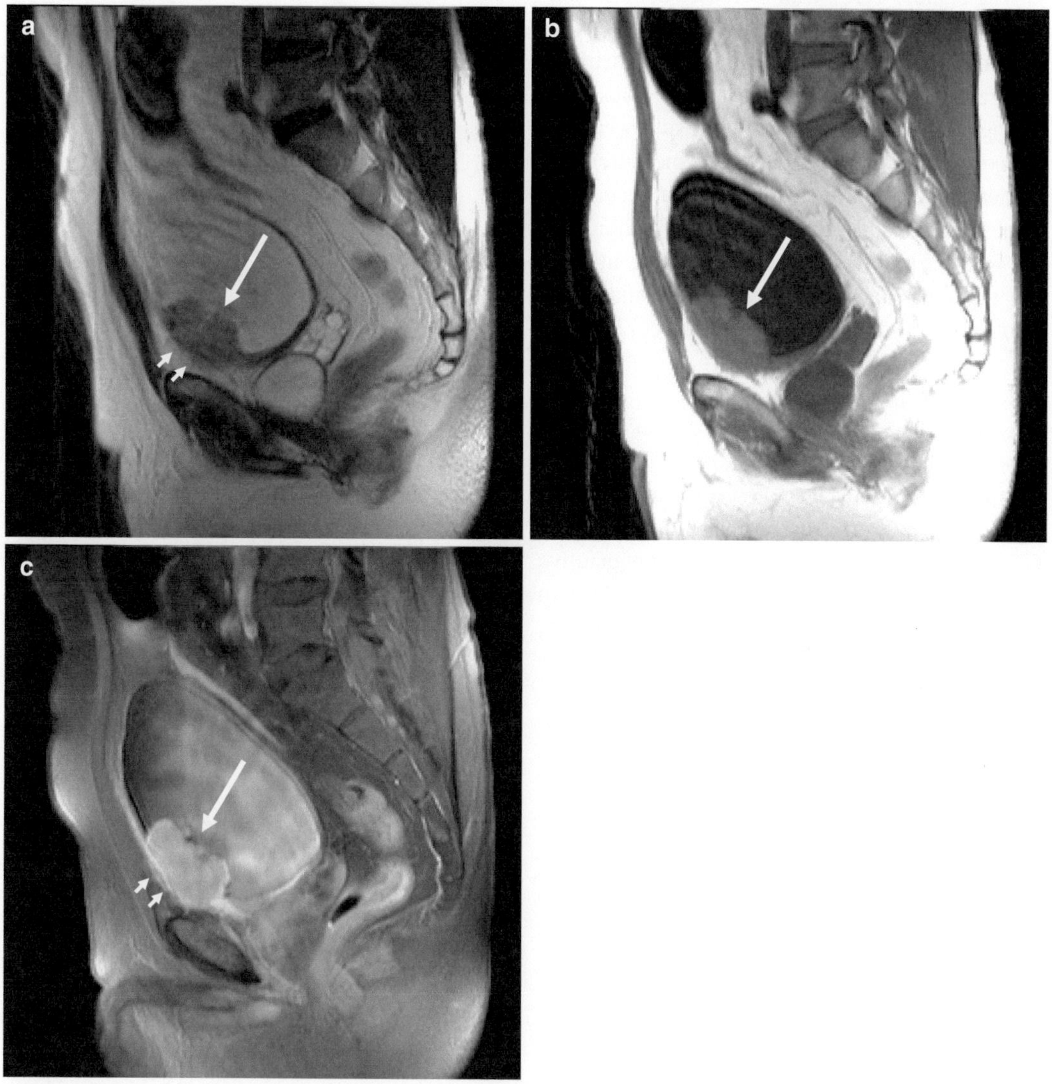

Fig. 2.3 A 57-year-old man with bladder cancer. (**a**) Sagittal T2-weighted MR image of tumor shows large mass with the bladder wall thickening (*arrow*). Perivesical stranding (*small arrows*) was confirmed to tumor spread at histopathologic examination. (**b**) Sagittal T1-weighted MR image shows mass in the bladder (*arrow*). Mass shows iso-signal intensity with adjacent muscle. (**c**) Sagittal contrast-enhanced T1-weighted MR image reveals enhancing mass in the bladder (*arrow*). Perivesical tumor spread is seen (*small arrows*)

The bladder wall does not show early enhancement on the gadolinium-enhanced images. In the early phase (20 s after intravenous contrast injection), bladder TCCs show more enhancement than adjacent bladder muscle [23]. The bladder TCCs, mucosal, and submucosa have early enhancement, but bladder muscle shows late enhancement (60 s) [18]. Bladder TCCs show as filling defect in delayed (>5 min) image, but small lesion can be obscured due to contrast material in the bladder.

The bladder TCCs with increased cellular density show increased signal intensity on diffusion-weighted images and reduced signal intensity on apparent diffusion coefficient (ADC) maps [24]. Changes of signal intensity on diffusion-weighted images are more useful than ADC measurement, because there can be interobserver variation in ADC values in the bladder tumor in relatively thin bladder wall [25]. Diffusion-weighted image in bladder TCCs has shown improved differentiation of bladder TCCs from bladder muscle layer [26–29].

2.2.1.3 Staging

The clinical stage of the bladder cancer is determined by the depth of invasion of bladder wall by the tumor. The clinical staging, with using CT or MR imaging, often underestimates tumor extent. CT is standard imaging modality for preoperative staging. The accuracy of contrast-enhanced CT in the local staging of bladder TCCs is 40–60 % [30, 31]. The accuracy of contrast-enhanced MR imaging is 52–93 % [18, 32–35]. Microscopic perivesical spread (T3a) is not detectable in CT or MR imaging. Macroscopic perivesical disease (T3b) can be diagnosed at CT or MRI. However, perivesical edema or inflammation especially after bladder cancer treatment can mimic perivesical tumor spread. The TNM classification of the renal pelvis and ureter is tabulated in Table 2.1 [36].

Table 2.1 TNM classification of the bladder TCC

Stage	Findings
Tx	Primary tumor cannot be assessed
T0	No evidence of primary tumor
Ta	Papillary noninvasive carcinoma
Tis	Carcinoma in situ
T1	Tumor invades subepithelial connective tissue
T2	Tumor invades muscularis propria
T2a	Tumor invades the superficial muscularis propria (inner half)
T2b	Tumor invades the deep muscularis propria (outer half)
T3	Tumor invades perivesical tissue
T3a	Tumor invades perivesical tissue microscopically
T3b	Tumor invades perivesical tissue macroscopically (extravesical mass)
T4	Tumor invades any of the following: prostatic stroma, seminal vesicles, uterus, vagina, pelvic wall, abdominal wall
T4a	Tumor invades prostatic stroma, uterus, vagina
T4b	Tumor invades pelvic wall, abdominal wall
Nx	Regional lymph nodes cannot be assessed
N0	No regional lymph node metastasis
N1	Single regional lymph node metastasis in the true pelvis (hypogastric, obturator, external iliac, or presacral lymph node)
N2	Multiple regional lymph node metastases in the true pelvis (hypogastric, obturator, external iliac, or presacral lymph node)
N3	Lymph node metastases to the common iliac lymph nodes
M0	No distant metastasis
M1	Distant metastasis

T primary tumor, *N* regional lymph nodes, *M* distant metastasis

2.2.2 Transitional Cell Carcinoma: Kidney and Ureter

Upper urinary tract TCCs occur in the sixth and seventh decades of life and have male predominance [37]. TCCs are common in the urinary bladder, and 5 % of urothelial tumors arise from the renal pelvis or ureter, and they account for 10 % of tumors of the upper urinary tract [38, 39]. Smoking, chemical carcinogens (aniline, benzidine, aromatic amine, azo dyes), analgesic abuse, cyclophosphamide, and heavy caffeine consumption increased risk of TCCs [38, 40].

Upper urinary TCCs are histologically similar to bladder TCCs [41]. Low-grade tumors have superficial, papillary appearance with broad base, are usually small and slowly growing, and have good prognosis [42]. High-grade tumors are less common, pedunculated or diffusely infiltrating, and more aggressive [43].

Synchronous bilateral TCCs occur in 1–2 % of renal TCCs and 2–9 % of ureteral TCCs, and 11–13 % of upper urinary tract TCCs develop metachronous upper urinary tract TCCs [37]. About 50 % of upper urinary tract TCCs will develop bladder TCCs after surgical treatment [38, 44]. Two percent of bladder TCCs have synchronous upper urinary tract TCCs and 6 % will have metachronous upper tract tumor [45].

2.2.2.1 Intravenous Urography and Retrograde Pyelography

TCCs from the upper urinary tract are usually diagnosed with intravenous urography (IVU) in the patients with hematuria. These days, CT urography gradually replaces the IVU the noninvasive methods of choice in the diagnosis of TCCs from the upper urinary tract. The TCCs from the upper urinary tracts are well visualized. Calcifications can be seen in precontrast radiograph in 2–7 % of tumors, and they can be confused as urinary stone [37].

TCCs from renal pelvicalyceal system can be seen as a filling defect in IVU. These filling defects can be single or multiple and smooth, irregular, or stippled (Fig. 2.4). Contrast material dispersed in the papillary mass is shown as stippled appearance in IVU. This finding also can be seen in benign lesions such as blood clot and fungus ball. Some TCCs can show stricture-like

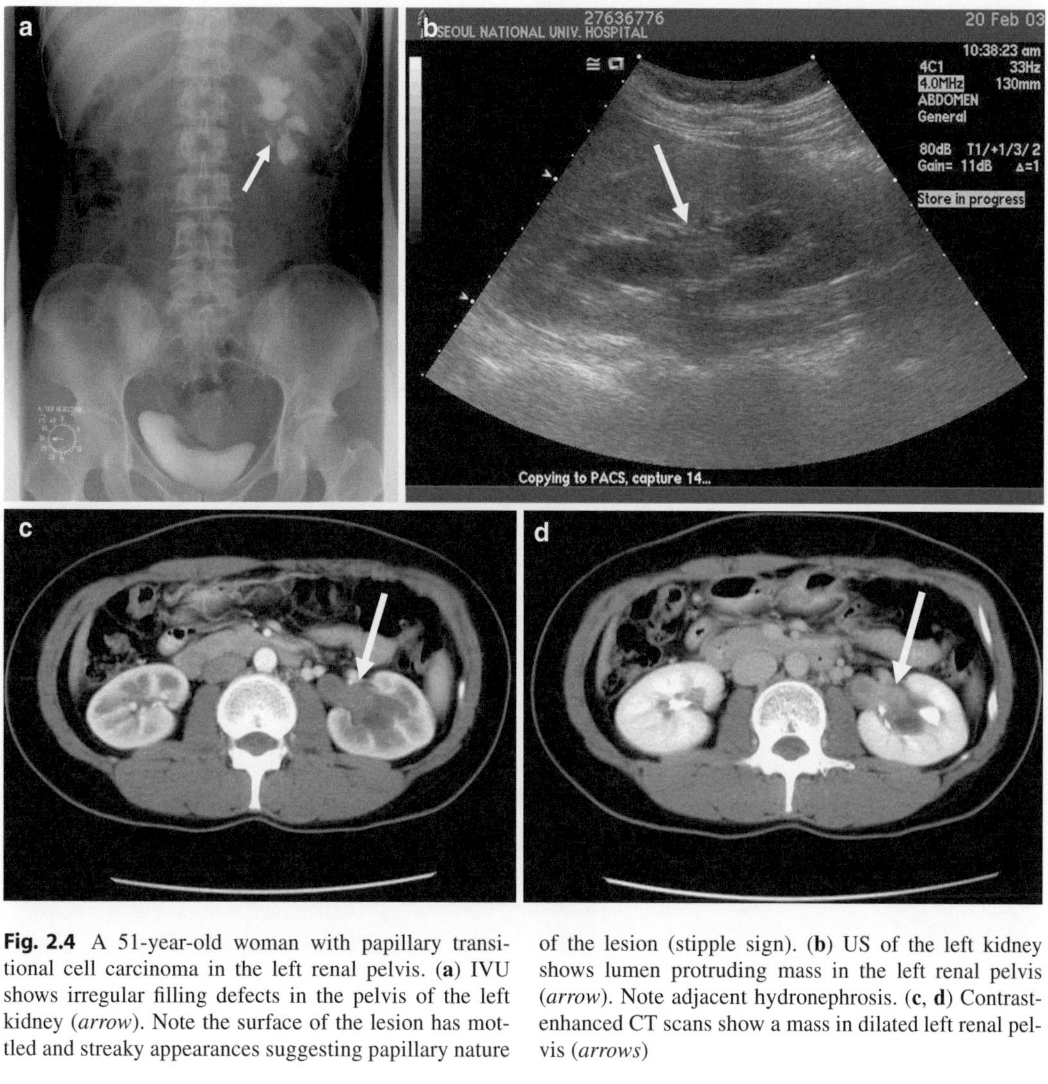

Fig. 2.4 A 51-year-old woman with papillary transitional cell carcinoma in the left renal pelvis. (**a**) IVU shows irregular filling defects in the pelvis of the left kidney (*arrow*). Note the surface of the lesion has mottled and streaky appearances suggesting papillary nature of the lesion (stipple sign). (**b**) US of the left kidney shows lumen protruding mass in the left renal pelvis (*arrow*). Note adjacent hydronephrosis. (**c**, **d**) Contrast-enhanced CT scans show a mass in dilated left renal pelvis (*arrows*)

lesions; these findings can be misinterpreted as renal tuberculosis [40]. When tumors obstruct renal infundibulum, affected calyx is not visualized in IVU and this is calyceal amputation. When calyx is not seen in IVU, we call it "phantom calyx" (Fig. 2.5).

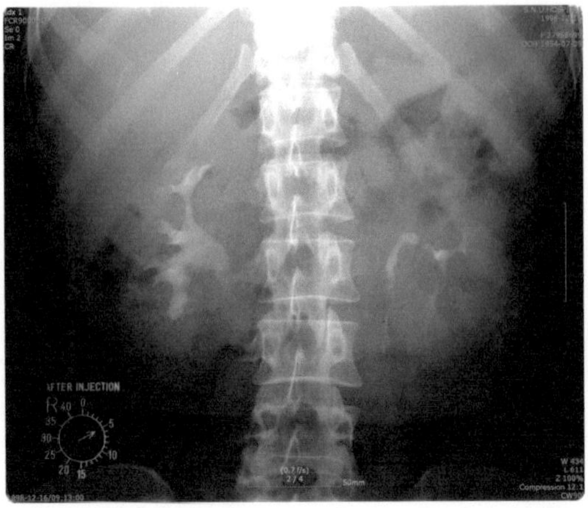

Fig. 2.5 A 54-year-old man with papillary transitional cell carcinoma in the left renal infundibulum. Upper polar calyx is not seen in IVU due to obstruction of infundibulum (phantom calyx)

TCCs from the ureter are seen as single or multiple filling defects. Stippling or proximal obstruction can be seen. When there are long-standing obstructions due to ureteric tumor, contrast excretion can be poor, and it may be hard to evaluate ureteric lesion. When this happens, contrast-enhanced CT or retrograde pyelography (RGP) can be done for further evaluation.

Retrograde pyelography is performed during cystoscopy, for further evaluation when upper urinary tract lesions are not well visualized during IVU or when patients are allergic to contrast materials. Although RGU is more invasive compared with IVU, it can aid confirmation of lesion detected in IVU and help biopsy or brushing during ureteroscopic examination.

Renal TCCs are irregular papillary or nodular mass in RGU (Fig. 2.6). Amputated calyx can be seen when TCCs invade and obstruct renal infundibulum. When tumor fills and distends calyx, we call it "oncocalyx."

Ureteral TCCs are usually seen as polypoid filling defect with proximal dilatation. Circumferential or eccentric ureteric strictures can be seen in TCC and sometimes they can be confused with benign

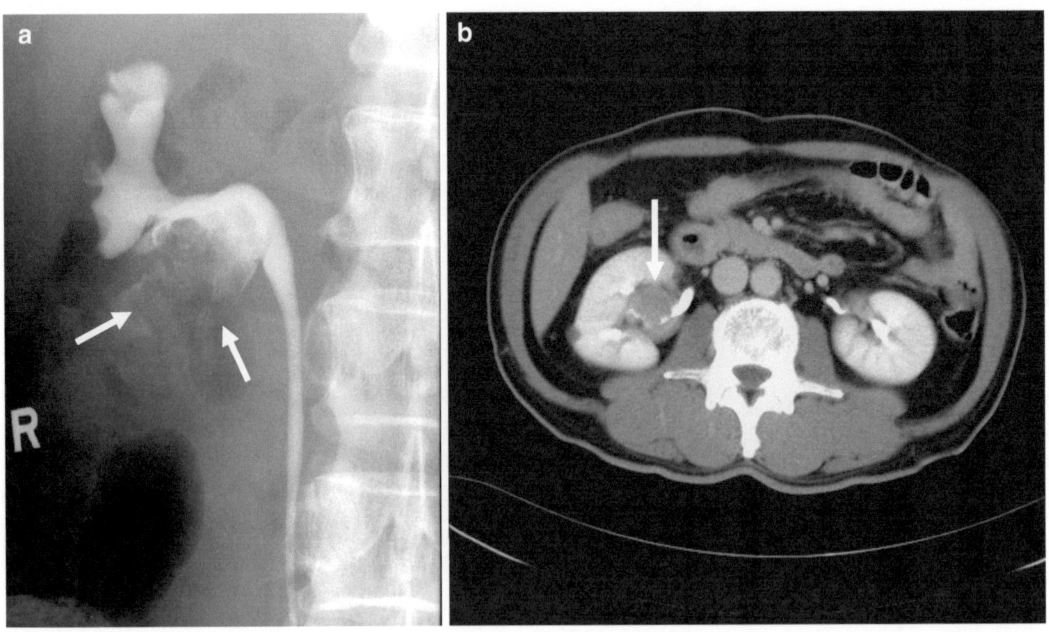

Fig. 2.6 An 84-year-old man with transitional cell carcinoma. (**a**) RGP shows a papillary filling defect in the right renal pelvis with amputation of the lower calyceal infundibulum (*arrows*). (**b**) Contrast-enhanced CT shows mass with irregular surface (*arrow*) in dilated renal pelvis in the left kidney

strictures. In malignant stricture, there are usually ureteric fixation and nontapering margin [37]. In RGP, dilatation of the ureter distal to ureteral mass is seen, and this is called "goblet" sign (Fig. 2.7).

2.2.2.2 CT

CT is useful in the diagnosis of upper urinary tract TCCs. With CT urography, a small renal pelvis mass and urinary tract mass can be detected. CT urography is superior to IVU in that urothelium, renal parenchyma, and adjacent tissue can be evaluated at a time.

There have been multiple different CT urography protocols: single-bolus technique, split-bolus technique, and triple-bolus technique. Among them single-bolus technique is most commonly used in practice. In single-bolus technique, precontrast scan is acquired from kidney to symphysis pubis. After that one bolus of contrast is injected and early, parenchymal, and excretory phase scan is acquired [46]. The advantage of this technique over the other technique (split-bolus and triple-bolus technique) is that it can provide optimal opacification and distension of the renal pelvis and ureter. In addition, small renal cell carcinomas can be more easily detected compared with

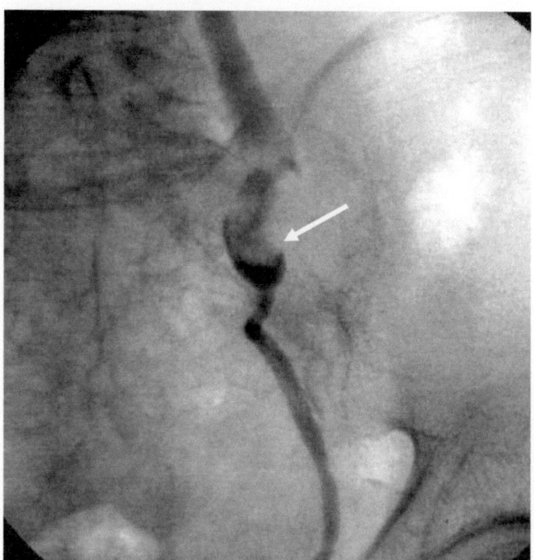

Fig. 2.7 An 88-year-old man with ureter transitional cell carcinoma. RGP shows a filling defect in the left midureter. Note smooth concavity of the ureter just beneath the tumor, which is "goblet sign" (*arrows*)

other technique. The major disadvantage of this technique is increased radiation dose due to multiple imaging phases. In split-bolus technique, contrast injection is divided into two sessions and imaging is acquired in combined nephrogenic and excretory phase. The advantage of this technique is decreased radiation due to reduced imaging phase [47, 48]. However, there are some questions about the optimal opacification of distal ureter due to half dose of contrast for excreted contrast [47, 48]. Triple-bolus technique splits dose of contrast into three boluses and acquires combined early-nephrogenic phase [49]. With this technique, the radiation dose can be reduced, but the opacification and distension of ureter are also questionable in this technique. In addition, detectability of small renal lesion (such as small renal cell carcinoma) can be decreased.

In performing CT urography, ancillary techniques, such as abdominal compression, intravenous (IV) saline, IV furosemide, and prone positioning, should be considered [46]. Abdominal compression is done for opacification of proximal urinary tract. But, the usefulness is in doubt [50]. IV saline injection is suggested in some studies to distend distal ureters [50]. IV diuretic injection improves distension and opacification of ureter [5]. But there are some difficulties in IV injection of diuretics in daily practice, because of allergy or hypotension.

Single-bolus technique is most commonly used because of optimal distension of the ureter and higher sensitivity in the detection of renal mass [46]. To decrease beam-hardening artifact, which can interfere detection of small lesions, delayed images after 5 min are recommended [51]. When there is obstruction, more delayed image acquisition for excretory phase is needed.

Renal TCCs are seen as filling defect renal pelvis wall thickening in the excretory phase (Fig. 2.4). Other findings are pelvicalyceal irregularity, oncocalyx, or obstructed calyx (Fig. 2.6). Early TCCs are separated from renal parenchyma. Advanced TCCs extend to renal parenchyma. Sometimes renal TCCs have mass-like appearance, mimicking centrally located renal cell carcinoma (RCC) (Fig. 2.8). Imaging features for renal TCCs are as follows: mass epicenter in the

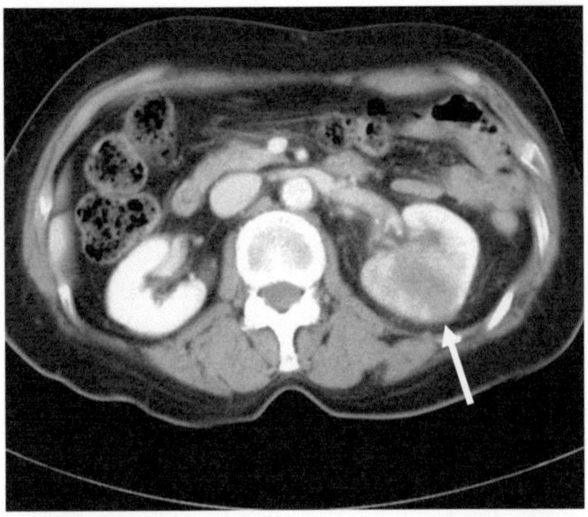

Fig. 2.8 A 77-year-old man with transitional cell carcinoma in the renal pelvis invading renal parenchyma. Contrast-enhanced CT shows extensive parenchymal invasion (*arrows*) of the left kidney. Note, the left kidney conserves reniform contour and mass shows homogeneous and solid feature

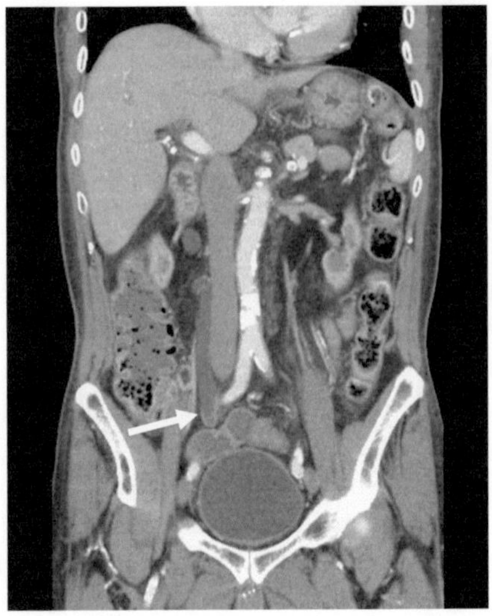

Fig. 2.9 Transitional cell carcinoma of the distal ureter in a 77-year-old man. Coronal reformation image of contrast-enhanced CT shows irregular wall thickening of the right midureter (*arrows*)

renal pelvis or calyx, presence of focal filling defect in collecting system, reniform contour preservation, mainly solid feature, homogeneous attenuation, moderate enhancement, and extension of tumor to ureteropelvic junction.

Ureteral thickening is the most common manifestation of ureteral TCCs (Fig. 2.9) [50]. To detect thickening of ureter in ureter TCCs, meticulous check of all three phase is needed because subtle urothelial thickening can be seen in all three phases. Not only irregular and eccentric but also circumferential and smooth wall thickening can be seen in ureteral TCCs [52]. TCCs show early enhancement so early phase is important phase in the detection of ureteral TCCs (Fig. 2.10) [52]. Enhancement pattern is usually focal and eccentric. Care should be taken for evaluation of ureteral enhancement because this can also be seen in inflammatory lesions [53]. Calcification can be seen ureteral TCCS. Calcification is usually located eccentrically or in the wall. This should be differentiated urinary stone which is located in the central lumen of ureter. Periureteral fat stranding can be seen in urinary TCCs. Usually cancer-related periureteral fat stranding is persistent after treatment; this is differential point from inflammation-related periureteral fat stranding. Filling defects are findings of ureteral TCCs. But, when mass size is small, sometimes it is difficult to detect tumor in excretory phase due to beam-hardening artifact. Some of these lesions can be seen in the early or nephrogenic phase [54]. Ureteral TCCs can accompany hydronephrosis or hydroureter. Dilatation of proximal ureter can be seen even when ureteral TCCs are no visible. So when there is ureteral dilatation proximal to suspected stricture without definite mass, ureteroscopic examination should be done not to miss small ureteral TCCs [52].

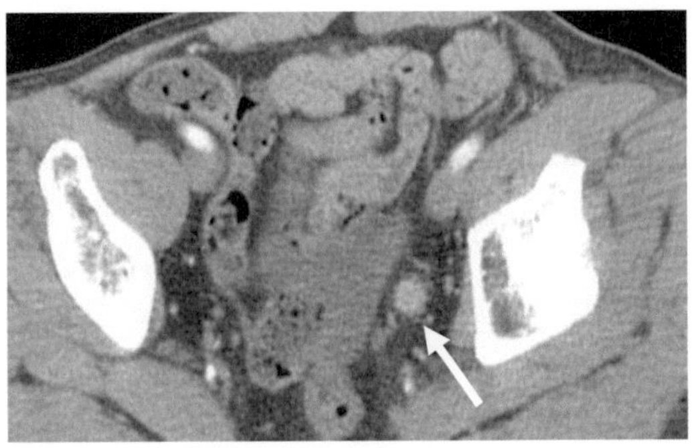

Fig. 2.10 Transitional cell carcinoma of the distal ureter in a 73-year-old man. Contrast-enhanced CT shows an enhancing soft tissue lesion (*arrow*) in the right distal ureter. Note non-opacification of both external iliac veins, indicating that this image is early phase after contrast injection

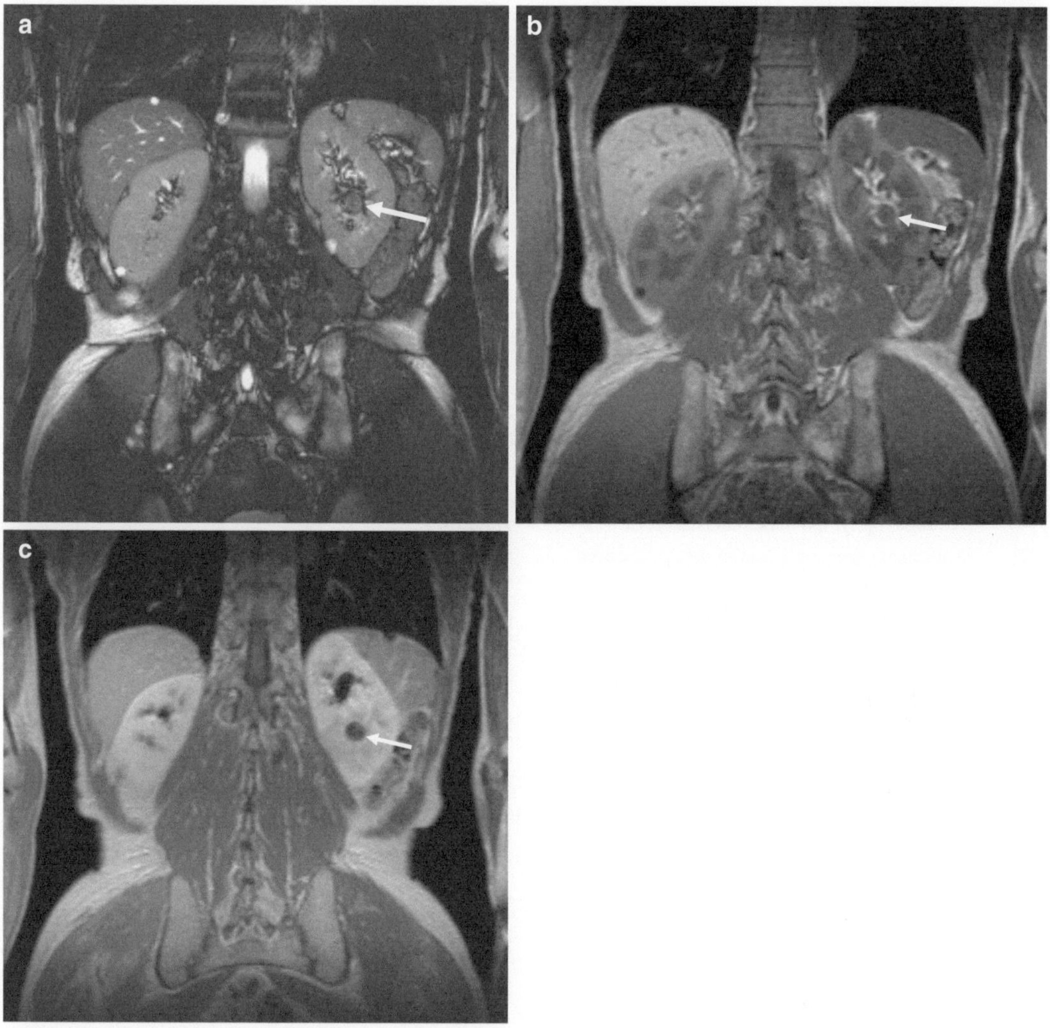

Fig. 2.11 An 82-year-old man with transitional cell carcinoma of the renal pelvis. (**a**) T2-weighted MR image shows hypointense mass in the left renal pelvis (*arrow*). Mass is confined to the renal pelvis. (**b**) T1-weighted MR image shows iso-attenuated mass in the left renal pelvis (*arrow*). (**c**) Contrast-enhanced T1-weighted image shows relatively less enhancement compared with renal parenchyma (*arrow*)

2.2.2.3 MRI

MR imaging is infrequently used in the evaluation of upper urinary tract TCCs. Generally, MR imaging is less commonly used compared with CT urography due to more time for acquiring image and more motion-related artifacts. However, when the patients have a contraindication to CT contrast agent, MRI can be an option. MR imaging has high soft tissue contrast, is independent to renal function, and allows multiplanar imaging.

TCC shows lower-signal intensity than urine in T2-weighted images and tumors are well visualized. In gadolinium contrast-enhanced images, TCCs show moderate enhancement (Fig. 2.11) [55]. MR urography is used in the evaluation of the upper urinary tract. At MR urography, ureteric TCCs are shown as irregular mass. Sometimes differentiation between stone and small TCCs is difficult in MR urography. Usually ureter stone has sharp margin but ureter TCCs usually have irregular margins.

2.2.2.4 Staging

The TNM classification of the renal pelvis and ureter is tabulated in Table 2.2 [36].

Table 2.2 TNM classification of the renal pelvis and ureter TCC

Stage	Findings
Tx	Primary tumor cannot be assessed
T0	No evidence of primary tumor
Ta	Papillary noninvasive carcinoma
Tis	Carcinoma in situ
T1	Tumor invades subepithelial connective tissue
T2	Tumor invades the muscularis
T3	Renal pelvis: tumor invades beyond muscularis into peripelvic fat or the renal parenchyma
	Ureter: tumor invades beyond muscularis into periureteric fat
T4	Tumor invades adjacent organs or through the kidney into the perinephric fat
Nx	Regional lymph nodes cannot be assessed
N0	No regional lymph node metastasis
N1	Metastasis in a single lymph node, ≤2 cm in greatest dimension
N2	Metastasis in a single lymph node, >2 cm but not >5 cm in greatest dimension; or multiple lymph nodes, none >5 cm in greatest dimension
N3	Metastasis in a lymph node, >5 cm in greatest dimension
M0	No distant metastasis
M1	Distant metastasis

T primary tumor, *N* regional lymph nodes, *M* distant metastasis

2.3 Nonurothelial Tumors

2.3.1 Squamous Cell Carcinoma

Squamous cell carcinoma consists less than 5 % of bladder tumors [1]. Symptoms are gross hematuria and irritation during voiding. Risk factors are nonbilharzial region residency, cyclophosphamide, intravesical BCG, smoking, bladder stone, or chronic infection. Paraplegic patients usually have both bladder stone and infection [1, 56]. Tumors are high grade and locally aggressive with muscle invasion [57]. They usually occur at the trigone and bladder lateral wall and diverticula [58]. Metastases are present in 10 % of cases at diagnosis and involve the regional lymph node, bone, lung, and bowel [59]. Muscle invasion is present in 80 %, and extravesical invasion is extensive [60]. Prognosis is generally poor because it presents with advanced stage. Death is usually from local failure, with metastasis (8–10 %) [61].

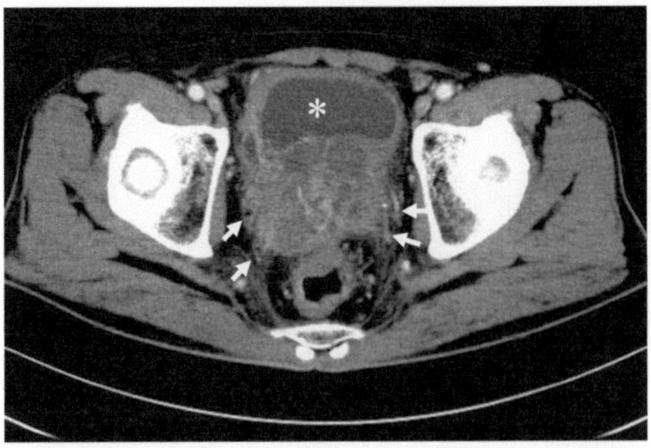

Fig. 2.12 A 72-year-old man with squamous cell carcinoma of the bladder. Contrast-enhanced CT shows diffuse bladder wall thickening with mass formation in the posterior wall of the bladder (*asterisk*). Note perivesical infiltration (*arrows*), which was histologically confirmed to tumor spread

Bladder squamous cell carcinoma has nonspecific imaging findings. Tumors show focal or diffuse bladder wall thickening or single enhancing bladder mass (Fig. 2.12) [60]. Diverticular squamous cell carcinomas are soft tissue masses and occasionally surface calcification may coexist [58]. Bladder squamous cell carcinoma shows sessile growth pattern compared to papillary growth pattern of TCCs. Bladder wall thickening or calcification can be seen.

2.3.2 Adenocarcinoma

Adenocarcinoma is a uncommon bladder neoplasm (less than 2 %) [1]. It can be classified as primary (nonurachal and urachal) and secondary. The mean age of diagnosis is 60 years, and urachal cancer occurs 10 years earlier. Nonurachal adenocarcinoma has male predominance, but urachal adenocarcinoma has equal prevalence in men and women. Hematuria and irritation are common symptoms. In 25 % mucous secreted in urine [62]. Umbilical discharge can be seen in urachal cancer.

Bladder adenocarcinoma is associated with bladder exstrophy and persistent urachus. Other risk factors are chronic mucosal irritation associated with intestinal metaplasia, urinary diversion, and pelvic lipomatosis associated with cystitis glandularis.

Metastatic adenocarcinoma of the bladder is more common than primary bladder adenocarcinoma. Adenocarcinoma is most common histologic type of secondary bladder neoplasms. Primary sites include direct invasion from colon, prostate, rectum, and pelvic tumors [63]. Hematogenous metastases from the stomach, breast, and lung are less common. Differentiation of primary and secondary bladder adenocarcinomas is important in deciding treatment plan. When bladder metastases occur, usually there are locally invasive primary malignancies.

Although urine cytology is useful, sensitivity is limited when tumor is located beneath mucosal layer. At cystoscopy, adenocarcinoma is usually single nodular lesion occurring at bladder base (58–67 %) and urachus. Primary adenocarcinoma is histologically same with colon adenocarcinoma, and it is difficult to distinguish primary adenocarcinoma from metastatic adenocarcinoma, even with special stain [63].

Nonurachal adenocarcinoma shows diffuse bladder wall thickening at CT (75 %) and stranding of surrounding fat (88 %) [64]. Distant metastases (38 %), lymph node metastasis (25 %), rectus muscle invasion (25 %), and peritoneal seeding were observed.

Urachus is a midline remnant of the cloaca and allantois. It is located extraperitoneally and is bounded by the transverse fascia and parietal peritoneum. This area is called "Retzius space" [65]. In fetal life, urachus is regressed to a fibrous band and becomes medial umbilical ligament. This extend anterior dome of the bladder to umbilicus. Incomplete regression of the urachus causes four anomalies: urachal sinus, patent urachus, urachal diverticulum, and urachal cyst. Among them, urachal cyst is the most common (30 %) [66]. Most urachal tumors are adenocarcinomas (90 %). Because urachal remnant is lined by transitional epithelium, the suggested pathogenesis is metaplasia of urachal mucosa into columnar epithelium and malignant transformation [65]. In urachal cancer, mucin stain is positive [62]. Urachal cancer has male predominance and occurs between 40 and 79 years old [65, 67].

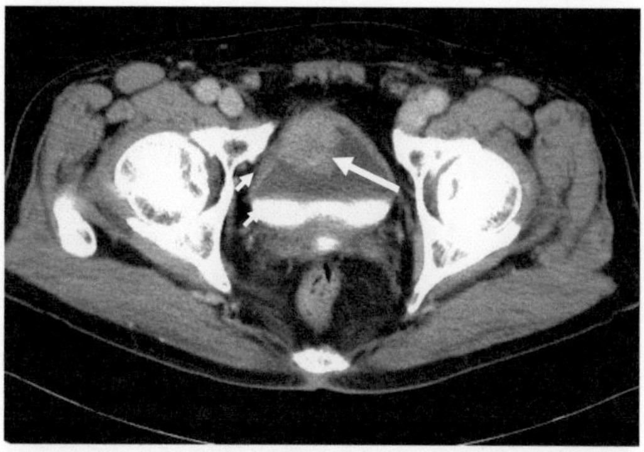

Fig. 2.13 A 57-year-old man with adenocarcinoma of the bladder. Contrast-enhanced CT shows well-enhancing mass (*arrow*) in the anterior wall of the bladder. There are irregularities in the outer margin of the tumor indicating perivesical tumor extension

Common symptoms are hematuria, dysuria, abdominal pain, suprapubic mass, and discharge from the umbilicus [17, 68].

In IVU or cystography, urachal adenocarcinoma is seen as a filling defect or extrinsic compression in the dome of the bladder. Tumor can be detected with ultrasound (US) as a fluid-filled, mixed echogenic solid mass with or without calcification adjacent to abdominal wall. But these imaging findings are nonspecific.

CT and MR imaging are more accurate imaging modalities for evaluation of both local staging and distant metastases. CT feature is a midline mass anterior superior to the dome of the bladder with mixed solid and cystic appearance (Fig. 2.13) [65]. The cystic component is mucin. Peripheral punctate or stippled or curvilinear calcification is present in 50–70 %, and they are considered pathognomonic for urachal carcinoma [65, 68–70]. Urachal adenocarcinoma is outside of the bladder in 88 % [70]. In contrast to bladder TCCs, extravesical tumor spread is common (Fig. 2.14). Bladder wall invasion is present in 92 % and metastases are present in 48 % [70, 71]. Pseudomyxoma peritonei rarely occurs.

MR imaging is the best technique for evaluation of urachal adenocarcinoma. On T2-weighted images, there are focal high-signal-intensity lesions suggestive of mucin [65]. On T1-weighted images, tumor shows iso-signal intensity and enhances with contrast material.

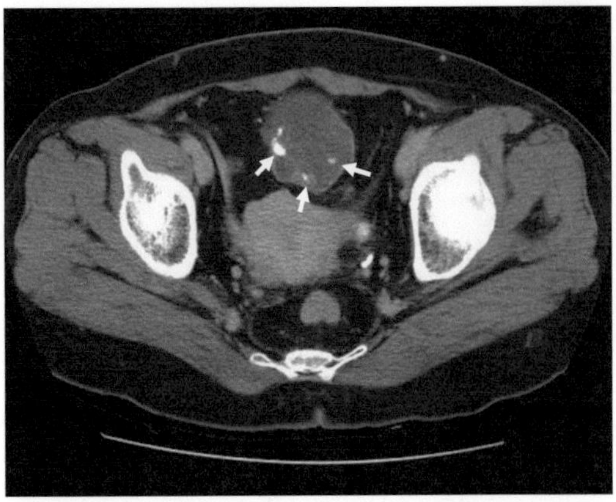

Fig. 2.14 A 62-year-old woman with urachal adenocarcinoma. Contrast-enhanced CT scan shows a mixed cystic and solid midline mass with punctate calcification anterocranial to the bladder (*arrows*)

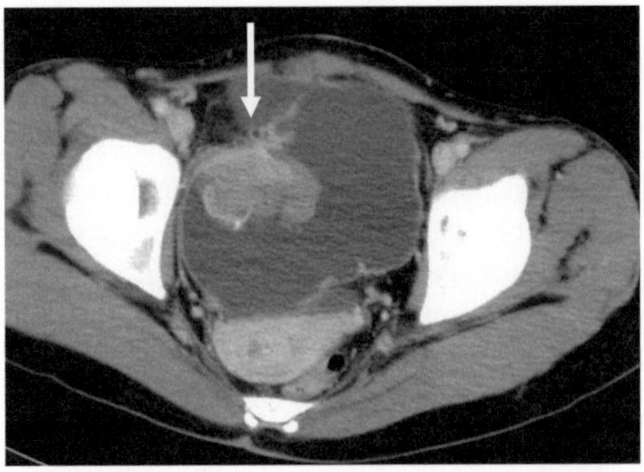

Fig. 2.15 Small cell carcinoma of the bladder in a 65-year-old woman. Contrast-enhanced CT scan shows broad-based, large mass (*arrow*), which is not distinguishable from other bladder tumors. Note perivesical infiltration

Most tumors are advanced at diagnosis, and due to extravesical location, urachal tumors are clinically silent until they get bigger [1]. Prognosis is poor for invasive tumors (20–40 % survival at 5 years) [1].

2.3.3 Small Cell Tumors

Small cell bladder tumor is a rare tumor (0.5 % of bladder tumor) [72, 73]. This tumor is an aggressive tumor with advanced stage at diagnosis. Presenting symptom is hematuria (88 %) and patients usually have smoking history (65 %). Patient's age has a wide range (20–90 years old); there is male predominance (male-female = 3-5:1) [72, 73].

Small cell bladder tumor arises from neuroendocrine cells. They are sheets of small cells with round hyperchromatic nuclei, sparse cytoplasm, and mitotic figure in histology. Majority have mixed tumor histology.

Cystoscopically, tumors are large and polypoid or nodular with ulcerative surface, mimicking other high-grade bladder cancer. The most common site is the lateral bladder wall [73]. On CT images, tumor has wall invasion, central necrosis, or cystic change (Fig. 2.15). Mass size is from 3 to 8 cm [74]. Calcification is not common. Tumor shows patchy enhancement unlike bladder TCCs [74]. Metastases occur rapidly, and the metastatic sites are the peritoneum, liver, bone, lung, and lymph nodes (66 %) [1].

2.3.4 Lymphoma

Lymphoma involvement of the bladder is much more often secondary rather than primary. Secondary involvement of the bladder is present in 10–25 % of lymphoma patients [75]. In secondary lymphoma, lymphadenopathy in abdomen and pelvis is usually found. It is common in middle-aged women with nonspecific urinary symptom (hematuria or mass effect). The cell type is B-cell mucosa-associated lymphoid tissue type or diffuse large B-cell type [75]. Hodgkin lymphoma is rare.

Imaging findings are well-defined bladder masses without infiltration (Fig. 2.16) [17]. They can mimic TCCs and cannot be differentiated from other primary bladder masses [76].

2.3.5 Leiomyoma

Bladder leiomyoma is a benign mass arising from the smooth muscle of the bladder and the most common benign bladder tumor [76]. Histologically, leiomyoma is noninfiltrative smooth muscle tumors

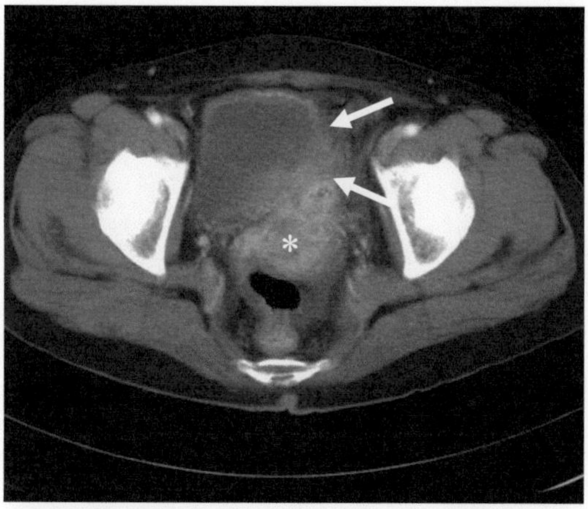

Fig. 2.16 Non-Hodgkin lymphoma of the bladder in a 49-year-old woman. Contrast-enhanced CT scan shows a homogeneously enhancing diffuse bladder wall thickening (*arrows*). Note enlargement of the uterus suggesting lymphoma involvement (*asterisk*)

lacking mitotic activity, cellular atypia, and necrosis. It is more common in women [77]. Two third of them grow externally, one third internally, and rarely grow intramurally [78]. Most are small and asymptomatic and discovered incidentally. Most of them have no symptoms, but sometimes, pressure from mass, urinary obstruction, hesitancy, dribbling, and hematuria can occur [79]. Although it is a benign tumor without malignant potential, histologic evaluation is needed to exclude possibility of well-differentiated leiomyosarcoma. They are benign and grow noninvasively and focal excision of the mass is the treatment of choice. However, sometimes they can recur after surgical treatment. At cystoscopy, leiomyoma is covered with normal bladder mucosa. They are well-circumscribed, solid, homogeneous, and smooth mass from the bladder wall. Cystic components indicate degeneration. MR imaging is superior to CT in characterizing leiomyoma, demonstrating the submucosal origin of the tumor and the preservation of the muscle layer.

Imaging findings of bladder are similar to those of uterine myoma. On T1-weighted image, they show iso-signal intensity, and on T2-weighted image, they show low signal intensity (Fig. 2.17). They can show heterogeneous high signal intensity on T2-weighted image if there are degeneration [79]. They show variable enhancement on contrast-enhanced image, with degenerated areas lacking enhancement [17]. A pedunculated luminal leiomyoma can be differentiated from bladder TCCs in that it has low signal intensity on T2-weighted images. A preoperative suggestion of leiomyoma is invaluable in alerting the surgeon to benign and preventing radical cystectomy.

2.4 Pathologic Consideration

2.4.1 Urothelial Tumors

2.4.1.1 Papillary Urothelial Lesion

Urothelial Papilloma

Pathologically, urothelial papilloma is exophytic papillary mass lined by benign, normal-looking urothelium with normal thickness (Fig. 2.18). Urothelial lining shows normal polarity, and umbrella layer is well developed. Cytologic atypia is absent or minimal. Branching of papillary architecture is minimal. Papillary core of urothelial papilloma is thin and slender, but occasionally is edematous. Most urothelial papillomas are solitary.

Inverted Papilloma

Inverted papilloma is benign urothelial tumor showing inverted growth pattern. Grossly inverted papilloma is small polypoid lesion with smooth surface. Microscopically inverted papilloma reveals invagination of urothelium into submucosa with cord or trabecular pattern (Fig. 2.19). Cytologic atypia of the urothelium is absent or minimal.

Papillary Urothelial Neoplasm of Low Malignant Potential

Papillary urothelial neoplasm of low malignant potential resembles urothelial papilloma but shows increased thickness of urothelial layers with minimal or no cytologic atypia (Fig. 2.20). The polarity of the urothelium is preserved, and the umbrella layer is often normally present. Papillary core is thin and delicate. Branching and complexity of papillae are limited.

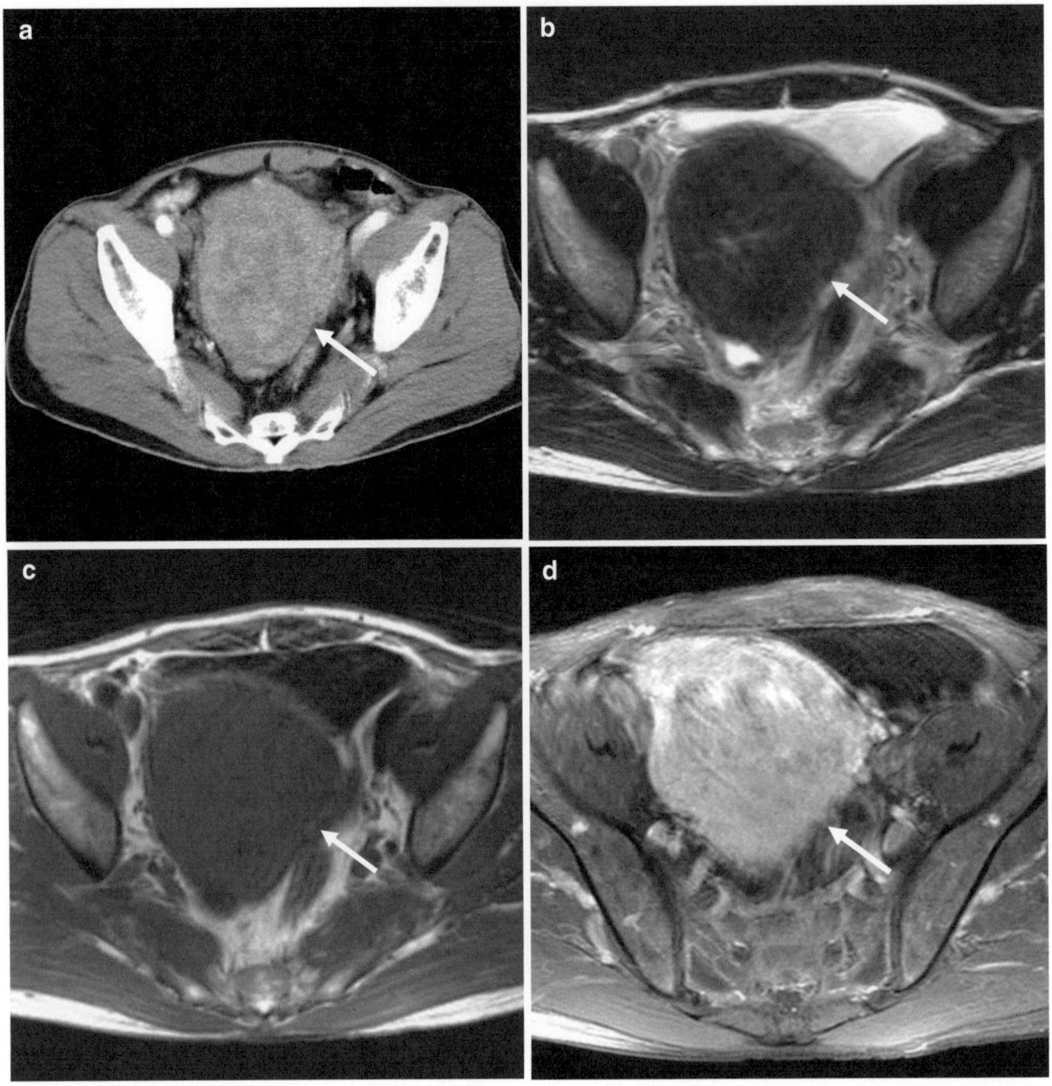

Fig. 2.17 Leiomyoma of the bladder in a 52-year-old man. (**a**) Contrast-enhanced CT images show a homogeneously enhancing, soft mass in the lower abdomen (*arrow*). (**b**) T2-weighted MR image shows low-signal-intensity mass from the posterior wall of the bladder (*arrow*). (**c**) T1-weighted MR images shows intermediate signal intensity mass (*arrow*). (**d**) Contrast-enhanced T1-weighted image shows strong enhancement of the mass (*arrow*)

Low-Grade Papillary Urothelial Carcinoma

Low-grade papillary urothelial carcinoma shows architectural disorganization and low-grade cytologic atypia. Grossly, this tumor is solitary or multiple exophytic papillary mass. Microscopically low-grade papillary urothelial carcinoma reveals more complex papillary architecture with thickened urothelial layers. Tumor cells also show loss of polarity with mild cytologic atypia and nuclear size variations (Fig. 2.21). But there is no marked nuclear pleomorphism. Mitotic figures are relatively rare.

High-Grade Papillary Urothelial Carcinoma

High-grade papillary urothelial carcinoma shows more complex architecture than low-grade papillary urothelial carcinoma. Tumor cells commonly show higher degree of nuclear atypia such as nuclear pleomorphism, hyperchromasia, and nuclear enlargement (Fig. 2.22).

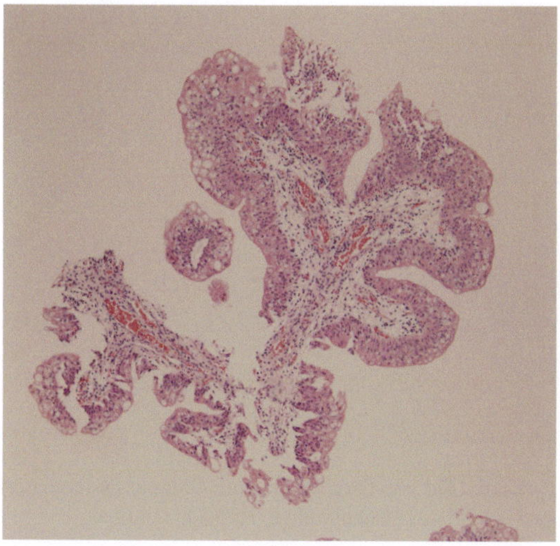

Fig. 2.18 Urothelial papilloma has fibrovascular core lined by normal-looking urothelium with normal thickness. Umbrella layer is well defined

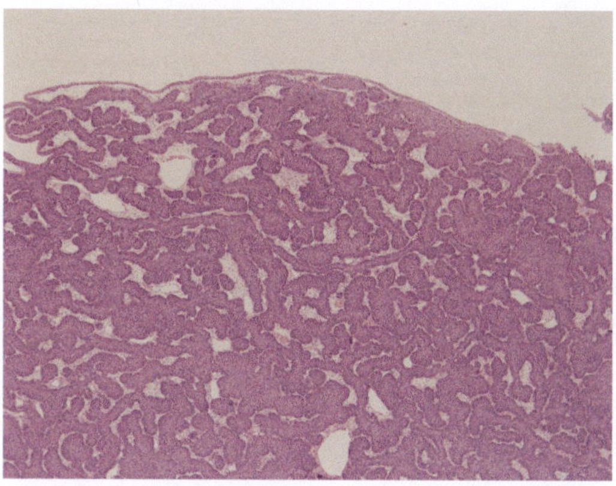

Fig. 2.19 Inverted papilloma shows endophytic growth of normal-looking urothelium with trabecular architecture. Overlying urothelium is normal

Mitoses are frequently observed. Tumor cells frequently reveal discohesion and denudation. High-grade papillary urothelial carcinoma can be admixed with low-grade area.

2.4.1.2 Fat Urothelial Lesion

Urothelial Dysplasia

Urothelial dysplasia is a premalignant lesion with poor reproducibility [80–82]. Microscopically, urothelial layer shows loss of polarity and cytologic atypia, but those are not enough to make diagnosis of urothelial carcinoma in situ (Fig. 2.23) [81, 82].

Urothelial Carcinoma In Situ

Urothelial carcinoma in situ can be defined as flat urothelial lesion composed of malignant urothelial cells without invasion. Grossly involved urothelial surface appears to be erythematous or edematous. Microscopically, tumor cells show high-grade atypia such as nuclear pleomorphism, hyperchromasia prominent nucleoli, or nuclear enlargement (Fig. 2.24a). Mitosis can be frequent. Occasionally, cellular discohesion and urothelial denudation can be prominent and only a few tumor cells can be found in denuded urothelium. Urothelial carcinoma in situ can be divided into several morphologic patterns, such as small cell, large cell, clinging (Fig. 2.24b), and pagetoid (Fig. 2.24c) [83]. Immunohistochemistry for CK20, CD44, and p53 can be helpful to make diagnosis of urothelial carcinoma in situ (Fig. 2.24d, e) [84].

Invasive Urothelial Carcinoma

Invasive urothelial carcinoma is defined as malignant urothelial tumor with invasion beneath the basement membrane. Invasive urothelial carcinoma can be developed from papillary urothelial carcinoma or urothelial carcinoma in situ. Grossly invasive urothelial carcinoma can be papillary, polypoid, or nodular. Microscopically, small nests, clusters, or single cells of malignant urothelial cells are found in subepithelial stroma, proper muscle layer, or perivesical soft tissue (Fig. 2.25a). Most invasive urothelial carcinomas are high grade. Focal glandular or squamous differentiation can be found in some cases (Fig. 2.25b, c) [85–88]. Some variants of urothelial carcinoma are present. Nested variant is composed of infiltration of small nests with relatively low cytologic atypia (Fig. 2.25d) [89]. Plasmacytoid variant consists of malignant urothelial cells that resemble plasma cells (Fig. 2.25e) [90]. Micropapillary variant shows small papillary configurations with surrounding retracted empty spaces (Fig. 2.25f). This micropapillary variant is known to have aggressive behavior [91, 92]. Sarcomatoid urothelial

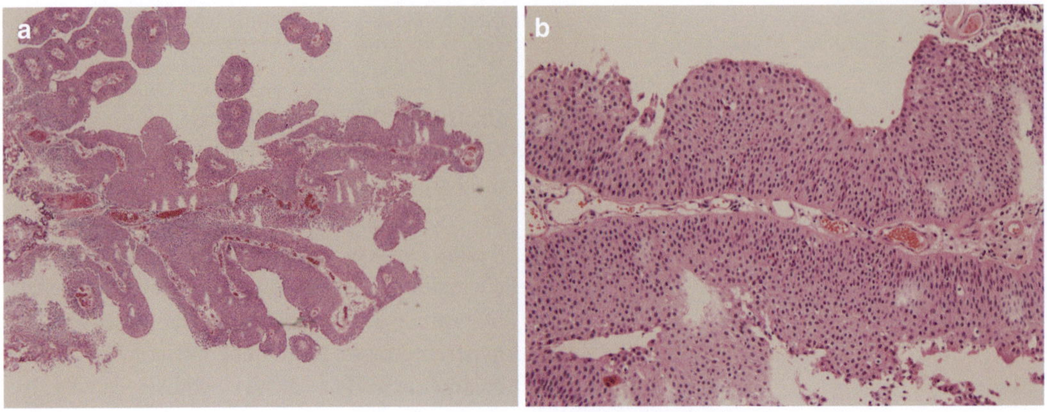

Fig. 2.20 (**a**) Papillary urothelial neoplasm of low malignant potential has papillary architecture with mildly increased branching and hyperplastic urothelial lining. (**b**) Urothelial layer is increased, but cytologic atypia is minimal

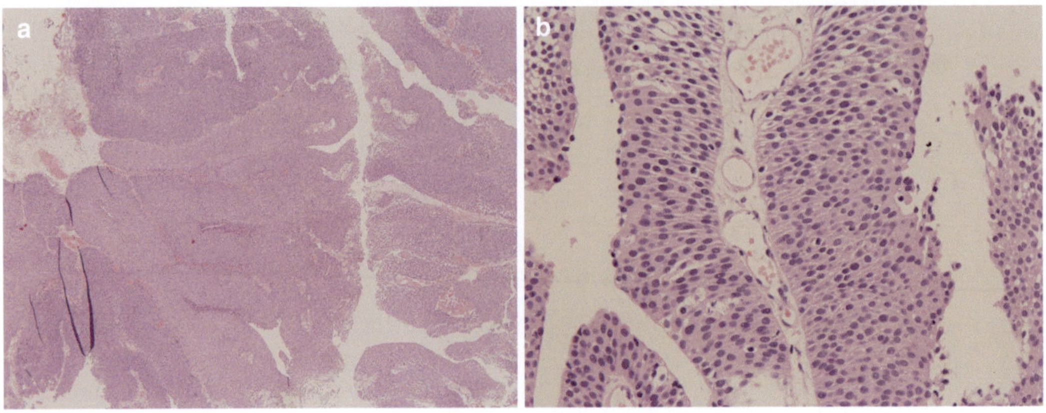

Fig. 2.21 (**a**) Low-grade papillary urothelial carcinoma shows more complex papillary architectures and thickening of urothelial layer with frequent branching and fusion of papillae. (**b**) Mild cytologic atypia and some mitotic figures are found

carcinoma is urothelial carcinoma having both epithelial and mesenchymal differentiation [93]. Microscopically, this tumor is composed of urothelial carcinoma and spindle cell sarcoma or other types of sarcoma such as osteosarcoma and chondrosarcoma (Fig. 2.25g).

2.4.2 Nonurothelial Tumors

2.4.2.1 Squamous Cell Carcinoma

Squamous cell carcinoma of the urinary bladder is a malignant epithelial neoplasm composed of pure squamous cell component. One of the major risk factors is schistosomiasis infection [94]. Grossly squamous cell carcinoma is often white-tan fungating mass. Occasionally nonneoplastic urothelium shows white discoloration due to squamous metaplasia (Fig. 2.26a). Microscopic features of squamous cell carcinoma of the urinary bladder are identical to those of squamous cell carcinoma of other sites (Fig. 2.26b). Urothelial carcinoma component cannot be found in primary squamous cell carcinoma of the urinary bladder by definition. Squamous metaplasia of nonneoplastic urothelium is occasionally found (Fig. 2.26c).

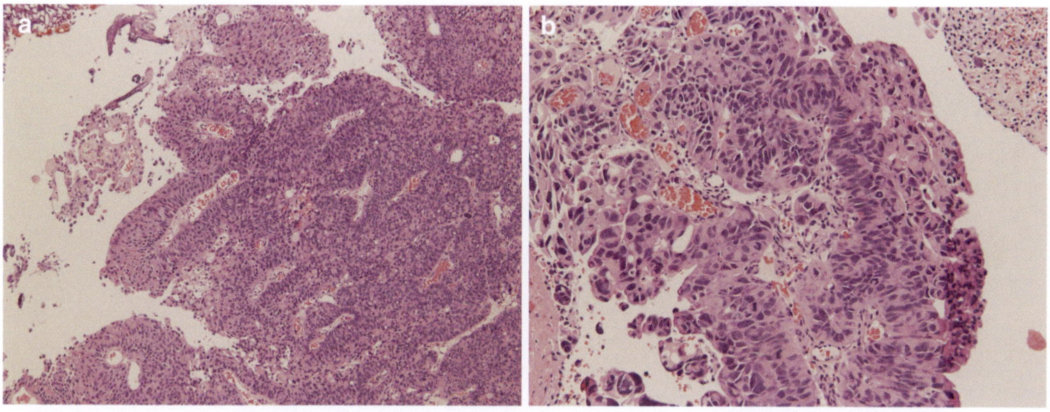

Fig. 2.22 (**a**) High-grade papillary urothelial carcinoma shows complex papillary architecture with occasional large atypical nuclei. (**b**) High-power view reveals prominent nuclear pleomorphism and frequent mitotic figures

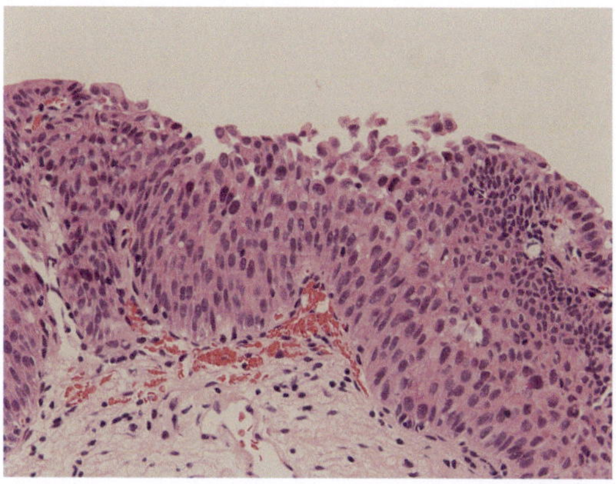

Fig. 2.23 Urothelial dysplasia shows mild nuclear atypia but not enough to make diagnosis of urothelial carcinoma in situ

2.4.2.2 Urachal Carcinoma

Urachal adenocarcinoma is an adenocarcinoma arising in the urachus. Grossly urachal adenocarcinoma is a protruding mass generally located in the dome of the urinary bladder (Fig. 2.27a) [95]. Urothelial mucosa is often intact due to its deep location in the bladder wall. Microscopically, urachal adenocarcinoma shows varying morphology such as enteric, mucinous, or signet ring cell adenocarcinoma. Occasionally, urachal remnant can be found and its presence is an evidence of its urachal origin. Massive mucin production with extensive mucin pool is occasionally found (Fig. 2.27b).

2.4.2.3 Metastatic Tumor

Common origins of metastatic or secondary carcinoma to urinary bladder are prostatic adenocarcinoma, colorectal adenocarcinoma, or carcinoma from the gynecologic tract [96]. These tumors must be differentiated from primary adenocarcinoma of urinary bladder. Immunohistochemical staining and history can help the differential diagnosis.

2.4.2.4 Neuroendocrine Tumors

Carcinoid

Carcinoid is rarely reported in the urinary bladder. Its microscopic features are similar to those of other sites [97–99]. Tumor cells have abundant cytoplasm with round- to oval-shaped uniform nuclei. The nuclei shows finely granular chromatin pattern. Tumor cells are arranged in acinar, trabecular, or pseudoglandular pattern (Fig. 2.28a). In immunohistochemical staining, tumor cells are positively stained with neuroendocrine markers such as synaptophysin and chromogranin (Fig. 2.28a).

Small Cell Carcinoma

Small cell carcinoma is a rare aggressive malignant neuroendocrine neoplasm composed of small cells [100]. Its morphology is identical to pulmonary counterpart. Microscopically, this tumor is composed of nests or sheets of

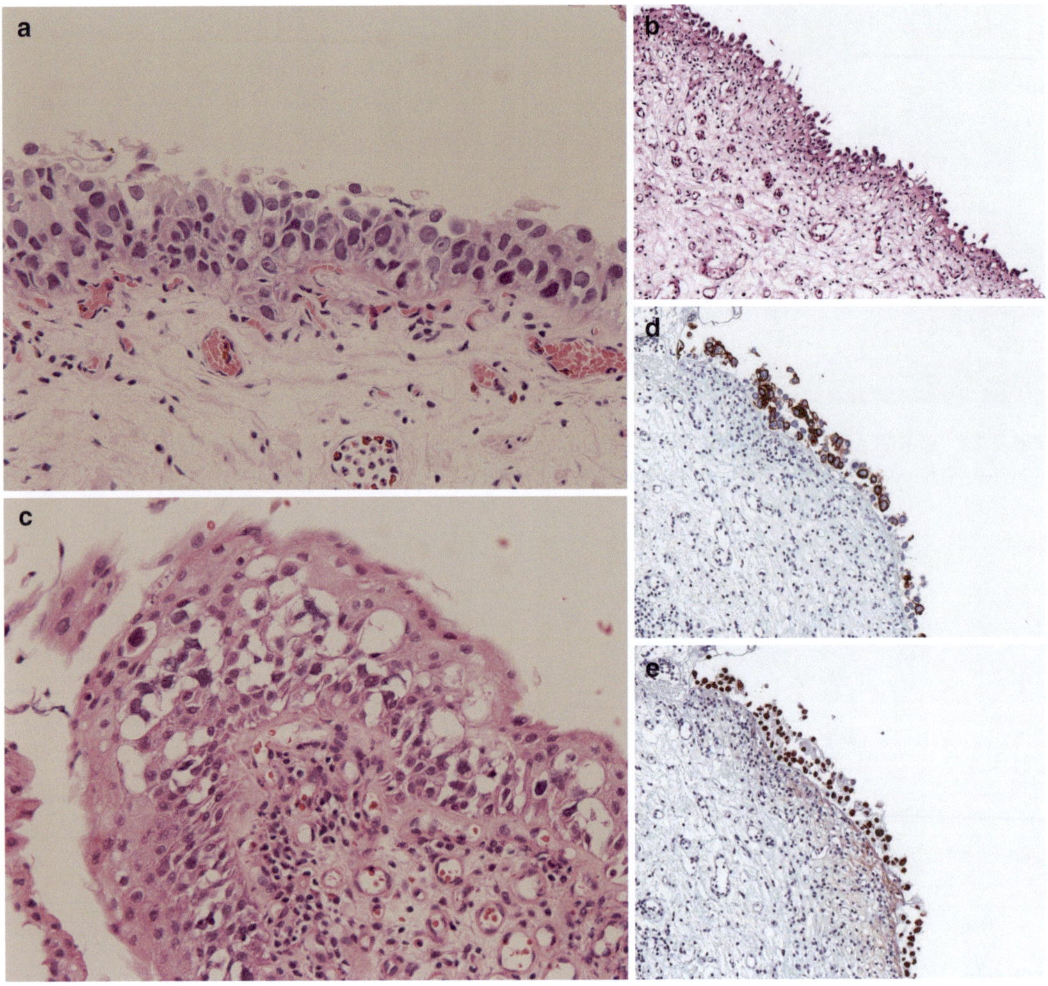

Fig. 2.24 (**a**). Tumor cells of urothelial carcinoma in situ show large hyperchromatic and pleomorphic nuclei with occasional prominent nucleoli. (**b**) Urothelial carcinoma in situ with clinging pattern. (**c**) Urothelial carcinoma in situ with pagetoid pattern. (**d**, **e**) CK20 (**d**) and p53 (**e**) immunohistochemical staining reveal strong positivity in urothelial carcinoma in situ cells

small tumor cells with scanty cytoplasm and finely granular nuclear chromatin (Fig. 2.29a). Other epithelial malignancy such as urothelial carcinoma or squamous cell carcinoma can be admixed (Fig. 2.29b). Tumor cells express the neuroendocrine markers (Fig. 2.29c). Urothelial carcinomas containing small cell carcinoma component show more aggressive behavior [72].

2.4.2.5 Lymphoma

Primary lymphoma of the urinary bladder is rare. MALT lymphoma is the most frequent lymphoma of the urinary bladder [75, 101]. Other lymphomas such as Burkitt lymphoma, T-cell lymphoma, or Hodgkin lymphoma have been reported.

2.5 Therapeutic Consideration

2.5.1 Surgical Treatment of Bladder Cancer

2.5.1.1 Transurethral Resection of Bladder Tumor

Proper endoscopic evaluation and transurethral resection are the cornerstones of diagnosis and treatment for bladder cancer management.

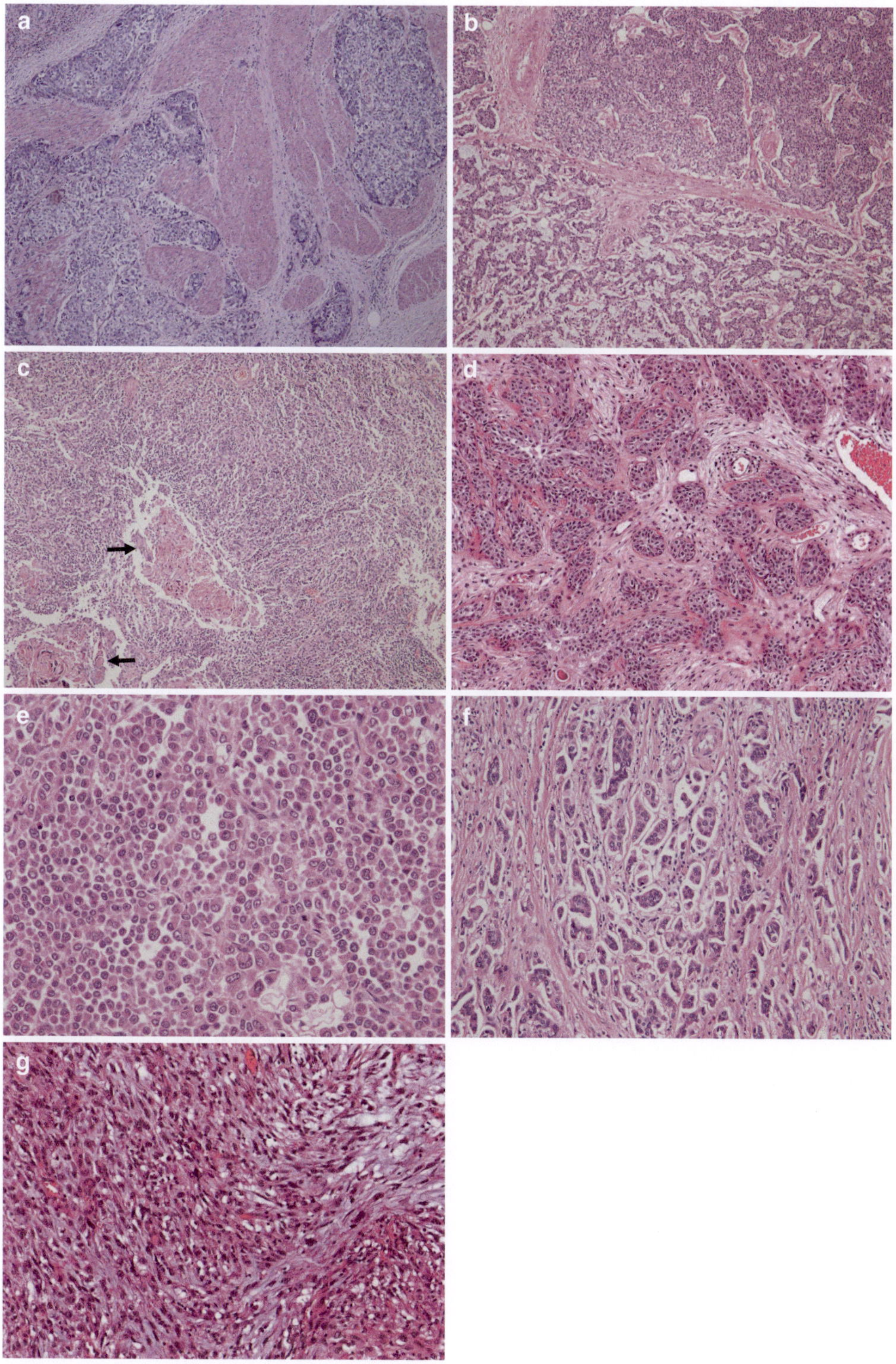

Fig. 2.25 Microscopic findings of invasive urothelial carcinoma. (**a**) Urothelial carcinoma invades into proper muscle layer. (**b**) Glandular differentiation of urothelial carcinoma is found in lower half of this photograph. (**c**) Squamous differentiation of urothelial carcinoma is found in the center and left lower (*arrow*). (**d**–**g**) Variants of urothelial carcinoma. (**d**) Nested variant. (**e**) Plasmacytoid variant. (**f**) Micropapillary variant. (**g**) Sarcomatoid change of urothelial carcinoma shows malignant spindle cells

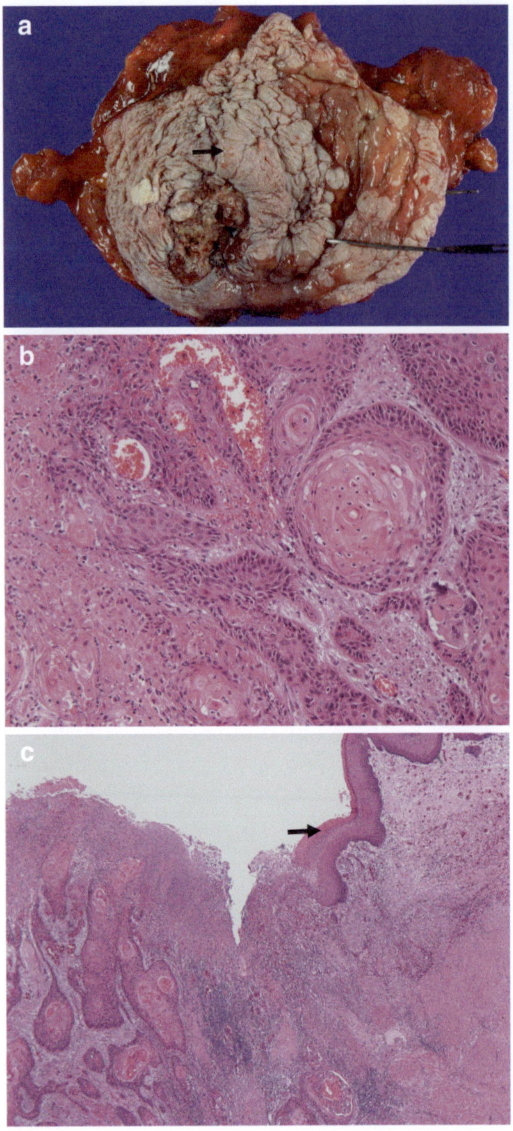

Fig. 2.26 Pathologic findings of squamous cell carcinoma of the urinary bladder. (**a**) Gross photograph of squamous cell carcinoma of the urinary bladder shows white to tan-colored ulcerofungating mass. *Whitish* discoloration of nonneoplastic mucosa of the urinary bladder indicating squamous metaplasia (*arrow*) is widely noted. (**b**) Microscopically well-differentiated squamous cell carcinoma invades to submucosa. (**c**) Squamous metaplasia (*arrow*) of mucosa is found adjacent to squamous cell carcinoma

The main goals of TURBT are to obtain adequate tissue specimens for pathologic examination and to achieve a complete resection with removal of all macroscopic visible tumor tissue and of associated CIS, if present [102]. Muscle should be included in the specimen for accurate staging.

Before endoscopy, with the patient fully anesthetized, a bimanual examination should be performed. The surgeon should estimate the size and number of tumors and should determine the position of tumors in reference to the bladder neck and ureteral orifices. The configuration of visible lesion is also important, and a determination should be made as to whether they are papillary or sessile, broad-bases, or pedunculated. Low-grade, low-stage (Ta) tumors appear papillary and frondular, with a stalk and normal surrounding urothelium. For tumors that may be high-grade or invasive (T1-T3), adequate resection is needed to obtain lamina propria and muscle. These tumors may appear nodular, sessile, or ulcerated. Areas of bladder mucosa remote from the tumor should be examined carefully for changes suggestive of CIS, which is generally described as a velvety erythematous area [103, 104]. The area of erythema suspicious for CIS can be sampled by cold cup biopsy. Blood from a ureteral orifice or tumors surrounding the orifice may be an indication for upper urinary tract evaluation.

2.5.1.2 Partial Cystectomy

The primary advantages cited in the use of partial cystectomy in the treatment of patients with bladder cancer include a full-thickness resection of cancerous tissue with adequate margins and a capability to sample regional nodal tissue while retaining physiologic bladder function, continence, and potency [105]. The primary disadvantage is the historically high local recurrence rate for this procedure.

The full-thickness segment of a bladder wall and tumor with adjacent perivesical fat is sent for frozen section pathologic inspection to verify tumor-free margins. The tumor is excised with a 2-cm margin. The tumor can be excised in a robotic and laparoscopic approach. A bilateral pelvic lymph node dissection should be performed.

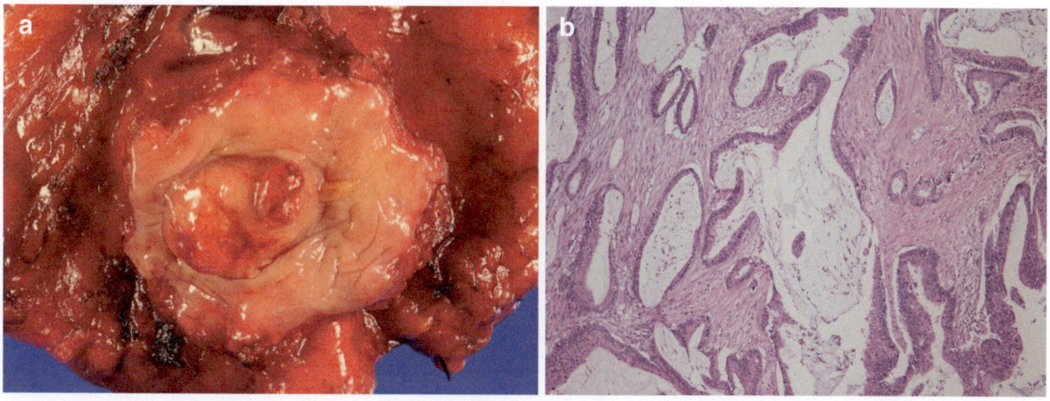

Fig. 2.27 (**a**) Grossly urachal carcinoma is a protruding mass located in the dome of the urinary bladder in this partial cystectomy specimen. (**b**) Microscopically, this tumor is adenocarcinoma with profound mucin production

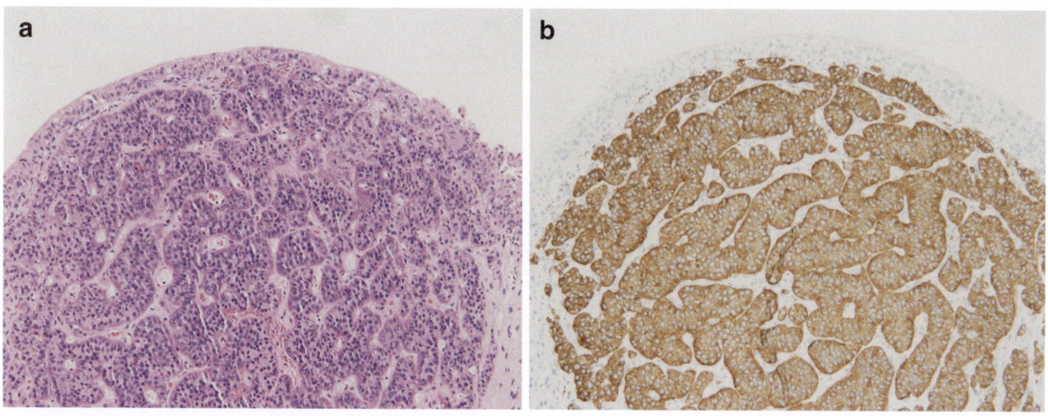

Fig. 2.28 (**a**) A case of carcinoid tumor of the urinary bladder shows trabecular pattern. (**b**) Tumor cells express synaptophysin

2.5.1.3 Radical Cystectomy with Urinary Diversion

Radical cystectomy is the treatment of choice for high-risk, recurrent, noninvasive bladder cancer as well as muscle-invasive bladder cancer.

Pelvic Lymph Node Dissection

Although the diagnostic and the therapeutic value of PLND have clearly been established, there is still debate about the optimum extent. Bilateral pelvic lymph node dissection is performed by removing all fibrous, fatty, and lymphatic tissue from an area bordered laterally by the genitofemoral nerve and medially by the bladder wall. An extended LND basically reaches the aortic bifurcation, and a superextended LND extends to the level of the inferior mesenteric artery [106].

Robotic and laparoscopic lymphadenectomy is started with lateral freeing of the external iliac vessels. The obturator fossa is entered and the obturator nerve is visualized. The superficial and deep obturator fossa is completely freed from all lymphatics and fatty tissue (Fig. 2.30).

Radical Cystectomy in Male Patients

The ureters are divided where they cross the iliac vessels. The dorsomedial pedicle is resected along the pararectal and presacral plane on the tumor-bearing side. The first major branch off the anterior surface of the hypogastric artery is

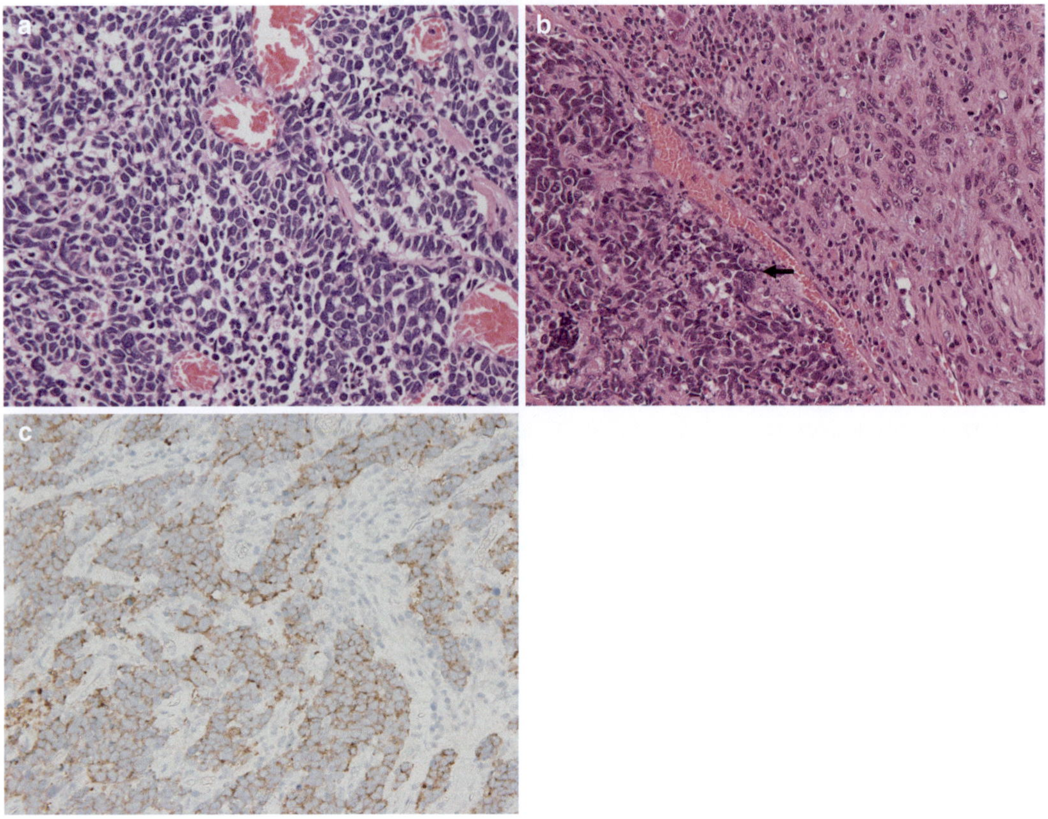

Fig. 2.29 (**a**) Small cell carcinoma of the urinary bladder is morphologically identical to those of other sites such as the lung. (**b**) Small cell carcinoma (*left side*, *arrow*) can be admixed with conventional urothelial carcinoma (*right side*). (**c**) Small cell carcinoma expresses neuroendocrine markers such as synaptophysin

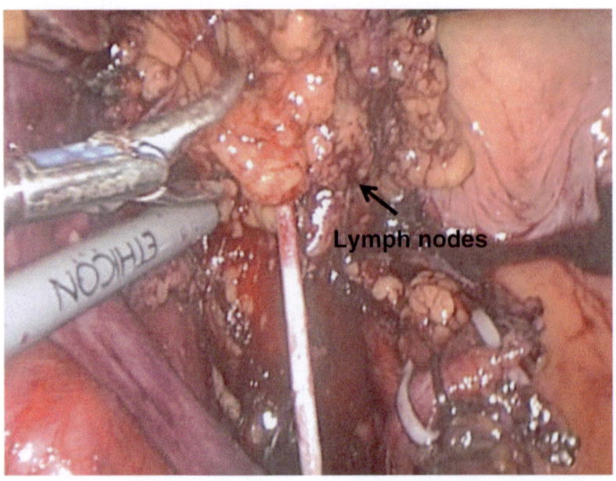

Fig. 2.30 Laparoscopic pelvic lymph node dissection; last stage of the lymphadenectomy. Careful diathermy at the base of the obturator fossa is necessary to ensure hemostasis

the obliterated umbilical artery/superior vesical branch. On this side, the dissection along the dorsolateral wall of the seminal vesicle is stopped at the base of the prostate. Santorini's plexus is then divided, and the membranous urethra is transected as close as possible to the apex of the prostate by excavating it out of the donut-shaped apex. When an orthotopic bladder substitution or potency-sparing approach is being performed, meticulous dissection of the prostate apex is particularly important.

Robotic and laparoscopic radical cystectomy is an attractive minimally invasive alternative to conventional open radical cystectomy, as it duplicates the open technique, yet is associated with decreased blood loss, and possibly better patient recovery [106].

The posterior peritoneum is incised, and then the plane between seminal vesicles and the anterior surface of the rectum is developed. Continued dissection brings the posterior layer of Denonvilliers' fascia, which reveals the prerectal fat posterior to

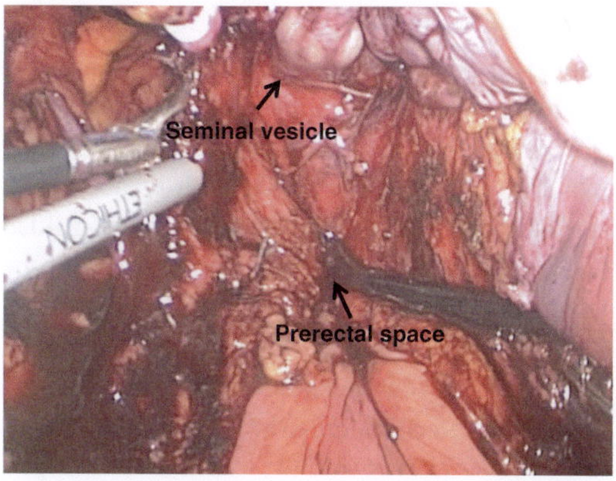

Fig. 2.31 Laparoscopic posterior dissection; prerectal fat posterior to the prostate. With this maneuver, a window is developed encompassing the dorsal aspect of the prostate

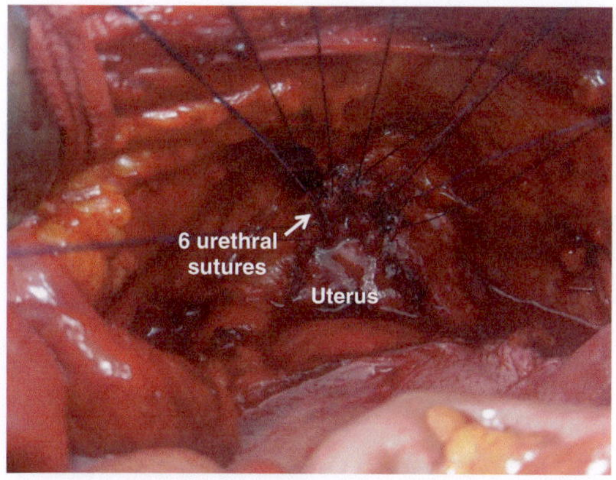

Fig. 2.32 Female radical cystectomy; circumferential 6 urethral sutures. In this organ-preserving approach, it is necessary to carefully dissect along the anterolateral vaginal wall and then close to the bladder neck distally, to spare the paravaginal tissue containing autonomic nerve fibers. Note the generous stump length of urethra to facilitate anastomosis to neobladder neck

the prostate. Blunt dissection is used to develop the rectovesical cul-de-sac (Fig. 2.31).

The space between the bladder and the lateral pelvic wall is developed bluntly. The lateral pedicles are clearly identified. The lateral pedicles are divided down to the endopelvic fascia. The endopelvic fascia is incised down to the region of the dorsal vein complex.

The levator muscle fibers are gently pushed away from the lateral side of the bladder. After exposing the anterior surface of the prostate, the superficial dorsal vein is coagulated, and the puboprostatic ligaments are divided. The dorsal vein complex is identified and transected with a laparoscopic endovascular GIA. The membranous urethra is transected with cold endoshears.

Radical Cystectomy in Female Patients

Radical cystectomy in women implies the en bloc removal of the pelvic organs anterior to the rectum, including the bladder, urachus, ovaries, fallopian tubes, uterus, cervix, vaginal cuff, and anterior pelvic peritoneum. Performing the LND before cystectomy can facilitate identification and dissection of the vesical and uterine vessels later during surgery [107].

The ureters are mobilized and divided below the iliac bifurcation. The vagina is opened circumferentially at the cervical insertion after incising the peritoneum in the pouch of Douglas. In an organ-preserving approach, the peritoneal incision is carried through the vesicouterine pouch (rather than the pouch of Douglas). It is usually no problem to enter the dissection plane between the anterior vaginal wall and bladder [108]. If an orthotopic bladder substitution is planned, it is important to spare the distal 1–3 cm of anterior vaginal wall to avoid the formation of urethro-vesical fistula [107]. To prevent fistula formation, a tubularized omental flap may be interposed between the anterior aspect of the vagina and the anastomosis of the urethra and the neobladder. The dorsal vein is ligated and divided. The endopelvic fascia is incised immediately lateral to the posterior urethra at the urethral vesical junction. If an orthotopic bladder substitution is planned, careful dissection around the bladder neck is paramount to preserve autonomic nerve fibers supplying the remnant urethra. Six urethral sutures are then placed circumferentially (Fig. 2.32). The urethra is reanastomosed in a tension-free, mucosa-to-mucosa fashion to the neobladder at the end of the procedure.

Urinary Diversion

Most surgeons favor construction from ileum because it affords greater compliance [109]. Four methods of urinary diversion are used after cystectomy: incontinent cutaneous, continent cutaneous, orthotopic, and rectosigmoid diversions.

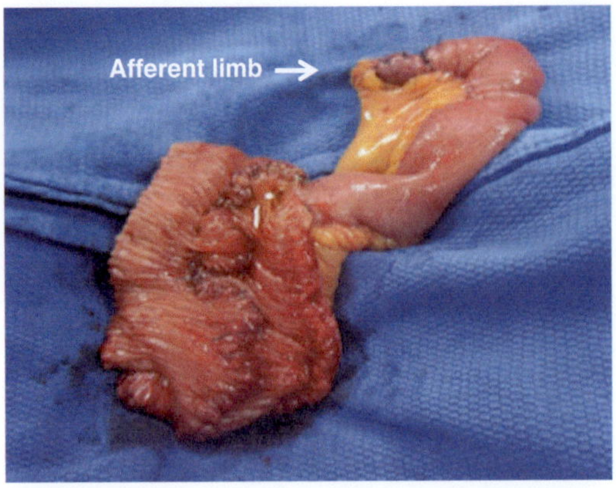

Fig. 2.33 Construction of the reservoir; folded bottom of U. This effectively creates a low-pressure spherical shaped reservoir

Laparoscopic and robot-assisted laparoscopic intracorporeal construction of urinary diversion is feasible but is currently considered experimental because of the limited number of cases reported, the absence of long-term oncologic and functional outcome data, and a possible selection bias [110]. In our institute, ileal conduit and orthotopic neobladder have been generally used. Construction of an ileal conduit or neobladder is performed through a 7 cm midline incision. We describe a simple method to construct an ileal conduit and orthotopic neobladder.

2.5.1.4 Ileal Conduit

The ileal segment 15 cm long is selected, beginning about 15 cm from the ileocecal valve and bowel continuity is restored. The ureteroileal anastomosis is performed at the proximal end of loop. A 2.5 cm hole is cut into the skin at the predetermined stoma site. The subcutaneous tissue and fat are incised down to the fascia. A cruciate incision is made in the rectus fascia. Four fascial sutures are placed from each quadrant of the fascia to the serosa of the bowel. The rosebud nipple is created by everting the intestinal mucosa and suturing the serosa of the bowel to the fascia and subcuticular skin.

2.5.1.5 Ileal Neobladder (Studer Type)

An ileal segment 45 cm long is isolated approximately 20 cm proximal to the ileocecal valve. The ureters are split and anastomosed by two running sutures using the Nesbit technique in an open end-to-end fashion to the proximal unopened part of the ileal segment to form the afferent tubular segment, which is 15 cm long. The bottom of the U is folded over between the two ends of the U (Fig. 2.33), thus resulting in a spherical reservoir consisting of four cross-folded ileal segment. The most dependent portion of the reservoir is the midway point on the right side. This will form the new bladder neck. Rotate the pouch 90° counterclockwise so that the new bladder neck aligns with the urethra.

2.5.2 Surgical Treatment of Upper Tract Carcinoma

Upper tract (UT) urothelial carcinomas (UC) are uncommon and account for only 5–10 % of UCs [111]. UTUCs that invade the muscle wall usually have a very poor prognosis. The 5-year cancer-specific survival is <50 % for pT2/pT3 and <10 % for pT4 [112, 113]. Radical nephroureterectomy (RNU) with bladder cuff excision remains the gold standard treatment for UTUC. However, endoscopic advancements have achieved favorable treatment outcomes and renal preservation rates in selected cases [114].

2.5.2.1 Radical Nephroureterectomy (RNU)

RNU consists of the removal of the entire kidney and ureter, along with excision of the ipsilateral bladder cuff [115]. It can be performed through a single midline incision, thoracoabdominal incision, or flank incision in conjunction with a Gibson or Pfannenstiel for removal of the bladder cuff. Excision of the bladder cuff is mandatory in invasive or high-risk noninvasive UTUC. Although a variety of techniques have been described for the management of the bladder cuff, it is imperative that complete removal is performed. During surgery, care has to be taken to avoid tumor spillage or positive surgical margins [116]

Laparoscopic RNU has emerged as minimally invasive alternative to open RNU, with advantages in terms of less blood loss, shorter length of hospital stay, and shorter convalescence. Modern variants of the laparoscopic approach include hand-assisted RNU, robotic-assisted laparoscopic RNU, retroperitoneoscopic RNU, and laparoendoscopic single-site RNU [117].

The patient is positioned in the usual nephrectomy position. Laparoscopic RNU is commended with a transperitoneal approach with pots positioned. After mobilization of the colon, the hilar anatomy is delineated before renal pedicle control. Hilar control is achieved using an Endo-GIA universal stapler. The kidney is then isolated with combination of cautery and blunt dissection. Bladder cuff excision is performed through a lower abdominal incision.

Recently, the da Vinci™ robot system (Intuitive Surgical, Sunnyvale, CA, US) was introduced to perform laparoscopic operations more easily by reducing the technical difficulty of intracorporeal suturing. In addition, the extra degrees of freedom and articulation of the robotic wrists make the isolation of the distal ureter and bladder closure less technically challenging [118].

The ureter is carefully dissected over the iliac vessels and down to the bladder. The detrusor muscle is identified and dissected until the bladder mucosa is tenting, allowing a wide margin of bladder cuff to be exposed. The cuff is dissected and removed, en bloc, along with the kidney and ureter (Fig. 2.34). The bladder is closed by running sutures in a watertight fashion with full-thickness closure of the defect.

In patients with clinically infiltrating UTUC, regional lymph node dissection (LND) is considered a part of the procedure [115]. As patients with histologically confirmed lymph node-negative UTUC exhibit improved survival compared with those with lymph node-positive disease [119], the diagnostic significance of LND is beyond question. However, the therapeutic role of LND at RNU and the appropriate extent of LND according to primary tumor location are not well defined [120].

2.5.2.2 Ureteroscopy

Evaluation of suspected UTUC includes imaging, urine cytology, and cystoscopy to rule out concomitant bladder tumors. However, the most accurate technique for diagnosis of UT lesions

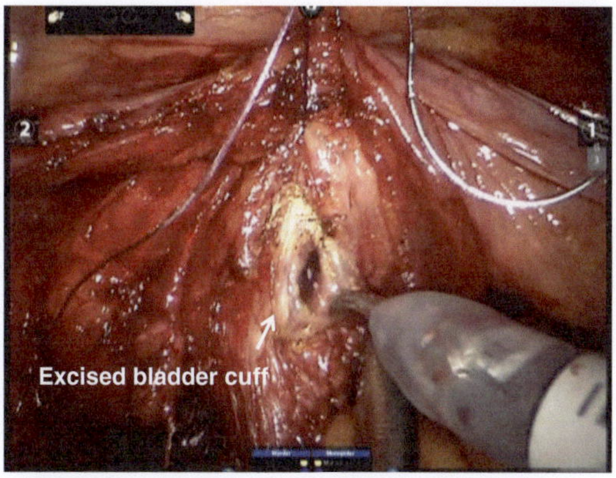

Fig. 2.34 Robot-assisted laparoscopic bladder cuff excision. Note the bladder cuff resected by en bloc circumferential excision

has been ureteroscopy with biopsy. The most commonly used biopsy devices are biopsy forceps and stainless steel flat wire basket. Ureteroscopic biopsies can determine tumor grade in 90 % of cases with a low false-negative rate regardless of the size of the sample [121], although sampling sufficient tissue for pathologic evaluation remains challenging.

Conservative management of UTUC can be considered in imperative or elective cases for low-grade, low-stage tumors [115]. The principal advantage of ureteroscopy is its low morbidity while maintaining urothelial integrity [122]. Available management options can include mechanical debulking (forceps or basket), electrofulguration, electroresection, laser photocoagulation, or ablation [123]. Narrow caliber flexible holmium:YAG and neodymium:YAG laser fibers permit ureteroscopic ablation of tumors using either rigid or flexible instruments while maintaining adequate hemostasis [124]

2.5.2.3 Segmental Resection

Segmental ureteral resection provides adequate pathologic specimens for definitive staging and grade analysis while preserving the ipsilateral kidney [115]. Complete distal ureterectomy and neocystostomy are indicated for noninvasive low-grade tumors in the distal ureter that cannot be removed completely by endoscopic means and for high-grade locally invasive tumors [125, 126].

Robot and laparoscopic procedures can also be properly used for treatment of tumors of the distal ureter. A transverse curvilinear incision is made on the anterior wall of the bladder. A suture is placed through the psoas tendon and then through the most superior and ipsilateral portion of the bladder. Next, the ureter is spatulated to prepare for the ureteroneocystostomy. To create an anti-refluxing anastomosis, the bladder mucosa is dissected off. The anastomosis is completed.

2.5.3 Radiation Therapy

Radiotherapy has been used for the treatment of muscle-invading transitional cell carcinoma (TCC) in the bladder. Along with concurrent chemotherapy, RT is an important component of bladder preservation treatment. Selecting patients for bladder preservation requires meticulous clinical staging by TURB and imaging studies to rule out node-positive or metastatic diseases. CT of abdomen and pelvis is mandatory to evaluate bladder cancer. Accurate definition of target volume is crucial for RT. Bladder map by urologists and CT/MRI provide important information on tumor spread in the bladder. Any extravesical tumor extension suspected or documented on CT/MRI images should guide target volume definition. Any bladder-specific imaging studies, if possible, should be performed before TURB to avoid postsurgical changes. After bladder preservation treatment, CT or MRI scanning as well as cystoscopy should be performed regularly lest salvage cystectomy is delayed if needed.

2.6 Chemotherapy in Advanced Urothelial Carcinoma

2.6.1 Introduction

The standard treatment for muscle-invasive bladder cancer (MIBC) is radical cystectomy (RC) combined with pelvic lymph node dissection. However, despite the improvement of surgical skill such as orthotopic neobladder formation, long-term survival after radical surgery is not enough to high. In cases of pT3/T4 or lymph node-positive disease, 5-year overall survival rate after RC shows from 25 to 35 %. In addition, about half of patients undergoing RC may develop distant metastasis, which is finally attributed to death from bladder cancer. Therefore, to early control micrometastatic disease at the time of surgery, it may be considered to conduct preoperative (neoadjuvant) or postoperative (adjuvant) chemotherapy in high-risk MIBC patients [110].

2.6.2 Chemotherapy Regimens

2.6.2.1 Single-Agent Chemotherapy

Urothelial carcinoma (UC) is known to be moderately chemosensitive tumor. However, the overall response rate (RR) to single chemotherapeutic agent seems to be generally poor. Cisplatin, most commonly used single agent, shows approximately 17 % RR. In case of carboplatin, RR only ranges from 12 to 14 % in a phase II trial [127]. Other agents, such as ifosfamide, lobaplatin, trimetrexate, gemcitabine, and taxanes (paclitaxel and docetaxel), has been suggested as possible single chemotherapeutic agents for bladder cancer. However, compared to combination chemotherapy, single-agent chemotherapy shows lower RR (10 ~ 30 %), rare complete remission. Therefore, single-agent chemotherapy should be only considered in MIBC patients who cannot receive combination chemotherapy owing to poor general performance status.

2.6.2.2 Combination Chemotherapy

In advanced UC, combination chemotherapy has been reported to be superior to single-agent chemotherapy in terms of clinical response and survival benefit. In particular, among cisplatin-based combination chemotherapy regimens (Table 2.1), MVAC (methotrexate, vinblastine, adriamycin, cisplatin) and GC (gemcitabine, cisplatin) are recommended as the first-line chemotherapeutic regimens according to current guidelines [128].

MVAC Regimen

The MVAC regimen was developed at the Memorial Sloan Kettering Cancer Center (MSKCC) in 1983, and the first preliminary results were published in 1985 [129]. This phase II study reported a 71 % overall response rate (CR 36 %). The efficacy of the MVAC regimen has been evaluated subsequently in several randomized studies and found to be superior to single-agent cisplatin [127] and combination chemotherapy with cisplatin, cyclophosphamide, and doxorubicin (CISCA) [130] and also methotrexate, carboplatin, and vinblastine (MCAVI) [131]. In these phase III studies, the overall response for MVAC regimen has varied between 39 and 65 %, with median survivals up to 16 months [127, 130, 131]. Therefore, chemotherapy using MVAC regimen has been considered as the "gold standard" in chemotherapy for advanced bladder cancer for a number of years. However, administration of MVAC may be limited due to severe toxicity and poor long-term survival outcome and therefore is not appropriate for all patients with advanced bladder cancer. The most significant side effects (grades 3 and 4) include myelosuppression (anemia, neutropenia, and thrombocytopenia), mucositis, alopecia, nausea, vomiting, infection, and diarrhea. MVAC-induced toxicity-related mortality rates range from 2 to 4 % [132]. In order to minimize severe toxicity and improve poor long-term survival associated with conventional MVAC regimen, high-dose-intensity MVAC (HD-MVAC) regimen, which simultaneously administers both MVAC and G-CSF or GM-CSF, is devised. According to phase III trial of EORTC genitourinary group, HD-MVAC supported with G-CSF has been compared with conventional MVAC in 263 patients [133]. The reported response rates were better for the HD-MVAC, with overall response rates of 61 % versus 50 %. The complete and partial response rates were 21 % and 55 % for HD-MVAC versus 9 % and 41 % for conventional MVAC, respectively. Interestingly, there was no statistically significant difference in survival or time to progression, though progression-free survival was superior in the high-dose arm. The toxic death rates were comparable, being 3 % for HD-MVAC versus 4 % for conventional MVAC.

GC Regimen

Cisplatin has been demonstrated to have a synergistic interaction with gemcitabine [134], and GC regimen has been shown to be safe and effective in the treatment of advanced urothelial carcinoma [135–137]. Von der Maase et al. compared GC regimen with conventional MVAC regimen as first-line therapy in a multicenter randomized phase III trial, comparing six cycles of each of the regimens, given to 405 patients with T4b and/or node-positive and/or distant metastatic disease. At a median follow-up of 19 months, the regimens were not statistically different in terms of overall survival, time to disease progression, or response rate. However, GC regimen was superior in terms of tolerability and effects on quality of life. In particular, GC resulted in a lower incidence of treatment-related mortality and fewer episodes of complicated myelosuppression, oral mucositis, and alopecia (resulting in fewer dose adjustments) and lesser effects on weight, performance status, and fatigue [137]. As a result, GC regimen is now widely considered to be a (second) standard of care, along with MVAC, for patients with advanced bladder cancer. Certainly, the GC regimen is now employed at many institutions as first-line therapy.

Carboplatin-Based Chemotherapy

The single-agent data favor cisplatin in terms of activity, but the administration of cisplatin is associated with nephrotoxicity. Carboplatin shows lower toxicity profiles relative to cisplatin. Therefore, carboplatin-based combination regimens have the advantage of being suitable for patients with renal impairment. In an analysis of 66 evaluable patients in a randomized phase II trial of cisplatin/gemcitabine versus carboplatin/gemcitabine, a response rate of 66 % in patients treated with cisplatin/gemcitabine compares favorably with a response rate of 35 % for carboplatin/gemcitabine, with similar toxicity profiles [138]. Based on previous studies, carboplatin-based combination chemo-regimen should be considered only in advanced UC patients who are inappropriate for the use of cisplatin.

2.6.3 Timing of Chemotherapy

2.6.3.1 Neoadjuvant Chemotherapy (NACH)

Advantages of NACH prior to RC are that chemotherapy is delivered when the burden of micrometastatic disease is low and chemosensitivity can be better observed; in addition, tolerability of chemotherapy is expected to be better before cystectomy than after. Indeed, responders to NACH, especially complete responders, show a significantly improved OS [139]. However, overtreatment of nonresponders and overtreatment of patients without micrometastases remain major limitations, and delayed cystectomy in nonresponders might compromise final outcome. Unfortunately, molecular profiling of the tumor is not yet able to identify responders. Also, imaging during treatment does not allow firm conclusions about response [140]. Another disadvantage is that only clinical staging is available in case of NACH, with known limitations of staging accuracy in 70 % of patients [141] and staging errors more common in cT2 tumors than in cT3–4 tumors. Even if this situation is a potential problem, there is no negative impact of NACH on the percentage of performable cystectomies. In the combined Nordic trials ($n=620$), cystectomy frequency was 86 % in the NAC arm and 87 % in the control arm. [142] Three meta-analyses were conducted to determine the survival advantage of NACH [143–145]. All three meta-analyses showed an increase in OS of 5 %. Of note, only combinations with cisplatin resulted in a meaningful benefit [143, 144]. A recent update of the largest trial, with a median follow-up of 8 years, confirmed an improvement in 10-year survival from 30 to 36 % with neoadjuvant cisplatin, methotrexate, and vinblastine but without any locoregional benefit [146].

2.6.3.2 Adjuvant Chemotherapy (ACH)

Advantages ACH following RC include the availability of accurate pathologic staging, which implies that treatment can be reserved for high-risk patients (extravesical and/or node-positive disease), and no delay in local surgical treatment in patients who are not sensitive to chemotherapy. Disadvantages include the absence of a measurable tumor and a delay of chemotherapy because of postoperative morbidity. Data on ACH are limited, with five published randomized trials with several limitations and one meta-analysis with only 491 patients [147]. In all, the data are not convincing enough to provide an unequivocal recommendation for the use of immediate adjuvant chemotherapy as compared with chemotherapy at the time of relapse.

2.6.4 Conclusions

Bladder cancer is a moderately chemosensitive disease, and a role for combination chemotherapy in improving disease-free survival in patients with advanced disease and good performance status is now well established. In patients with good renal function, regimen should be cisplatin-based combinations. For those not considered suitable for cisplatin-containing regimens, chemotherapy may be based around carboplatin or newer agents. Cisplatin-based combination NACH has been demonstrated in several meta-analyses to improve survival in advanced MIBC. Therefore, the use of cisplatin-based NACH is currently recommended as the standard of care in patients with advanced MIBC (T2-T4). Whereas ACH in bladder cancer is controversial because neither randomized trials nor a meta-analysis has provided sufficient data to support the routine use of adjuvant chemotherapy.

References

1. Murphy WM GD, Perman EJ. Tumors of the kidney, bladder, and related urinary structures. Washington, DC: American Registry of Pathology; 2004. p. 394.
2. Jemal A, Siegel R, Xu J, Ward E. Cancer statistics. CA Cancer J Clin. 2010;60:277–300.
3. Zeegers MP, Tan FE, Dorant E, van Den Brandt PA. The impact of characteristics of cigarette smoking on urinary tract cancer risk: a meta-analysis of epidemiologic studies. Cancer. 2000;89:630–9.
4. Saad A, Hanbury DC, McNicholas TA, Boustead GB, Morgan S, Woodman AC. A study comparing

various noninvasive methods of detecting bladder cancer in urine. BJU Int. 2002;89:369–73.
5. Sadow CA, Silverman SG, O'Leary MP, Signorovitch JE. Bladder cancer detection with CT urography in an Academic Medical Center. Radiology. 2008;249:195–202.
6. Pashos CL, Botteman MF, Laskin BL, Redaelli A. Bladder cancer: epidemiology, diagnosis, and management. Cancer Pract. 2002;10:311–22.
7. Kawashima A, Vrtiska TJ, LeRoy AJ, Hartman RP, McCollough CH, King Jr BF. CT urography. Radiographics. 2004;24 Suppl 1:S35–54; discussion S55-38.
8. Ng CS. Radiologic diagnosis and staging of renal and bladder cancer. Semin Roentgenol. 2006;41:121–38.
9. Hall TMVA. Imaging of bladder cancer. Imaging. 2001;13:1–10.
10. Tsampoulas C, Tsili AC, Giannakis D, Alamanos Y, Sofikitis N, Efremidis SC. 16-MDCT cystoscopy in the evaluation of neoplasms of the urinary bladder. AJR Am J Roentgenol. 2008;190:729–35.
11. Beer A, Saar B, Link TM, et al. Virtual endoscopy of the urinary tract from T(2)-weighted and gadolinium-enhanced T(1)-weighted MR urographic images. Rofo. 2001;173:997–1005.
12. Bernhardt TM, Rapp-Bernhardt U. Virtual cystoscopy of the bladder based on CT and MRI data. Abdom Imaging. 2001;26:325–32.
13. Verma S, Rajesh A, Prasad SR, et al. Urinary bladder cancer: role of MR imaging. Radiographics. 2012; 32:371–87.
14. Jimenez RE, Gheiler E, Oskanian P, et al. Grading the invasive component of urothelial carcinoma of the bladder and its relationship with progression-free survival. Am J Surg Pathol. 2000;24:980–7.
15. Shinagare AB, Sadow CA, Sahni VA, Silverman SG. Urinary bladder: normal appearance and mimics of malignancy at CT urography. Cancer Imaging. 2011;11:100–8.
16. McPartlin DS, Klausner AP, Nottingham CU, et al. Is cystoscopy indicated for incidentally identified bladder wall thickening? Can J Urol. 2013;20: 6615–9.
17. Wong-You-Cheong JJ, Woodward PJ, Manning MA, Sesterhenn IA. From the archives of the AFIP: neoplasms of the urinary bladder: radiologic-pathologic correlation. Radiographics. 2006;26:553–80.
18. Tekes A, Kamel I, Imam K, et al. Dynamic MRI of bladder cancer: evaluation of staging accuracy. AJR Am J Roentgenol. 2005;184:121–7.
19. Lawler LP. MR imaging of the bladder. Radiol Clin North Am. 2003;41:161–77.
20. Barentsz JO, Ruijs SH, Strijk SP. The role of MR imaging in carcinoma of the urinary bladder. AJR Am J Roentgenol. 1993;160:937–47.
21. Hood MN, Ho VB, Smirniotopoulos JG, Szumowski J. Chemical shift: the artifact and clinical tool revisited. Radiographics. 1999;19:357–71.
22. Semelka R. Abdominal-pelvic MRI. Hoboken: Wiley-Blackwell; 2010.
23. Neuerburg JM, Bohndorf K, Sohn M, Teufl F, Guenther RW, Daus HJ. Urinary bladder neoplasms: evaluation with contrast-enhanced MR imaging. Radiology. 1989;172:739–43.
24. Sato C, Naganawa S, Nakamura T, et al. Differentiation of noncancerous tissue and cancer lesions by apparent diffusion coefficient values in transition and peripheral zones of the prostate. J Magn Reson Imaging. 2005;21:258–62.
25. Koh DM, Takahara T, Imai Y, Collins DJ. Practical aspects of assessing tumors using clinical diffusion-weighted imaging in the body. Magn Reson Med Sci. 2007;6:211–24.
26. Abou-El-Ghar ME, El-Assmy A, Refaie HF, El-Diasty T. Bladder cancer: diagnosis with diffusion-weighted MR imaging in patients with gross hematuria. Radiology. 2009;251:415–21.
27. El-Assmy A, Abou-El-Ghar ME, Mosbah A, et al. Bladder tumour staging: comparison of diffusion- and T2-weighted MR imaging. Eur Radiol. 2009; 19:1575–81.
28. Takeuchi M, Sasaki S, Ito M, et al. Urinary bladder cancer: diffusion-weighted MR imaging--accuracy for diagnosing T stage and estimating histologic grade. Radiology. 2009;251:112–21.
29. Watanabe H, Kanematsu M, Kondo H, et al. Preoperative T staging of urinary bladder cancer: does diffusion-weighted MRI have supplementary value? AJR Am J Roentgenol. 2009;192:1361–6.
30. Beyersdorff D, Zhang J, Schoder H, Bochner B, Hricak H. Bladder cancer: can imaging change patient management? Curr Opin Urol. 2008;18: 98–104.
31. Zhang J, Gerst S, Lefkowitz RA, Bach A. Imaging of bladder cancer. Radiol Clin North Am. 2007; 45:183–205.
32. Scattoni V, Da Pozzo LF, Colombo R, et al. Dynamic gadolinium-enhanced magnetic resonance imaging in staging of superficial bladder cancer. J Urol. 1996;155:1594–9.
33. Hayashi N, Tochigi H, Shiraishi T, Takeda K, Kawamura J. A new staging criterion for bladder carcinoma using gadolinium-enhanced magnetic resonance imaging with an endorectal surface coil: a comparison with ultrasonography. BJU Int. 2000;8 5:32–6.
34. Narumi Y, Kadota T, Inoue E, et al. Bladder tumors: staging with gadolinium-enhanced oblique MR imaging. Radiology. 1993;187:145–50.
35. Barentsz JO, Jager G, Mugler 3rd JP, et al. Staging urinary bladder cancer: value of T1-weighted three-dimensional magnetization prepared-rapid gradient-echo and two-dimensional spin-echo sequences. AJR Am J Roentgenol. 1995;164:109–15.
36. Edge SBBD, Compton CC, editors. AJCC cancer Staging manual. New York: Springer; 2010.
37. Wong-You-Cheong JJ, Wagner BJ, Davis Jr CJ. Transitional cell carcinoma of the urinary tract: radiologic-pathologic correlation. Radiographics. 1998;18:123–42; quiz 148.

38. Kirkali Z, Tuzel E. Transitional cell carcinoma of the ureter and renal pelvis. Crit Rev Oncol Hematol. 2003;47:155–69.
39. Hall MC, Womack S, Sagalowsky AI, Carmody T, Erickstad MD, Roehrborn CG. Prognostic factors, recurrence, and survival in transitional cell carcinoma of the upper urinary tract: a 30-year experience in 252 patients. Urology. 1998;52:594–601.
40. Lee TY, Ko SF, Wan YL, et al. Unusual imaging presentations in renal transitional cell carcinoma. Acta Radiol. 1997;38:1015–9.
41. Melamed MR, Reuter VE. Pathology and staging of urothelial tumors of the kidney and ureter. Urol Clin North Am. 1993;20:333–47.
42. Urban BA, Buckley J, Soyer P, Scherrer A, Fishman EK. CT appearance of transitional cell carcinoma of the renal pelvis: part 1. Early-stage disease. AJR Am J Roentgenol. 1997;169:157–61.
43. Buckley JA, Urban BA, Soyer P, Scherrer A, Fishman EK. Transitional cell carcinoma of the renal pelvis: a retrospective look at CT staging with pathologic correlation. Radiology. 1996;201:194–8.
44. Keeley FX, Kulp DA, Bibbo M, McCue PA, Bagley DH. Diagnostic accuracy of ureteroscopic biopsy in upper tract transitional cell carcinoma. J Urol. 1997;157:33–7.
45. Herranz-Amo F, Diez-Cordero JM, Verdu-Tartajo F, Bueno-Chomon G, Leal-Hernandez F, Bielsa-Carrillo A. Need for intravenous urography in patients with primary transitional carcinoma of the bladder? Eur Urol. 1999;36:221–4.
46. Raman SP, Horton KM, Fishman EK. Transitional cell carcinoma of the upper urinary tract: optimizing image interpretation with 3D reconstructions. Abdom Imaging. 2012;37:1129–40.
47. Maheshwari E, O'Malley ME, Ghai S, Staunton M, Massey C. Split-bolus MDCT urography: upper tract opacification and performance for upper tract tumors in patients with hematuria. AJR Am J Roentgenol. 2010;194:453–8.
48. Chow LC, Kwan SW, Olcott EW, Sommer G. Split-bolus MDCT urography with synchronous nephrographic and excretory phase enhancement. AJR Am J Roentgenol. 2007;189:314–22.
49. Kekelidze M, Dwarkasing RS, Dijkshoorn ML, Sikorska K, Verhagen PC, Krestin GP. Kidney and urinary tract imaging: triple-bolus multidetector CT urography as a one-stop shop--protocol design, opacification, and image quality analysis. Radiology. 2010;255:508–16.
50. Caoili EM, Inampudi P, Cohan RH, Ellis JH. Optimization of multi-detector row CT urography: effect of compression, saline administration, and prolongation of acquisition delay. Radiology. 2005; 235:116–23.
51. Johnson PT, Horton KM, Fishman EK. Optimizing detectability of renal pathology with MDCT: protocols, pearls, and pitfalls. AJR Am J Roentgenol. 2010;194:1001–12.
52. Browne RF, Meehan CP, Colville J, Power R, Torreggiani WC. Transitional cell carcinoma of the upper urinary tract: spectrum of imaging findings. Radiographics. 2005;25:1609–27.
53. Bechtold RB, Chen MY, Dyer RB, Zagoria RJ. CT of the ureteral wall. AJR Am J Roentgenol. 1998;170:1283–9.
54. Caoili EM, Cohan RH, Inampudi P, et al. MDCT urography of upper tract urothelial neoplasms. AJR Am J Roentgenol. 2005;184:1873–81.
55. Pretorius ES, Wickstrom ML, Siegelman ES. MR imaging of renal neoplasms. Magn Reson Imaging Clin N Am. 2000;8:813–36.
56. Stein JP, Skinner EC, Boyd SD, Skinner DG. Squamous cell carcinoma of the bladder associated with cyclophosphamide therapy for Wegener's granulomatosis: a report of 2 cases. J Urol. 1993;149: 588–9.
57. Serretta V, Pomara G, Piazza F, Gange E. Pure squamous cell carcinoma of the bladder in western countries. Report on 19 consecutive cases. Eur Urol. 2000;37:85–9.
58. Dondalski M, White EM, Ghahremani GG, Patel SK. Carcinoma arising in urinary bladder diverticula: imaging findings in six patients. AJR Am J Roentgenol. 1993;161:817–20.
59. Tekes A, Kamel IR, Chan TY, Schoenberg MP, Bluemke DA. MR imaging features of non-transitional cell carcinoma of the urinary bladder with pathologic correlation. AJR Am J Roentgenol. 2003;180:779–84.
60. Wong JT, Wasserman NF, Padurean AM. Bladder squamous cell carcinoma. Radiographics. 2004;24: 855–60.
61. Shokeir AA. Squamous cell carcinoma of the bladder: pathology, diagnosis and treatment. BJU Int. 2004;93:216–20.
62. Sheldon CA, Clayman RV, Gonzalez R, Williams RD, Fraley EE. Malignant urachal lesions. J Urol. 1984;131:1–8.
63. Bates AW, Baithun SI. Secondary neoplasms of the bladder are histological mimics of nontransitional cell primary tumours: clinicopathological and histological features of 282 cases. Histopathology. 2000;36:32–40.
64. Hughes MJ, Fisher C, Sohaib SA. Imaging features of primary nonurachal adenocarcinoma of the bladder. AJR Am J Roentgenol. 2004;183:1397–401.
65. Brick SH, Friedman AC, Pollack HM, et al. Urachal carcinoma: CT findings. Radiology. 1988;169: 377–81.
66. Yu JS, Kim KW, Lee HJ, Lee YJ, Yoon CS, Kim MJ. Urachal remnant diseases: spectrum of CT and US findings. Radiographics. 2001;21: 451–61.
67. Ashley RA, Inman BA, Sebo TJ, et al. Urachal carcinoma: clinicopathologic features and long-term outcomes of an aggressive malignancy. Cancer. 2006;107:712–20.

68. Mohile SG, Schleicher L, Petrylak DP. Treatment of metastatic urachal carcinoma in an elderly woman. Nat Clin Pract Oncol. 2008;5:55–8.
69. Narumi Y, Sato T, Kuriyama K, et al. Vesical dome tumors: significance of extravesical extension on CT. Radiology. 1988;169:383–5.
70. Thali-Schwab CM, Woodward PJ, Wagner BJ. Computed tomographic appearance of urachal adenocarcinomas: review of 25 cases. Eur Radiol. 2005;15:79–84.
71. Rafal RB, Markisz JA. Urachal carcinoma: the role of magnetic resonance imaging. Urol Radiol. 1991;12:184–7.
72. Cheng L, Pan CX, Yang XJ, et al. Small cell carcinoma of the urinary bladder: a clinicopathologic analysis of 64 patients. Cancer. 2004;101(5):957–62.
73. Sved P, Gomez P, Manoharan M, Civantos F, Soloway MS. Small cell carcinoma of the bladder. BJU Int. 2004;94:12–7.
74. Kim JC, Kim KH, Jung S. Small cell carcinoma of the urinary bladder: CT and MR imaging findings. Korean J Radiol. 2003;4:130–5.
75. Bates AW, Norton AJ, Baithun SI. Malignant lymphoma of the urinary bladder: a clinicopathological study of 11 cases. J Clin Pathol. 2000;53:458–61.
76. Dighe MK, Bhargava P, Wright J. Urinary bladder masses: techniques, imaging spectrum, and staging. J Comput Assist Tomogr. 2011;35:411–24.
77. Maya MM, Slywotzky C. Urinary bladder leiomyoma: magnetic resonance imaging findings. Urol Radiol. 1992;14:197–9.
78. Metzdorf MM, Schmidt JD. Urinary bladder leiomyoma associated with pulmonary lymphangioleiomyomatosis. Urology. 2008;71:755.e3–4.
79. Cornella JL, Larson TR, Lee RA, Magrina JF, Kammerer-Doak D. Leiomyoma of the female urethra and bladder: report of twenty-three patients and review of the literature. Am J Obstet Gynecol. 1997;176:1278–85.
80. Eble JN, Sauter G, Epstein JI, et al. Pathology and genetics of tumours of the urinary system and male genital organs. Lyon: International Agency for Research on Cancer (IARC); 2004.
81. Hodges KB, Lopez-Beltran A, Davidson DD, et al. Urothelial dysplasia and other flat lesions of the urinary bladder: clinicopathologic and molecular features. Hum Pathol. 2010;41(2):155–62.
82. Lopez-Beltran A, Montironi R, Vidal A, et al. Urothelial dysplasia of the bladder: diagnostic features and clinical significance. Anal Quant Cytopathol Histpathol. 2013;35(3):121–9.
83. McKenney JK, Gomez JA, Desai S, et al. Morphologic expressions of urothelial carcinoma in situ: a detailed evaluation of its histologic patterns with emphasis on carcinoma in situ with microinvasion. Am J Surg Pathol. 2001;25(3):356–62.
84. McKenney JK, Desai S, Cohen C, et al. Discriminatory immunohistochemical staining of urothelial carcinoma in situ and non-neoplastic urothelium: an analysis of cytokeratin 20, p53, and CD44 antigens. Am J Surg Pathol. 2001;25(8):1074–8.
85. Billis A, Schenka AA, Ramos CC, et al. Squamous and/or glandular differentiation in urothelial carcinoma: prevalence and significance in transurethral resections of the bladder. Int Urol Nephrol. 2001; 33(4):631–3.
86. Lee YJ, Moon KC, Jeong CW, et al. Impact of squamous and glandular differentiation on oncologic outcomes in upper and lower tract urothelial carcinoma. PLoS One. 2014;9(9):e107027.
87. Lopez-Beltran A, Requena MJ, Alvarez-Kindelan J, et al. Squamous differentiation in primary urothelial carcinoma of the urinary tract as seen by MAC387 immunohistochemistry. J Clin Pathol. 2007;60(3):332–5.
88. Wasco MJ, Daignault S, Zhang Y, et al. Urothelial carcinoma with divergent histologic differentiation (mixed histologic features) predicts the presence of locally advanced bladder cancer when detected at transurethral resection. Urology. 2007;70(1):69–74.
89. Dhall D, Al-Ahmadie H, Olgac S. Nested variant of urothelial carcinoma. Arch Pathol Lab Med. 2007;131(11):1725–7.
90. Ricardo-Gonzalez RR, Nguyen M, Gokden N, et al. Plasmacytoid carcinoma of the bladder: a urothelial carcinoma variant with a predilection for intraperitoneal spread. J Urol. 2012;187(3):852–5.
91. Kwon GY, Ro JY. Micropapillary variant of urothelial carcinoma. Adv Urol. 2011;2011:217153.
92. Samaratunga H, Khoo K. Micropapillary variant of urothelial carcinoma of the urinary bladder; a clinicopathological and immunohistochemical study. Histopathology. 2004;45(1):55–64.
93. Cheng L, Zhang S, Alexander R, et al. Sarcomatoid carcinoma of the urinary bladder: the final common pathway of urothelial carcinoma dedifferentiation. Am J Surg Pathol. 2011;35(5):e34–46.
94. Sharfi AR, el Sir S, Beleil O. Squamous cell carcinoma of the urinary bladder. Br J Urol. 1992;69(4):369–71.
95. Gopalan A, Sharp DS, Fine SW, et al. Urachal carcinoma: a clinicopathologic analysis of 24 cases with outcome correlation. Am J Surg Pathol. 2009;33(5):659–68.
96. Velcheti V, Govindan R. Metastatic cancer involving bladder: a review. Can J Urol. 2007;14(1):3443–8.
97. Chen YB, Epstein JI. Primary carcinoid tumors of the urinary bladder and prostatic urethra: a clinicopathologic study of 6 cases. Am J Surg Pathol. 2011;35(3):442–6.
98. Martignoni G, Eble JN. Carcinoid tumors of the urinary bladder. Immunohistochemical study of 2 cases and review of the literature. Arch Pathol Lab Med. 2003;127(1):e22–4.
99. Yang CH, Krzyzaniak K, Brown WJ, et al. Primary carcinoid tumor of urinary bladder. Urology. 1985; 26(6):594–7.

100. Zhao X, Flynn EA. Small cell carcinoma of the urinary bladder: a rare, aggressive neuroendocrine malignancy. Arch Pathol Lab Med. 2012;136(11):1451–9.
101. Kempton CL, Kurtin PJ, Inwards DJ, et al. Malignant lymphoma of the bladder: evidence from 36 cases that low-grade lymphoma of the MALT-type is the most common primary bladder lymphoma. Am J Surg Pathol. 1997;21(11):1324–33.
102. Wiesner C, Jäger W, Thüroff JW. Surgery illustrated – surgical atlas. BJU Int. 2010;105:1610–21.
103. Althausen AF, Prout Jr GR, Daly JJ. Non-invasive papillary carcinoma of the bladder associated with carcinoma in situ. J Urol. 1976;116:575–80.
104. Lamm DL. Carcinoma in situ. Urol Clin North Am. 1992;19:499–508.
105. Sweeney P, Kursh ED, Resnick MI. Partial cystectomy. Urol Clin North Am. 1992;19:701–11.
106. Challacombe BJ, Bochner BH, Dasgupta P, Gill I, Guru K, Herr H, Mottrie A, Pruthi R, Redorta JP, Wiklund P. The role of laparoscopic and robotic cystectomy in the management of muscle-invasive bladder cancer with special emphasis on cancer control and complications. Eur Urol. 2011;60:767–75.
107. Schilling D, Horstmann M, Nagele U, Sievert KD, Stenzl A. Cystectomy in women. BJU Int. 2008; 102:1289–95.
108. Hautmann RE. The ileal neobladder to the female urethra. Urol Clin North Am. 1997;24:827–35.
109. Benson MC, Olsson CA. Urinary diversion. Urol Clin North Am. 1992;19:779–95.
110. Witjes JA, Compérat E, Cowan NC, De Santis M, Gakis G, Lebret T, Ribal MJ, Van der Heijden AG, Sherif A, European Association of Urology. EAU guidelines on muscle-invasive and metastatic bladder cancer: summary of the 2013 guidelines. Eur Urol. 2014;65(4):778–92.
111. Siegel R, Naishadham D, Jemal A. Cancer statistics, 2012. CA Cancer J Clin. 2012;62:10–29.
112. Abouassaly R, Alibhai SM, Shah N, Timilshina N, Fleshner N, Finelli A. Troubling outcomes from population-level analysis of surgery for upper tract urothelial carcinoma. Urology. 2010;76:895–901.
113. Jeldres C, Sun M, Isbarn H, Lughezzani G, Budäus L, Alasker A, Shariat SF, Lattouf JB, Widmer H, Pharand D, Arjane P, Graefen M, Montorsi F, Perrotte P, Karakiewicz PI. A population-based assessment of perioperative mortality after nephroureterectomy for upper-tract urothelial carcinoma. Urology. 2010;75:315–20.
114. Grasso M, Fishman AI, Cohen J, Alexander B. Ureteroscopic and extirpative treatment of upper urinary tract urothelial carcinoma: a 15-year comprehensive review of 160 consecutive patients. BJU Int. 2012;110:1618–26.
115. Rouprêt M, Babjuk M, Compérat E, et al. European guidelines on upper tract urothelial carcinomas: 2013 update. Eur Urol. 2013;63:1059–71.
116. Zigeuner RE, Hutterer G, Chromecki T, et al. Bladder tumour development after urothelial carcinoma of the upper urinary tract is related to primary tumour location. BJU Int. 2006;98:1181–6.
117. Ristau BT, Tomaszewski JJ, Ost MC. Upper tract urothelial carcinoma: current treatment and outcomes. Urology. 2012;79:749–56.
118. Zargar H, Krishnan J, Autorino R, Akca O, Brandao LF, Laydner H, Samarasekera D, Ko O, Haber GP, Kaouk JH, Stein RJ. Robotic nephroureterectomy: a simplified approach requiring no patient repositioning or robot redocking. Eur Urol. 2014;66: 769–77.
119. Cha EK, Shariat SF, Kormaksson M, et al. Predicting clinical outcomes after radical nephroureterectomy for upper tract urothelial carcinoma. Eur Urol. 2012;61:818–25.
120. Kondo T, Hashimoto Y, Kobayashi H, et al. Template-based lymphadenectomy in urothelial carcinoma of the upper urinary tract: impact on patient survival. Int J Urol. 2010;17:848–54.
121. Rojas CP, Castle SM, Llanos CA, Santos Cortes JA, Bird V, Rodriguez S, Reis IM, Zhao W, Gomez-Fernandez C, Leveillee RJ, Jorda M. Low biopsy volume in ureteroscopy does not affect tumor biopsy grading in upper tract urothelial carcinoma. Urol Oncol. 2013;31:1696–700.
122. Raman JD, Scherr DS. Management of patients with upper urinary tract transitional cell carcinoma. Nat Clin Pract Urol. 2007;4:432–43.
123. Park BH, Jeon SS. Endoscopic management of upper urinary tract urothelial carcinoma. Korean J Urol. 2013;54:426–32.
124. Bagley DH, Grasso 3rd M. Ureteroscopic laser treatment of upper urinary tract neoplasms. World J Urol. 2010;28:143–9.
125. Lughezzani G, Jeldres C, Isbarn H, Sun M, Shariat SF, Alasker A, Pharand D, Widmer H, Arjane P, Graefen M, Montorsi F, Perrotte P, Karakiewicz PI. Nephroureterectomy and segmental ureterectomy in the treatment of invasive upper tract urothelial carcinoma: a population-based study of 2299 patients. Eur J Cancer. 2009;45:3291–7.
126. Jeldres C, Lughezzani G, Sun M, Isbarn H, Shariat SF, Budaus L, Lattouf JB, Widmer H, Graefen M, Montorsi F, Perrotte P, Karakiewicz PI. Segmental ureterectomy can safely be performed in patients with transitional cell carcinoma of the ureter. J Urol. 2010;183:1324–9.
127. Loehrer PJ, Einhorn LH, Elson PJ, Crawford ED, Kuebler P, Tannock I, et al. A randomized comparison of cisplatin alone or in combination with methotrexate, vinblastine, and doxorubicin in patients with metastatic urothelial carcinoma: a cooperative group study. J Clin Oncol. 1992;10:1066–73.
128. Calhoun A, Pohar K. Guideline-based management of muscle-invasive bladder cancer: NCCN, ICUD, and EAU. In: Konety BR, Chang SS, editors. Management of bladder cancer. New York: Springer; 2015. p. 457–63.
129. Sternberg C, Yagoda A, Scher H, Watson R, Ahmed T, Weiselberg L, et al. Preliminary results of M-VAC (methotrexate, vinblastine, doxorubicin and cisplatin) for transitional cell carcinoma of the urothelium. J Urol. 1985;133:403–7.

130. Logothetis CJ, Dexeus FH, Finn L, Sella A, Amato RJ, Ayala AG, et al. A prospective randomized trial comparing MVAC and CISCA chemotherapy for patients with metastatic urothelial tumors. J Clin Oncol. 1990;8:1050–5.
131. Bellmunt J, Ribas A, Eres N, Albanell J, Almanza C, Bermejo B, et al. Carboplatin-based versus cisplatin-based chemotherapy in the treatment of surgically incurable advanced bladder carcinoma. Cancer. 1997;80:1966–72.
132. von der Maase H, Hansen S, Roberts J, Dogliotti L, Oliver T, Moore M, et al. Gemcitabine and cisplatin versus methotrexate, vinblastine, doxorubicin, and cisplatin in advanced or metastatic bladder cancer: results of a large, randomized, multinational, multicenter, phase III study. J Clin Oncol. 2000;18: 3068–77.
133. Sternberg CN, de Mulder PHM, Schornagel JH, Théodore C, Fossa SD, van Oosterom AT, et al. Randomized phase III trial of high–dose-intensity methotrexate, vinblastine, doxorubicin, and cisplatin (MVAC) chemotherapy and recombinant human granulocyte colony-stimulating factor versus classic MVAC in advanced urothelial tract tumors: European Organization for Research and Treatment of Cancer Protocol no. 30924. J Clin Oncol. 2001;19:2638–46.
134. Peters GJ, Bergman AM, Ruiz vHV, Veerman G, Kuiper CM, Braakhuis B. Interaction between cisplatin and gemcitabine in vitro and in vivo. Semin Oncol. 1995;22:72–9.
135. Kaufman D, Raghavan D, Carducci M, Levine EG, Murphy B, Aisner J, et al. Phase II trial of gemcitabine plus cisplatin in patients with metastatic urothelial cancer. J Clin Oncol. 2000;18:1921–7.
136. Moore MJ, Winquist EW, Murray N, Tannock IF, Huan S, Bennett K, et al. Gemcitabine plus cisplatin, an active regimen in advanced urothelial cancer: a phase II trial of the National Cancer Institute of Canada Clinical Trials Group. J Clin Oncol. 1999;17:2876–81.
137. Von der Maase H, Andersen L, Crino L, Weinknecht S, Dogliotti L. Weekly gemcitabine and cisplatin combination therapy in patients with transitional cell carcinoma of the urothelium: a phase II clinical trial. Ann Oncol. 1999;10:1461–5.
138. Carteni G, Dogliotti L, Crucitta E, Martoni A, Siena S, Onat H, et al. Phase II randomised trial of gemcitabine plus cisplatin (GP) and gemcitabine plus carboplatin (GC) in patients (pts) with advanced or metastatic transitional cell carcinoma of the urothelium (TCCU). Proc Am Soc Clin Oncol. 2003;22:384.
139. Rosenblatt R, Sherif A, Rintala E, Wahlqvist R, Ullén A, Nilsson S, et al. Pathologic downstaging is a surrogate marker for efficacy and increased survival following neoadjuvant chemotherapy and radical cystectomy for muscle-invasive urothelial bladder cancer. Eur Urol. 2012;61:1229–38.
140. Nishimura K, Fujiyama C, Nakashima K, Satoh Y, Tokuda Y, Uozumi J. The effects of neoadjuvant chemotherapy and chemo-radiation therapy on MRI staging in invasive bladder cancer: comparative study based on the pathological examination of whole layer bladder wall. Int Urol Nephrol. 2009;41:869–75.
141. Sternberg CN, Pansadoro V, Calabro F, Schnetzer S, Giannarelli D, Emiliozzi P, et al. Can patient selection for bladder preservation be based on response to chemotherapy? Cancer. 2003;97:1644–52.
142. Sherif A, Holmberg L, Rintala E, Mestad O, Nilsson J, Nilsson S, et al; Nordic Urothelial Cancer Group. Neoadjuvant cisplatinum based combination chemotherapy in patients with invasive bladder cancer: a combined analysis of two Nordic studies. Eur Urol. 2004;45:297–303.
143. Collaboration ABCM-a. Neoadjuvant chemotherapy in invasive bladder cancer: update of a systematic review and meta-analysis of individual patient data advanced bladder cancer (ABC) meta-analysis collaboration. Eur Urol. 2005;48:202.
144. Vale C, Collaboration ABCM-a. Neoadjuvant chemotherapy in invasive bladder cancer: a systematic review and meta-analysis. Lancet. 2003;361:1927–34.
145. Winquist E, Kirchner TS, Segal R, Chin J, Lukka H. Neoadjuvant chemotherapy for transitional cell carcinoma of the bladder: a systematic review and meta-analysis. J Urol. 2004;171:561–9.
146. International Collaboration of Trialists. International phase III trial assessing neoadjuvant cisplatin, methotrexate, and vinblastine chemotherapy for muscle-invasive bladder cancer: long-term results of the BA06 30894 trial. J Clin Oncol. 2011;29:2171.
147. Collaboration ABCM-a. Adjuvant chemotherapy in invasive bladder cancer: a systematic review and meta-analysis of individual patient data Advanced Bladder Cancer (ABC) Meta-analysis Collaboration. Eur Urol. 2005;48:189.

3 Prostatic Tumors

Hak Jong Lee, Jeong Yeon Cho, Gi Jeong Cheon, Cheol Kwak, Hyung Suk Kim, and Jin Ho Kim

3.1 Introduction

Prostate cancer is the second most frequently diagnosed cancer worldwide and the sixth leading cause of cancer death in men, accounting for 14 % of total new cancer cases and 6 % of total cancer deaths [1]. In Europe and America, prostate cancer is the most common neoplasm occupying about two or three times more than lung and colorectal cancer [2, 3]. The cancer shows highest prevalence in men occupying 417,000 cases and 22.8 % of all incidental cases in Europe [4].

According to the reports from National Cancer Institute in the United States, the number of new cases of prostate cancer in 2014 was 233,000 patients, and the number of deaths due to prostate cancer is 29,480 [5]. For the diagnosis of prostate cancer, one million prostate biopsies are performed annually in United States [6]. About one in seven men is affected by the disease during his lifetime [7]. The incidence of prostate carcinoma increases with age, and in autopsy studies, 71 % of men between 80 and 89 years have latent prostate carcinoma [8]. The incidence is still rising as well as Asian countries including Japan and Korea. In Korea, the incidence was increased seven times during recent 10 years [9].

The most common tools for the diagnosis of prostate cancer are serum prostate-specific antigen (PSA) level measurement and physical examination by digital rectal examination (DRE) [10, 11]. However, DRE has a very low positive predictive value and a low interobserver agreement among clinicians [12]. When prostate cancer is suspected with elevated PSA levels and abnormal DRE, transrectal ultrasound (TRUS)-guided biopsy is needed for confirmation of

H.J. Lee (✉)
Department of Radiology, Seoul National University Bundang Hospital, Seoul National University College of Medicine, Gyeonggi-do, Republic of Korea
e-mail: hakjlee@snu.ac.kr

J.Y. Cho (✉)
Department of Radiology, Seoul National University, Seoul, Korea
e-mail: radjycho@snu.ac.kr

G.J. Cheon
Department of Nuclear Medicine, Seoul National University Hospital, Seoul National University College of Medicine, Seoul, Republic of Korea

C. Kwak • H.S. Kim
Department of Urology, Seoul National University Hospital, Seoul National University College of Medicine, Seoul, Republic of Korea

J.H. Kim
Department of Radiation Oncology, Seoul National University Hospital, Seoul National University College of Medicine, Seoul, Republic of Korea

S.H. Kim, J.Y. Cho (eds.), *Oncologic Imaging: Urology*, DOI 10.1007/978-3-662-45218-9_3

cancer. Magnetic resonance imaging (MRI) is an alternative assessment technique that has been shown to be highly accurate for the detection of clinically significant prostate cancer as well as tumor staging.

The mortality of prostate cancer has been declining due to early diagnosis and improvements in treatment techniques [1]. The prognosis of patients with prostate cancer depends on several factors including disease extent, histological aggressiveness, Gleason score, and PSA [13]. It has been estimated that about 50 % of the asymptomatic men, in whom prostate cancer is detected by prostate biopsy following PSA measurement, do not require active treatment [7].

3.2 Anatomy

A clear understanding of the prostatic anatomy is very important for adequate interpretation of imaging studies and helps the clinical communications with referring urologists [14]. The volume of normal prostate ranges from 18 to 20 ml. The shape of prostate is very similar to inverted cone on coronal images. On coronal images, the prostate is divided into base, midgland, and apex. The apex and base refer to the most caudal and cranial aspects of the prostate, respectively. The prostate is surrounded by bladder ventrally and by seminal vesicles dorsally. The urogenital diaphragm surrounds the inferior border of prostate. The prostate is separated from the rectum posteriorly by fascia known as Denonvillier's fascia. The Santorini plexus of veins and the pubic symphysis border the prostate anteriorly. The lateral border of prostate is surrounded by levator ani and obturator internus muscles.

The prostate is two components: glandular and nonglandular components. The nonglandular components include anterior fibromuscular stroma and prostatic urethra. The anterior fibromuscular stroma is located anterior to the urethra. The proximal part of the prostatic urethra begins from prostate base and meets bilateral ejaculatory ducts at verumontanum. The ejaculatory ducts are originated from inferomedial aspect of the seminal vesicle and extend within the midline of the peripheral zone. The preprostatic and distal prostatic sphincters are largely responsible for urinary continence. The distal sphincter starts from the prostate apex and continues through the urogenital diaphragm [15].

The glandular components of the prostate include peripheral zone, central zone, transition zone, and periurethral glandular tissues (Fig. 3.1). The peripheral zone occupies about 70 % of the prostate in young males. It surrounds the posterolateral aspect of the prostate and extends to the anterior fibromuscular stroma anterolaterally. Seventy to 75 % of prostate cancers arise in the peripheral zone. Because there is much water content, the peripheral zone shows high signal intensity in T2-weighted image of prostate MR.

The central zone is located in the upper anterior portion of the peripheral zone and surrounds the ejaculatory ducts. The central zone occupies about 20–25 % of the prostate. The immunohistologic features in central zone is quite different from the remaining part of the prostate. The reason is thought that the central zone is originated from the Wolffian duct, not urogenital sinus.

The transition zone occupies about 5 % of total prostate. As benign prostate hyperplasia (BPH) develops, the transition zone becomes the predominant components. The enlarged transition zone condenses the surrounding central zone into a thin rim. This rim serves as the pseudocapsule used as the plane for surgical treatment of BPH. BPH nodules very often demonstrate a thin, well-defined rim of low T2 signal intensity. Lack of this capsule has been described as a sign associated with central-gland cancers.

The periurethral glandular tissue represents less than 1 % of the volume of the prostate.

The signal characteristics of BPH on T2-weighted MR imaging are largely related to the composition of the BPH nodules. The BPH nodules with predominantly stromal and collagen components show hypointense signal intensity, and highly glandular BPH nodules show high signal intensity on T2-weighted MR image (Fig. 3.2).

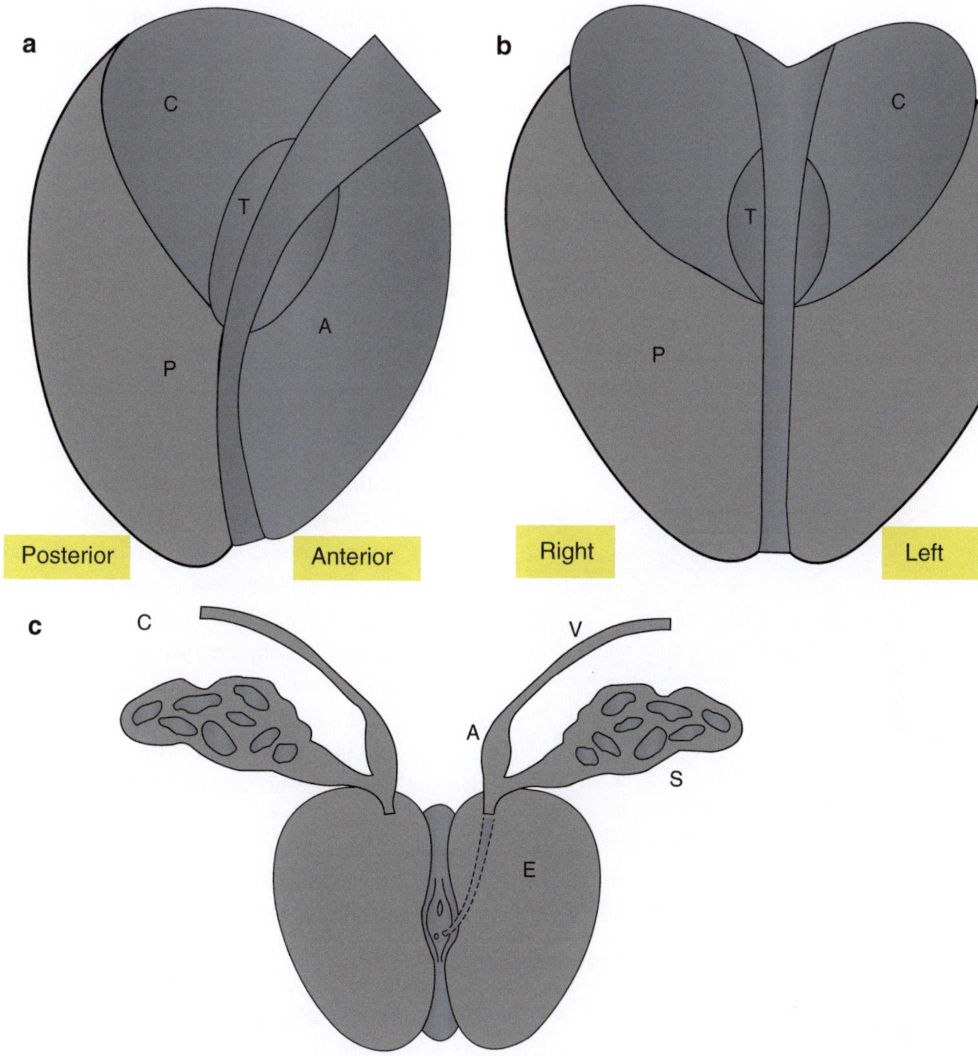

Fig. 3.1 Schematic drawing of prostate. Sagittal (**a**) and coronal (**b**) schematic drawings of prostate show anterior fibromuscular stroma (*A*), transitional zone (*T*), central zone (*C*), and peripheral zone (*P*). The upper part of prostatic urethra is surrounded by transitional zone and central zone, and the lower part of prostatic urethra is surrounded by peripheral zone. (**c**) Schematic drawing from posterior aspect of prostate shows seminal vesicle (*S*), vas deferens (*V*), and ampullary portion of vas deferens (*A*). Vas deferens forms ampullary portion with communication of seminal vesicle and connects ejaculatory duct (*E*). The ejaculatory duct communicates with prostatic urethra on verumontanum

The seminal vesicles are paired lobulated glands found immediately superior and posterior to the prostate base. They can be well demonstrated on axial and coronal T2-weighted MR images. The seminal vesicles have elongated, multi-septated, and fluid-filled structures mimicking bundle of grapes (Fig. 3.3).

3.3 US

3.3.1 Conventional US

For the ultrasound evaluation of the prostate, transrectal, transabdominal, and transperineal approaches are possible; however, TRUS is the most common method for evaluation of prostate due to high image quality. It provides excellent images of the gland, its boundaries, the adjacent bladder, seminal vesicles, and anterior rectal wall (Figs. 3.4 and 3.5).

The main purposes of TRUS are calculating prostate volume; evaluating prostate, BPH, and prostatitis; and seeking the etiology of male infertility. Besides prostate evaluation, TRUS can be also used to evaluate the seminal vesicle, vas deferens, bladder, distal ureter, and urethra and to find out the etiology of hematospermia.

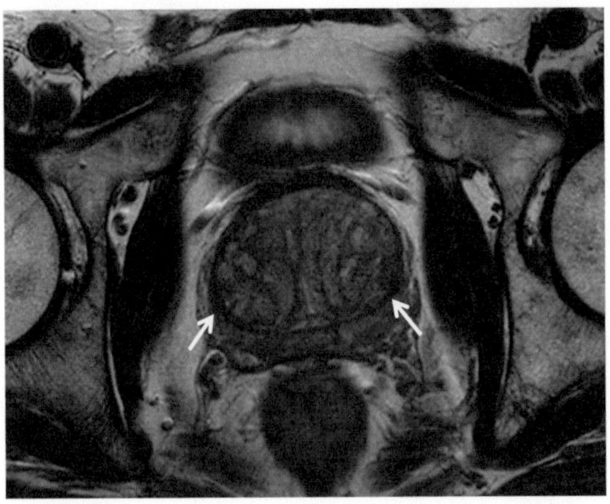

Fig. 3.2 MR imaging of benign prostate hyperplasia (BPH). T2-weighted axial image shows well-marginated low signal intensity lesion replaced transitional zone (*arrows*)

TRUS-guided procedures such as TRUS-guided biopsy or drainage are also commonly used. In case of lower urinary tract symptom, the evaluation of prostate volume is important for the diagnosis of BPH. The prostate volume is easily obtained by prolate ellipse volume calculation ($\pi/6 \times$ transverse diameter $\times$ anteroposterior diameter $\times$ longitudinal diameter). Transverse diameter and anteroposterior diameter can be commonly obtained from axial TRUS scan, and longitudinal diameter can be obtained from sagittal scan.

Typically the prostate gland is scanned in the axial plane, from the apex to the base (Fig. 3.4). The seminal vesicles are identified bilaterally, using an oblique sagittal view that also demonstrates the ampulla of the vas deferens (Fig. 3.5) [14]. In normal prostate, the peripheral zone shows high echogenicity and is routinely distinguished from the central gland, which is typically hypoechoic and heterogeneous owing to BPH (Fig. 3.6). Prostate cancer is characteristically identified as a round or oval focus of low echogenicity in the peripheral zone (Fig. 3.7); however, they may be isoechoic or hyperechoic [16, 17].

About 37–50 % of cancers are isoechoic or only slightly hypoechoic when compared with the peripheral zone [18]. The positive predictive value of the biopsy of a peripheral hypoechoic lesion is 25–30 % [16]. The differential diagnosis in evaluating the low echoic focal lesion includes

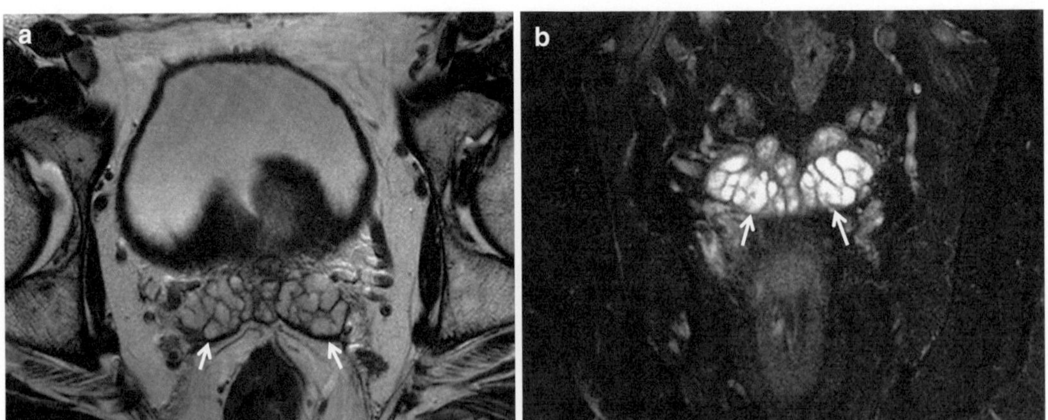

Fig. 3.3 Normal appearance of seminal vesicle on MR. T2-weighted axial (**a**) and coronal (**b**) image shows elongated, multiseptated, fluid-filled structures mimicking bundle of grapes

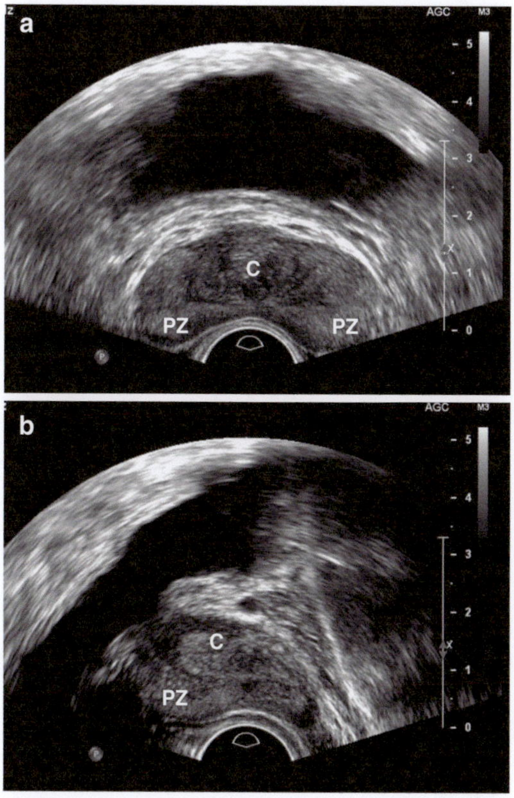

Fig. 3.4 Normal transrectal ultrasound (TRUS) findings of prostate. Transrectal axial (**a**) and sagittal (**b**) image show normal anatomy of prostate. The peripheral zone (PZ) shows relatively homogenous slightly high echogenicity, whereas the central zone (C) shows relatively heterogeneous and low echogenicity

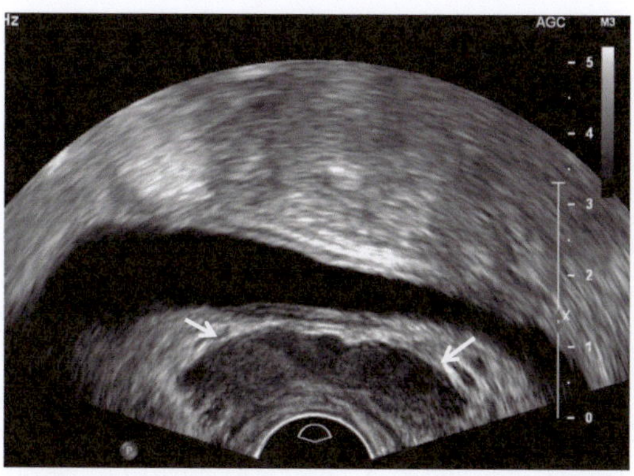

Fig. 3.5 Normal TRUS findings of seminal vesicle. Axial TRUS image reveals bundle of grapes appearance representing seminal vesicle

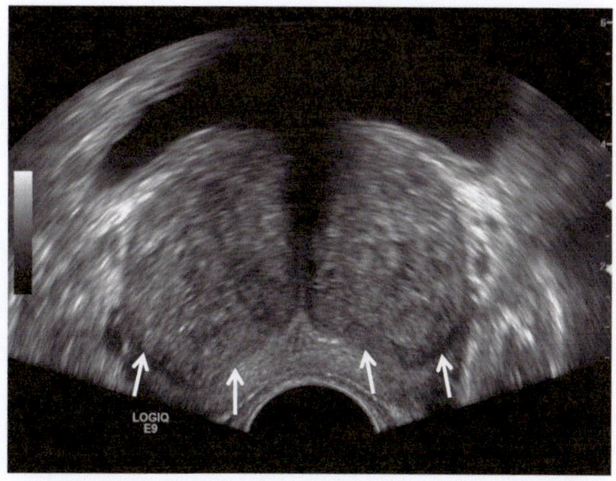

Fig. 3.6 TRUS findings of benign prostate hyperplasia (BPH). TRUS image shows round low echoic area suggesting benign prostate hyperplasia (BPH) arising from transitional zone (*arrows*)

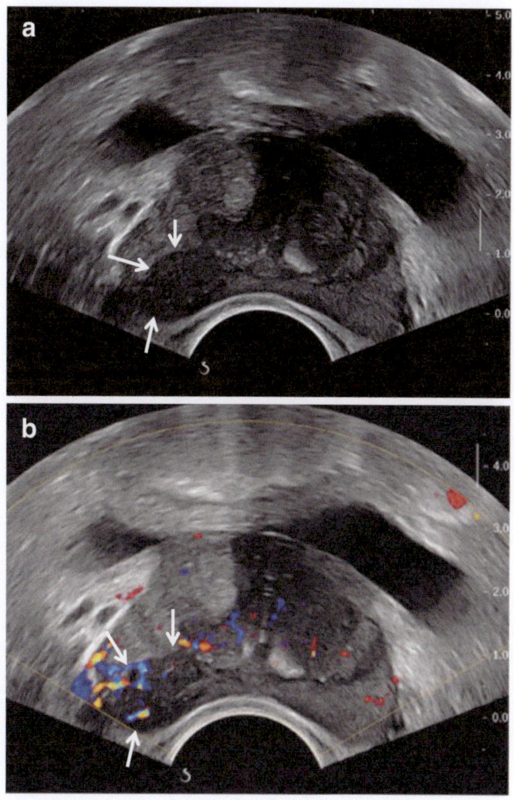

Fig. 3.7 Prostate cancer shown as focal hypoechoic lesion on TRUS. (**a**) TRUS axial scan reveals well-marginated low echoic nodular lesion on left portion of prostate. (**b**) Color Doppler image shows definitely increased vascularity on the focal lesion

inflammation, fibrosis, infarction, or benign prostate hyperplasia nodules [19].

B-mode TRUS has very limited ability to identify tumors in the central gland. It has been shown that some prostate cancers demonstrate increased flow on color Doppler, a feature that is also used to guide biopsies (Fig. 3.7) [9].

According to the study of Onur et al. [20], out of 3,912 consecutive patients who performed TRUS-guided biopsies, prostate cancer was detected in 25.5 % with a hypoechoic lesion and in 25.4 % without a hypoechoic lesion. The percentage of core detection was 9.3 % for hypoechoic and 10.4 % for isoechoic areas. Over the past decade, there has been a trend to obtain larger numbers of biopsy specimens, with most clinicians taking 8- to 12-core biopsies; most current studies are recommending a 12-core biopsy scheme [21].

Other attempts were tried. Lee et al. [22] tried to evaluate the imaging findings of focal hypoechoic lesions seen on TRUS with several parameters of shape, margin irregularity, vascularity, and the location of the lesion. They concluded that the positive predictive value was up to 80 % when the focal lesion located in peripheral portion showed nodular and irregular marginated hypoechoic lesion with increased vascularity.

In spite of these results, many reports showed that the simple hypoechoic lesion showed low sensitivity and specificity of grayscale ultrasound for the detection of prostate cancer. And there is limited value for grayscale-targeted biopsies. However, due to the high-quality images and the inexpensive and simple procedure, it is still the most optimal technique for guiding prostate biopsies [23].

Besides, recently, new emerging technologies in TRUS-guided prostate biopsy such as image fusion, elastography, and contrast-enhanced ultrasound were introduced and showed high potential in the diagnosis of prostate cancer. Ultrasound contrast agent studies can provide the information regarding vascularity of the lesion. New novel technologies for the synthesis of new microbubbles with specific ligand are introduced and visualize the presence of specific marker. The advent of ultrasonic molecular imaging may provide a new diagnostic method for the early diagnosis of prostate cancer.

Elastography is an emerging ultrasound technique that can provide the information regarding tissue elasticity and stiffness. The image fusion, which can show the information both from multiparametric magnetic resonance imaging (mpMRI) and TRUS imaging, will have a potential modality in performing targeted biopsy.

3.3.2 US Elastography

Elastography is an ultrasound imaging technique based on the concept that significant differences exist between elastic properties of benign and malignant tissue [24]. It is an emerging ultrasound technique that can visualize tissue elasticity and stiffness [25]. It is based on the assumptions that if force is applied to the unit area (stress), relative displacement of points (strain) will be proportional to the applied force and is represented by well-described Young's modulus. Tumors are usually stiffer than normal tissue because of its increased cellular density. Prostatic cancer is normally 5–28 times stiffer than the surrounding soft tissue [26]. This change of local stiffness is the background of digital rectal exam of prostate gland. However, digital rectal exam is subjective to the examiner, and only part of the prostate is palpable.

In elastography, there are two types, using strain and shear wave technology. Strain forces are generated by manual compression by transducers, while shear wave is a technique that uses a sonographic push pulse to generate a shear wave in the tissues (Figs. 3.8 and 3.9) [27].

Soft tissues tend to exhibit higher strain (deformation) than stiffer areas when compression is applied. Strain elastography of the prostate is based on the analysis of tissue deformation in a region, generated by compression of the tissue by the transrectal transducer. A speckle comparison, before and after compression, yields to a color map of local tissue deformation or strain called elastogram [28]. Because tissue stiffness is estimated by visualizing the differences in strain between adjacent regions, there is no quantitative elasticity.

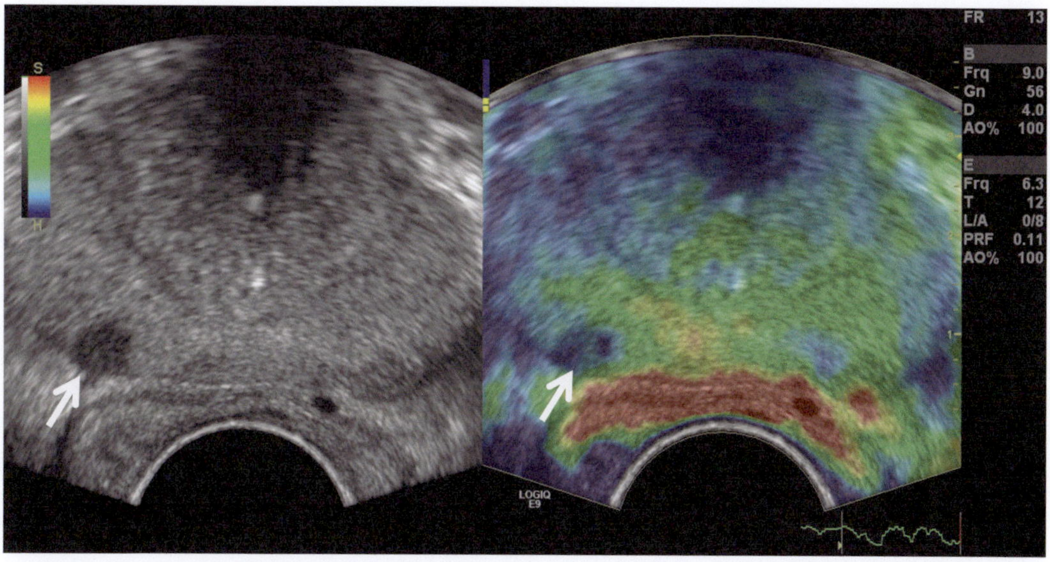

Fig. 3.8 Elastography using strain forces. Elastography shows relatively focal lesion showing low elasticity (*arrows*). This lesion is well matched with the focal lesion on grayscale TRUS

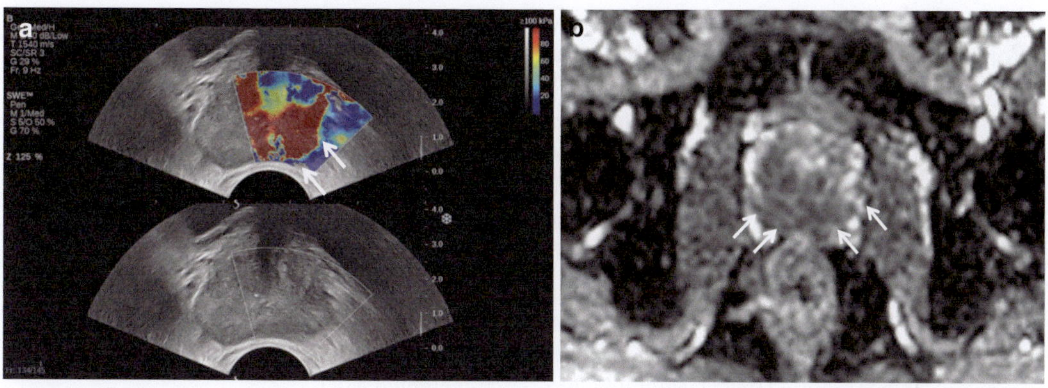

Fig. 3.9 Prostate cancer of shear wave elastography. (**a**) Elastography shows area of low elasticity in left peripheral zone of prostate (*arrows*), which is not definite on grayscale TRUS. Pathologic report revealed that prostate cancer was in this lesion. (**b**) Apparent diffusion coefficiency (ADC) map image shows diffuse signal drops in whole prostate, suggesting diffuse prostate cancer

The ROI can be placed on abnormal lesion and the other areas of the prostate. Semiquantitative information can be derived by measuring strain ratio between two ROI (usually one considered "normal" and the other "abnormal"). The strain for each pixel is color coded and displayed as overlay on the B-mode image (Fig. 3.8). Because the stiffness color scale is automatically distributed from the lowest to the highest strain found in the image plane, it may induce some variability [29]. Elastography permits depiction of the cancer of isoechogenecity on grayscale ultrasound, otherwise can be missed by conventional TRUS.

Shear wave elastography (SWE) is another type of elastography, which can provide quantitative information on tissue elasticity. The basic principle of SWE relies on two successive steps; a shear wave is remotely induced by the endorectal transducer in the prostate, using the acoustic radiation force of a focused ultrasonic beam, and the shear wave propagation is captured by

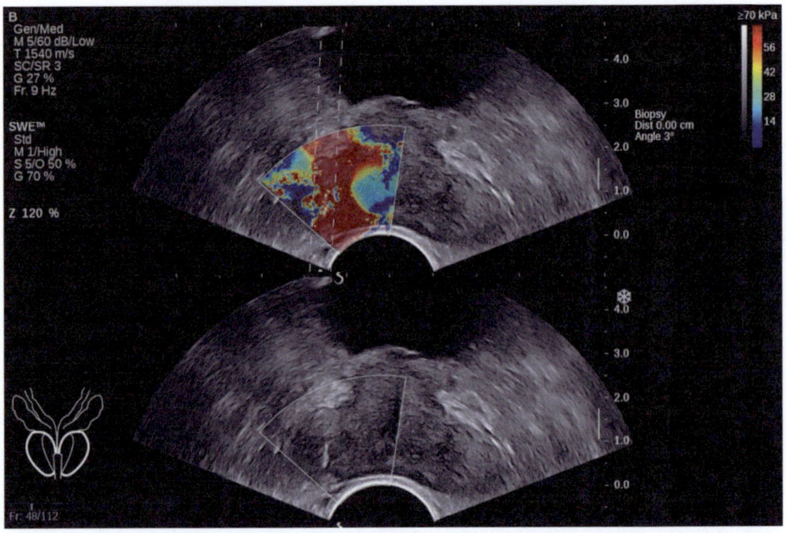

Fig. 3.10 Figure showing shear wave elastography-guided biopsy. TRUS image shows shear wave elastography-guided biopsy. The guide indicates that the lesion with low elasticity

imaging the prostate. By measuring the shear wave propagation velocity, shear modulus can be derived. The shear wave speed (in meter per second) or the Young's modulus (in kilopascal) is color mapped on the images in B-mode [29].

Unlike strain elastography, SWE requires no compression on the rectal wall to produce elastograms (Fig. 3.9). SWE is based on the measurement of shear wave velocity propagating through the tissues [30]. This technique has advantages of providing a quantitative map of elastic characteristics in real time, which can be displayed either in kilopascal or in meter per second.

Several studies reported that elastography provides useful additional information to conventional TRUS for prostate cancer detection. There are several applications of elastography. It can be used in characterization of region detected by grayscale imaging, color Doppler US, or MRI (Fig. 3.9). It can be also used for the characterization of lesions which were not detected on conventional US, and it can be used for biopsy targeting (Fig. 3.10) [31].

A meta-analysis study using strain elastography reported sensitivity in the range of 71–82 % and a specificity of 60–95 % with reference standard of radical prostatectomy specimen [28]. Elastography-guided prostate biopsies in patients with cancer were 2.9-fold more likely to detect prostate cancer than systemic biopsy [32].

Another prospective study of elastography by Brock et al. reported that overall prostate cancer detection rate was significantly higher in patients who underwent biopsy with the elastography-guided approach compared to the grayscale ultrasound-guided biopsy (51.1 % vs. 39.4 %) [33]. However, the sensitivity of elastography did not reach levels to omit a systematic biopsy approach.

The comparison of elastography with T2-weighted conventional MRI was reported by Aigner et al. [34]. Overall sensitivities and specificities were similar between elastography and T2-weighted MRI.

The drawback of strain elastography is that quantification of tissue elasticity is not achievable. Semiquantitative stiffness evaluation using a strain index (strain ratio of tissue over normal tissue) is introduced to overcome this limitation and reported to be useful in the evaluation of prostate cancer [35]. However, these studies are all based on region of interest drawing, which have some difficulties in reproducibility and standardization.

With SWE, during evaluation, the transducer should be kept in steady-state position for several seconds until stabilization of the signals. Usually, stiff tissues are color coded in red, while soft tissues appear in blue color [29]. Hypoechoic lesions with stiff elasticity are suspicious for malignancy. The absolute value of elasticity can be obtained for each ROI. In young men without prostate disease, the elasticity values are below 30 kPa. Typical prostate cancer nodules in the peripheral zone are stiffer, showing more than 35 kPa [29].

The advantage of SWE over strain elastography is that SWE does not require compression by the transducer, which means that measurement is operator independent. A few initial reports showed very promising results for SWE, including high sensitivities and specificities over 90 % for prostate cancer [27, 36]. However, the sensitivity and specificity were decreased to be 50–60 % in another recent study by Woo et al. [37]. Nevertheless, SWE parameters of mean stiffness and mean stiffness ratio are significantly different between prostate cancer and benign tissue and correlate with Gleason score.

For the evaluation of diagnostic accuracy or feasibility, more validation studies beyond the initial reports will be required with prospective trials and/or radical prostatectomy specimen basis.

Elastography is rapidly maturing and now produces excellent and diagnostically useful images of prostate. By measuring the stiffness, it may help for the characterization of the focal lesion seen on TRUS and for guiding the prostate biopsy.

3.3.3 Contrast-Enhanced TRUS

Microbubble contrast agents are composed of tiny bubbles of gas contained within a supporting shell. The shell may be composed of albumin, galactose, lipids, or polymers ranging from 10 to 200 nm [38]. The inner space is filled with gases having a high molecular weight and low solubility such as perfluorocarbon or sulfur hexafluoride which has characteristics of prolonging the agents' existence in the blood pool [39].

Ultrasound contrast agents are mainly used as intravascular contrast media, although they can be instilled into the urinary bladder to evaluate ureteric reflux or into the uterus to look out for tubal patency [40, 41]. The size of microbubbles is nearly equal to that of red blood cells, and they behave as intravascular blood pool agents (Fig. 3.11). They are able to better show the neovascularity and increased vascular density that has been correlated to the presence of prostate cancer, cancer stage, metastasis, and postoperative biochemical failure [42, 43].

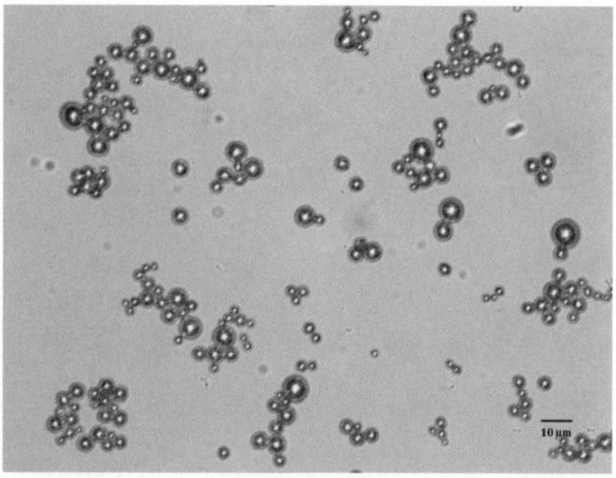

Fig. 3.11 Figure showing microbubble. Microscopic image shows bubble like structures with the size less than 10 µm

The echogenicity of an individual microbubble is dependent on the elasticity of the shell, the compressibility of the core, the length of time that the bubble will remain in circulation, and the amount of acoustic energy that the microbubbles can absorb before breaking down [44].

Prostate cancer, like other solid organ malignancy, has been demonstrated to have measurable neovascularity and tumor-associated angiogenesis. The tumor growth and metastasis require angiogenesis, the growth of new blood vessels. These abnormal blood vessels may represent a possible marker for the presence of cancer [42]. The measure of tumor angiogenesis correlates with the microvessel density (MVD) and metastasis in various malignancies [45]. Hence, microbubbles have considerable potential for imaging of tumor angiogenesis as intravascular contrast agents. According to preclinical study in xenograft prostate cancer model using PC-3 prostate tumor cells, maximum intensity was positively correlated with the MVD with statistical significance (Figs. 3.12 and 3.13) [46]. In clinical study, Weidner et al.

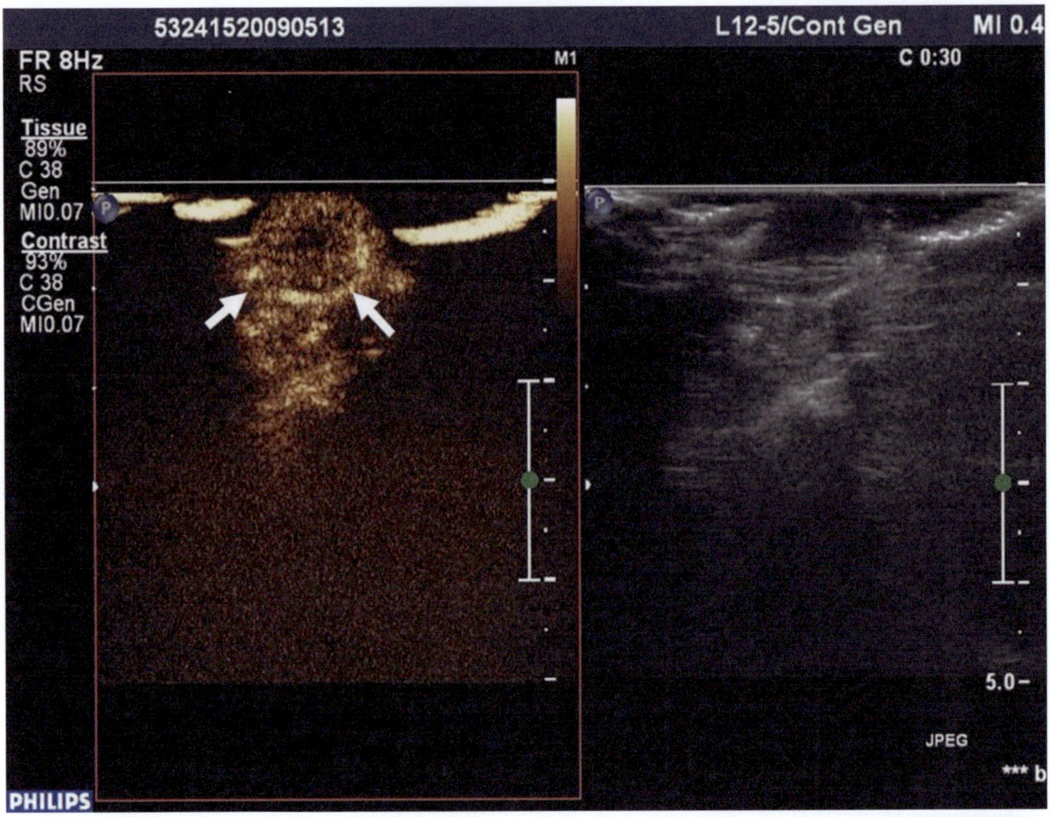

Fig. 3.12 Xenograft animal study showing microbubbles for angiogenesis assessment. Contrast-enhanced US shows well-enhancing solid mass on PC-3 xenograft mouse model (Published with kind permission of Korean Society of Ultrasound in Medicine *J Korean Soc Ultrasound Med* 2009;28:139–145)

reported that microvessel counts increased with increasing Gleason score in prostatectomy specimen [45]. Sedelaar et al. showed that ultrasound contrast-enhanced areas had a 1.93 times higher MVD as compared to the nonenhanced areas (Fig. 3.14) [47].

For the contrast-enhanced ultrasound, various imaging strategies including grayscale, Doppler, harmonic imaging, maximum intensity projection, and flash replenishment techniques can be used. Harmonic imaging uses the distortion produced by the microbubble contrast agent on the sound wave reflection, in harmonic multiples of the incident frequency [38]. Maximum-intensity projection adds the information between ultrasound frames, allowing tracking of microvessel morphology.

In clinical practice, contrast-enhanced sonography has many advantages in that it can be performed on patients safely, easily, and repeatedly without any radiation. However, it has disadvantages in its lack of objectivity in determining the extent of enhancement because the image qualities are affected by many factors. Also the results are sometimes operator dependent. However, these disadvantages may be overcome by development of dedicated software for analysis.

For the evaluation of TRUS-guided biopsy using ultrasound contrast agents, many clinical studies were performed. The detection rate of prostate cancer was higher when they use contrast-enhanced color Doppler-targeted biopsy comparing 10 systemic biopsies in 690 men (26 % vs. 20 %). And, the Gleason score was also higher in contrast-enhanced targeted biopsy than that of systemic biopsy (mean, 6.8 vs. 5.4) [48]. In a recent report published by Jiang, the peak

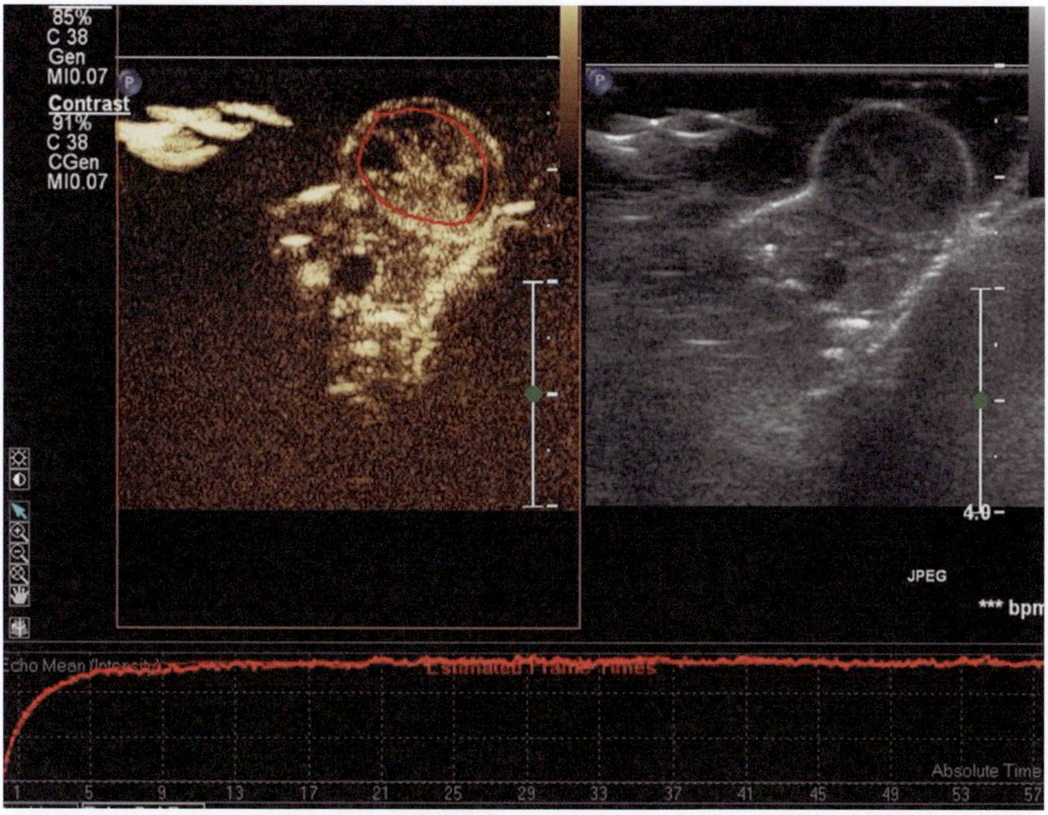

Fig. 3.13 Quantitative evaluation of tumor angiogenesis. Time-intensity curve can be obtained with software. Several quantitative parameters can be calculated based on time-intensity curve. Published with kind permission of Korean Society of Ultrasound in Medicine

intensity on contrast-enhanced ultrasound correlated with Gleason score and MVD in 147 prostate cancer patients [49].

According to the meta-analysis regarding the diagnostic performance of contrast-enhanced ultrasound in patients with prostate cancer, the pooled sensitivity and specificity were 0.7 and 0.74 from 2,624 patients [50]. At present, contrast-enhanced ultrasound is a promising tool in the detection of prostate cancer, but it cannot completely replace systematic biopsy under the present circumstances.

Targeted microbubbles have additional ligand molecules that bind to the specific sites. Possible receptor targets for prostate cancer are those that are upregulated during the process of angiogenesis. Most research regarding targeted microbubbles has been focusing on the vascular endothelial growth factor (VEGF) receptors [51]. For contrast-enhanced imaging of the high expression of VEGF receptor 2 (VEGFR2) in tumor neovasculature, VEGFR2 receptor-loaded targeted microbubbles were introduced [52].

Recently, there are other novel technologies for targeting prostate cancer cells using nanoscale ultrasound contrast agents. Among prostate cancer biomarkers, prostate-specific membrane antigen (PSMA) is considered to be the most important protein target in diagnostic-specific immunolocalization imaging and immune-directed therapy [53, 54]. PSMA is a type II transmembrane glycoprotein in the prostate cell membrane. The levels of PSMA expression are different in normal prostate tissue, benign prostatic hyperplasia, and prostate cancer epithelial tissue, respectively. And it is also known that positive PSMA expression rate in hormone-refractory prostate cancer and metastases are

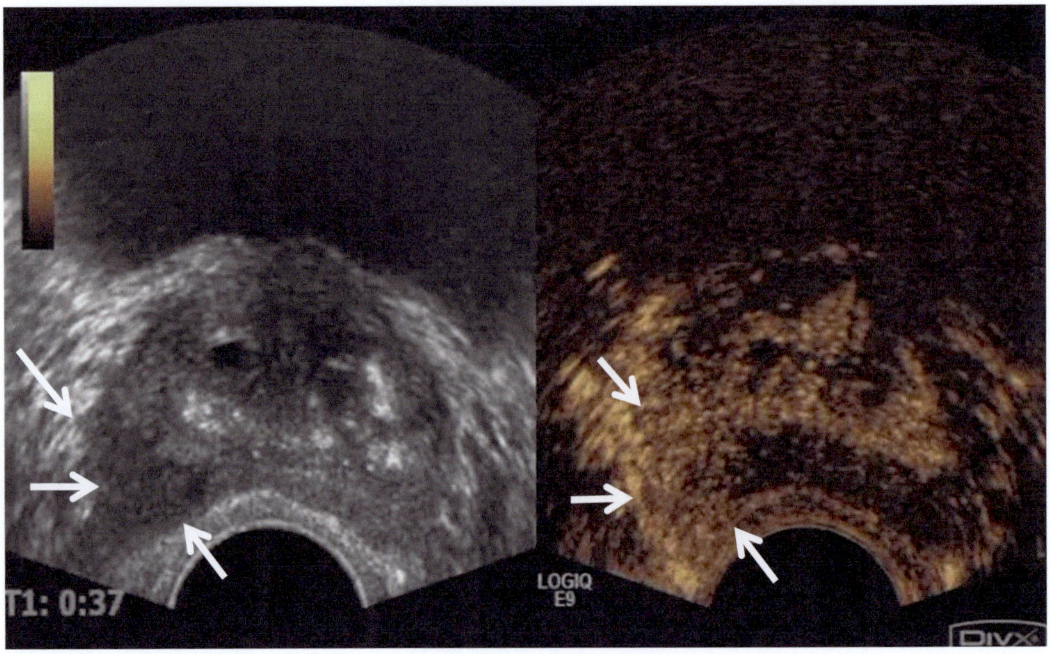

Fig. 3.14 Contrast-enhanced TRUS showing prostate cancer. Contrast-enhanced TRUS shows well-enhancing lesion on right peripheral zone of prostate (*arrows*). The lesion showed prostate adenocarcinoma after TRUS-guided biopsy

significantly higher than that of the normal or benign tissue [53]. Wang et al. [54] reported in vitro and in vivo results of PSMA-targeted nanoscale microbubbles in prostate cancer. They synthesized stable PSMA monoclonal antibody-loaded MBs and investigated their in vitro target-binding capability with the selected prostate cancer cells. Besides, targeted contrast enhancement and specificity were also examined with a xenograft prostate tumor models. The results showed that targeted microbubbles can significantly increase peak intensity and duration of contrast enhancement than that in control microbubbles [54]. These targeted ultrasound contrast agents, which are on the way of development, would be very potential methodologies not only for prostate cancer-specific imaging but also for targeted ultrasound-guided prostate biopsy.

3.3.4 Image Fusion

TRUS plays a crucial role in the screening imaging study and guidance of the biopsy of the prostate glands. However, overall detection rate of TRUS for prostate cancer remains approximately 50 %, and biopsies yield at least one positive biopsy in only 25 % of the patients [55, 56]. Moreover, over detection of the clinically insignificant cancer is another important issue, which leads to overtreatment. Therefore, detection of highest grade or representative cancer tissue in the prostate gland is required to decide treatment plan. Several potential benefits of MRI-targeted biopsy were reported in the literature. The accurate localization of significant cancer before biopsy may correct the limitations of systematic random biopsy [6].

Introduction of high-field MRI in clinical field impacts improved image quality due to increased signal-to-noise ratio (SNR). Still there remain some controversies, but the use of uncomfortable endorectal coil is not obligatory for the prostate MRI because of its increased SNR of 3.0 Tesla MRI [57].

Application of stronger magnet and multiparametric MRI (mpMRI) from morphologic and functional MRI technique enables to detect more cancers. T2-weighted MRI is excellent in the evaluation of anatomy and detection

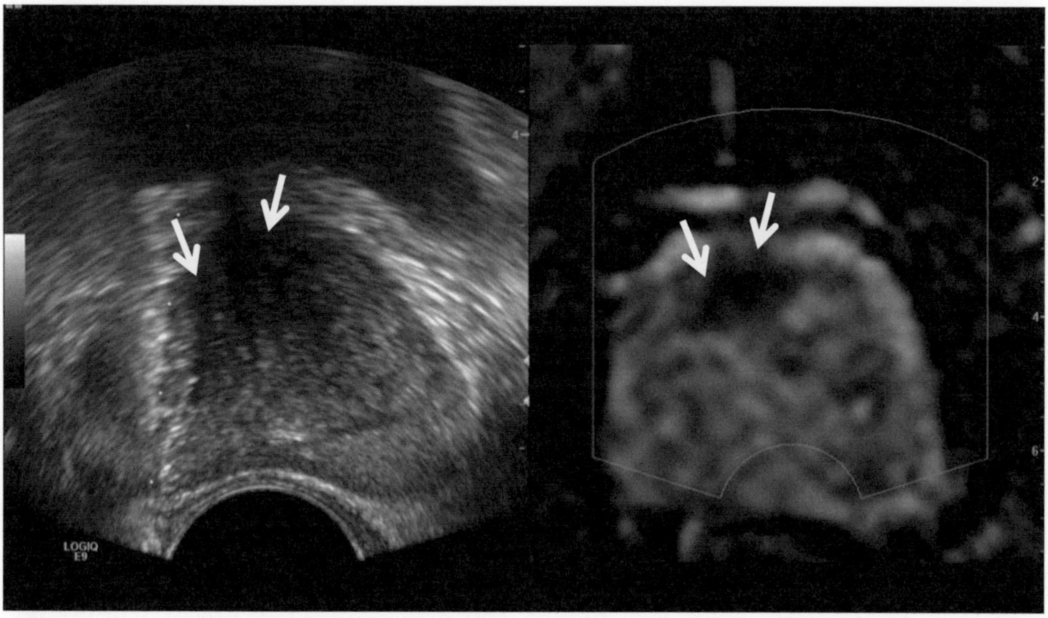

Fig. 3.15 Image showing MRI-TRUS fusion. TRUS-MR fusion image-guided biopsy can cover the most suspicious lesion seen on ADC map. TRUS guide biopsy was performed on the suspicious lesion seen on ADC map in anterior portion of transitional zone, and pathologic report revealed prostate cancer with Gleason score of 8 (*arrows*)

of peripherally located cancer. However, T2-weighted image has limited value in the detection of central-gland cancer. In addition, T2-weighted images are very susceptible to post-biopsy hemorrhage, which shows low signal intensity and interferes tumor detection [58].

Functional techniques including apparent diffusion coefficient (ADC) map from diffusion-weighted imaging, dynamic contrast-enhanced MRI with fast imaging, and magnetic resonance spectroscopy (MRS) are very helpful in the diagnosis of prostate cancer. The detection rates of prostate cancer are increased with these techniques, and even centrally located cancer can be more easily and confidently diagnosed [59]. For the staging of prostate cancer, mpMRI is superior to detect extracapsular extension and seminal vesicle invasion. To monitor treatment effect, mpMRI significantly improves the assessment of patients with suspected recurrence after treatment [60].

ADC map can discriminate cancers with Gleason score over 7 (4+3) from cancer with lower Gleason score [59]. Because of this superior detectability of cancer with highest Gleason score with MRI, MRI-guided prostate biopsy is introduced. Although it has great advantage of reducing the number of core biopsy, it has limited value due to increased procedure time and costs [61].

The simplest way to MRI-guided biopsy is visual estimation of MRI during TRUS-guided biopsy. Visual estimation allows the adaptation of MRI-targeted biopsy in clinical practice without significant cost, but it needs a significant learning curve and lacks real-time feedback regarding accuracy [6]. The current studies about TRUS-guided biopsy with MR visual estimation suggest improved accuracy and efficiency compared to systematic biopsy but also demonstrated that visual estimation biopsy varies by operator experiences [62, 63].

MR-US fusion image by co-registration software can be another powerful option for guidance of prostate biopsy (Fig. 3.15). Image fusion is the process of combining image information from two or more images into a single image, and the resulting image provides more information than any input image alone. Image fusion of prostate refers to the superimposition of stored prostate MRI images and real-time TRUS images, when prostate biopsy is performed [64]. The fused image gives the operator the advantages of the tumor-detecting value of MRI with the ease of use of TRUS.

A number of commercial platforms for image fusion have become available [6]. These applications vary by co-registration technologies including mechanical, electromagnetic, or real time. Hardware platform to align the biopsy is different.

Reduction of time and cost of direct MRI guidance without sacrificing diagnostic accuracy can be achievable. Sonn et al. [61] reported that targeted biopsy with MR-US fusion was three times more likely to identify cancer than a systematic biopsy (27 % vs. 7 %). Out of the men with Gleason score 7 or greater cancer, 38 % had disease detected only on targeted biopsies. Fusion biopsy can provide improved detection of prostate cancer in men with prior negative biopsies and elevated PSA levels [65]. Fusion software co-registration potentially overcomes the limitation of cognitive fusion through reproducible methods of identifying MRI lesions on ultrasound. MR-US fusion biopsy potentially has greater reproducibility because it involves less operator dependence and provides real-time feedback of actual biopsied locations.

There is still some technical issue to be solved in MR-US fusion. Precise registration of MRI and US is the key for the successful image fusion. However, the shape of prostate in MR and TRUS is different because the prostate is displaced and deformed due to ultrasound probe. Nonrigid registration of the prostate gland for this elastic deformation is needed, but still many fusion techniques are based on rigid registration which cannot reflect elastic deformation by transducer. However, this issue can be overcome by development of fusion techniques [66]. Disadvantages also include a high cost for the image fusion software/device, dependence on the software for accuracy, and the associated learning curve and operator training.

Among the patients with no previous biopsy, the role of image fusion is poorly defined, but it has the potential to reduce false-negatives contributing to reduce repeated biopsies and to get the representative information regarding patients' cancer. The patients with a previous negative biopsy but persistent clinical suspicion have the potential for increased cancer detection and reduced further repeated biopsy. With development of MRI technologies for depicting the prostate cancer, image fusion may have more important role in prostate cancer patients.

3.3.5 TRUS-Guided Biopsy

The diagnosis, management, and prognosis of prostate cancer are largely dependent on histopathological features obtained by TRUS and TRUS-guided biopsy [14]. Traditionally, the decision to perform prostate biopsy has been based on abnormal digital rectal examination (DRE) or increased PSA level. TRUS-guided biopsy uses B-mode and/or color Doppler imaging to localize the prostate, target suspicious areas, and systematically obtain anywhere from 6- to more than 40-core biopsy using 18-gauge needles.

Because of these sampling errors, however, the reported false-negative rate of TRUS-guided biopsy reaches up to 30 % [67]. In addition, Gleason scores established through TRUS-guided biopsy are often discordant with prostatectomy specimens. TRUS-guided biopsy underestimates the score of cancer in up to 38 % of patients, therefore misrepresenting tumor aggressiveness [68]. The volume of disease can be estimated based on the number of positive core biopsies and on the percentage of tumor seen in positive cores. According to Park et al., among several parameters from prostate biopsy, the maximum cancer length was found to be the most reliable predictor of disease staging [69]. In other studies, multiple risk-stratification schemes are available to predict prognosis and plan treatment [70, 71]. These criteria rely heavily on the histopathologic findings of Gleason grade and extent of tumor seen in the TRUS-guided core biopsy specimens.

Although there is no absolute cutoff value for prostate biopsy, general agreement is that PSA higher than 4 ng/ml is suggestive of the presence of prostate cancer for TRUS-guided biopsy [31]. In other reports, a PSA threshold of 2.6 ng/ml doubles cancer detection rates in men younger than 60 years with little loss in specificity [72]. There are several other factors to consider in proceeding to biopsy, potentially including PSA velocity, % free PSA, PSA density (PSAD), age, family history, ethnicity, and comorbidities.

The National Comprehensive Cancer Network (NCCN) in the United States recommends the use of a PSA velocity of 0.35 ng/ml/year or greater as indication for biopsy in men with PSA 2.5 ng/ml or less [73]. The use of % free PSA as an alternative indication of initial biopsy was also suggested. The % free/total PSA ratio can be used to recommend biopsy if the value is less than 10 %, and prostate biopsy is not recommended if the value is greater than 25 % [31]. PSAD and age-referenced PSA have been investigated but are still controversial [73]. Several predictive models have been developed to reduce unnecessary biopsies and still detect most clinically important cancers and are available on the internet.

Pain control is one of the important issues in the aspect of patient care. Periprostatic nerve block (PPNB) with 1 % lidocaine is considered the standard anesthetic technique. And many protocols and researches were reported to reduce the pain during TRUS-guided biopsy [74, 75]. The most common site of injection is bilaterally at the junction of the base of the prostate and seminal vesicles, because neural pathway originates from the inferior hypogastric plexus located at the tip of seminal vesicles and passes between the prostate and rectum [76]. Various sites of infiltration were studied including the apex-only [77, 78] bilateral neurovascular bundles [79, 80], apex and neurovascular regions [81, 82], or three locations of base, mid, and apex [82]. Ismail et al. reported that combined bilateral neurovascular bundles with apical infiltration resulted in more effective reduction in pain associated with TRUS biopsy than bilateral neurovascular infiltration alone, especially in younger patients [83]. Lee et al. reported that intraprostatic anesthesia and periprostatic nerve block are effective and useful techniques tolerated by the patient based on randomized, double-blinded study [84]. In other respect, for the relieving pain related to probe insertion, Cormio et al. reported that lidocaine-prilocaine cream was most effective in probe-related pain for prostate biopsy [81].

The number of cores from TRUS-guided biopsy is also important because it is related with the patient's discomfort or the accuracy of prostate cancer diagnosis. Recently, TRUS-guided biopsy with 12 cores is considered the standard procedure for cancer detection. Several studies have reported the higher yield of an extended prostate biopsy versus the old standard sextant biopsy, without an increase in the detection of insignificant cancer [75, 85]. The studies regarding the number of core biopsy have demonstrated sextant prostate biopsy sensitivities at 30 %, with increasing sensitivity with increasing numbers of core biopsies, 36–58 % for 12-core biopsies and 53–58 % for 18-core biopsies [86]. On the other hand, it has been shown that the saturation technique as an initial prostate biopsy strategy does not improve cancer detection. Jones et al. had suggested that further efforts at extended biopsy strategies beyond 10–12 cores are not appropriate as initial biopsy strategy [87]. Eichler et al. showed that there is no significant benefit in taking more than 12 cores and methods requiring more than 18 cores have a poor side-effect profile [21]. Sampling accuracy tends to decrease progressively with an increasing prostate volume. In addition to the number of cores and prostate volume, the site of core biopsy is also important. Because the apex and the base of the peripheral gland are the most common cancer sites, it is advised that biopsies should be directed to apex and base of peripheral zone. The parasagittal biopsies have been shown to have the lowest possibility of prostate cancer at the initial biopsy. The American Urological Association (AUA) has recently completed a white paper confirming that a 12-core systematic biopsy is optimal and that there was not compelling evidence that individual site-specific labeling of cores benefits clinical decision making regarding the initial management of prostate cancer [31]. Studies of repeat prostate biopsy after negative extended prostate biopsy indicate that up to 30 % of patients have cancers that were not previously diagnosed [88, 89]. Repeated biopsy seems to be recommended in patients with an initial negative biopsy but persistent suspicion of prostate cancer based on age, comorbidities, DRE findings, PSA measurements, other PSA derivatives (% free PSA, PSAD, PSA velocity), or urinary prostate cancer antigen 3 (PCA3) score [28].

While MRI-targeted biopsy and MR-TRUS fusion biopsy have the potential to overcome the limitations of standard TRUS-guided biopsy, they need further studies regarding the accuracy in prostate cancer detection, cost-effectiveness analysis, and improvements in technical limitations [6].

The complications of prostate biopsy include urinary tract infection, hematuria, bleeding per rectum, hematospermia, and acute urinary tract obstruction. In case of bleeding, clinically significant hematuria was developed only in 1–2 % of patients who underwent prostate biopsy. Desmond et al. reported that out of 670 patients who underwent prostate biopsy, about 0.6 % showed gross hematuria and 0.1 % of patients needed management [90]. Azjen et al. reported that 1 % of the patients showed transient hematuria [91]. In larger scales, Berger et al. showed hematospermia (36.3 %), hematuria (14.5 %), and rectal bleeding less than 48 h (2.3 %); however, most cases need no management. They reported that only 0.7 % of patients showed fever immediately after biopsy, 0.6 % showed severe rectal bleeding, and 0.2 % showed acute urinary retention [92]. Infections after prostate biopsy are urinary tract infection, prostatitis, epididymitis, prostatic abscess, or sepsis. To avoid significant infection, it is important to use prophylactic antibiotics before biopsy and to detect the symptoms and signs of infection earlier.

3.4 CT

Computed tomography (CT) is one of the most commonly used modality in abdomen and pelvis imaging; however, it gives little information regarding prostate and has a very limited role in prostate cancer staging [93]. CT shows little contrast between prostate and adjacent organs including seminal vesicle. However, it may be considered for the staging of men with high-risk prostate cancer. High risk is usually defined as total serum PSA greater than 20.0 ng/ml, locally advanced disease on clinical assessment such as positive findings on DRE, or Gleason score greater than or equal to 8 [14]. CT of prostate cancer is almost used for assessing potential metastasis in lymph nodes, soft tissues, or bones of advanced prostate cancer patient (Fig. 3.16). The most common sites for lymph node metastasis in prostate cancer include anterior or lateral route of pelvic

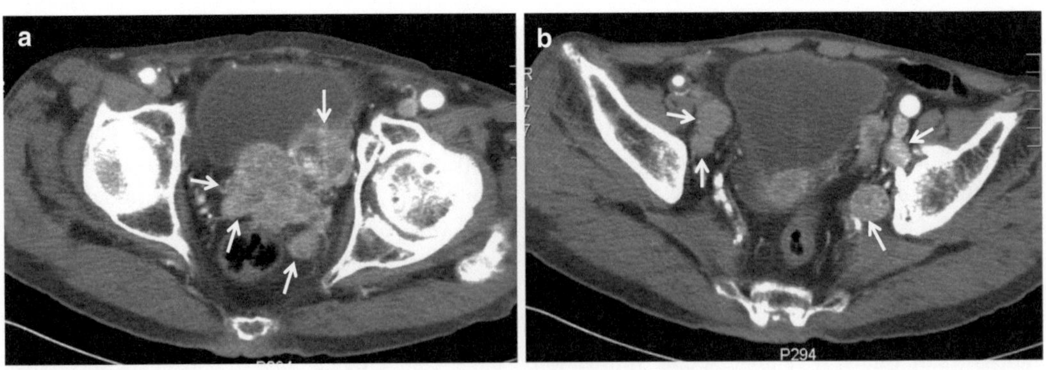

Fig. 3.16 CT findings of multiple metastasis of prostate cancer. (**a**) Post-contrast CT scan shows bulky mass involving prostate and posterior bladder wall (*arrows*). (**b**) At the higher level, CT scan shows multiple metastatic lymphadenopathies (*arrows*)

pathway (external iliac lymph nodes), internal iliac route (internal iliac lymph nodes), and sometimes presacral route (presacral lymph nodes). Even in patients with high-risk cancer, the sensitivity of CT scanning for detecting positive nodes is only about 35 % [14].

For the diagnosis of bone metastasis, bone scan is significantly more sensitive than CT, and many patients with normal CT findings show positive radionuclide scan findings. Although osseous metastases can be identified on CT, CT is usually used to follow up patients with known metastatic disease rather than to diagnose it.

3.5 MRI

3.5.1 Conventional MRI

Usually, prostate MRI studies combine anatomic images from high-resolution T2-weighted (T2W) images and functional information obtained from diffusion-weighted imaging (DWI), dynamic contrast-enhanced imaging (DCEI), and MRS, in a multiparametric approach.

High-resolution T2-weighted images are used for prostate cancer detection, localization, and staging. Many institutions obtain T2-weighted sagittal, axial, and coronal planes. Fast-spin echo T2-weighted image provides high signal-to-noise ratio (SNR) and high spatial resolution images with significant T2 contrast. High-contrast T2-weighted images allow the depiction of subglandular structures located mainly in the peripheral zone.

In T2-weighted images, the normal peripheral zone of the prostate has hyperintense signal, whereas the central and transition zones have low signal intensity, allowing the zonal anatomy of the prostate to be clearly demonstrated (Fig. 3.17). The prostate capsule is demonstrated as a thin line of low signal intensity surrounding the gland [94]. The nodular, glandular, stromal, and cystic changes of BPH can be clearly visualized [95]. For T2W imaging without functional sequences, the sensitivity and specificity for prostate cancer are approximately 57–83 and 62–82 % [96, 97].

Normal peripheral zone consists primarily of glandular lumen lined with secretory epithelium, all of which is embedded within a stromal matrix [98, 99]. In normal structures, macromolecular water content and free water content are low in stroma and high in luminal space on T2-weighted images. These characteristics result from relatively long T2 values and unrestricted water diffusion with high ADCs in the peripheral zone. Peripheral zone prostate cancer typically shows low signal intensity nodule on T2-weighted images, but imaging findings can be changed according to the tumor growth pattern and the aggressiveness of the tumor. In case of tumors with densely packed malignant glands, T2-weighted image shows low-signal-intensity mass usually on the peripheral zone (Fig. 3.18). However, in case of tumors with sparse malignant glands intermixed with normal tissue, the signal intensity of the tumor is not significantly different from the surrounding normal tissue and is not readily detected on MRI [100]. Sometimes it is difficult to differentiate prostate cancer from other benign lesions showing low signal intensity on T2-weighted image. For focal low signal intensity on the T2-weighted images, wedge-shaped and diffused extension without mass effect are the best predictors of benignity, whereas mass effect and irregular margin suggest malignancy [101]. A few benign conditions of the prostate, including chronic prostatitis, scars, and post-biopsy hemorrhage, can result in low-signal-intensity areas on the T2W images and can be confused with cancer [102]. In case of prostatitis, the glandular luminal space is replaced by the inflammatory cells. These inflammatory changes with scar formation due to the thickening of the ductal walls contribute to shorter T2 values, which reveal subsequently hypointense regions on T2-weighted image [103]. Sometimes age-related changes in the prostate show increase in ADC in the peripheral zone [104].

The detection of tumors located in the transition zone is more difficult. Because the signal intensities of BPH and prostate cancer usually overlap on the T2-weighted images, other imaging features such as homogeneous low

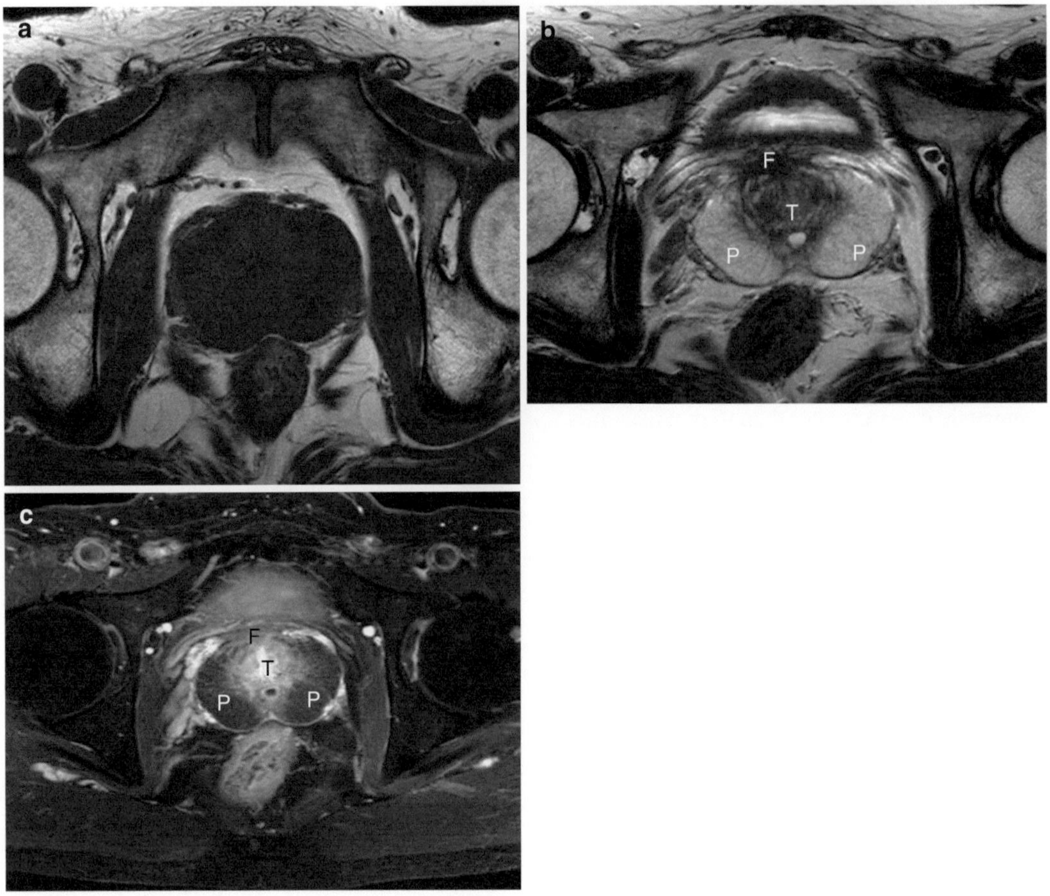

Fig. 3.17 Normal findings of prostate in 45-year-old man. (**a**) T1-weighted axial image shows homogenous low signal intensity of prostate. (**b**) T2-weighted axial image shows bright signal intensity of peripheral zone. Also note low signal intensity transitional zone (*T*) and anterior fibromuscular stroma (*F*) in central and anterior portion of prostate. (**c**) Post-contrast MR image shows relatively well-enhancing transitional zone (*T*) and anterior fibromuscular stroma (*F*). Also note the peripheral zone shows little enhancement due to prominent glandular portion (*P*)

T2W signal intensity, ill-defined margins, lack of capsule, lenticular shape, and extension into the fibromuscular stroma may help for the suspicion of prostate tumor [105].

Although post-biopsy hemorrhage may give us confusion, sometimes the hemorrhage can support the detection of a suspected lesion known as "hemorrhage exclusion sign." It is noted when the tumor composed of compact tumor cells presents as an isointense area on the T1-weighted images, surrounded by hyperintense hemorrhage in normal tissue [106] (Fig. 3.18).

To avoid unnecessary diagnostic difficulties due to biopsy hemorrhage, prostate MRI is usually recommended at least 6–8 weeks after biopsy; however, post-biopsy hemorrhage can also persist for several months [95]. It is presumed that the anticoagulative effects of the citrate which is highly concentrated in normal prostate tissue but is low in cancer tissue results in increased bleeding. Prostate cancer tissue is probably also a better site of degradation for hemorrhage than normal prostate tissue.

3.5.2 Diffusion-Weighted Image (DWI)

One of the most important recent advances in prostate cancer imaging is the use of diffusion-weighed

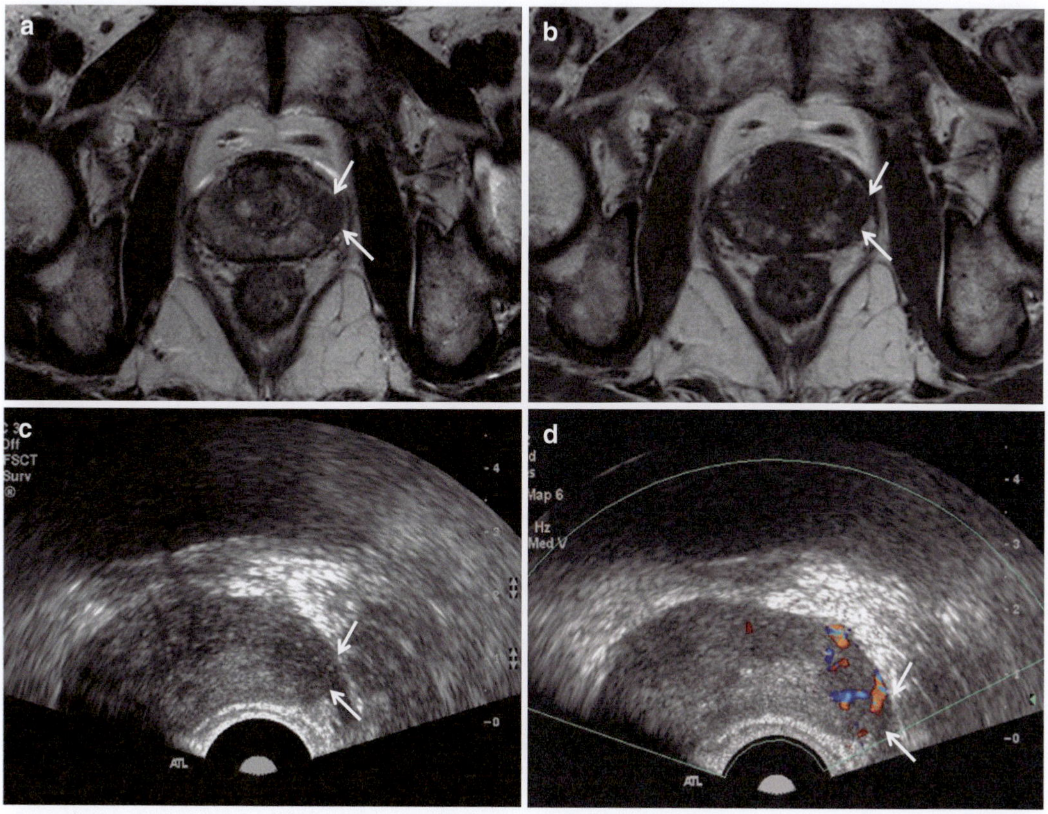

Fig. 3.18 Typical findings of prostate cancer. (**a**) T2-weighted axial scan shows well-marginated low signal intensity lesion located in left peripheral zone (*arrows*). (**b**) T1-weighted image also shows low signal intensity in left peripheral zone (*arrows*). Also note high signal intensity lesions in peripheral zone suggesting hemorrhage probably due to previous biopsy. (**c**) TRUS shows relatively irregular marginated low echoic lesion in same area (*arrows*). (**d**) Color Doppler image shows increase vascularity. The pathologic report after prostatectomy showed prostatic adenocarcinoma

imaging technique for characterizing prostate tissues and localizing the prostate cancer. DWI reflects the Brownian molecular motion of water. DWI has become an important part of oncological imaging since most of malignant tumors show different Brownian motion of water comparing normal tissue [107].

Recently, the technological developments of echo-planar imaging (EPI), high-amplitude gradients, multichannel coils, and the introduction of parallel imaging have extended the applications of DWI from neuroimaging to the abdomen and pelvis [108].

On DWI, the prostate cancers show high signal intensity on b values of 800–1000 s/mm^2. The sensitivity of the DWI sequence to molecular motion can be modified by changing the "b value" parameter. The b value depends on the amplitude, duration, and time interval between the paired gradients used to generate the DWI sequence [100].

An optimal b value for prostate imaging has not yet been established. Increased b values over 1000 s/mm^2 can increase tumor visibility, especially in the transition zone. However, increased b values also lead to an increase in the scan time and more pronounced image distortion artifacts. In 2012, the European Society of Urogenital Radiology (ESUR) suggests the use of the b values of 0, 100, and 800–1000 s/mm^2 [57].

The signal intensity on the DWI images reflects the amount of restriction of water to diffusion but also the T2-weighted characteristics of the tissue, which is the so-called "T2 shine through" effect. Apparent diffusion coefficient (ADC) can be calculated from the diffusion-weighted image data. The ADC map is obtained by using data from DWI trace images with at least two different b values and does not reflect T2W characteristics.

In the ADC maps, areas with diffusion restriction such as cancer show low signal intensity. The ADC levels are significantly lower in prostate cancer tissue than in noncancerous prostate, which enables the localization of prostate cancer [109]. Prostate cancer demonstrates high signal intensity on the DWI at high b values and has low signal intensity on the ADC map (Fig. 3.19). For detecting prostate cancer on diffusion-weighted imaging study, both DWI and the ADC map should be assessed because some tumors are diagnosed only on the ADC maps, and others are visible only on the DWI images [110]. Most studies showed that DWI is a very useful and it can increase sensitivity by 10–25 % in the diagnosis of prostate cancer [111–113]. From the point of view about technical aspect, to optimize the discrimination of prostate cancer from benign tissue using ADC, Kim et al. and Metens et al. suggested b values of 1000 to 1500 s/mm^2 to be the most helpful [114, 115].

Because ADC values are lower in BPH, usually located in transition zone, than in the peripheral zone, the accuracy for detection of prostate cancer in the transition zone is significantly lower and even lower in the prostate base [116]. And DWI must be evaluated together with T2-weighted imaging especially when assessing the central portions of the prostate gland to avoid confusing the BPH and prostate cancer [112].

Several studies showed that DWI can also reflect the information regarding the aggressiveness of prostate cancer. They have shown a correlation between the ADC and the Gleason score [117, 118]. ADC value in cancer has a negative correlation with the Gleason score, and low ADC values were seen primarily in high-grade aggressive prostate cancers [111, 119]. Some researchers reported that DWI may play a potential role in differentiating low-grade tumor with Gleason score of 6 from high-grade tumor with Gleason score of more than 7 (4+3) [117, 120, 121].

In conclusion, DWI is a fast and simple technique in the point of not only increasing accuracy

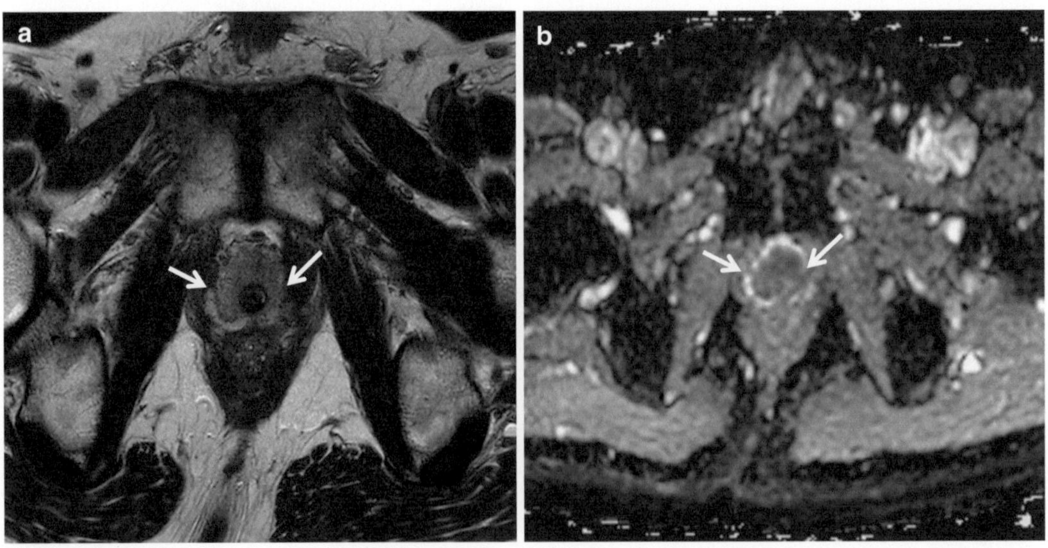

Fig. 3.19 Apical prostate cancer seen on diffusion-weighted imaging. (**a**) T2-weighted axial scan shows irregular marginated low signal intensity lesion surrounding prostatic urethra (*arrows*). (**b**) Apparent diffusion coefficient (ADC) map image shows signal drops of prostate apex (*arrows*). This lesion was confirmed as prostate cancer after prostatectomy

in detection but also providing additional quantitative information that correlates with aggressiveness of prostate cancer.

3.5.3 Dynamic Contrast-Enhanced MRI

Dynamic contrast-enhanced (DCE) MRI is a fast T1-weighted imaging technique that dynamically measures a bolus pass of an intravenously administrated MR contrast agent through the prostate and cancer [13]. The goal of DCE imaging is to capture the passage of contrast material into and out of the prostate using T1WI with high temporal resolutions. In DCE acquisition, the temporal resolution is fast enough to capture the rapid increase of signal within the first 30 s of contrast administration.

Contrast-enhanced MRI sequences can be used to assess the vascularity and permeability of tissues. Usually fast T1-weighted gradient echo sequences with a temporal resolution of 4–10 s are used in prostate imaging [57]. Prostate cancers are characterized by early washin (early peak enhancement) and early washout compared to normal prostate tissue [122].

For its nutrient and oxygen supply, a tumor rapidly forms new networks of tumor vessels named of neo-angiogenesis. In tumor tissue, these vessels made from tumor angiogenesis are often leaky or incomplete, which makes it easier for a contrast agent to extravasate into the extravascular extracellular space. In this extracellular space, the gadolinium-based contrast agent increases the signal intensity of T1-weighted images.

DCE-MRI measures the time-intensity curves passing through the prostate by repeatedly acquiring T1-weighted images at high temporal resolution with the order of seconds (Fig. 3.20). These time-intensity curves can be described semiquantitatively or modeled into pharmacokinetic parameters. The parameters of semiquantitative measurement include the start of enhancement, washin gradient, maximum enhancement, time to peak, washout gradient, and area under the gadolinium curve. And the pharmacokinetic parameters after the fitting to a pharmacokinetic model include

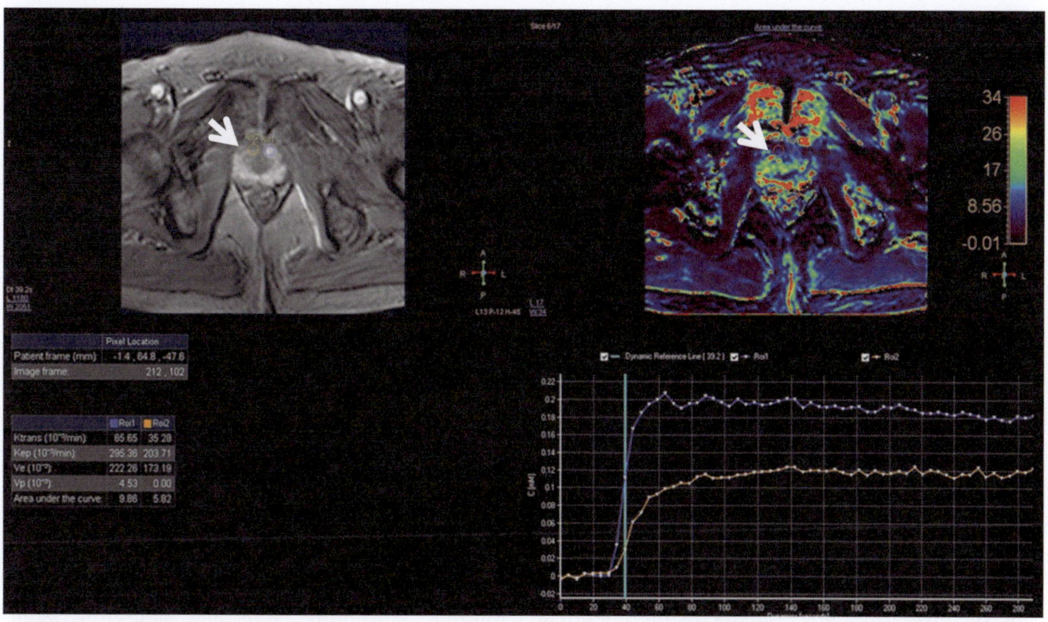

Fig. 3.20 Dynamic contrast-enhanced (DCE) MRI of prostate cancer. DCE images show early enhancing lesion in apex (*arrows*) comparing contralateral portion

forward leakage rate, washout rate constant, and leakage space [123].

For example, on the basis of enhancement curves, gadolinium concentrations in tissue and tissue transport constants in the direction of the tumor interstitium (K_{trans}) and back in the direction of the blood plasma (K_{ep}) can be calculated using two-compartment Tofts model [124].

For an accurate assessment of the model parameters, an arterial input function is needed that describes the shape of the contrast bolus arriving at the prostate. Tumor tissue of the prostate is characterized by increased pharmacokinetic parameters compared with healthy tissue.

DCE-MRI has been shown to be of use in detection and staging of prostate cancer within a multiparametric protocol [97, 125, 126] and is especially useful in follow-up after systemic treatment [127, 128]. Even though the currently available studies do not provide a clear conclusion regarding the improvement of prostate cancer detection via DCE, some studies were able to show an improvement of the diagnostic accuracy of conventional MRI (T2-weighted and T1-weighted images) when supplemented by DCE imaging [129, 130].

As with other imaging technologies, DCE also has a problem in differentiating hyperplastic nodules in BPH from prostate cancer. Because BPH nodules can enhance and wash out quickly like prostate cancer, K_{trans} and K_{ep} can be increased and limit the sensitivity and specificity of DCE in diagnosing prostate cancer [131]. In addition, inflammation can often have greater vascularity and tissue permeability, which confuse the diagnosis of prostate cancer.

In spite of these limitations, using DCE, the local staging of prostate cancer and the detection of local tumor relapses after definitive therapy can be significantly improved with good temporal resolution [127, 132].

3.5.4 MR Spectroscopy

MR spectroscopy (MRS) analyzes the chemical substances in an organ. The normal prostate gland produces citrate-containing secretion, resulting in high citrate content and a low choline level. A high concentration of citrate is unique to the prostate, and it plays an important role in normal physiological function of the gland [30]. Measured in parts per million (ppm), citrate, creatine, and choline-containing compounds appear at 3.2, 3.0, and 2.6 ppm with respect to the water resonance at 4.7 ppm [93]. In prostate cancer, the choline level is significantly elevated, and the citrate content is reduced due to the metaplastic processes of the cell membranes (Fig. 3.21). Increased concentrations of choline-containing metabolites are related to an increased cell turnover and have also been associated with the presence and progression of prostate cancer [133]. The relationship between these two metabolites can be used as a measure of malignancy [134]. At common clinical field strengths, even though it is difficult to differentiate choline peaks from creatine peaks on the spectra, the ratio of choline plus creatine to citrate is used as a metabolic biomarker for prostate cancer [135].

MRS increases the diagnostic accuracy of the morphological MRI examination from 52 to 75 % [136]. The European Society of Urogenital Radiology (ESUR) suggested Prostate MR Guidelines 2012 using either a qualitative or a quantitative approach for interpreting prostate MRS. The qualitative approach is based on visual analysis of the citrate and choline/creatine peaks. If the choline/creatine peak is higher than the citrate peak in at least three adjacent voxels, prostate cancer is suspected. In the quantitative approach, the areas of the peaks are measured, and choline plus creatine-to-citrate ratios higher than 0.72 in at least two adjacent voxels are considered to indicate malignant tissue, whereas ratios between 0.58 and 0.72 are considered ambiguous [57].

For the good spectral resolution, a homogeneous magnetic field and sufficient suppression of the fat and water signal during the measurement is needed in MRS measurements. In addition to sequence adjustments, MRS usually requires multiple shimming steps and saturation bands around the prostate for optimal information. Evaluation and interpretation of MRS are very

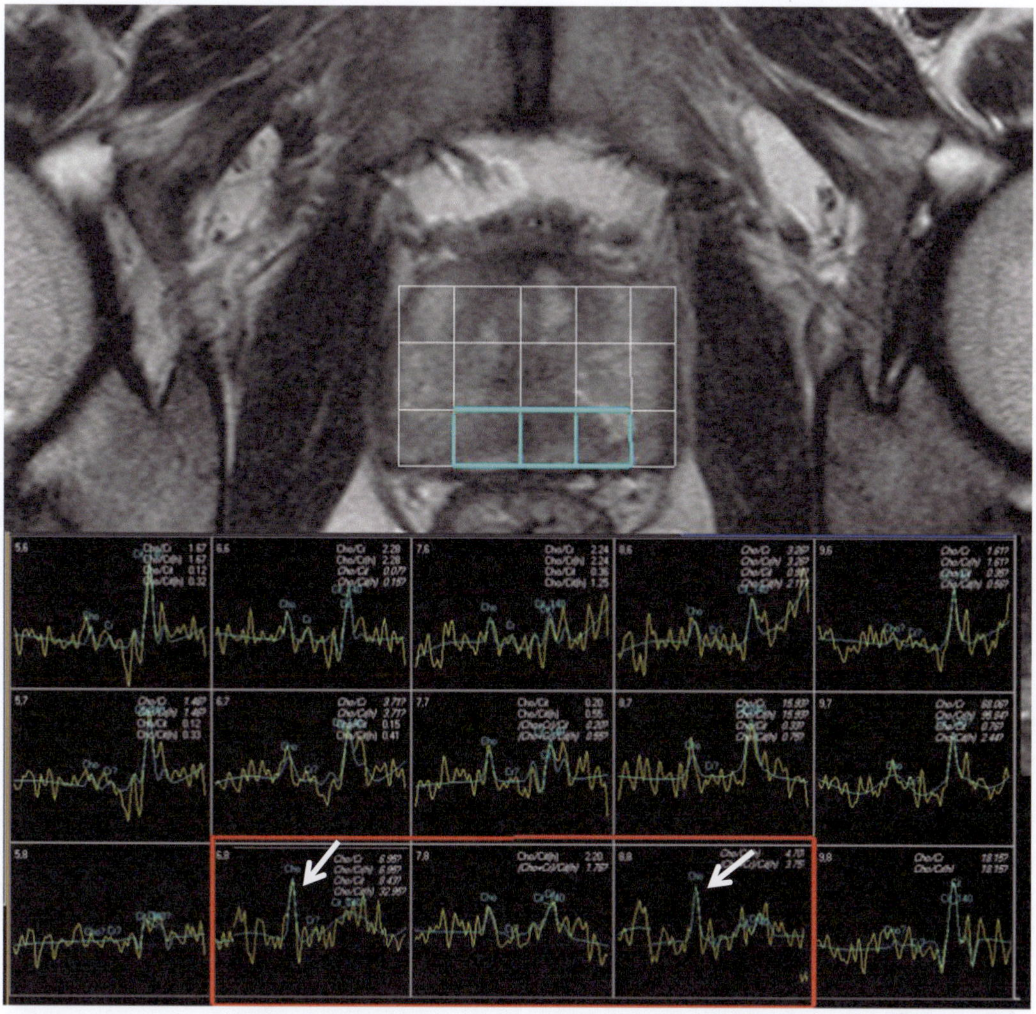

Fig. 3.21 MR spectroscopy (MRS) of prostate cancer. Note that the choline peak is increased in the box area (*arrows*). The lesion was confirmed as prostate cancer (Gleason score, 7) after prostatectomy (Courtesy of prof. Chan Kyo Kim, Samsung Medical Center)

complex and often only possible after appropriate physical adjustments. Because of these technical requirements, complexity of interpretation, and significant time investment, MR spectroscopy will remain limited in its daily use.

3.5.5 Multiparametric MRI

Multiparametric MRI incorporates several different imaging modalities including T2WI, DWI, and DCE to assess potential lesions in the prostate (Fig. 3.22). In prostate MR imaging, no single technique is able to adequately detect and characterize prostate cancer. T2-weighted image shows the best tissue contrast for the detection, localization, and staging of prostate cancer, which has shorter T2 comparing normal prostate tissues. However, other process such as prostatitis or BPH can also show T2 shortening. Although the image quality is not so good as T2-weighted image, DWI provides the information regarding Brownian motion of water molecules. Because free water motion is generally restricted within cancer tissue, DWI is an essential component of mpMRI (Fig. 3.22).

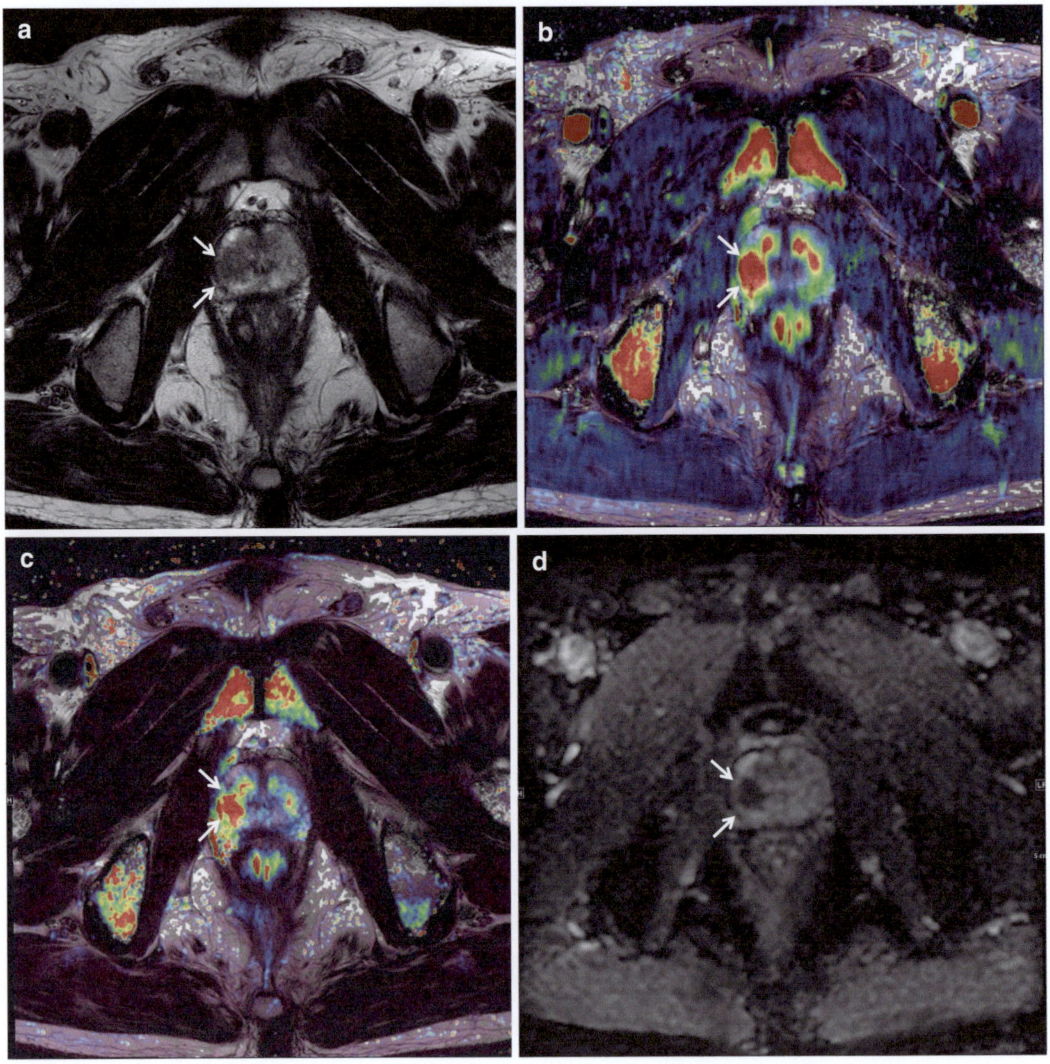

Fig. 3.22 Multiparametric MR images of prostate cancer. T2-weighted (**a**), Kep map (**b**), Ktrans map (**c**), and ADC map (**d**) images show focal abnormal lesion on right peripheral zone of prostate (*arrows*). This patient underwent radical prostatectomy and confirmed as prostate cancer with Gleason score of 7 (Courtesy of prof. Chan Kyo Kim, Samsung Medical Center)

Modern MRI studies often incorporate a combination of the several MR techniques including T2-weighted imaging, DWI, DCE, and MRS. The combination of anatomic T2W images and the functional techniques has been shown to increase the predictive power of MRI for detection and staging of prostate cancer [93]. ESUR prostate MR guideline suggests the use of T2W images plus two functional techniques [137].

There are several reports about the clinical results of mpMRI. Tanimoto et al. reported a significant increase in the area under the receiver operating curve (AUC) for the detection of prostate cancer as they evaluated a protocol with T2W images only (AUC = 0.711), a protocol combining T2W imaging and DWI (AUC = 0.905), and finally a more complete protocol including T2W imaging, DWI, and DCE (AUC = 0.966) [138]. Turkbey and colleagues also reported a higher sensitivity for the combination of T2W images, MRS, and DCEI than for each sequence alone [139].

The advantages of mpMRI are achieved by combining the information obtained with the various techniques. Software for the evaluation of two or more multiparametric images in one view is developed for the integrated interpretation of anatomic and functional findings. In addition, supportive techniques such as computer-aided diagnosis are needed to achieve fast and reliable diagnosis from large complex data [140–142]. For the more common usage of mpMRI, the education, experience, and dedications of radiologists are essential [143].

3.5.6 MR PI-RADS

In 2012, the ESUR created the magnetic resonance prostate imaging reporting and data system (MR PI-RADS) as part of its MRI guidelines for prostate imaging [57]. They suggested a standardized method for reporting mpMRI of the prostate for the detection of prostate cancer.

Based on criteria according to PI-RADS, every lesion suspicious for tumor within the prostate is assigned a point value between 1 and 5 for mpMRI, usually consisting of T2W, DWI, and DCE. A value 1 means that a lesion is probably benign, while a value 5 indicates a high probability of malignancy. Total point value is calculated for every lesion suspicious for tumor [144]. Thus, a probability statement regarding the presence of a clinically significant prostate cancer should be possible. Many studies reported good and reproducible diagnosis accuracy [145–147]. In 2015, they revised PI-RADS to PI-RADS v2. The difference point of PI-RADS v1 and v2 is that the primary determining sequence is different according to the zone in v2. According to PI-RADS v2, for the peripheral zone, DWI is the primary determining sequence; on the contrary, for the transition zone, T2-weighted image is the primary determining sequence.

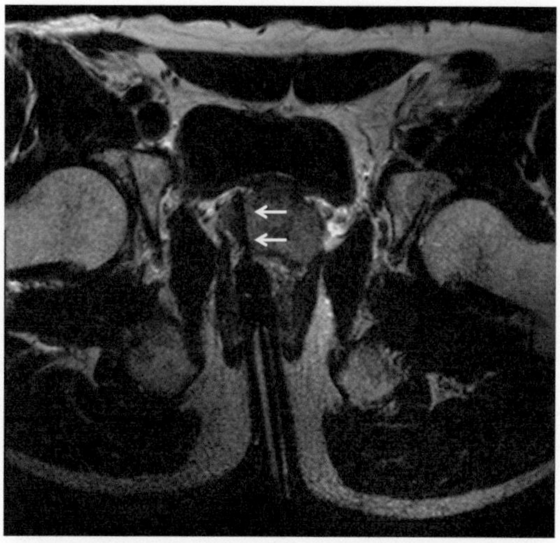

Fig. 3.23 MR-guided biopsy using MR-compatible device in the magnet. MR compatible endorectal device is inserted into the rectum, and the location of the needle can be confirmed in MR magnet (*arrows*) (Courtesy of Prof. Chan Kyo Kim, Samsung Medical Center)

3.5.7 MRI-Guided Biopsy

If patients have negative results after TRUS-guided biopsy with clinically suspicion of prostate cancer, MRI can be used to detect suspicious areas to be targeted during TRUS-guided biopsies. Three different methods are suggested in MR-guided biopsy. The first one is to use fusion software for MRI and TRUS images during TRUS-guided biopsy procedure, which is the most common method using MRI. The second one is direct targeting in the magnet using MRI compatible devices (Fig. 3.23). The last one is cognitive targeting in which the operator reviews the MRI images before TRUS-guided prostate biopsy and tries to target the suspected area during the TRUS-guided biopsy [10].

Many literatures about image-guided biopsy of prostate using MRI images revealed that most studies reported superior performance than random systematic biopsies [100]. Haffner et al. reported a higher diagnostic accuracy for the detection of significant cancer than random systematic biopsies when they used cognitively targeted biopsies (0.98 vs. 0.88, respectively) [148].

In random systematic biopsies, the tumors located at low apical and anterior prostate are difficult to detect. Anteriorly located prostate tumors account for about 21 % of all prostate cancers and are more often missed on systematic biopsies [149]. A study using mpMRI-targeted biopsy revealed that the accuracy of prostate biopsy on anterior tumors was about 98 %, comparing 46 % in random systematic biopsies [150]. Clinically, under the situation of elevated PSA and a negative biopsy, the option to perform the repeat biopsy using direct or indirect MRI-guiding can be suggested.

3.5.8 MRI for Active Surveillance

Active surveillance is defined as the initial expectant management, with close follow-up and selective delayed intervention for the subset of patients reclassified over time as at higher risk for progression, based on clinical, pathological, or molecular parameters [151]. The criteria of active surveillance include Gleason ≤6, PSA <10 ng/ml, and fewer than three positive biopsies. All core biopsies should not contain more than 50 % cancer involvement. mpMRI can play a significant role in identifying suitable patients [152].

Recently, as alternatives to the prostatectomy, a number of minimally invasive, focal, organ-preserving methods have been introduced. These methods include focal tumor ablation using cryoablation, high intensity-focused ultrasound (HIFU), or laser-induced ablation [153]. The main advantages of these treatments are to avoid postoperative complications such as incontinence and impotence. Advanced imaging technologies including mpMRI made it possible to determine the exact location of relevant tumor foci and to guide focal therapies [153].

3.5.9 MR Imaging of Treated Prostate Cancer

The treatment options of prostate cancer include radical prostatectomy, radiation therapy, androgen-deprivation therapy, or focal therapy such as cryotherapy or HIFU. Radical prostatectomy has been performed for more than a century and the most common treatment choice in patients with organ-confined disease [154]. MRI after radical prostatectomy reveals low signal intensity at anastomotic site. These lesions suggest postoperative scarring. Sometimes the remained seminal vesicles are observed in about 20 % of patients after prostatectomy [155]. The presence of soft tissue showing iso-signal intensity on T1-weighted image and slightly hyperintense signal intensity on T2-weighted image at prostatectomy site strongly suggests the tumor recurrence. The most common site of prostate cancer recurrence is around vesicourethral anastomosis around urinary bladder and membranous urethra [127]. In most cases, it is possible to differentiate the tumor recurrence at anastomotic site and postoperative fibrosis. On DCE-MRI, recurrent tumor tends to early enhancement and early washout pattern, while postoperative changes tend to show no enhancement or mild enhancement in the venous phase (Fig. 3.24).

Radiation therapy is another option alternative to prostatectomy. It is known that about 25 % of patients with prostate cancer undergo radiation therapy [156]. Three-dimensional conformal RT is introduced [157]. The computer modifies the radiation beams to focus the region of the prostate. Intensity-modulated radiation therapy is one of the most sophisticated types of radiation therapy. Brachytherapy, in which radioactive seeds or needles are implanted directly into the prostate gland and sometimes into the surrounding tissues, is one of radiation therapy. After radiation therapy, MR study reveals that the entire prostate and seminal vesicles show marked decreased size and low signal intensity on T1- and T2-weighted images. The whole prostate, including central zone, transitional zone, and peripheral zone, is not distinct and shows low signal intensities. The recurrent tumor after radiation therapy typically shows a nodular lesion of lower signal intensity than adjacent normal prostate [158]. Restricted diffusion on DWI or rapid enhancement on DCE-MRI suggests the presence of tumor recurrence [158].

Androgen deprivation therapy has been used in patients with metastasis, increasing PSA levels after local treatment or advanced disease.

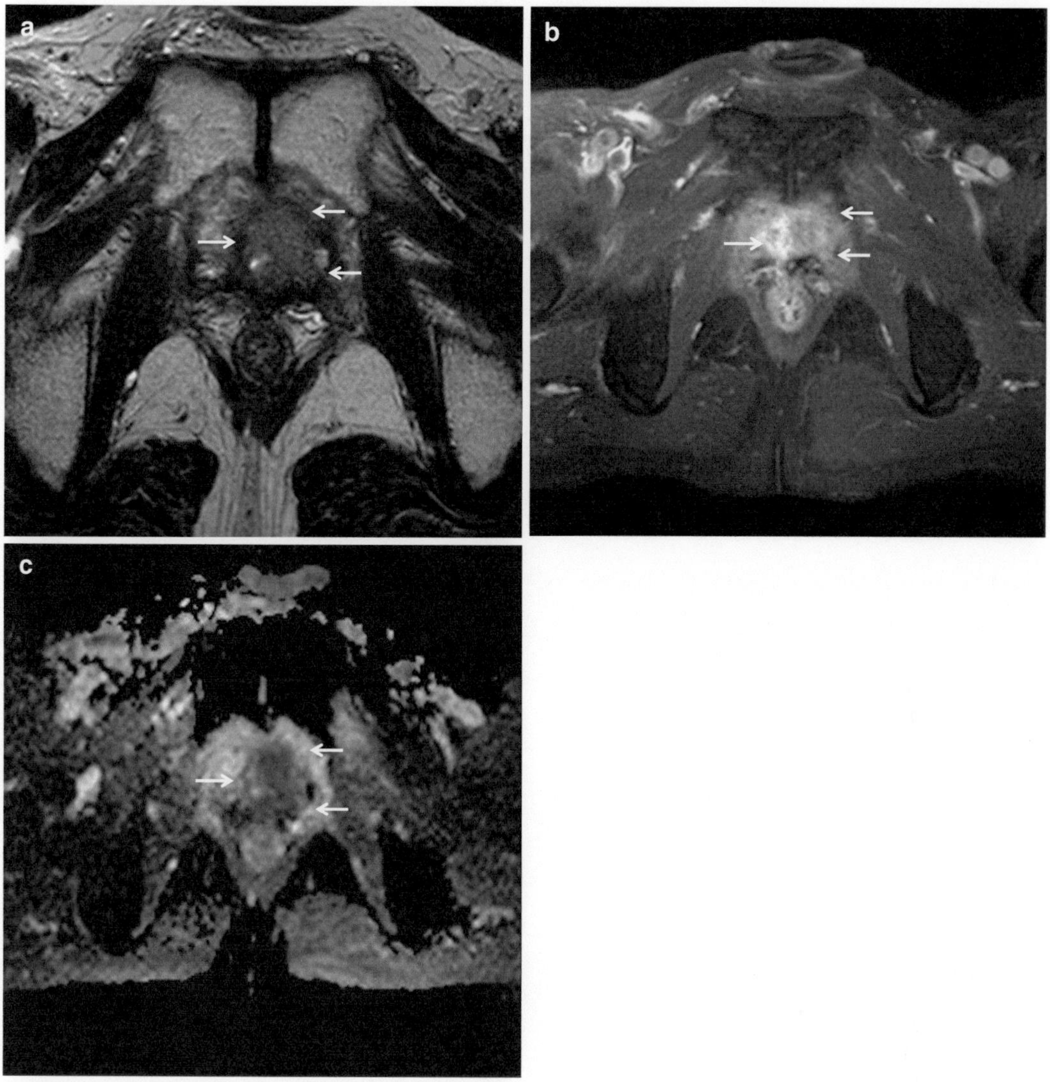

Fig. 3.24 Prostate cancer recurrence after prostatectomy. (**a**) T2-weighted axial scan shows slightly high signal intensity lesion at anastomotic site (*arrows*). (**b**) Post-contrast T1-weighted image shows well-enhancing mass-like lesion at anastomotic site (*arrows*). (**c**) ADC map shows decreased signal intensity lesion at anastomotic site. TRUS-guided biopsy revealed that this lesion was prostate cancer with Gleason score of 9

Androgen deprivation therapy can be performed surgically or pharmacologically [159]. The MRI findings of after-androgen-deprivation therapy are similar to those after radiation therapy. The size and the signal intensity of prostate are decreased (Fig. 3.25). However, the radiation therapy-induced changes in adjacent organs are not definite [158].

Especially, MRI plays an important role not only in localized prostate cancer but also in evaluating the recurrence after prostatectomy, radiation therapy, or androgen-deprivation therapy.

3.5.10 Hyperpolarized MRI

Hyperpolarized ^{13}C MRI is a new technique that enhances signal tens of thousandfold [160]. For ^{13}C imaging, the polarization mixture typically contains the ^{13}C-enriched substrate, free radical,

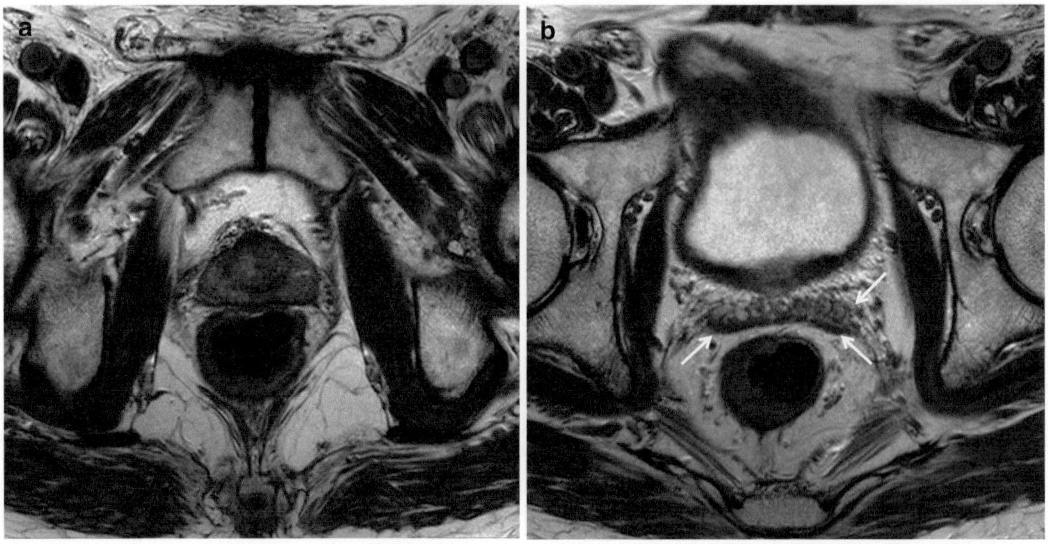

Fig. 3.25 Prostate MR imaging after hormone therapy. This 85-year-old man underwent hormone therapy for 1 year since he was diagnosed as prostate cancer. (**a**) T2-weighted axial scan shows atrophic changes of prostate. The signal intensity of prostate is low regardless of the zone. (**b**) The seminal vesicle also shows atrophic changes and obliteration of seminal vesicle lumen (*arrows*)

gadolinium, and glassing material. Chen et al. reported their initial experience about hyperpolarized ^{13}C metabolic imaging of mice with transgenic adenocarcinoma of the prostate (TRAMP) using hyperpolarized ^{13}C-pyruvate. They found that highly elevated lactate signal in later-stage prostate tumors. In case of advanced prostate cancer, the level of lactate signal is increased with tumor progression and correlated with histologic grade [160].

3.5.11 The Future of Prostate MR

There are a number of ongoing technical developments that may have an impact on the evaluation of prostate. The development of ultrahigh-field MR systems such as 7 T showed the possibilities for potentially higher spatial and spectral resolution [137], diffusion tensor imaging (DTI) [161], and multi-b-factor approaches to access multicomponent diffusion information. Hyperpolarized ^{13}C MRI showed the potentials for direct observation and measurement of dynamics within the biochemical pathways in normal and abnormal prostate metabolism [162]. MR elastography that combines the principles of ultrasound elasticity and MRI to make measures of the "elasticity or stiffness" of prostate tissues has been demonstrated [163, 164]. Even though these techniques have technical challenges, they show potentials for exact localization of the prostate cancer by advanced techniques and for getting the representative prostate tissue by advanced image-guided biopsy techniques.

3.6 PET-CT

PET/CT is a widely used molecular imaging modality. ^{18}F-FDG, glucose metabolism targeting radiotracer, is the main radiotracer for oncologic study. Enhanced glucose metabolism, Warburg effect, is one of the hallmarks in cancer [165], though it is not a cancer-specific phenomenon. The clinical utility of oncology PET using FDG has been proven in staging and restaging of malignant tumors such as the head and neck, lung, breast, and colorectal cancers, malignant lymphoma, and melanoma [166]. FDG-PET is capable of visualizing malignant tumors and

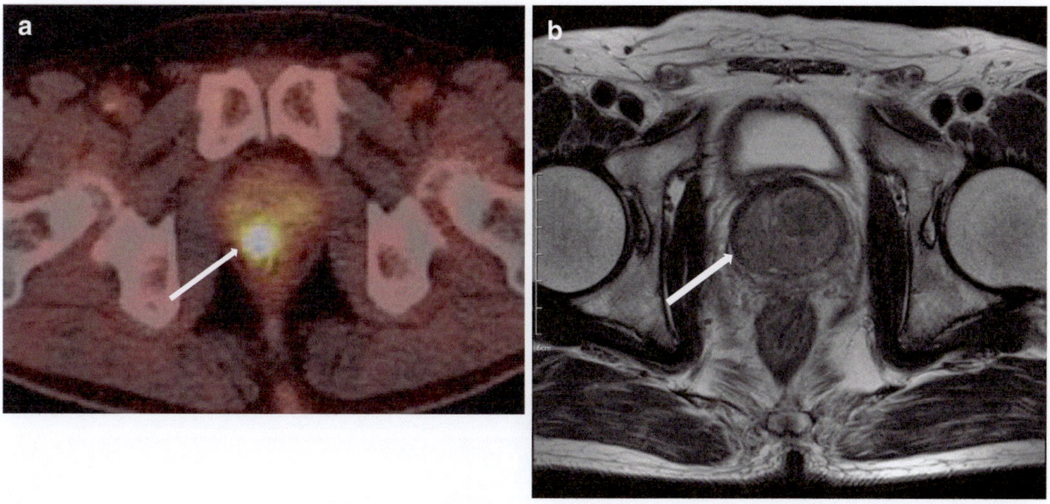

Fig. 3.26 FDG-PET has a limited role in detecting malignant tumors of the prostate. However, it may be helpful in patients with suspected poorly differentiated prostate cancer and higher serum PSA levels. A 64-year-old man presented with nocturia/hematuria and elevated serum PSA level of 19.7 ng/mL. FDG-PET/CT (**a**) shows focal hypermetabolism (3.7 of SUVmax, *arrow*) corresponding the lesion of low signal intensity (*arrow*) on T2-weighted MRI (**b**). Prostate adenocarcinoma was confirmed on pathology with Gleason score of 7 (4 + 3)

associated lymph nodes and distal metastatic sites in a single test. However, ^{18}F-FDG-PET has a limited role in primary diagnosis and staging of the prostate cancer due to not only overlap accumulation of normal and abnormal prostate tissue but also the intrinsic metabolic alteration of prostate cancer itself [167]. There is limited data on the use of FDG-PET/CT in initial staging of prostate cancer because of the general low avidity of FDG for the primary prostate cancer [168]. But, FDG-PET is not generally recommended in the diagnosis or staging of clinically organ-confined disease due to overlap of uptake among normal, benign, and tumor tissues and the high excreted radiotracer in the adjacent urinary bladder [169]. However, FDG-PET may be useful in patients with suspected poorly differentiated primary tumors (Gleason sum score above 7) and higher serum PSA level [170] (Figs. 3.1 and 3.26). In the early analysis of the National Oncologic PET Registry (NOPR) data in the Unites States for initial staging of prostate cancer, FDG-PET/CT had an impact on clinical management in 32 % (95 % CI: 30.0–34.1 %) [171].

In recent years, lipogenesis targeting radiotracer, such as ^{11}C-choline or ^{11}C-acetate upregulated in malignant cells, has shown potential usefulness in brain, prostate, and esophageal cancers because of enhanced synthesis of membrane phospholipids [172]. Both ^{11}C-choline and ^{18}F-fluorocholine (FCH) have been studied for prostate cancer. ^{11}C-choline has the advantage of low excreted urine activity. ^{18}F-fluorocholine has the advantage of longer half-life that facilitates regional tracer distribution without the need of on-site cyclotron and radiochemistry facilities [173]. ^{18}F-FCH PET/CT reveals promising but limited evidence for primary prostate cancer staging and has been known to be useful for detection of locoregional and distant metastasis of recurred prostate cancer [172, 174] (Fig. 3.27). A systematic review and meta-analysis by Umbehr et al. of ^{11}C-choline and ^{18}F-fluorocholine PET for the initial staging of prostate cancer reported a pooled sensitivity and specificity of 84 % and 79 % on a per-patient basis (10 studies, $n=637$ patients, respectively) [175, 176]. The uptake of choline tracers in prostate cancer is higher than that of prostate hyperplasia, but there is still overlap between the prostate cancer and benign disease [177].

Other kinds of molecular imaging targets have been proposed in order for more specific to prostate cancer. Anti-1-amino-3-^{18}F--

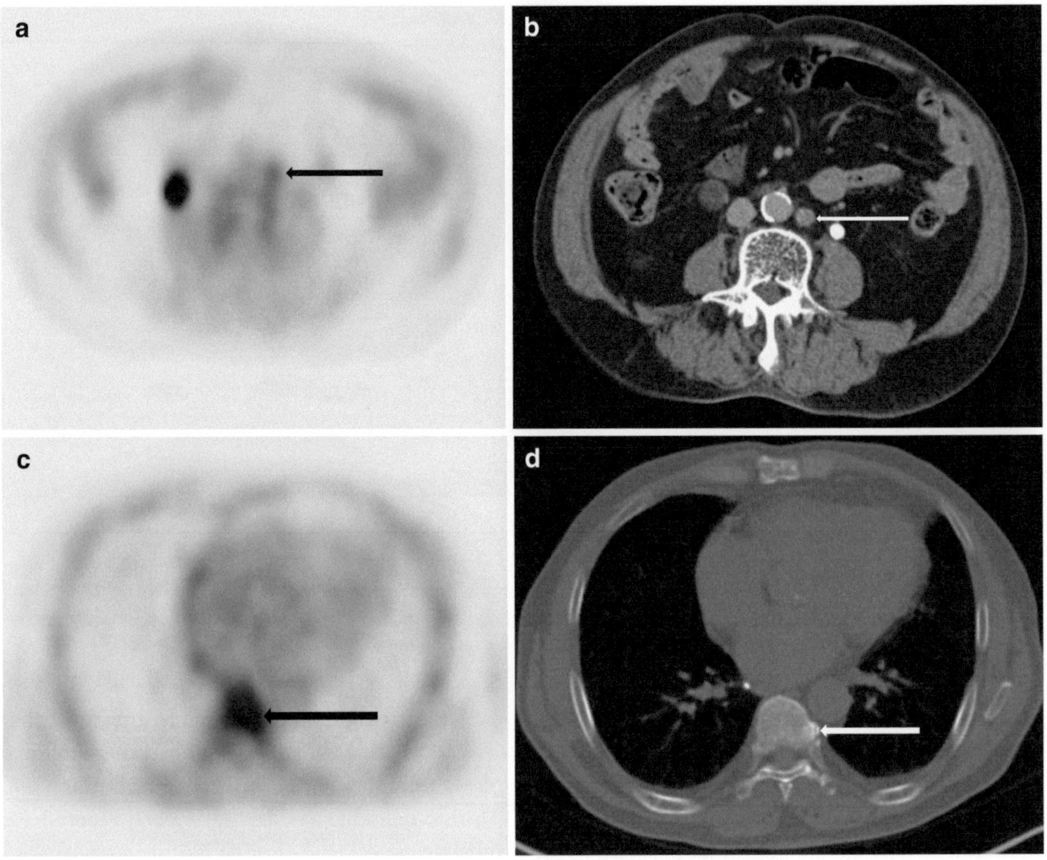

Fig. 3.27 A 84-year-old patient performed 18F-FCH PET/CT in suspicion of prostate cancer recurrence. Serum prostate-specific antigen (PSA) level increased from 2.3 to 57.3 ng/ml. On 18F-FCH PET/CT, paraaortic lymph nodes metastasis (**a, b**, *arrow*) and T8 spine metastasis (**c, d**, *arrow*) are detected

fluorocyclobutane-1-carboxylic acid (anti-^{18}F-FACBC) is a synthetic non-metabolized amino acid analog that accumulates in prostate cancer via overexpression of the ASC (alanine, serine, and cysteine) transport system and other amino acid transport systems [178]. ^{18}F-fluoro-5α-dihydrotestosterone (^{18}F-FDHT) is a labeled analog targeting the androgen receptor, which plays an important role in the development, growth, and maintenance of the prostate gland [179]. PSMA is a type II cell surface transmembrane glycoprotein (also known as folate hydrolase I or glutamate carboxypeptidase II) upregulated in prostate cancer, providing a promising molecular target for diagnostic imaging and directed therapy labeled with radionuclide such as ^{177}Lu or ^{90}Y [180].

Another approach is to use the multimodal, multiparametric imaging for the prostate cancer. Simultaneous PET/MRI has been developed lately and expected to be a better diagnostic imaging modality by combining functional, molecular, and morphological information. Moreover, it is expected to be valuable than PET/CT in the aspect of one-stop imaging with low radiation exposure and good soft tissue contrast resolution [181]. Combined PET/MR imaging could facilitate the use of MRI-assisted metabolic parameters or PET-guided multiparametric imaging analysis for the precise identification of targeted lesions and appropriate method for diagnosis and therapy planning of the primary prostate cancer [182] (Fig. 3.28). Simultaneous acquisition of multiparametric

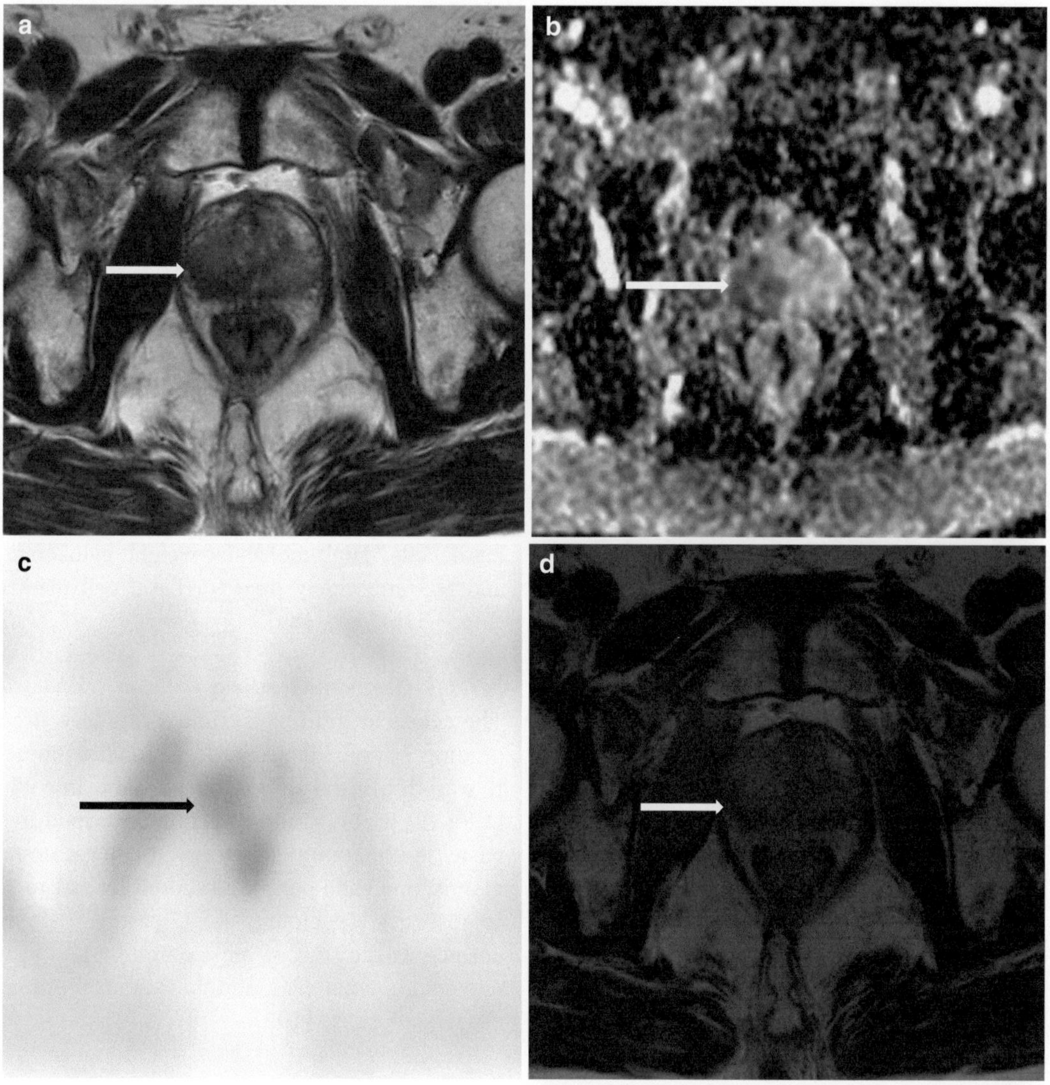

Fig. 3.28 A 77-year-old patient performed 18F-FCH PET/MRI for initial staging of prostate cancer. Axial T2-weighted MRI (**a**) shows low signal intensity (*arrow*) in the prostate cancer, with diffusion restriction (*arrow*) on the ADC map (**b**). 18F-FCH PET (**c**) and PET/MRI (**d**) demonstrated concordant results (*arrow*) with a possible application of MRI-assisted metabolic-volumetric PET quantification

MR and PET images with an appropriate radiotracer may be particularly valuable for identifying high-yield candidate biopsy sites that could reduce false-negative initial and repeated biopsies [183, 184].

In summary, FDG-PET has been evaluated with promising and disappointing results in the field of urologic cancer [166, 168]. PET as molecular imaging and PET/MRI with dual tracers and multiparametric approaches are challenging fields to be applicable to all clinical phases of prostate cancer with the concept of precision and personalized medicine [173, 182]. Additional potential applications may include not only the assessment but also the deciphering of new insights into the biologic changes induced by various novel therapies [176].

3.7 Pathology of Prostate Cancer

3.7.1 Acinar Adenocarcinoma

3.7.1.1 Macroscopy

Grossly prostatic adenocarcinoma is a hard, yellow, or whitish nodule (Fig. 3.29). But frequently, prostatic adenocarcinoma is not distinguishable grossly, and tumor border is also not evident. Prostatic acinar adenocarcinoma mainly arises in the peripheral zone (posterior and posterolateral side) and is frequently multifocal [185–187].

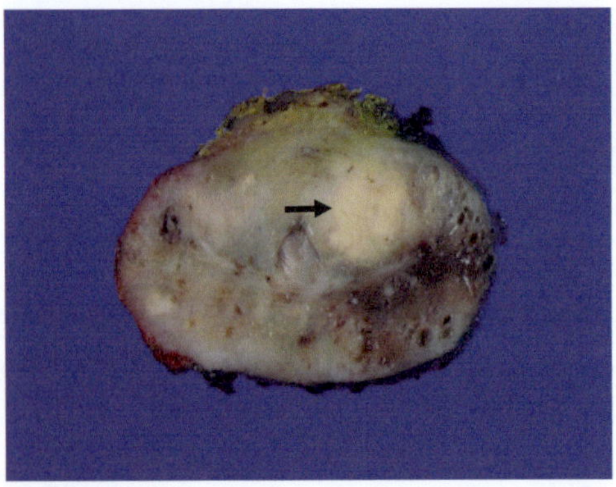

Fig. 3.29 On the cut surface of prostatectomy specimen, a vague yellow to whitish nodule (*arrow*) is found in the left lobe. Grossly prostatic adenocarcinomas are frequently ill-defined

3.7.1.2 Microscopy

Microscopic appearance of acinar adenocarcinomas varies according to their differentiation. Well-differentiated tumors show aggregation of well-formed small glands with infiltration between benign glands (Fig. 3.30a). Poorly differentiated tumors reveal poorly formed glands, glandular fusion, cribriform glands, single cells, cords, or solid tumor nests (Fig. 3.30b).

Two differences between malignant and benign prostatic glands help the pathological diagnosis of prostatic adenocarcinoma. First, malignant glands have prominent nucleoli. Second, basal cells are not present in malignant glands (Fig. 3.31a). Loss of basal cells is readily identifiable by immunohistochemical staining for basal cells. High-molecular-weight cytokeratin and p63 are widely used for basal cell marker (Fig. 3.31b) [188, 189].

3.7.1.3 Gleason Grading

The Gleason grading system is widely used grading system of prostatic adenocarcinoma. It was firstly developed by Gleason in 1966 [190, 191]. This grading system described five basic architectural patterns of carcinoma glands, and each pattern is scored from 1 to 5. In resection specimen, the Gleason grade is defined as the sum of most common and second common patterns, and this sum is reported as Gleason score [192].

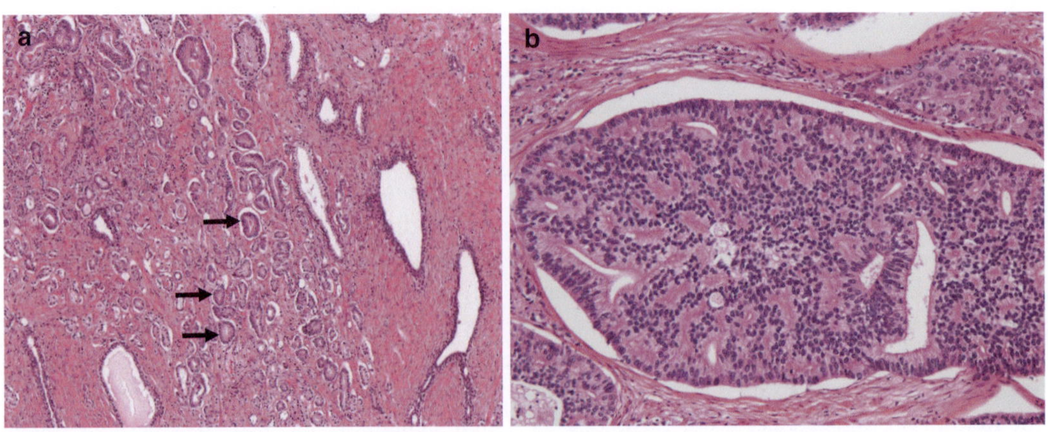

Fig. 3.30 (**a**) Infiltrations of small well-formed carcinoma glands (*arrows*) between normal glands are found in well-differentiated adenocarcinoma. (**b**) Poorly differentiated adenocarcinoma shows cribriform glands

This grading system has been modified several times. Recently, International Society of Urological Pathology (ISUP) 2005 consensus conference proposed some modification in Gleason grading system. This modification includes criteria of Gleason pattern, grading of variants of prostatic adenocarcinoma, and reporting of secondary and tertiary pattern.

According to the 2005 ISUP modified Gleason system [192], Gleason patterns are defined as below:

Pattern 1 is defined as a well-circumscribed nodule of closely packed, well-formed, medium-sized, round to oval glands. The glands are usually larger than pattern 3, and there is no infiltration into adjacent benign glands. This pattern is very rare. Pattern 2 is defined as fairly circumscribed nodule with minimal infiltration (Fig. 3.32a). The tumor glands shows more size variation and are more loosely arranged than pattern 1. Pattern 3 is defined as well-formed individually discrete glands with infiltration between benign glands (Fig. 3.32b). More size variation is present than pattern 1 or 2. Small cribriform glands with smooth margin are also included in this pattern. Pattern 3 is the most common pattern. Pattern 4 includes fused microacinar glands (Fig. 3.32c), ill-defined glands with inconspicuous lumina (Fig. 3.32d), and large cribriform glands (Fig. 3.32e). Pattern 5 is defined as tumors with no glandular differentiation. It consists of solid sheets (Fig. 3.32f), cords, or aggregation of single cells (Fig. 3.32g). Cribriform pattern with central comedonecrosis is also included in pattern 5 (Fig. 3.32h).

3.7.1.4 Variants of Acinar Adenocarcinoma

Some morphologic variants are present such as atrophic variant (Fig. 3.33a, b), pseudohyperplastic variant (Fig. 3.33c, d), and foamy gland variant (Fig. 3.33e).

3.7.1.5 High-Grade Prostatic Intraepithelial Neoplasia

High-grade prostatic intraepithelial neoplasia consists of atypical cells confined to preexisting prostatic duct or acini (Fig. 3.34a, b). The abnormal cells resemble adenocarcinoma cells frequently showing prominent nucleoli. This lesion has intact basal cell layer, and is frequently found around prostatic adenocarcinoma. High-grade prostatic intraepithelial neoplasia is regarded as a precursor for prostatic adenocarcinoma.

3.7.2 Other Carcinomas

3.7.2.1 Ductal Adenocarcinoma

Histologic feature of ductal adenocarcinoma is somewhat different from acinar adenocarcinoma. This tumor shows large papillary or cribriform

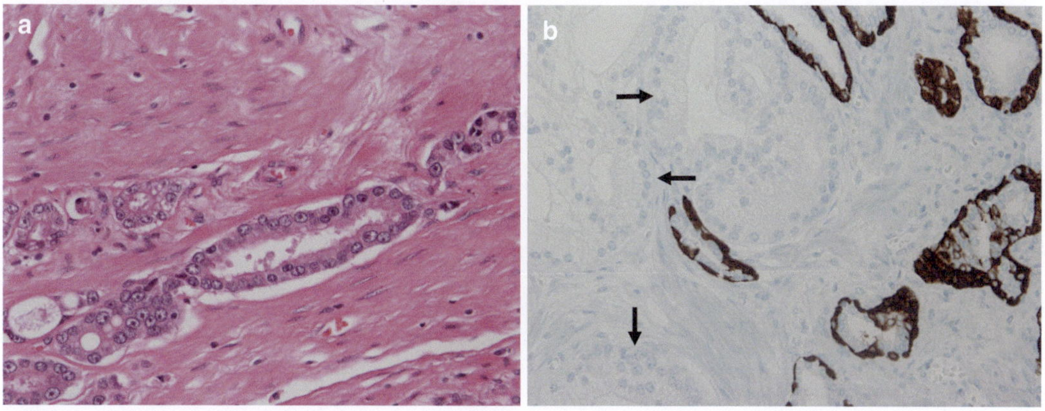

Fig. 3.31 (**a**) Malignant glands of prostate show prominent nucleoli and loss of basal cells. (**b**) Immunohistochemical staining for basal cell markers (high molecular weight cytokeratin and p63 cocktail) shows loss of basal cells in carcinoma glands (*arrows*). Adjacent normal glands have basal cells positively stained with basal cell markers

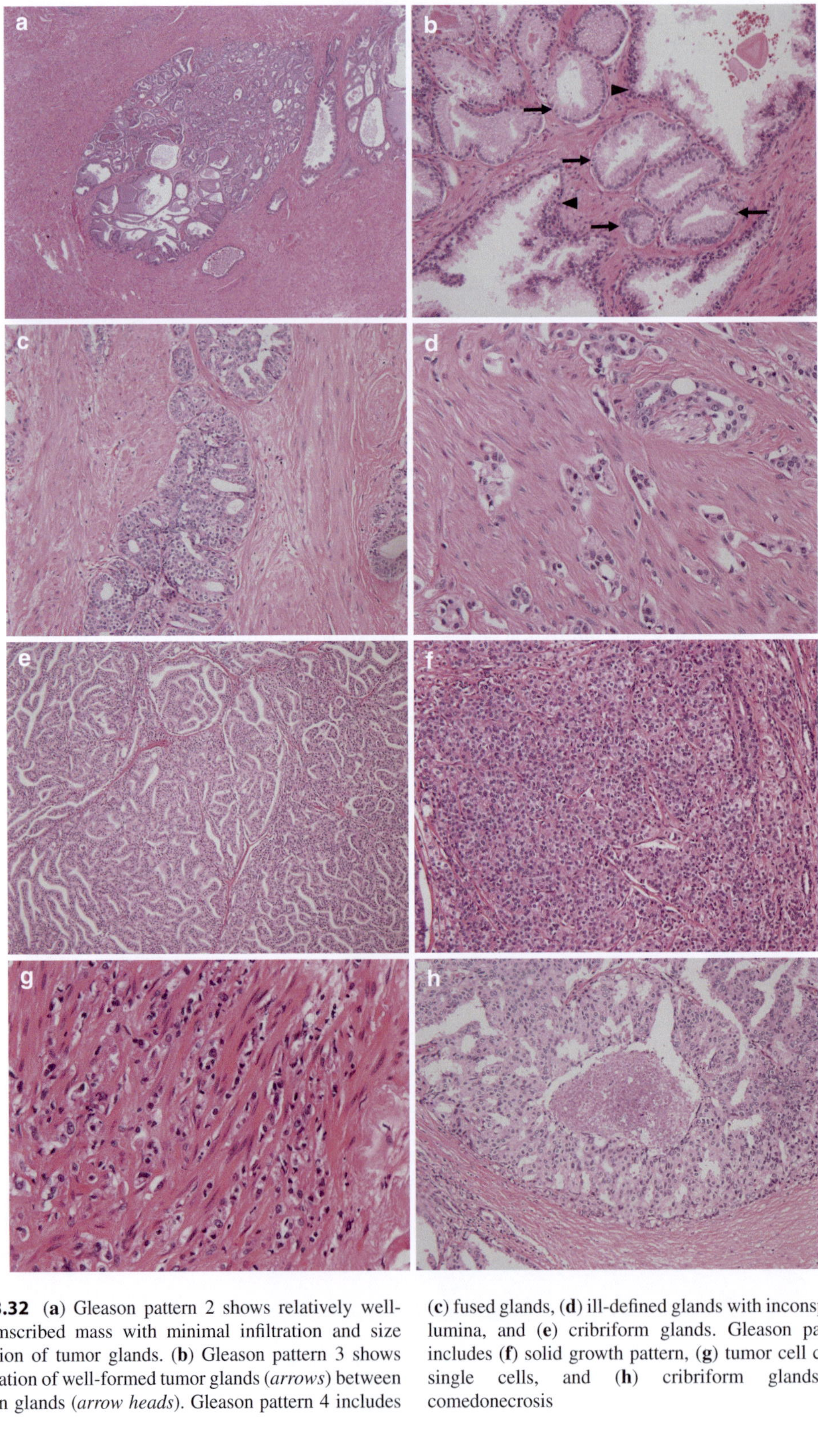

Fig. 3.32 (**a**) Gleason pattern 2 shows relatively well-circumscribed mass with minimal infiltration and size variation of tumor glands. (**b**) Gleason pattern 3 shows infiltration of well-formed tumor glands (*arrows*) between benign glands (*arrow heads*). Gleason pattern 4 includes (**c**) fused glands, (**d**) ill-defined glands with inconspicuous lumina, and (**e**) cribriform glands. Gleason pattern 5 includes (**f**) solid growth pattern, (**g**) tumor cell cords or single cells, and (**h**) cribriform glands with comedonecrosis

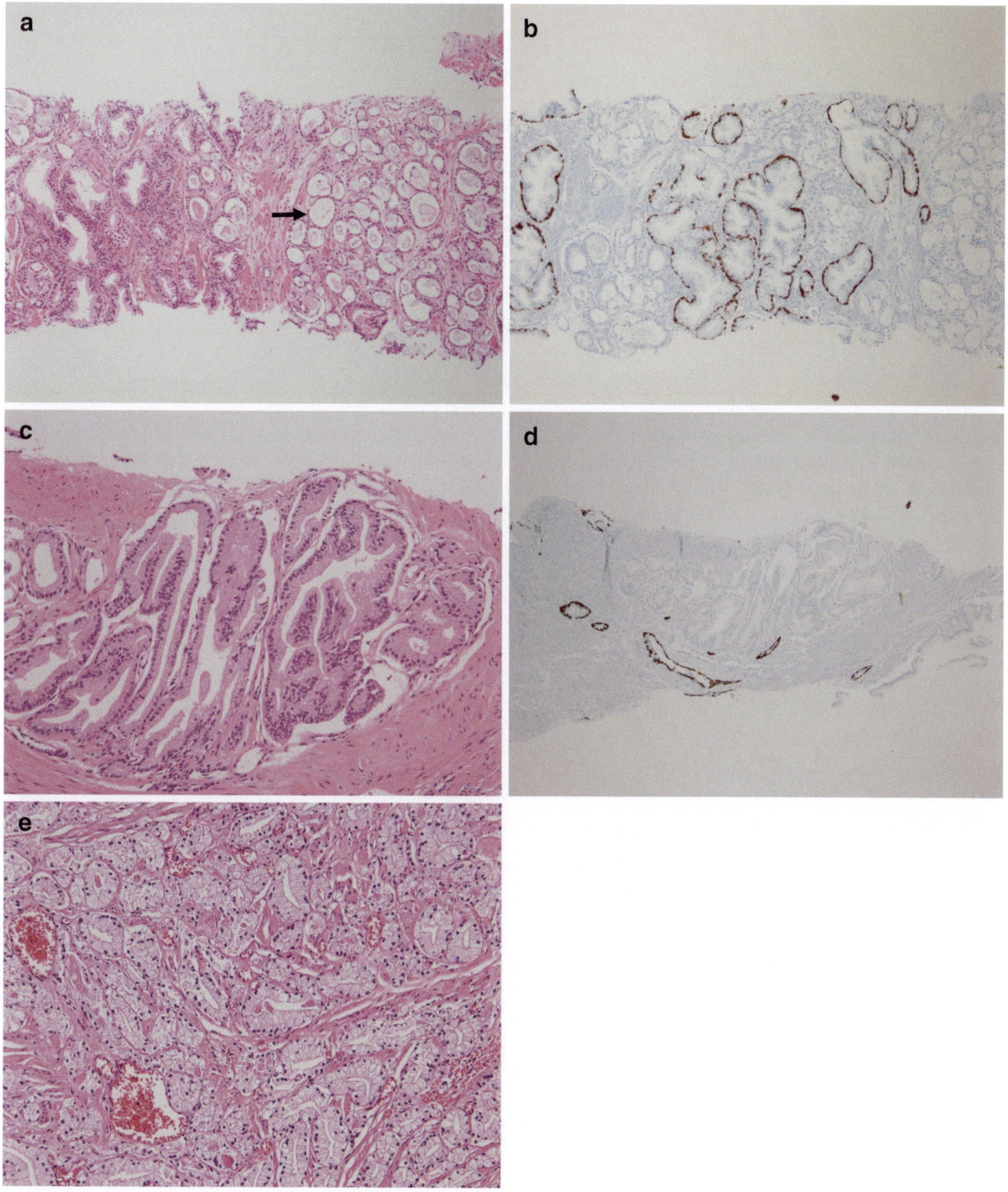

Fig. 3.33 Variants of prostatic adenocarcinoma. (**a**, **b**) Atrophic variant shows malignant tumor glands with scanty cytoplasm (*arrow*) (**a**), and these glands reveal the loss of basal cells in immunohistochemistry for basal cell markers, indicating their malignant feature (**b**). (**c**, **d**) Pseudohyperplastic variant shows large glands with papillary infoldings mimicking benign hyperplastic glands (**c**), but loss of basal cells in immunohistochemical staining for basal cell markers confirms the diagnosis of adenocarcinoma (**d**). (**e**) Foamy gland carcinoma reveals characteristic abundant foamy cytoplasm with relatively small nuclei

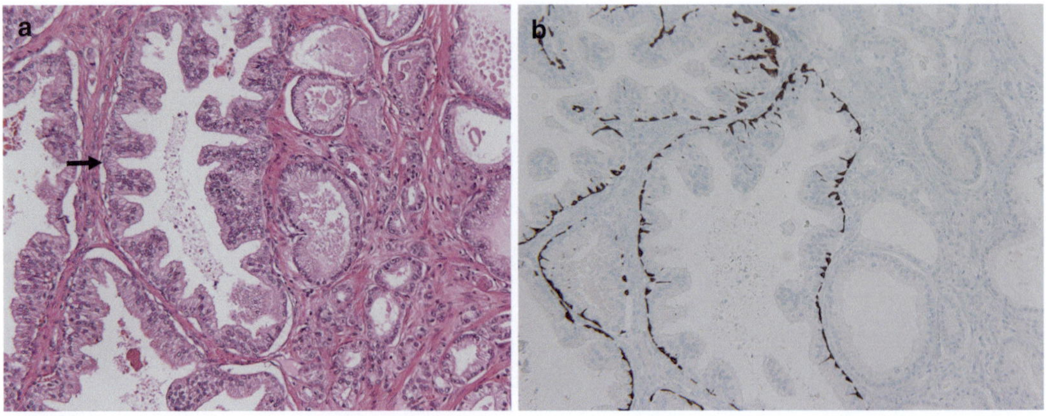

Fig. 3.34 Microscopic findings of high-grade prostatic intraepithelial neoplasia (HGPIN). (**a**) HGPIN in this photograph shows large glands with papillary infoldings (*arrow*). The lining cells occasionally show prominent nucleoli. Adenocarcinoma glands are found adjacent HGPIN. (**b**) Immunohistochemical staining for basal cells shows preserved basal cell layer in HGPIN

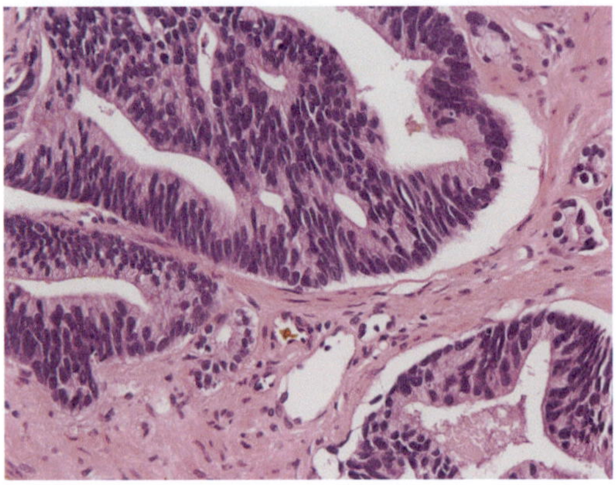

Fig. 3.35 Ductal adenocarcinoma consists of tall columnar cells with pseudostratification. This case shows cribriform pattern

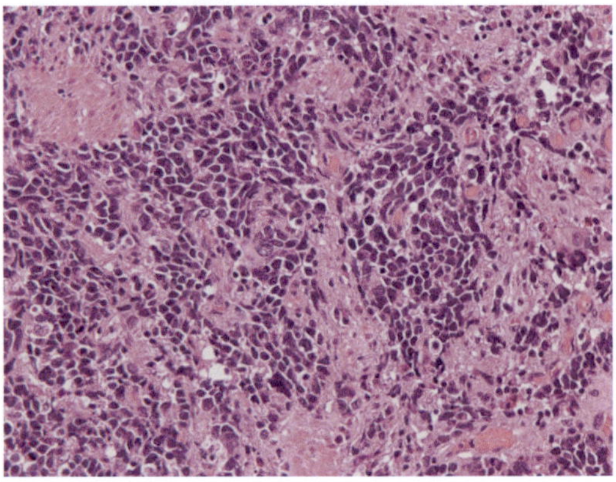

Fig. 3.36 Small cell carcinoma of prostate shows identical morphology to small cell carcinoma of other sites

architecture (Fig. 3.35). The tumor cells are tall columnar cells with pseudostratification. Basal cells are not present. This tumor is classified as Gleason pattern 4.

3.7.2.2 Urothelial Carcinoma

Urothelial carcinoma of prostate is developed in prostatic urethra or periurethral glands. Morphologic features are identical to bladder urothelial carcinoma.

3.7.2.3 Small Cell Carcinoma

Small cell carcinoma can be developed in prostate. Histologic features of small cell carcinoma of prostate are similar to small cell carcinoma of other sites. Microscopically tumor cells have scanty cytoplasm with round nuclei and "salt and pepper" nuclear chromatin pattern (Fig. 3.36). Necrosis is quite common. Tumor cells express the neuroendocrine markers.

3.8 Staging

The information about the staging is essential because it influences the treatment plans and guessing the prognosis and disease spread. The clinical parameters such as pretreatment PSA

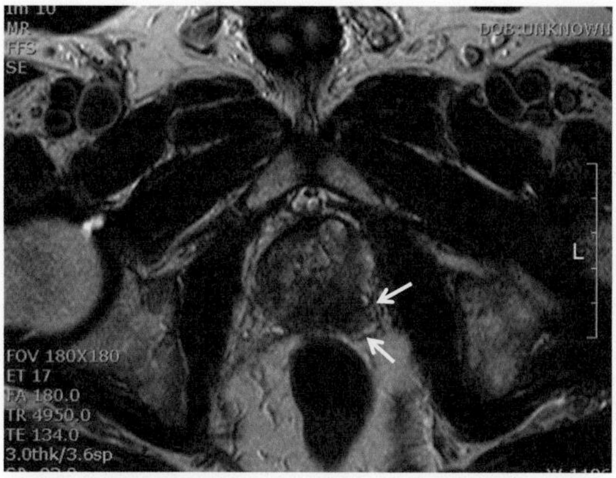

Fig. 3.37 Prostate cancer with periprostatic invasion. T2-weighted axial image shows irregular contour bulging lesion in left peripheral zone, suggesting periprostatic invasion (*arrows*)

level, rate of rise or doubling time, Gleason score, clinical T staging, and volume of disease detected on biopsy are also important in evaluating stages. Imaging modalities commonly used for the prostate include MR, CT, radioisotope bone scan, and positron emission tomography (PET). Local staging about periprostatic invasion is usually performed by digital rectal examination (DRE) and MRI (Fig. 3.37). Regional staging in pelvic area is performed by either CT or MRI. And CT or bone scan are used for the evaluation of distant metastasis, metastatic lymphadenopathy, or bone metastasis (Fig. 3.38). In addition, clinical or laboratory data including PSA level or Gleason score can also yield useful information for evaluating tumor stage.

For the staging of prostate cancer, the evaluation of seminal vesicle seen on MR is very important (Fig. 3.39). For the evaluation of seminal vesicle invasion, MR is the most commonly used modality. Jung et al. suggested six categories according the shape of seminal vesicle. Among six groups, the groups with apparent mass with destructive architecture or focal asymmetric low signal intensity lesion within the seminal vesicle without definite mass showed high positive predictive values [193].

The American Joint Committee on Cancer (AJCC) staging is a widely used staging system in prostate cancer [194]. Stage T1 is clinical staging defined as "clinically inapparent tumor neither palpable nor visible by imaging." Pathologic stage T2 means tumors confined to prostate. pT3 includes extraprostatic extension (pT3a) (Fig. 3.40a) and seminal vesicle invasion (pT3b) (Fig. 3.40b). pT4 is tumors with invasion of an adjust organ such as the rectum, levator muscle, or pelvic wall.

3.9 Treatment of Prostate Cancer

3.9.1 Active Surveillance

3.9.1.1 Introduction

Widespread prostate cancer screening, which uses DRE and PSA, has led to increase the detection of low-volume, low-grade disease, namely, clinically insignificant prostate cancer (CIPC) [195]. Immediate definitive treatment for CIPC may give rise to unnecessary complications related to treatment. In the light of these points of view, active surveillance (AS) can redeem the problems of overdiagnosis and overtreatment resulting from early diagnosis of prostate cancer [196]. Therefore, AS has been universally considered to be a therapeutic modality in low-risk-localized prostate cancer. Given that active intervention is performed if there is clear evidence of progression of the cancer during observation period, AS is a distinct therapeutic modality from previous expectant management or watchful waiting [197]. In other words, the objective of AS is to conduct a definitive therapy with curative intent in patients who show clear signs of cancer progression and to reduce treatment-related complications in patients with a low possibility of progression during observation period.

3.9.1.2 Definition of CIPC

CIPC generally refers to "low-risk" prostate cancer. Many physicians and patients take into account AS for selected low-risk prostate cancers. In fact, one of the major controversies in AS may be a definition of the CIPC [198]. The criteria stratifying the risk of prostate cancer have been suggested by several investigators

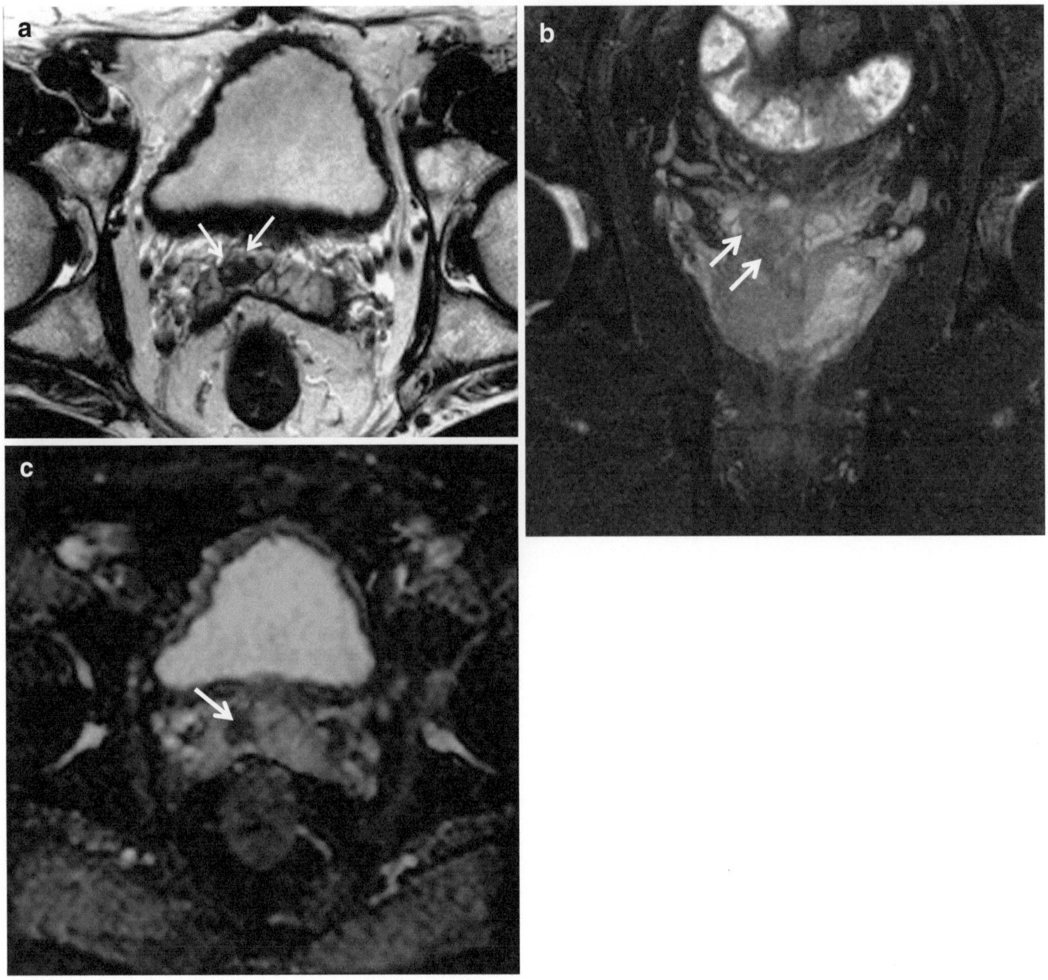

Fig. 3.38 Prostate cancer with SV invasion. T2-weighted axial scan (**a**) and coronal scan (**b**) reveals destruction of seminal vesicle wall and mass-like low signal intensity lesion in left seminal vesicle (*arrows*). (**c**) ADC image also reveals signal drop, suggesting diffusion restriction

(Table 3.1). However, caution should be taken when assessing the CIPC using these criteria. In several studies utilizing the postoperative pathologic findings, it was reported that approximately 8 % of prostate cancers which were classified as CIPC on the basis of Epstein criteria were not localized within the prostate [199, 200]. The consensus, which early detected CIPC as a result of serum PSA testing has no significant effect on clinical outcomes of the patients with life expectancy of less than 20 years, has been reached among NCCN guideline panels [201].

3.9.1.3 Selection of Patients and Triggers for Intervention in AS

There have not been standardized criteria for reclassification of patients requiring definitive treatment during AS period, and different criteria among institutions have been applied. The examples of various AS protocols are summarized in Table 3.2. Generally, the definition for disease progression during follow-up period is determined on the basis of serum PSA value (i.e., PSA doubling time (PSADT) of 3 years or less) and histologic (i.e., Gleason sum of 4 + 3 or

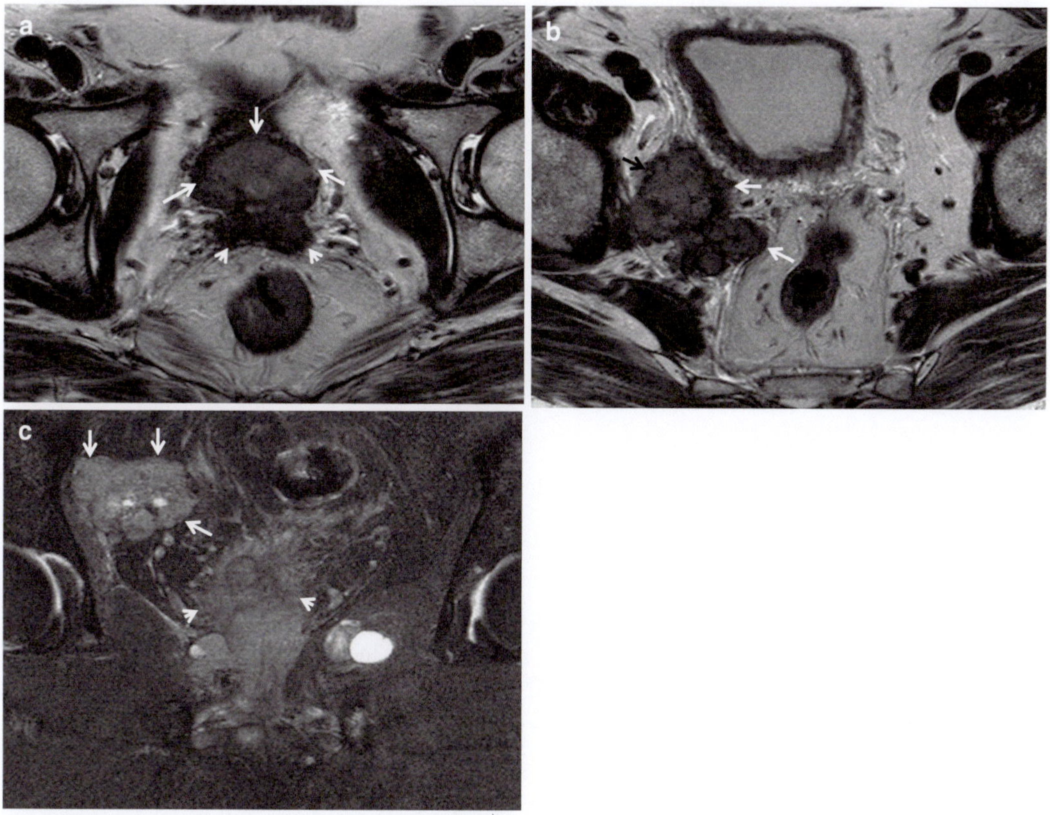

Fig. 3.39 Advanced prostate cancer with multiple metastatic lymphadenopathies. (**a**) T2-weighted axial scan shows the whole prostate is replaced by low signal intensity lesion (*arrows*). Also note that the low signal intensity lesion invades the bilateral seminal vesicles, suggesting seminal vesicle invasion (*arrowheads*). (**b**) T2-weighted axial scan at bladder level shows irregular-shaped large mass, suggesting conglomerated metastatic lymphadenopathy (*arrows*). (**c**) T2-weighted coronal image show irregular-shaped lymphadenopathy (*arrows*). Also note ill-defined prostate mass, suggesting prostate cancer (*arrowheads*)

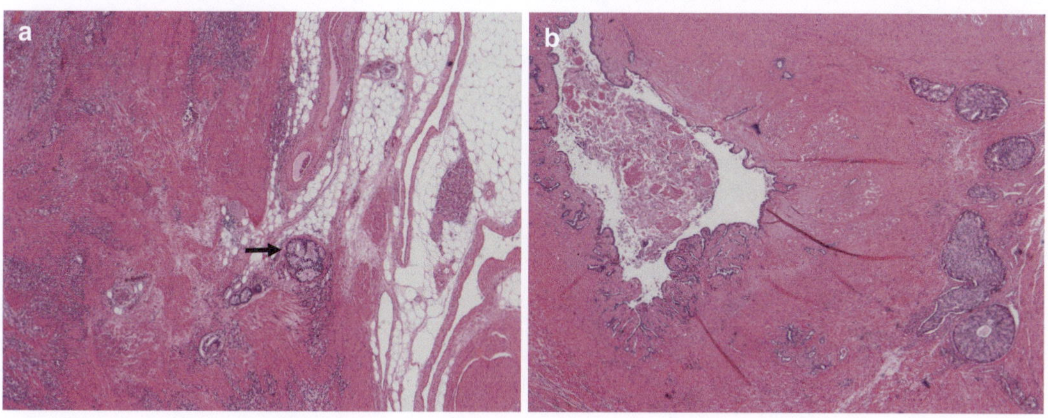

Fig. 3.40 (**a**) Extraprostatic extension of prostatic adenocarcinoma (pT3a) is defined as infiltration into soft tissues beyond fat plane (*arrow*). (**b**) Prostatic adenocarcinoma with cribriform pattern invades into the seminal vesicle (pT3b)

Table 3.1 Definition of insignificant prostate cancer

Epstein criteria for CIPC [71, 202]	D'Amico low-risk prostate cancer [203]	NCCN risk stratification [201]
1. Clinical stage T1c 2. Gleason score ≤6 3. A third or less core biopsies positive 4. 50 % or less involvement of any 1 core 5. PSA density <0.15 ng/ml/g	1. Gleason score <6 2. PSA <10 ng/ml 3. Clinical stage T1	1. Very low risk (a) Clinical T1c (b) Gleason score ≤6 (c) PSA <10 ng/ml (d) Fewer than 3 prostate core biopsy positive, ≤50 % cancer in any core (e) PSA density <0.15 ng/ml/g 2. Low risk (a) Clinical T1-T2a (b) Gleason score ≤6 (c) PSA <10 ng/ml

higher on repeat biopsy of the prostate) and clinical evidence of disease progression (i.e., more than a doubling of the product of the maximum perpendicular diameters of the primary lesion as measured by DRE, local progression of prostate cancer requiring transurethral resection of the prostate, development of ureteral obstruction, or radiologic or clinical evidence of distant metastasis) [204–208]. NCCN has recommended an initiation of curative treatment in case of patients with Gleason grade 4 or 5, increased tumor number, or volume on repeat biopsy, PSADT <3years [201].

3.9.1.4 Methods of AS

The aim of AS is to detect a portion of patients of completely curable state with biologically aggressive features within appropriate period. In general, serum PSA and DRE are measured every 3–6 months, but there have been differences with reference to manner and interval of repeat prostate biopsy from institution to institution (Table 3.2). Further additional study regarding optimal biopsy interval and number will be required to minimize biopsy-related complications and detect prostate cancer with more possibility of progression requiring radical therapy [213, 214]. According to AS program of 2011 NCCN guideline, serum PSA and DRE should be examined every 3 months (at least 6 months) and 6 months (at least 12 months), respectively. Besides, repeat prostate biopsy is recommended within 6 months in case of initial core biopsy <10 [201].

3.9.1.5 Conclusions

AS may be a safe alternative to immediate treatment in men with a low risk of cancer progression, and it appears to be feasible in many men diagnosed with prostate cancer. Major areas of future study include identifying appropriate baseline clinical parameters in selecting men for AS, confirming the role of imaging in diagnosing low-risk prostate cancer, identifying additional circulating and tissue markers defining risk, and developing appropriate follow-up regimens and definitions of progression. Repeat prostate biopsy appears to be critical to defining progression, and PSADT has been widely employed, although its accuracy requires confirmation. With appropriate selection of patients, close follow-up, and the selective use of local therapies in those with local cancer progression, AS may be an acceptable choice for the management of selected patients with low-risk, early-stage prostate cancer.

3.9.2 Focal Therapy

3.9.2.1 Introduction

Owing to introduction of PSA screening, it has been possible to detect prostate cancer at early stage, and frequency of small-sized prostate cancer involving less than 5–10 % of prostate volume has been increased [215, 216]. Radical prostatectomy (RP), external beam, or interstitial radiotherapy has been generally performed for the treatment of localized prostate cancer, but focal therapies, including cryosurgery and high

Table 3.2 Various active surveillance protocols

Variables	University of Toronto [207]	Johns Hopkins [208, 209]	Multicenter European study (PRIAS) [210]	University of California [206]	University of Miami [211]	Multicenter Japanese Study [212]
1. Patients selection criteria						
(a) Clinical stage	T1c	T1c	T1c or T2	T1 or T2a	NI	T1c
(b) PSA (ng/ml)	≤10–15	NI	≤10	≤10	NI	≤20
(c) Gleason score	≤6(3+3)	≤6(3+3)	≤6(3+3)	NI	NI	NI
(d) PSA density (ng/ml)	NI	≤0.15	<0.2	NI	NI	NI
(e) Number of positive cores	NI	2 (core total not specified) and <50 % of cancer in any core	2 (of 8–12 cores)	<33 % cores biopsy and <50 % of cancer in any core	≤2 (of 10 cores minimum) and ≤20 % of cancer in any core	2 (6–12 cores) and <50 % of cancer in any core
2. AS methods						
(a) PSA and DRE monitoring	3 monthly PSA and 6 monthly DRE for 2 years; 6 monthly PSA and annual DRE thereafter	6 monthly PSA and DRE	3 monthly PSA and 6 monthly DRE	3 monthly PSA with TRUS at 6–12-month intervals	3–4 monthly PSA and DRE for 2 years; 6 monthly thereafter	2 monthly PSA for 6 months; 3 monthly thereafter; DRE with TRRUS at least every 6 months
(b) Re-biopsy	6–12 months in the first year and then every 2–3 years	Annually	At 1, 2, and 7 years or cT3 or PSADT ≤3 years (changed to ≤10 years in recent years)	Every 1–2 years	Annually or triggered by PSA or DRE change	At 1 year
3. Trigger for curative intervention	PSADT <3 years	Surveillance biopsy breaching selection criteria; patient request	Gleason score ≥7;>2 positive cores on re-biopsy	Gleason upgrade; increase in PSA velocity of 0.75 ng/ml per year	Gleason upgrade; increase in tumor volume; >2 positive cores on biopsy	PSADT ≤2 years; pathological change breaching selection criteria

intensity-focused ultrasound (HIFU), have been emerging as alternative treatments of localized prostate cancer [217–220]. Focal therapy of prostate cancer is an attractive trial in terms of preservation of prostate function and selective removal of only tumor portion.

3.9.2.2 Cryosurgery

Freezing of the prostate is conducted by using a multi-probe cryosurgical device. Multiple hollow-core probes are placed percutaneously under TRUS guidance. In addition, thermo-sensor is placed at external urethral sphincter and bladder neck, and warming device is located at the urethra to minimize urethral sloughing and prevent urinary incontinence. Commonly used gases are argon for cooling and helium for heating. Two freeze-thaw cycles are usually performed in all patients, and if the iceball does not adequately extend to the apex of the prostate, the cryoprobes are pulled backward into the apex, and additional freeze-thaw cycles are undertaken. The temperature at the edge of the iceball is 0 to −2 °C, while actual cell destruction requires −25 to −50 °C.4,6 Therefore, actual tissue destruction occurs within a few millimeters inside the iceball edge and cannot be monitored precisely by ultrasound imaging.

Thanks to development of third-generation cryosurgical device and advancement of gas-driven and transrectal probes, the outcomes of cryosurgery have been gradually improved [221–226]. However, the objective evaluation with regard to treatment outcomes of cryosurgery is difficult on account of the application of different PSA threshold concerning treatment and recurrence among institutions. The biochemical recurrence-free survival rates (BFSR) in patients receiving cryosurgery have been reported ranging from 36 to 92 % and shows a difference depending on PSA nadir level defined as post-treatment failure and risk group.

Compared to other local therapy, the frequency of erectile dysfunction (ED) is higher following cryosurgery [221–226]. Although some series have reported rates ranging from 40 to 47 %, more contemporary series report the rates between 50 and 90 % [222–224]. The high incidence of ED following cryosurgery may be due to the use of multiple freeze-thaw cycles and extension of the iceball beyond the prostate, into the areas adjacent to the neurovascular bundles. ED has been also reported as approximately 80 % in third-generation cryotherapy [219, 223]. The incidence of urinary incontinence varies among institutions, with rates ranging from 2 to 27 %, but in the third-generation cryosurgery using microprobes, the incidence of incontinence decreased up to less than 2 % [221–226]. Rectourethral fistula formation may occur in less than 3 %, and its incidence becomes much higher if there is a history of radiation therapy [221, 223, 226]. Other complications included perineal or pelvic pain, penile paresthesia, penile and scrotal swelling, and urethral stricture [221–226].

3.9.2.3 HIFU

HIFU is different from cryotherapy in that the focal zone is extremely discrete with little or no tissue effects in areas immediately adjacent to the treatment zone [227]. HIFU uses high-energy ultrasound waves to destroy the tissue at the focal point of a transducer without injuring the intervening tissue. Strong ultrasound waves in the inaudible sound range and approximately 10,000 times stronger than diagnostic ultrasound are generated by a transducer with a parabolic configuration. This parabolic configuration focuses these sound waves into a discrete focal point measuring approximately 3 mm × 3 mm × 11 mm. This focal point is located 3–4 cm distant from the transducer, and its size and shape depend on the energy emitted by the transducer, the geometric configuration of the transducer, and the characteristics of the tissue. At the focal point of the transducer, ultrasound energy is concentrated, is absorbed by the tissue, and generates temperatures that can exceed 80 °C, resulting in coagulative necrosis and the destruction of tissue [227].

Since HIFU was introduced for the treatment of prostate cancer in 1993, a number of relevant studies have been reported. Early studies reported a low BCR-free survival of 30 %, but recent studies have reported a BCR-free survival of 60–90 %, owing to the development of equipment and accumulation of relevant skills [228–234]. PSA nadir value is the most important factor for predicting the success of treatment [235, 236]. The probability of treatment failure may be high if PSA value following HIFU is more than 0.2 ng/ml or does not reach to nadir level within 6 months [235, 236]. HIFU has been considered as alternative therapeutic modality to active surveillance in carefully selected localized prostate cancer. Besides, in cases of local recurrence after RT or vesicourethral anastomotic recurrence following RP, the application of HIFU as salvage therapy has been reported [230–234]. However, because there were not yet prospectively randomized control trials and appropriate standard of biochemical recurrence (BCR), the use of HIFU in real clinical practice is currently indistinct.

The complications of HIFU include acute urinary retention (4–22 %), urethral stricture, urinary tract infection, and urinary incontinence [228, 231, 234]. However, owing to the development of equipment and skill, the frequency of complications has been decreasing. The most severe complication is rectourethral fistula whose frequency was reported as 0.6–0.9 % [237–241]. Erectile dysfunction (18–54 %) can be developed. Other complications included chronic perineal discomfort, hematospemia, and perineal edema.

3.9.3 Conclusion

Cryotherapy is a possible alternative therapeutic modality in patients who are inoperable or have a life expectancy of 10 years or less. HIFU is still an experimental therapeutic method, and therefore further long-term observation may be required to apprehend the therapeutic role of prostate cancer. Currently, focal therapy of prostate cancer is still at an early stage; therefore, focal therapy cannot be recommended as the standard treatment of prostate cancer in clinical practice.

3.9.4 Radiation Therapy

Radiation therapy (RT) has been used as curative treatment for localized prostate cancer for nearly a century. The past two decades have witnessed important technological advances in methods of external beam RT resulting in wide availability of image-guided RT (IGRT) and intensity-modulated RT (IMRT). It is well known that escalation of radiation dose beyond 75 Gy improves survival free from biochemical failure [242, 243]. Without the conformal RT technique, prescription radiation doses usually fall short of 70 Gy due to concerns of radiation-associated bowel or bladder toxicities. Advent of IMRT makes the dose escalation possible without a commensurate increase in radiation-related toxicities. Thus, whenever possible, it is highly recommended to delivery 75 Gy or higher using IMRT. Imaging studies play crucial roles to select patients for radical RT. All patients should be screened using CT and/or MRI for nodal or distant metastases prior to consideration of definitive RT. Presence of extraprostatic extension (EPE) should be incorporated with target volume definition. MRI is useful to evaluate local tumor spread beyond the prostatic capsule. MRI performs superiorly to CT in revealing EPE. MRI is indispensable to detect tumor involvement of the seminal vesicles. Prostate is compactly juxtaposed by normal structures, such as the rectum, bladder, pelvic diaphragm, and penile bulb. Differentiation of those structures from the prostate is often difficult by CT images alone. Co-registration of planning CT and MRI may help to provide accurate relations of adjacent soft tissue structures with the prostate. Since 1920, brachytherapy has been used as monotherapy or in conjunction with EBRT to treat localized prostate cancer. Presence of macroscopic EPE should be evaluated before a decision to perform brachytherapy is made.

3.9.5 Surgical Management

3.9.5.1 Introduction

Radical prostatectomy (RP) is a surgical treatment suitable for localized prostate cancer, which aims to completely remove the tumor while preserving urinary continence and erectile function [244]. A study analyzing 15-year survival of 12,677 patients who underwent RP showed a cancer-specific mortality rate of 12 % and overall mortality rate of 38 % [245]. Patients with low-grade prostate cancer who did not receive surgical treatment had a cancer-specific mortality rate of less than 10 % over 20 years [246]. Thus, it is important to consider a patient's life expectancy and comorbidities when choosing the treatment modality, though age itself should not be the sole criteria for rejection of RP.

RP is the only treatment method shown to improve cancer-specific survival in a randomized controlled trial [245]. Retropubic and perineal approaches, as traditional open surgical methods, have been broadly applied over the last 30 years and offer high cure rates with minimal complications if performed by an experienced surgeon [247, 248]. In recent years, minimally invasive surgical modalities, including laparoscopic radical prostatectomy (LRP) and robot-assisted laparoscopic radical prostatectomy (RALP), have been broadly used. According to systemic reviews and meta-analysis, LRP and RALP have lower intraoperative blood loss and transfusion rates with comparable functional and oncological outcomes [249, 250], though some studies report contradictory results [251, 252]. Though traditional open RP has been substituted in favor of LRP or RALP in recent years, it is not clear whether LRP or RALP is superior in terms of functional and oncological outcomes and cost-effectiveness. A prospective clinical trial is therefore required.

3.9.5.2 Major Complications

Main complications following RP are urinary incontinence and erectile dysfunction, which have a tremendous impact on the patient's quality of life. However, recent advances in the understanding of surgical anatomy, especially in radical retropubic prostatectomy (RRP), have enabled dissection under excellent visual conditions. This allows preservation of the cavernous nerve and external sphincter, maintaining postoperative erectile function and urinary continence, respectively [253].

Urinary Continence

Recent studies have reported urinary continence rates of more than 80 % after RP, with recovery of urinary continence persisting over 24 months post-operation [254]. Postoperative urinary continence is influenced by various factors, which can be classified into preoperative factors, including age, weight/body mass index (BMI), preoperative voiding function, prostate volume, preoperative prostate-specific antigen level, clinical pathologic stage, and preoperative Gleason score, and intraoperative factors, including intraoperative blood loss, urethral stump length, nerve sparing technique, bladder neck-sparing technique, puboprostatic ligament sparing, and experience of the surgeon [254]. If performed by a highly trained surgeon, the rate of urinary continence recovery is considered to be more than 90 %.

Erectile Dysfunction

Most studies define potency following RP as the ability to maintain a rigid erection sufficient for penetration and sexual intercourse with or without the help of a PDE-5 inhibitor. Recent studies have reported an overall recovery rate of erectile function after RP of 48 % and about 50 % if the neurovascular bundle is spared [255].

3.9.5.3 Pelvic Lymph Node Dissection in Radical Prostatectomy

Pelvic lymph node dissection (PLND) is the most reliable method to determine the N stage, since preoperative imaging, including computed tomography and magnetic resonance imaging, cannot detect metastatic lymph nodes smaller than 5 mm. The decision of PLND is based on the probability of lymph node metastasis. Generally, PLND can be omitted in low-risk localized prostate cancer (PSA <10 ng/ml, Gleason score <7, clinical stage ≤T2a). The probability of lymph node metastasis can be estimated with a nomogram using variables such as the preoperative prostate-specific antigen (PSA), Gleason score, and clinical stage [256, 257]. The European Association of Urology (EAU) recommends extended PLND when the probability of lymph node metastasis is greater than 7 %. Some studies have shown that extended PLND can improve survival and eliminate micrometastases of prostate cancer [258–261].

3.9.5.4 Surgical Procedure and Anatomy

In this chapter, the surgical procedures and relevant anatomic structures of RRP and RALP, the most common open and minimally invasive surgical procedures, respectively, are introduced.

RRP

Starting from the symphysis pubis, a midline incision of about 12–15 cm is made in the skin. After incision of the anterior rectus fascia, the rectus muscle is divided in the midline in order to approach the retropubic space (Retzius space). After approaching the Retzius space, PLND is initiated, if necessary. PLND must be performed in an extended manner [262, 263] and must include the external iliac vein anteriorly, pelvic wall laterally, bladder wall medially, pelvic floor posteriorly, Cooper's ligament distally, and internal iliac artery proximally. A greater number of dissected lymph nodes are associated with more accurate staging. After PLND, the fibro-adipose tissue covering the anterior side of the prostate must be dissected to expose the prostate. This exposes the anterior side of the prostate, including the superior branch or dorsal vein, puboprostatic ligament, and endopelvic fascia (Fig. 3.41a).

The endopelvic fascia can be opened with scissors or electrocauterization. After opening of the fascia, the venous plexus of Santorini can be visualized. The opening of the endopelvic fascia is extended to the puboprostatic ligament. The puboprostatic ligament can be spared or completely divided. Sparing of the puboprostatic ligament can provide anterior support of the urethra [264]. Poore et al. reported the positive impact of puboprostatic sparing on the early recovery of urinary continence [265]. However, Deliverliotis et al. reported no effect on the final continence rate with puboprostatic ligament sparing [266]. The dorsal vein complex (DVC) is then ligated. To ligate the DVC, it is gathered with a clamp at the apex of the prostate and the junction between the bladder neck and prostatic base. DVC ligation is a very important step because complete ligation is essential for good visualization of the surgical field. After DVC ligation, apical prostate dissection is performed. This is a critical step in cancer control and functional outcome. After division of the DVC, dissection between the prostate and urethra must be performed precisely to avoid a positive surgical margin at the apex. During apical dissection, fixation of the length of the urethra is also important for postoperative recovery of urinary continence, as this may preserve more of the striated sphincter (Fig. 3.41b).

A urethral catheter is brought out through the opening of the prostatic urethra at the apex and pulled out and upward. Dissection of the seminal vesicle and vas deferens is performed. Following dissection of the seminal vesicle, pedicles along the posterolateral side of the prostate are divided and locked with a vascular clip.

After the procedure described above, the prostate is only attached to the bladder neck at the base of the prostate. The bladder neck is incised anteriorly, and the incision is extended to the posterior side of the prostate. The division of the posterior bladder neck is carefully performed, avoiding injury to the ureteral orifice. The bladder neck is reconstructed with eversion sutures for hemostasis and exposure of the bladder mucosa. If the bladder neck opening is too large, it can be suitably closed using tennis racket suturing. For vesicourethral anastomosis, five to six stitches are made at the urethral stump and the corresponding position in the bladder neck (Fig. 3.41c). After the urethral Foley catheter is indwelled, all sutures are tidied and knotted outside.

RALP

Since robot-assisted surgery was introduced in 2000, RALP has gradually replaced LRP as a popular surgical treatment option for organ-confined prostate cancer. Currently, the da Vinci surgical robot (Intuitive Surgical, Sunnyvale, CA) is the mainly used system, which provides 3-dimensional vision of the surgical field and multi-articular movement of the instruments, enabling delicate tissue manipulation and easy suturing. LRP and RALP offer similar surgical views to the surgeon, but a robotic system provides a more magnified view of the operation field than LRP. Here, the surgical procedure and relevant anatomy of RALP are described.

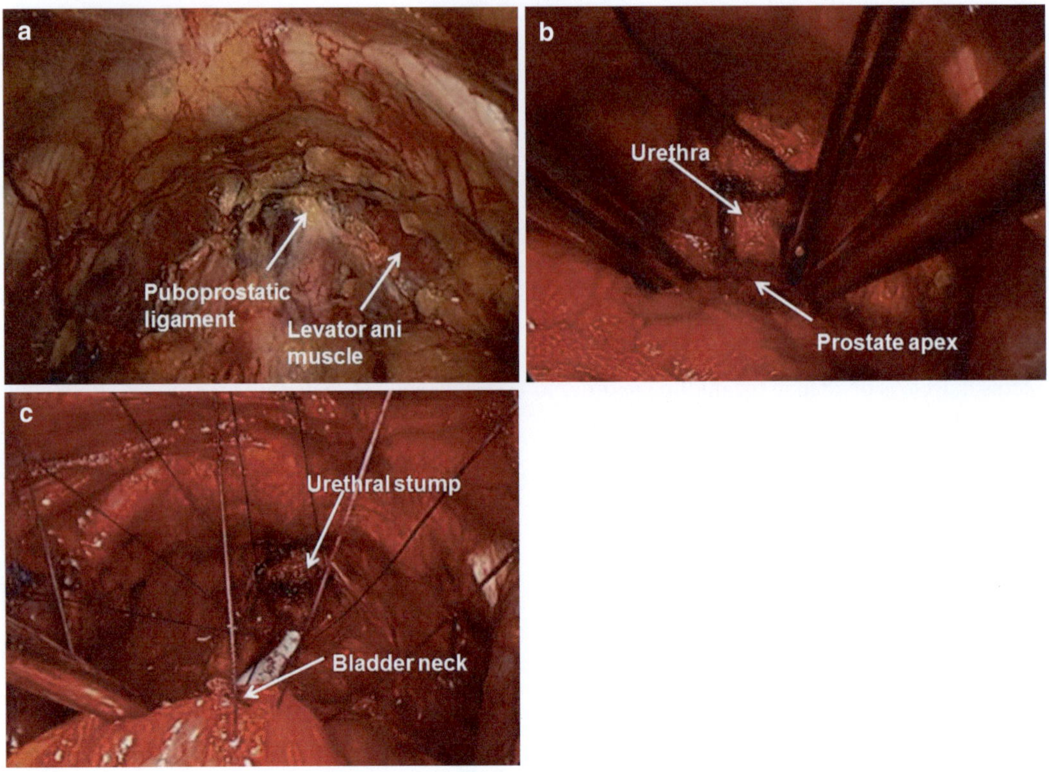

Fig. 3.41 (**a**) Anterior side of prostate, the fibro-adipose tissue covering the anterior side of the prostate is removed to expose the prostate. This exposes the anterior side of the prostate, including the superior branch or dorsal vein, puboprostatic ligament, and endopelvic fascia (**b**). Urethra and prostate apex, during dissection of prostatic apex, fixation of the length of the urethra is also important for postoperative recovery of urinary continence, as this may preserve more of the striated sphincter (**c**). Vesicourethral anastomosis, six stitches are made at the urethral stump and the corresponding position in the bladder neck. After the urethral Foley catheter is inserted, all sutures are tied and knotted outside

Both intraperitoneal and extraperitoneal laparoscopic approaches offer comparable perioperative outcomes. Intraperitoneal access is more commonly used. For an intraperitoneal approach, a pneumoperitoneum can be made using a Veress needle or the open Hasson technique. A 12 mm vertical incision is made superior to the umbilicus, and the Veress needle is introduced carefully into the peritoneal cavity. After the pneumoperitoneum is established, a 12 mm trocar is placed through the vertical incision. A robotic camera is introduced through the trocar, allowing the surgeon to inspect the intra-abdominal wall for subsequent trocar placement. In general, five additional trocars, used for the robotic arm and assistant instrument, are introduced into the peritoneal cavity. To access the Retzius space, the median umbilical ligaments and urachus are divided and an incision is made in the parietal peritoneum. The incision is extended to the lateral pelvic wall up to the vas deferens. Blunt dissection along the lateral pelvic wall allows visualization of the symphysis pubis, anterior side of bladder and prostate, puboprostatic ligament, and endopelvic fascia. After excision of the fibro-adipose tissue overlying the prostate, the anterior aspect of the prostate and superficial dorsal vein can be visualized (Fig. 3.42a).

The superficial dorsal vein is coagulated by bipolar electrocauterization at this step. The endopelvic fascias are divided, and the underlying levator muscle attached to the lateral portion of the prostate is bluntly dissected. At this step, the deep dorsal vein complex (DVC) overlying

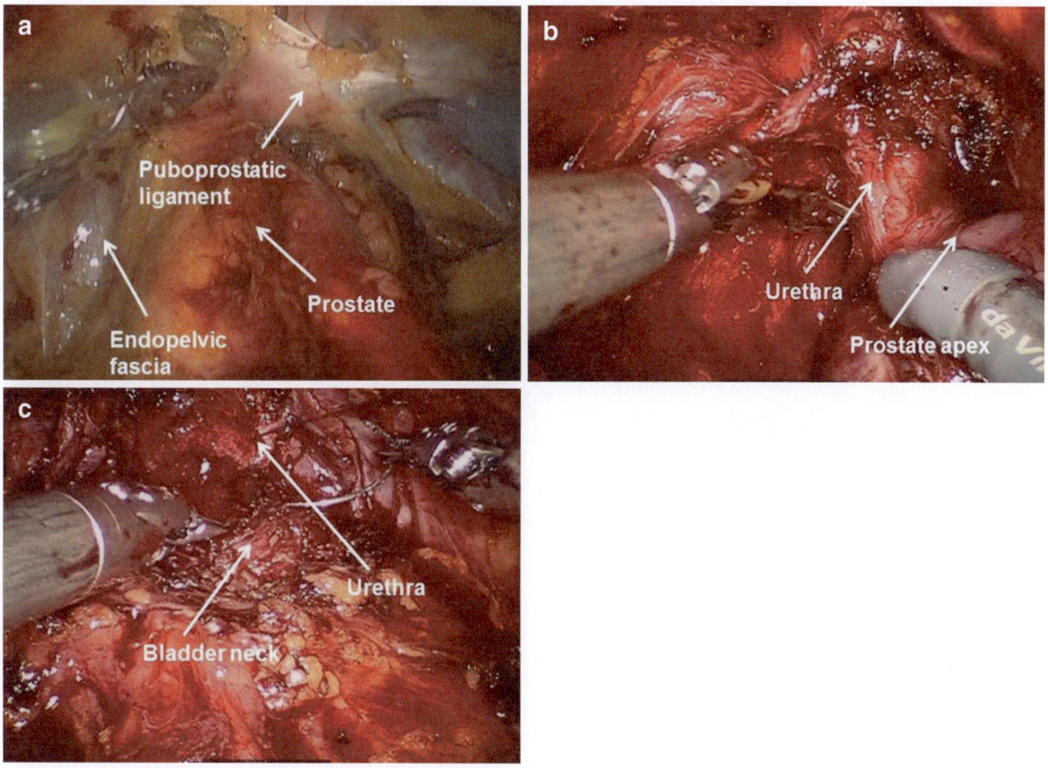

Fig. 3.42 RALP (**a**) Anterior aspect of prostate; after excision of the fibro-adipose tissue overlying the prostate, the anterior aspect of the prostate and superficial dorsal vein is visualized. (**b**) Apical dissection of the prostate, precise division between the apex of the prostate and urethra is also important for cancer control and postoperative continence in RALP. (**c**) Vesicourethral anastomosis, in RALP, continuous suturing (double-armed sutures) between urethra mucosa and bladder neck mucosa is usually applied for vesicourethral anastomosis

the urethra and apex of the prostate can be ligated by suture or coagulated or ligated at a later time. Caudal retraction of the preoperatively indwelled urethral Foley catheter allows the surgeon to reach the junction of the bladder neck and prostate base. A horizontal incision at the anterior side of the bladder neck is made at the junction of the bladder neck and prostate. The anterior bladder neck is divided until the urethral Foley catheter is visible. The tip of the urethral catheter is pulled out through the anterior bladder neck opening and the posterior bladder neck is divided. After division of the bladder neck, the vas deferens and seminal vesicle are dissected and divided. In this procedure, cold dissection is recommended, if possible, to avoid thermal damage to the adjacent neurovascular bundle. Following division of vas deferens and seminal vesicle, the posterior plane of the prostate is developed. Denonvilliers' fascia, derived from the peritoneum, covers the posterior aspect of the prostate and anterior aspect of the rectum. In general, the plane between Denonvilliers' fascia and the posterior lobe of the prostate is developed for neurovascular bundle (NVB) sparing, which is most commonly used and is known as the interfascial approach. Denonvilliers' fascia is separated from the posterior aspect of the prostate by blunt and sharp dissection to the apex. If NBV saving is not indicated, a wider resection plane including Denonvilliers' fascia must be made.

The parasympathetic nerve fibers, located at the periprostatic tissue, are important for erectile function [267], and the bundle of nerve fibers along the posterolateral side of the prostate, known as the NBV, are located between the lateral pelvic fascia and prostate capsule. In the interfascial approach, the plane between lateral pelvic fascia and prostate capsule is developed to spare the NBV. The lateral pelvic fascia is incised at the anterolateral side of the prostate, and the incision is extended to the prostate base and apex. Blunt dissection without thermal energy along the plane between the lateral pelvic fascia and prostate capsule is made, and the lateral pelvic fascia is released laterally. During posterior and lateral dissection, the vascular pedicle of the prostate is usually divided and secured by a locking clip. The accessory pudendal artery (APA) can often be seen traveling over the anterolateral side of the prostate. Presence of a visible APA has been reported in 4 % of men [268]. Lack of blood supply to the corpus cavernosum is one of the main reasons for postoperative erectile dysfunction. Injury of the APA during RP can cause postoperative arterial insufficiency of the corpus cavernosum. Remaining attachments between the prostate and lateral pelvic fascia are dissected with scissors. Following the procedure described above, the remaining attached sites are the DVC and urethra. The DVC is divided, and the urethra and apex of the prostate are visualized. Like the open radical prostatectomy, precise division between the apex of the prostate and urethra is important for cancer control and postoperative continence (Fig. 3.42b). After careful hemostasis, vesicourethral anastomosis is performed. In general, continuous mucosa to mucosa suturing is made using double-armed sutures secured together (Fig. 3.42c).

3.9.6 Hormonal Therapy

3.9.6.1 Introduction

Since Huggins and Hodges had reported the effect of surgical castration and oral estrogen medication at the progression of metastatic prostate cancer in 1941, androgen depravation therapy (ADT) has been recognized as a crucial therapeutic method for advanced prostate cancer [269, 270]. However, ADT has been used in combination with other treatment in patients who had non-metastatic early prostate cancer or recurrent cancer following radical therapy [271]. ADT can effectively improve patients' symptoms in advanced prostate cancer, but there has been currently no definite evidence of the extension of survival duration.

3.9.6.2 Hormonal Regulation of the Prostate

The growth, function, and proliferation of the prostate are physiologically dependent on androgen. Although androgens have no carcinogenic effect, it is essential for the growth and maintenance of tumor cell [272]. Testosterone, which is the main androgen, is made in the testis, and the remaining androgens are made in the adrenal gland. The secretion of testosterone is regulated by hypothalamus-pituitary-gonadal axis. The luteinizing hormone-releasing hormone (LHRH) stimulates the anterior lobe of the pituitary gland, secretes luteinizing hormone (LH) and follicle-stimulating hormone (FSH), and then LH stimulates the secretion of testosterone from Leydig cell of the testis. Testosterone within the prostate cell is converted into 5-a-dihydrotestosterone (DHT), which is tenfold stronger androgen stimulant than testosterone, by the action of 5-a reductase [273]. Circulating testosterone is aromatized to estrogen at the periphery and has a negative feedback on LH secretion at the hypothalamus. If there is no stimulation of androgen to the prostate, apoptotic process will occur.

3.9.6.3 Types of Hormonal Therapy

Simple Orchiectomy (Physical Castration)

Surgical castration is still the standard treatment of ADT and induces the immediate hypogonadism state following surgery. The criterion of castration is a serum testosterone level of 50 ng/dl or less. Bilateral orchiectomy is a simple and uncomplicated surgical method. It can be conducted under local anesthesia, and within 12 h after surgery, serum testosterone comes to castration level [274].

Estrogen Agent

Estrogen has a variety of effects including downregulation of LHRH secretion, inactivation of androgen, direct inhibition of Leydig cell function, and direct cytotoxicity to prostatic epithelial cells [275]. Diethylstilbestrol (DES) is commonly used estrogen agent in prostate cancer [275–277]. Oral medication of low-dose (1 and 3 mg) DES showed a similar therapeutic effect compared to bilateral orchiectomy, but 3 mg DES is associated with high cardiovascular toxicity [276]. Owing to concern of cardiovascular toxicity and advent of LHRH agonist and antiandrogen agent, DES is not nearly used currently.

LHRH Agonist

Long-acting LHRH agonists (goserelin, leuprolide, and triptorelin) have been already used as a main method of ADT 15 years ago [271, 278]. Long-term stimulation of LHRH agonist finally causes downregulation of LHRH receptor and inhibits LH and FSH secretion in pituitary gland and testosterone synthesis, and then serum testosterone level decreases to castration level within 2–4 weeks [279, 280]. Recent meta-analysis reported that LHRH agonist showed a similar effect with orchiectomy and DES [281]. Owing to psychological and physical discomfort of orchiectomy and cardiovascular side effect of DES, LHRH agonist is currently used as standard treatment of hormonal therapy. However, flare-up phenomenon may be a concerned problem. Combination therapy with antiandrogen can lower the prevalence of clinical recurrence. It was reported that the long-term use of LHRH agonist is associated with mini-flare phenomenon, but its clinical effect was unknown [282].

LHRH Antagonist

Contrary to LHRH agonist, LHRH antagonists (abarelix, degarelix) immediately combine with LHRH receptor and then can rapidly decline serum level of LH, FSH, and testosterone. However, because many LHRH antagonists have severe and life-threatening histamine-related complications, their use in clinical practice is limited [265–267]. According to several studies, LHRH antagonists were effective in light of castration, but showed no superior effect compared to LHRH agonists [283–285]. As LHRH antagonist should be administered every month, its use is limited compared with leuprorelin of 3 or 6 months interval method. Because most studies have been conducted for 1-year follow-up duration, long-term effect with respect to LHRH antagonist should be proved through further prospective study.

Antiandrogens

Antiandrogens combine with nucleus of prostatic cell competing with testosterone and DHT and then inhibit the growth of prostate cancer or facilitate the apoptosis of cancer cell [286]. Antiandrogens are divided into steroidal (cyproterone acetate) and nonsteroidal (nilutamide, flutamide, bicalutamide, abiraterone, enzalutamide). Steroidal antiandrogen, which is a synthetic extract of hydroxyprogesterone, not only blocks the androgen receptor but also inhibits secretion of LH and FSH and suppresses adrenal function. Although cyproterone acetate (CPA) is the first authorized antiandrogen drug, relevant studies are so limited that optimum dose and comparative result to standard castration method are insufficient. Nonsteroidal antiandrogen monotherapy has been developed on account of improvement of quality of life and compliance compared with physical castration method. These drugs can maintain sexual desire, general physical activity, and bone density with no effect to the secretion of testosterone [287]. In terms of nonpharmacological aspect, bicalutamide shows a better safety and tolerability than nilutamide or flutamide [279]. Abiraterone and enzalutamide, which are recently introduced antiandrogen agents, showed a survival benefit in patients with metastatic CRPC who received previous chemotherapy including docetaxel [288, 289].

Combination Hormonal Therapy

Several investigators insist that restraining both testicular and adrenal androgens (complete androgen blockade) allows for a better initial and a longer response compared with those methods that inhibit production of only testicular androgens. Complete androgen blockade can be attained by combining antiandrogen with LHRH agonist or orchiectomy. The patients with limited disease and a good performance status who are treated with combined androgen blockade (LHRH agonist and antiandrogen agent) seem to survive longer than those treated with an LHRH agonist alone [290]. However, another study comparing antiandrogen alone with antiandrogen plus orchiectomy failed to demonstrate a survival difference between the two groups [291]. A meta-analysis of monotherapy and complete androgen blockade for the treatment of advanced prostate cancer suggested that there might be a small survival advantage to complete androgen blockade [292].

Intermittent ADT Versus Continuous ADT

Ongoing trials are studying the use of intermittent androgen-deprivation (IAD) to determine whether this might result in a delay in the appearance of the hormone-refractory state. IAD, compared to continuous therapy, may be related to improved quality of life and reduced treatment cost and drug-related side effect because serum testosterone levels may be normalized during off-therapy duration [293]. However, currently, there is little definite evidence with regard to whether IAD can actually increase survival or delay progression to castration-resistant prostate cancer (CRPC).

Immediate ADT Versus Deferred ADT

There has been still controversy with regard to the timing of initial hormonal therapy in advanced prostate cancer, that is, immediate versus deferred ADT in localized prostate cancer and asymptomatic metastatic cancer. Several studies have reported that in patients who underwent ADT as primary therapy or adjuvant therapy following radical prostatectomy, immediate ADT markedly decreased a cancer progression and progression-related complication rate [277, 294, 295]. However, immediate ADT failed to improve cancer-specific survival and relatively showed a small benefit to overall survival with absolute risk reduction of 5.5 % 10 years later [296]. According to ASCO guideline, it is concluded that the initiation of hormone therapy is not recommended in asymptomatic advanced prostate cancer patients until the result of study regarding initial hormone therapy in androgen-sensitive metastatic, recurrent, or progressive prostate cancer is reported [296].

3.10 Imaging and Pathologic Finding of Unusual Tumors

More than 95 % of malignant tumors of the prostate are adenocarcinomas [297]. However, numerous rare morphologic variants of prostate carcinoma have been identified. These unusual tumors of the prostate may arise from the prostatic epithelium or stroma or from ectopically located cells within the prostate. Moreover, even though these tumors present with signs and symptoms that resemble those of typical prostate adenocarcinoma, they may show a variable prognosis. Several unusual prostate involving neoplasms have been described and characterized during recent years. In addition, benign prostate stromal hyperplasia also mimics a malignant tumor, and benign inflammatory lesions can also present as malignant-looking lesions. However, few reports about the imaging findings of these unusual tumor or tumorlike lesions have been published.

Unusual tumors or tumorlike lesions in the prostate may have prognoses that are quite unlike those of prostatic adenocarcinoma. Radiologic findings may overlap, and they have limited roles in the diagnoses of these entities. However, knowledge of these variable unusual tumors and tumorlike conditions is helpful when making accurate radiologic diagnoses, which have important clinical implications for treatment and prognosis.

Prostate tumors can be subdivided into epithelial, neuroendocrine, stromal, metastatic, mesenchymal, hematolymphoid, and miscellaneous tumors. The epithelial tumors that involve the prostate include glandular neoplasms such as adenocarcinoma, urothelial tumors, squamous tumors, and basal cell tumors. Neuroendocrine tumors include carcinoid tumors, small cell carcinoma, paraganglioma, and neuroblastoma. Mesenchymal tumors include leiomyosarcoma, rhabdomyosarcoma, chondrosarcoma, and malignant fibrous histiocytoma (MFH). In addition to hematolymphoid tumors such as lymphoma and leukemia, rare tumors like germ cell tumor and melanoma can also arise from the prostate.

3.10.1 Pathology of Stromal Tumor and Stromal Sarcoma

Mesenchymal tumors of prostate are uncommon. Well-known soft tissue tumors such as leiomyoma, leiomyosarcoma, rhabdomyosarcoma, or inflammatory myofibroblastic tumor can be developed in the prostate. In addition, mesenchymal tumors derived from specialized prostatic stroma are also found. These lesions specific to prostate can be classified into stromal tumors of uncertain malignant potential (STUMP) and stromal sarcoma [298, 299].

3.10.1.1 STUMP

Grossly STUMP is firm, solid, or partly cystic mass with white to tan-colored cut surface. Microscopically, STUMP can show four histologic patterns including degenerative atypia, hypercellular stroma, myxoid, and phyllodes type [298, 299].

3.10.1.2 Stromal Sarcoma

Grossly stromal sarcoma is solid or partly cystic mass with gray to tan color. Microscopically stromal sarcoma reveals stromal proliferation with hypercellularity, pleomorphism, and increased mitosis and necrosis. Biphasic pattern resembling phyllodes tumor of breast can be found [298, 299].

3.10.2 Epithelial Tumors

3.10.2.1 Mucinous Adenocarcinoma

Prostate mucinous adenocarcinoma is an uncommon variant of prostatic carcinoma occurring in 0.1–2 % of prostatic surgical specimens [297]. The diagnosis of mucinous adenocarcinoma requires that more than 25 % of an excised tumor consists of tumor cells and clusters of cells floating in lakes of mucin. Mucinous carcinomas demonstrate an accumulation of large amounts of extracellular mucin during histologic examinations. Moreover, the mucin within these tumors differs in chemical composition from that of normal prostatic tissue [297].

Because of mucin component, MR imaging appears as high signal intensity lesions on T2-weighted images. However, variable T2-weighted signal intensities may be observed due to a smaller mucin amount or a different chemical composition. Some articles have reported that mucinous adenocarcinoma signal intensity is similar to that reported for rhabdomyosarcoma of the prostate, although the clinical, morphologic, and histopathologic features of this tumor are distinctly different [300]. The differential diagnosis of these cystic mass includes cystic prostatic hyperplasia, abscesses, and cysts.

3.10.2.2 Squamous Cell Carcinoma

Primary squamous cell carcinoma of the prostate is very rare. It accounts for approximately 0.5–1 % of all prostate cancers [297]. Primary bladder urethral origin carcinoma should be excluded before a diagnosis of primary squamous cell carcinoma of the prostate is made. The common clinical presentations include prostate urethral obstruction, hematuria, or bone pain suggesting bone metastasis. Unlike sclerotic bone metastasis from adenocarcinoma, squamous cell carcinoma shows osteolytic lesion. Squamous cell carcinomas often arise in the setting of prior hormone or radiation therapy, and the prognosis of this tumor is very poor [166]. Pathologically squamous features of keratinization, squamous pearls, and intercellular bridges are characteristic [301]. Imaging findings of squamous cell carcinoma are similar to those of adenocarcinoma. TRUS shows low echoic hypervascular lesions, and MR shows low signal intensity lesion on T2-weighted image (Fig. 3.43). Lymph node metastasis can be seen in iliac, inguinal, obturator, and para-aortic lymph nodes, bladder, seminal vesicle, rectum, and lung [297].

3.10.2.3 Transitional Cell Carcinoma

Transitional cell carcinoma (TCC) of the prostate may originate from prostatic ducts or acini or may be due to synchronous or metachronous spread from transitional cell carcinoma in the bladder or urethra (Fig. 3.44). The primary prostate TCC is rare, occupying only 2–4 % of all prostate cancers, whereas secondary involvement of TCC in

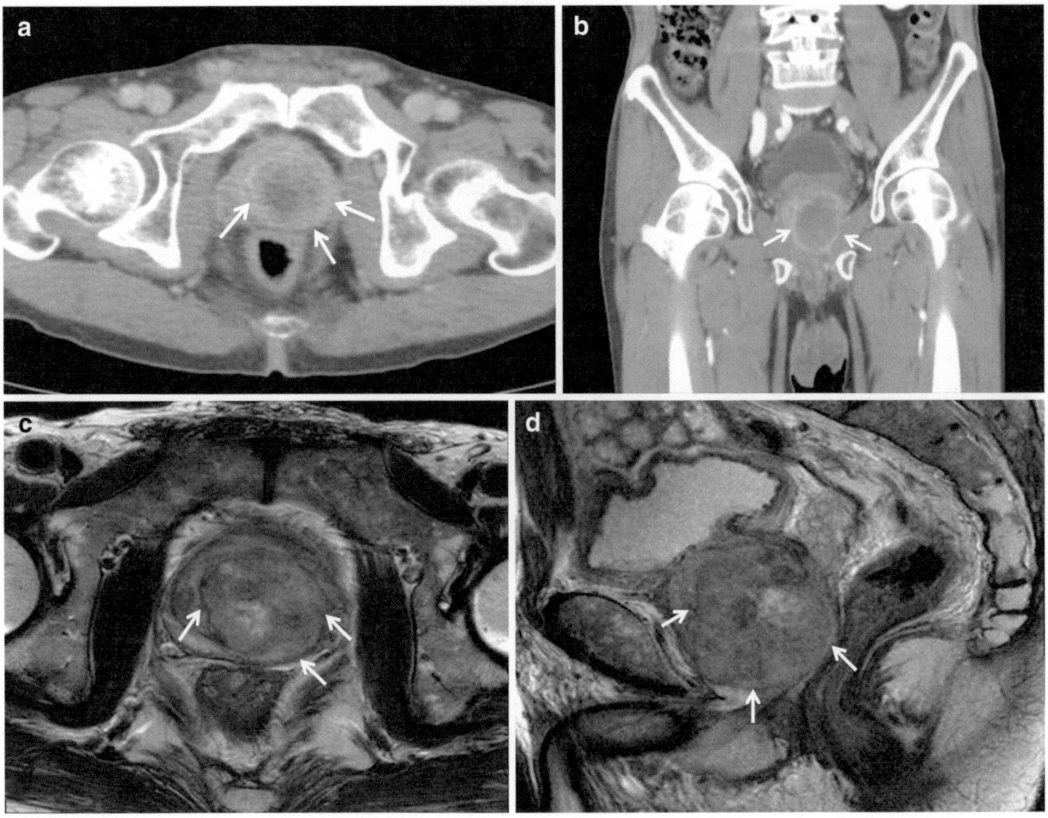

Fig. 3.43 Squamous cell carcinoma in a 70-year-old man. Axial (**a**) and coronal (**b**) CT scans show low-attenuated mass arising from prostate (*arrows*). T2-weighted axial (**c**) and coronal (**d**) images reveal sold looking mass in the prostate (*arrows*). The patient underwent prostatectomy and confirmed to have squamous cell carcinoma

bladder into the prostate is common, occurring in 7–43 % of men with bladder TCC. Whether primary or secondary, TCC of the prostate is traditionally believed to have a poor prognosis [297]. TRUS of prostate TCC reveals hypoechoic lesions involving the central portion of prostate, which is quite different from prostate adenocarcinoma [302]. CT scan shows a low attenuating lesion seen in central portion of prostate (Fig. 3.45).

3.10.3 Neuroendocrine Neoplasm

Neuroendocrine differentiation in prostatic carcinoma can be divided into three forms: focal neuroendocrine differentiation in conventional prostatic adenocarcinoma, carcinoid tumor, and small cell neuroendocrine carcinoma [303]. The most common type of neuroendocrine differentiation observed in prostate malignancy is focal, individual cell neuroendocrine differentiation. Small cell carcinomas and carcinoid tumors constitute a small percentage of prostatic malignancies, representing less than 5 % of all prostatic malignancies [297]. The incidence of prostatic tumors with neuroendocrine differentiation is increasing [304]. Because the treatment and prognosis may differ from that of typical adenocarcinoma, the presence of a neuroendocrine component can also affect clinical management.

3.10.3.1 Carcinoid Tumor

Carcinoid tumors of the prostate are exceedingly rare and show classic cytologic features of carcinoid tumors and diffuse neuroendocrine differentiation, for example, chromogranin A and synaptophysin immunoreactivity [303]. Carcinoid tumor is essentially negative for

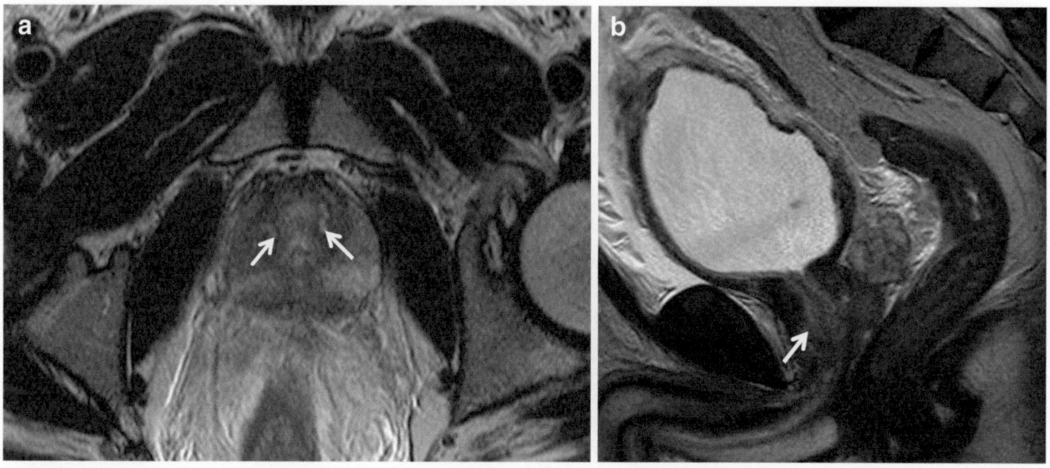

Fig. 3.44 MR findings of transitional cell carcinoma arising from prostatic urethra. T2-weighted axial (**a**) and sagittal (**b**) scan show ill-defined irregular lesion surround prostatic urethra (*arrows*)

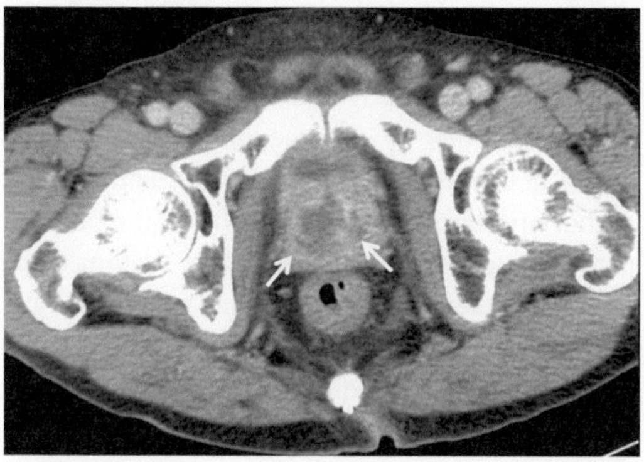

Fig. 3.45 CT findings of transitional cell carcinoma. Post-contrast CT scan of other patient reveals ill-defined low-attenuated lesion located in central portion of prostate (Published with kind permission of Korean Society of Ultrasound in Medicine *J Korean Soc Ultrasound Med* 2006;25:1–10)

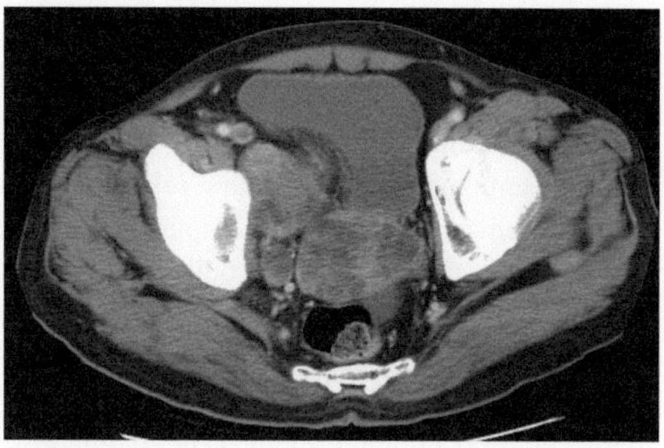

Fig. 3.46 CT findings of carcinoid tumor arising from prostate. Post-contrast CT scan shows heterogeneous-enhancing mass with multiple metastatic lymphadenopathies. TRUS-guided biopsy performed and confirmed as carcinoid tumor

PSA. Because the number of reported cases is small, the prognosis is uncertain. No image findings have been reported for carcinoid tumors of the prostate. In our case, TRUS showed a low echoic irregular outlined mass with increased vascularity, and CT revealed low attenuating mass with peripheral enhancement (Fig. 3.46).

3.10.3.2 Small Cell Carcinoma

Schwartz et al. reported that 44 % of patients with a clinically anaplastic clinical variant of prostate cancer show a small cell carcinoma component in the mass [304]. Anaplastic clinical variant is defined clinically by one or more of the following: a rapid progression of clinical symptoms, the presence of visceral metastasis, poor response to androgen ablation therapy, and relatively low serum prostate-specific antigen (PSA) levels. Small cell carcinoma has an aggressive clinical course characterized by widespread metastatic disease and a lack of response to hormone therapy [304].

The rapid onset of bladder outlet obstructive symptom is a common presentation. Distant metastases are generally observed at the time of diagnosis. The paraneoplastic syndromes of small cell carcinomas are occasionally observed

[297]. These tumors are morphologically identical to small cell carcinomas of the lung and other sites [304]. Currently, neuroendocrine tumor cells are thought to arise from a common stem cell or multipotent cell that can differentiate into multiple tissues [297]. This theory explains the heterogeneous cell population present in many prostate cancers and the observation that diagnosis of small cell carcinoma is often preceded by a diagnosis of adenocarcinoma of the prostate.

Imaging findings have rarely reported for small cell carcinoma of the prostate, but extensive bone metastasis and abdominal and pelvic lymphadenopathy are noted at CT [304]. CT may also show a well-enhanced lobulated contoured soft tissue mass in the prostate (Fig. 3.47).

3.10.4 Mesenchymal Tumors

3.10.4.1 Leiomyosarcoma

Leiomyosarcoma usually occurs relatively old age between 40 and 70 years comparing rhabdomyosarcoma and presents as a bulky tumor with diffuse infiltration of surrounding tissues [305]. Leiomyosarcoma is the second most common sarcoma involving the prostate following rhabdomyosarcoma occupying about 25 % of all prostate sarcoma. Comparing rhabdomyosarcoma, the speed of growing is relatively slow. Pathologically, leiomyosarcoma consists of interlaced bundles of spindle cells with blunted-end nuclei and eosinophilic cytoplasm by light microscopy [297]. Necrosis and hemorrhage are common in leiomyosarcoma. Even though the findings of leiomyosarcoma are very similar to those of rhabdomyosarcoma, the local extent of these sarcomas can be determined by CT or MR imaging [305] (Fig. 3.48). Both of these modalities can clearly delineate tumors from surrounding normal tissues. In leiomyosarcoma, local recurrence is frequent, and the most common metastatic sites are lung followed by bone and liver. Regional lymph nodal metastases occur infrequently [297].

3.10.4.2 Rhabdomyosarcoma

Rhabdomyosarcoma is the most common tumor of the lower genitourinary tract in young age in the first two decades. The etiology is uncertain and may arise from a primitive cell in any organ. It represents 5–10 % of all malignant solid tumors of childhood, ranking fourth in frequency after central nervous system neoplasms, neuroblastoma, and Wilms' tumor [306]. Genitourinary rhabdomyosarcoma usually involves the bladder, prostate, testis, penis, perineum, vagina, and uterus. Genitourinary rhabdomyosarcoma accounts for about 15–30 % of all rhabdomyosarcoma cases in children. In children, the age of presentation with rhabdomyosarcoma is approximately 7 years [306]. Histologically, more than 65 % are embryonal rhabdomyosarcomas and the 5 % are alveolar subtype. Just like leiomyosarcoma, rhabdomyosarcoma grows rapidly and invade adjacent soft tissues and the bladder.

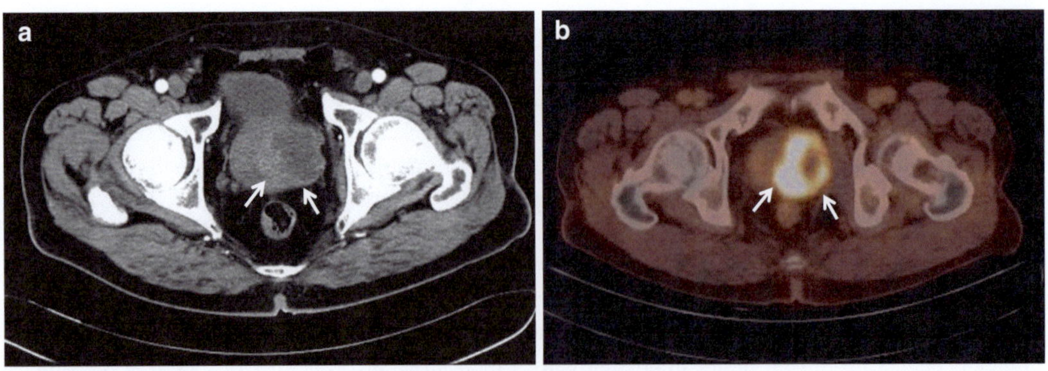

Fig. 3.47 Small cell carcinoma in prostate. (**a**) Post-contrast CT reveals ill-defined low-attenuated area involving left lobe of prostate (*arrows*). (**b**) PET-CT image reveals very hot uptake of glucose in same area (*arrows*)

The main symptoms of leiomyosarcoma include the bladder outlet obstruction, lower abdominal distension, dysuria, or signs of urinary tract infection [306]. The gross appearance of rhabdomyosarcoma is variable. The margins of tumor may be infiltrative or well defined by a compressible pseudocapsule. Grossly, cut sections of rhabdomyosarcoma typically appear firm, fleshy, and lobulated, and secondary hemorrhage and necrosis are also common findings. Calcification is rare [306]. TRUS reveals a hyperechoic or hypoechoic solid lesion showing hemorrhage or necrosis [306]. CT shows bulky pelvic mass with heterogeneous attenuation (Fig. 3.49). The mass may invade periprostatic, periurethral, and perivesical tissues, or it may also extend into the ischiorectal fossa. Sometimes the origin of the tumor is often confusing because primary prostate rhabdomyosarcoma may invade the bladder base or the prostate may have been invaded by a bladder rhabdomyosarcoma [306]. MR imaging can clearly show the site of origin as the central prostate area, and multiplanar image of MR permits accurate assessment of tumor extent [300].

3.10.4.3 Malignant Fibrous Histiocytoma (MFH)

MFH contains fibroblast-like cells in varying proportions in bone or soft tissues. A histologic examination reveals a mesenchymal proliferation of spindle cells with abundant eosinophilic cytoplasm [307]. MFH originated from prostate is very rare, and few case reports have been published. No specific findings are known for

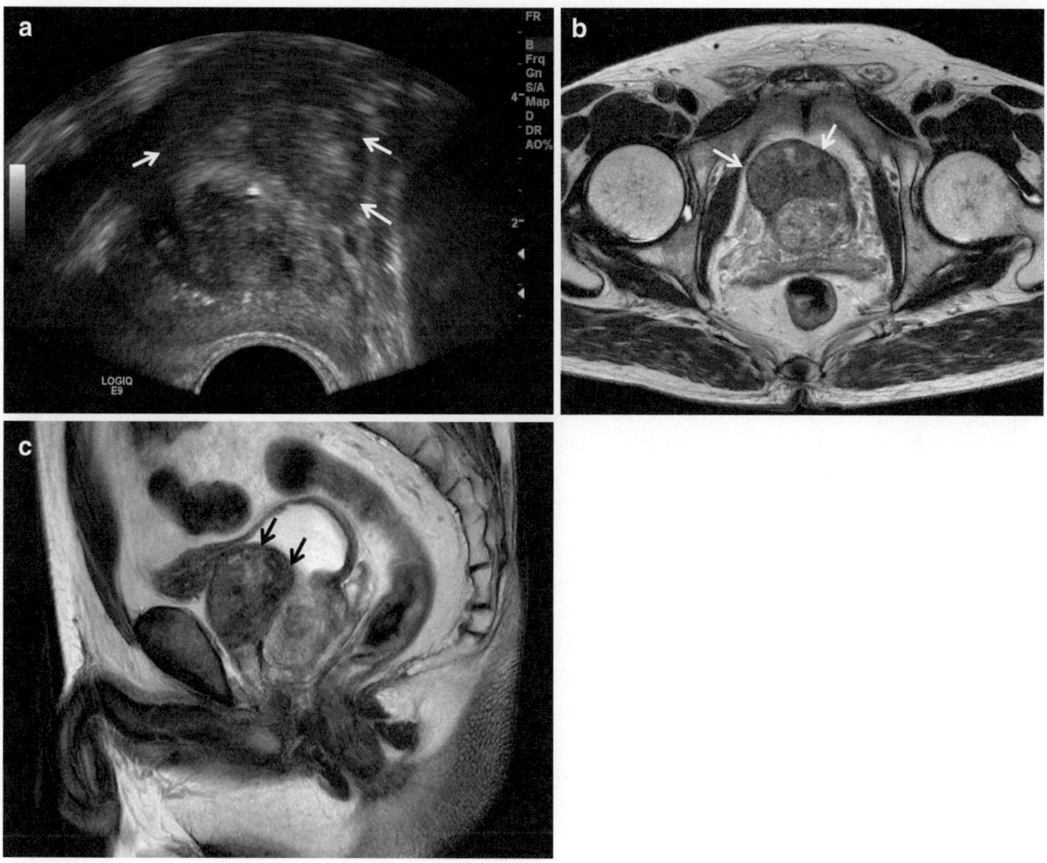

Fig. 3.48 Leiomyosarcoma in a 74-year-old man. (**a**) TRUS image shows well-defined low and heterogeneous echoic mass abutting prostate. T2-weighted axial (**b**) and coronal (**c**) image show relatively low signal intensity lesion arising from peripheral portion of prostate. TRUS-guided biopsy revealed that this lesion was spindle cell tumor favoring leiomyosarcoma

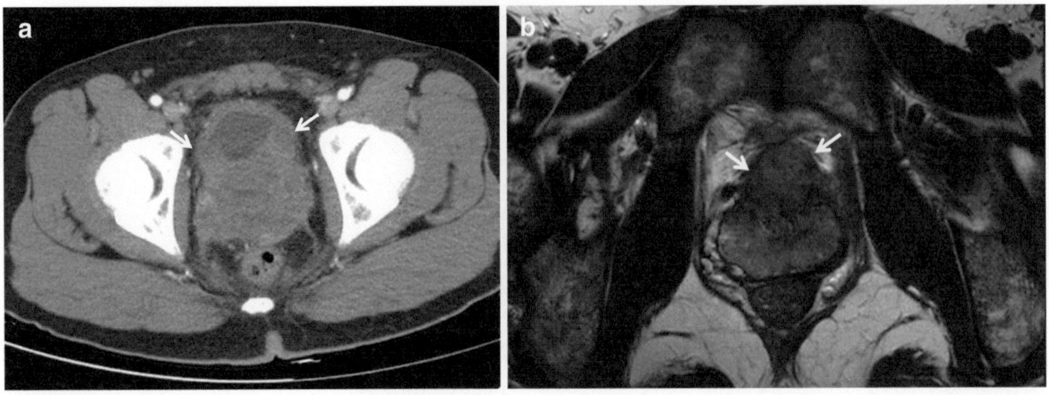

Fig. 3.49 Rhabdomyosarcoma in an 18-year-old boy. (**a**) Post-contrast CT scan shows ill-defined bulky mass arising from prostate. Also note that bladder is invaded by this mass (*arrows*). TRUS-guided biopsy revealed that this mass confirmed as rhabdomyosarcoma. (**b**) After chemotherapy, the size of the mass was decreased, showing low signal intensity mass occupying anterior portion of prostate on T2-weighted axial image (*arrows*)

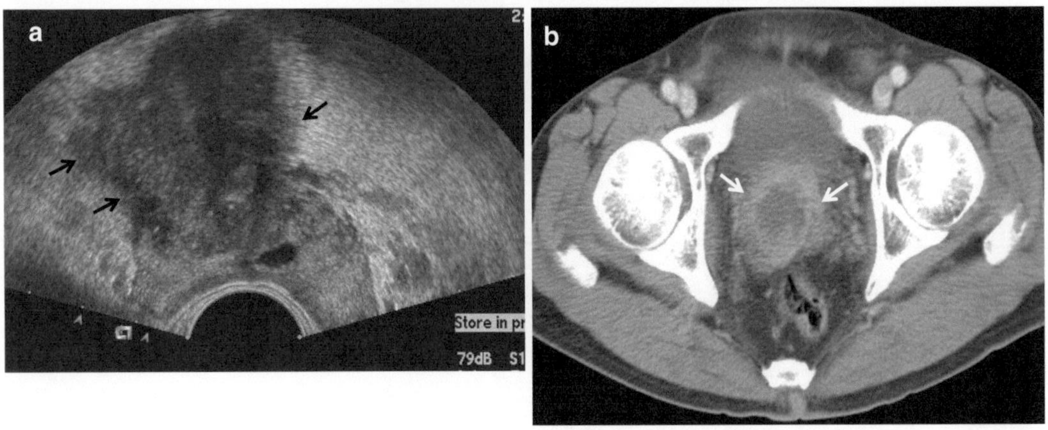

Fig. 3.50 Malignant fibrous histiocytoma in 71-year-old man. (**a**) TRUS shows relatively well-defined low echoic mass arising from prostate (*arrows*). (**b**) Post-contrast CT scan shows low-attenuated mass located in prostate (*arrows*) (Published with kind permission of Korean Society of Ultrasound in Medicine *J Korean Soc Ultrasound Med* 2006;25:1–10)

MFH in the prostate. And the differential diagnosis with rhabdomyosarcoma or other soft tissue sarcomas is very difficult. Our case showed a low echoic, contour bulging mass by TRUS just like rhabdomyosarcoma or leiomyosarcoma. In addition, strong, peripheral contrast enhancement of the soft tissue mass was noted on contrast-enhanced CT (Fig. 3.50).

3.10.4.4 Synovial Sarcoma

Synovial sarcoma is one of mesenchymal neoplasm that typically arises in para-articular soft tissues in young adults [308]. Distant pulmonary metastasis is common after primary tumor surgery. The involvement of the genitourinary tract of primary synovial sarcomas is extremely rare, and it can occur in a variety of locations such as the middle ear, orofacial or oropharyngeal region, esophagus, larynx, lung, pleura, heart, blood vessels, abdominal wall, and retroperitoneum [308]. The image findings of prostatic synovial sarcoma are not well reported (Fig. 3.51). In one case report by Shirakawa et al., T2-weighted MR image showed a high signal mass originating in the prostatic fascia [308].

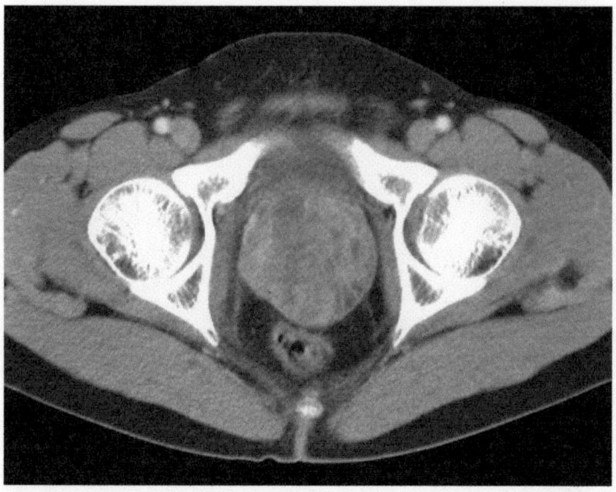

Fig. 3.51 Synovial sarcoma in a 36-year-old man. Postcontrast CT scan shows relatively well-defined mass arising from prostate. TRUS-guided biopsy revealed synovial sarcoma

3.10.5 Hematopoietic Malignancy

3.10.5.1 Lymphoma

Whether as a primary extranodal lymphoma or as a secondary spread to the prostate from other sites, the malignant lymphoma involving the prostate is rare. Primary prostatic lymphomas are much less common than secondary lymphomas, and primary lymphoma can be diagnosed when the lesions are located only in prostate and there is no evidence of systemic lymph node involvement by lymphoma cells [297]. When a young male presents with a large prostate mass, lymphoma of the prostate should be suspected. The systemic symptoms, which are usually presented in lymphoma patients, such as fever, chills, night sweats, and weight loss, are rarely observed. However, the patients with widespread lymphoma can present systematic symptoms. On physical examination, the prostate is usually diffusely enlarged and soft with a rubbery consistency [297]. TRUS reveals large hypoechoic masses located in both the central and peripheral zones and sometimes beyond the boundaries of the prostate in a young man. CT findings of lymphomas reveal soft tissue masses with relatively homogeneous enhancement in the vast majority of cases (Fig. 3.52). Additionally, MR imaging provides some information about the involvement of the bone marrow in patients with high-grade non-Hodgkin's lymphoma. Both CT and MR can assess the extent of the primary disease and associated lymph node enlargement [297].

3.10.6 Non-tumorous or Benign Condition Mimicking Malignancy

3.10.6.1 Benign Prostatic Hyperplasia (BPH)

BPH may be identified as a single, focal nodule or multiple nodules usually within the transition zone. The sonographic characteristics of these nodules vary, and they may show variable echogenicity. Nodules may be surrounded by a thin hypoechoic rim that clearly delineates them from the surrounding tissue [305]. On TRUS, it is difficult to differentiate these lesions from other pathologic processes common to the prostate such as prostate cancer or prostatitis because of the variable appearance of BPH. Moreover, because BPH nodules and prostate cancer may have a similar appearance and echogenicity, it is not possible to differentiate BPH nodules from prostate cancer reliably, based on sonographic characteristics alone (Fig. 3.53). Sometimes, Doppler US was tried to differentiate prostate cancer from benign prostatic hyperplasia. However, Arger et al. reported that quantitative vascularity does not correlate with malignancy [309], because both prostate cancer and benign prostatic hyperplasia can show increased vascularity.

3.10.6.2 Prostatitis and Prostatic Abscesses

The symptoms of acute prostatitis include fever, pain, tenderness on digital rectal examination, dysuria, urgency, and pyuria. Usually, the prostate is enlarged and has low echogenicity on TRUS. At Doppler US, the vascularity is increased [305]. In some cases, acute prostatitis can advance to prostate formation, particularly in diabetic and immunosuppressed patients. The

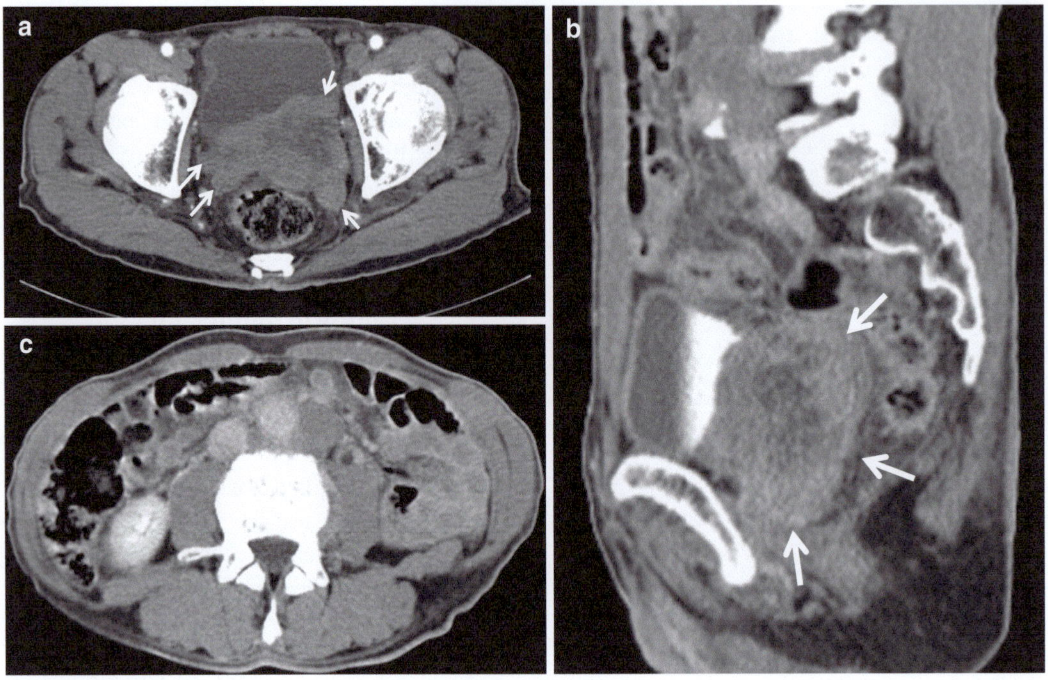

Fig. 3.52 Lymphoma in a 74-year-old man with hematuria. (**a**) CT scan shows ill-defined bulky mass involving prostate and posterior wall of urinary bladder (*arrows*). (**b**) Sagittal-reformatted image also shows bulky mass replacing whole prostate (*arrows*). (**c**) CT scan at right kidney lower pole level shows enlargement of lymph node. Transurethral resection of bladder (TUR-B) revealed diffuse large B cell lymphoma

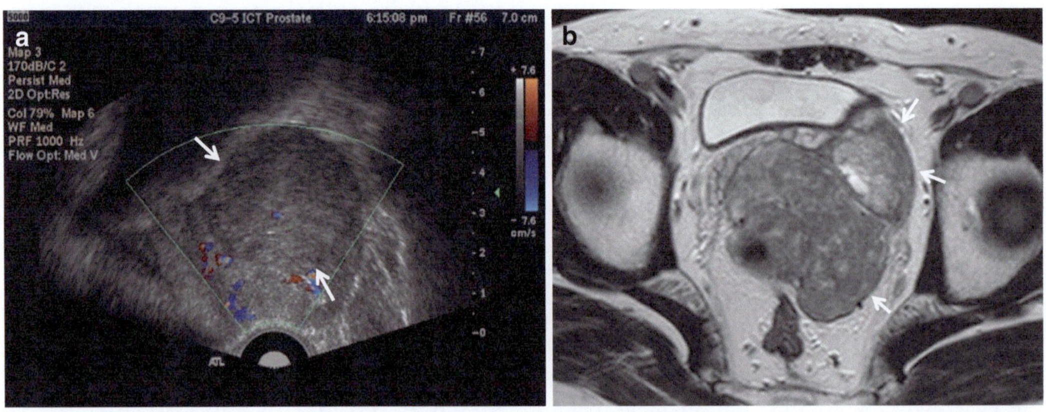

Fig. 3.53 Unusual benign prostate hyperplasia mimicking prostate cancer in a 56-year-old man. (**a**) TRUS image shows huge low and homogenous echoic mass abutting prostate (*arrows*). (**b**) T2-weighted axial scan shows huge heterogeneous signal intensity lesion in pelvic cavity (*arrows*)

organisms most frequently involved are Escherichia coli and Staphylococcus, whereas gonococcus is rarely encountered [310].

The TRUS findings of prostatic abscess include low echoic mass within the prostate, which are similar to those of prostate cancer, whereas CT reveals a low attenuating prostate lesion with peripheral enhancing rims [305] (Fig. 3.54).

Percutaneous transperineal or TRUS-guided aspiration is a useful therapy, because of the lower risk of complications as compared with surgery [305].

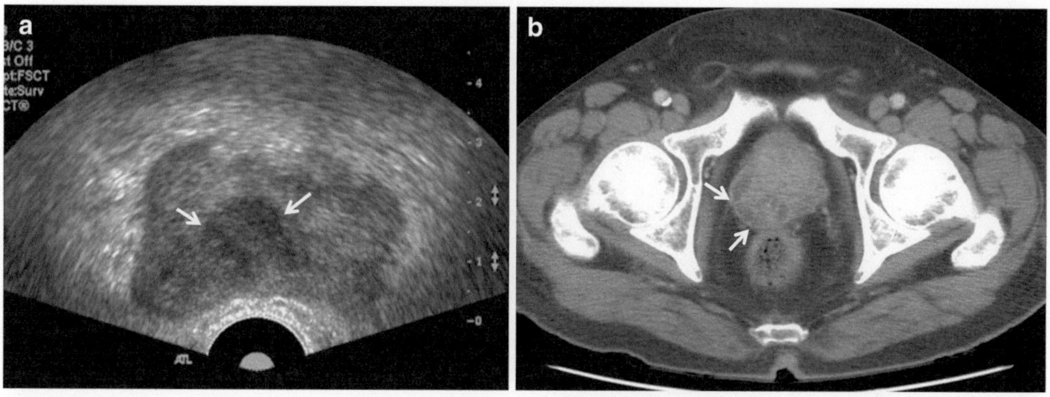

Fig. 3.54 Prostate abscess in a 65-year-old man. (**a**) TRUS image shows relatively well-marginated low echoic lesion in the prostate (*arrows*). (**b**) Post-contrast CT scan shows ill-defined abscess-like lesion involving prostate (*arrows*). The patient was Klebsiella sepsis patient and diagnosed as acute bacterial prostatitis (Published with kind permission of Korean Society of Ultrasound in Medicine *J Korean Soc Ultrasound Med* 2006;25:1–10)

3.10.6.3 Tuberculous Prostatitis

Tuberculosis can involve the prostate as a form of prostatitis or as an abscess [311]. Tuberculosis-related granulomatous prostatitis frequently occurs in cases of Bacillus Calmette-Guerin (BCG) therapy for superficial transitional cell carcinoma of the bladder. In a previous report, granulomatous prostatitis was identified in 75 % of patients who received intravesical BCG therapy.

TRUS in cases of tuberculous prostatitis reveals hypo-echogenic lesion or nodule with increased vascularity (Fig. 3.55). These findings are very similar to that of prostate cancer. Diffuse dystrophic calcifications can also be observed [311]. Post-contrast T1-weighted image shows peripheral enhancing lesion.

3.10.6.4 Prostatic Cystadenoma

Cystadenoma includes multilocular cyst or giant multilocular prostatic cystadenoma. It often presents with obstructive urinary symptoms, with or without a palpable abnormal mass. Histologically, this tumor is characterized by glands and cysts lined with cuboidal epithelium in a fibrous stroma. Positive immunohistochemical staining of epithelial cells for prostate-specific antigen confirms that the tumor is originated from prostate [312]. Usually, these tumors are well-circumscribed and mimic nodular hyperplasia with multiple cysts [285].

Image findings reveal a large multiseptated cystic mass without evidence of local invasion and some soft tissue components may be present (Fig. 3.56). Differential diagnosis includes parasitic hyperplasia, a phyllodes variant of atypical prostatic hyperplasia, and cystic carcinoma [312]. Cystic degeneration in benign prostatic hyperplasia or retention cysts can be differentiated by size. And prostatic abscess can be differentiated because they are usually accompanied by clinical symptoms and signs of infection.

3.10.6.5 Leiomyoma

Leiomyoma primarily originated from prostate is a very rare disease. It is believed to originate from smooth muscle elements of periglandular prostatic tissue, the prostatic capsule, or the Müllerian duct remnant. Just like other leiomyomas in other organs, it is defined specifically as a circumscribed or encapsulated mass of smooth muscle with the size of 1 cm or more in diameter, containing varying amounts of fibrous tissue [313].

Occasionally leiomyoma present as a large mass bulging into the rectum and produce rectal symptoms. TRUS reveals a circumscribed low echoic mass. On post-contrast CT images, leiomyoma appears to be a round heterogeneous attenuated mass (Fig. 3.57). MR reveals it as an isointense signal intensity mass with similar to that

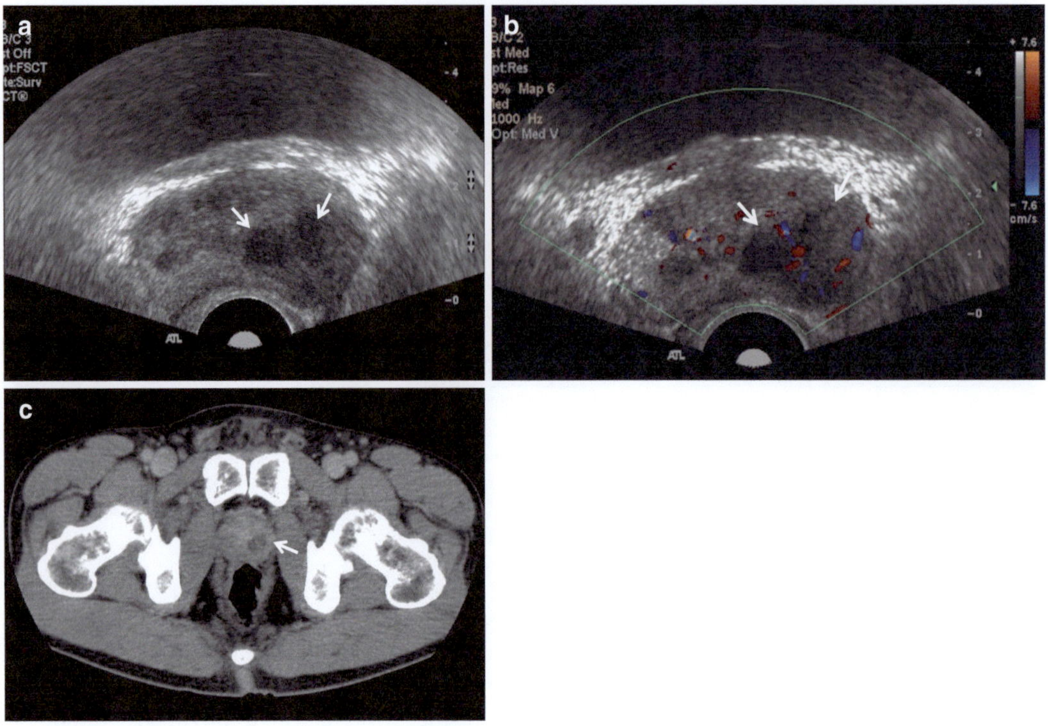

Fig. 3.55 Tuberculous prostatitis in a 64-year-old man. (**a**) TRUS shows low echoic mass-like lesion involving left lobe of prostate (*arrows*). (**b**) Color Doppler image shows increased vascularity on the lesion (*arrows*). (**c**) Post-contrast CT shows low-attenuated abscess-like lesion in left peripheral zone (Published with kind permission of Korean Society of Ultrasound in Medicine *J Korean Soc Ultrasound Med* 2006;25:1–10)

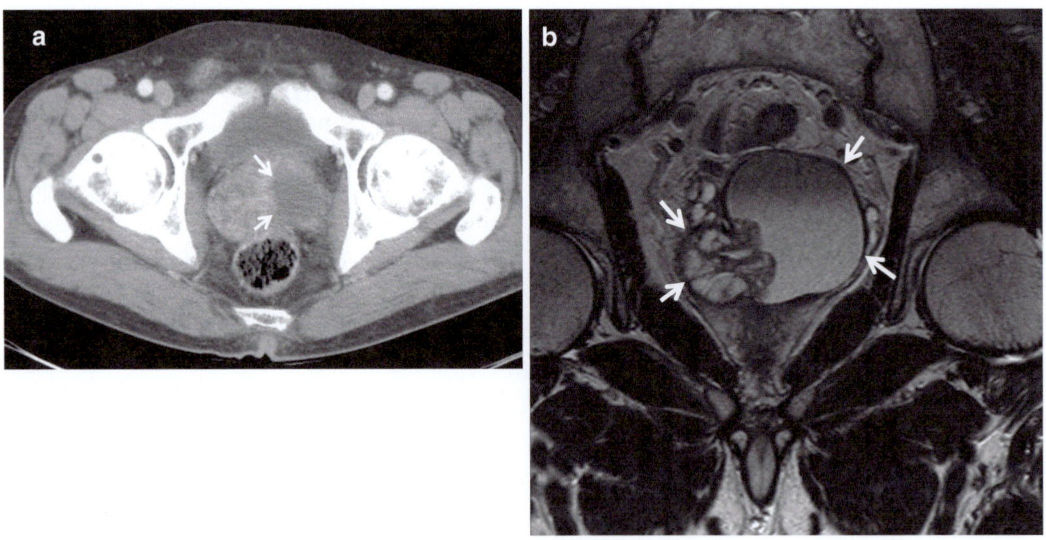

Fig. 3.56 Multilocular cystadenoma in a 64-year-old man. (**a**) Post-contrast CT scan shows relatively well-marginated cystic lesion involving left lobe of prostate (*arrows*). (**b**) T2-weighted coronal image shows multiseptated high signal intensity lesion (*arrows*) (Reprint permission is needed *J Korean Soc Ultrasound Med* 2006;25:1–10)

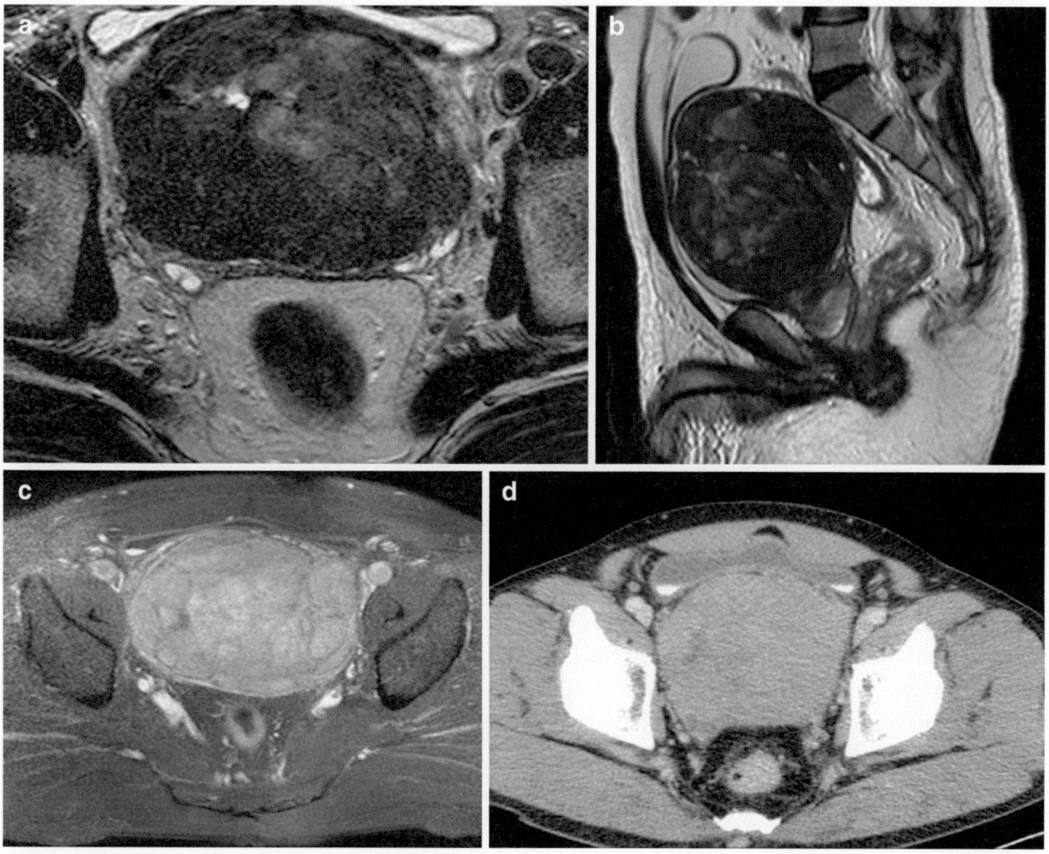

Fig. 3.57 Huge leiomyoma arising from prostate in a 52-year-old man. T2-weighted axial (**a**) and sagittal (**b**) images show dark signal intensity mass abutting prostate. The signal intensity is very similar to that of uterine leiomyoma in women. (**c**) Post-contrast T1-weighted axial scan also shows homogenously enhancing mass in pelvic cavity. (**d**) Post-contrast CT scan also reveals solid mass with homogenous attenuation. TRUS-guided biopsy revealed that this lesion was leiomyoma

of muscle on a T1-weighted images and as slightly hyperintense mass on T2-weighted images [314].

3.10.7 Summary

Many kinds of benign and malignant prostate tumor or tumorlike lesions present as low echoic focal lesions or nodules on TRUS. And they show different signal intensities or attenuations with enhancement patterns on MR or CT according to histologic type. Even though specific radiologic findings suggesting specific diagnosis are rare, knowledge about their radiologic and pathologic findings helps make an accurate radiologic diagnosis and understanding of clinical findings.

Conclusions

Grayscale TRUS is the first-line image modality in evaluating prostate. Also, it is an essential tool for TRUS-guided prostate biopsy. For a satisfactory sampling of the prostate, many tries were performed to increase diagnostic accuracy with small number of cores.

Using ultrasound contrast agents, microvascular abnormalities related to tumor angiogenesis in prostate cancer can be identified and guide an ideal biopsy target representing whole status of prostate. Besides, targeted microbubbles can show the future tool for the evaluation of prostate in the aspect of molecular imaging. Because shear wave elastography has several advantages in that it can provide quantitative information on tissue elasticity, it is a potential modality for evaluating prostate lesions. More validation studies will be needed for the evaluation about the role of elastography in the diagnosis of prostate cancer.

MR imaging is playing an increasing role in the clinical management of patients. From the clinical point of view, MR imaging provides good accuracy in the detection of clinically significant cancer. Especially DWI showed good correlation with tumor aggressiveness.

MP MRI, which includes T2-weighted image and functional images such as diffusion-weighted image, and dynamic contrast-enhanced image, gives us more information regarding the localization of prostate cancer. The MRI images can be used to guide TRUS-guided biopsy via image registration and fusion. However, the lack of standardization in obtaining images and interpreting MR findings is still a problem to be solved in the future.

References

1. Jemal A, Bray F, Center MM, et al. Global cancer statistics. CA Cancer J Clin. 2011;61(2):69–90.
2. Heidenreich A, Bellmunt J, Bolla M, et al. EAU guidelines on prostate cancer. Part 1: screening, diagnosis, and treatment of clinically localised disease. Eur Urol. 2011;59(1):61–71.
3. Watanabe H, Igari D, Tanahasi Y, et al. Development and application of new equipment for transrectal ultrasonography. J Clin Ultrasound. 1974;2(2):91–8.
4. Ferlay J, Steliarova-Foucher E, Lortet-Tieulent J, et al. Cancer incidence and mortality patterns in Europe: estimates for 40 countries in 2012. Eur J Cancer. 2013;49(6):1374–403.
5. National Cancer Institute. Available at: http://www.cancer.gov/cancertopics/types/prostate. Accessed 23 Jan 2015.
6. Bjurlin MA, Meng X, Le NJ, et al. Optimization of prostate biopsy: the role of magnetic resonance imaging targeted biopsy in detection, localization and risk assessment. J Urol. 2014;192(3):648–58.
7. National Institute for Health and Care Excellence (NICE). NICE CG58 prostate cancer: full guidance. London: NICE; 2008. URL: http://guidance.nice.org.uk/CG58/Guidance/pdf/English. Accessed June 2012.
8. Franks LM. Latent carcinoma of the prostate. J Pathol Bacteriol. 1954;68(2):603–16.
9. Yoon DK, Kim WJ, Kim CS, et al. The incidence of Urogenital tumor during recent five years in Korea. Korean J Urol. 2003;44:203.
10. Thompson I, Thrasher JB, Aus G, et al. Guideline for the management of clinically localized prostate cancer: 2007 update. J Urol. 2007;177(6):2106–31.
11. Ferlay J, Shin H, Bray F. Globocan 2008. Prostate cancer incidence, mortality and prevalence worldwide in 2008. 2008. Available at: http://globocan.iarc.fr. Accessed 18 Aug 2012.
12. Smith DS, Catalona WJ. Interexaminer variability of digital rectal examination in detecting prostate cancer. Urology. 1995;45(1):70–4.
13. Mowatt G, Scotland G, Boachie C, et al. The diagnostic accuracy and cost-effectiveness of magnetic resonance spectroscopy and enhanced magnetic resonance imaging techniques in aiding the localisation of prostate abnormalities for biopsy: a systematic review and economic evaluation. Health Technol Assess. 2013;17(20):1–281.
14. Jung AJ, Westphalen AC. Imaging prostate cancer. Radiol Clin North Am. 2012;50(6):1043–59.
15. Coakley FV, Hricak H. Radiologic anatomy of the prostate gland: a clinical approach. Radiol Clin North Am. 2000;38(1):15–30.
16. Rifkin MD, Dahnert W, Kurtz AB. State of the art: endorectal sonography of the prostate gland. AJR Am J Roentgenol. 1990;154(4):691–700.
17. Dahnert WF, Hamper UM, Eggleston JC, et al. Prostatic evaluation by transrectal sonography with histopathologic correlation: the echopenic appearance of early carcinoma. Radiology. 1986;158(1):97–102.
18. Vo T, Rifkin MD, Peters TL. Should ultrasound criteria of the prostate be redefined to better evaluate when and where to biopsy. Ultrasound Q. 2001;17(3):171–6.
19. Ismail M, Gomella LG. Ultrasound for prostate imaging and biopsy. Curr Opin Urol. 2001;11(5):471–7.
20. Onur R, Littrup PJ, Pontes JE, et al. Contemporary impact of transrectal ultrasound lesions for prostate cancer detection. J Urol. 2004;172(2):512–4.
21. Eichler K, Hempel S, Wilby J, et al. Diagnostic value of systematic biopsy methods in the investigation of prostate cancer: a systematic review. J Urol. 2006;175(5):1605–12.
22. Lee HY, Lee HJ, Byun SS, et al. Classification of focal prostatic lesions on transrectal ultrasound (TRUS) and the accuracy of TRUS to diagnose prostate cancer. Korean J Radiol. 2009;10(3):244–51.
23. Smeenge M, de la Rosette JJ, Wijkstra H. Current status of transrectal ultrasound techniques in prostate cancer. Curr Opin Urol. 2012;22(4):297–302.
24. Kapoor A, Kapoor A, Mahajan G, et al. Real-time elastography in the detection of prostate cancer in patients with raised PSA level. Ultrasound Med Biol. 2011;37(9):1374–81.
25. Ginat DT, Destounis SV, Barr RG, et al. US elastography of breast and prostate lesions. Radiographics. 2009;29(7):2007–16.

26. Zhang M, Nigwekar P, Castaneda B, et al. Quantitative characterization of viscoelastic properties of human prostate correlated with histology. Ultrasound Med Biol. 2008;34(7):1033–42.
27. Barr RG, Memo R, Schaub CR. Shear wave ultrasound elastography of the prostate: initial results. Ultrasound Q. 2012;28(1):13–20.
28. Aboumarzouk OM, Ogston S, Huang Z, et al. Diagnostic accuracy of transrectal elastosonography (TRES) imaging for the diagnosis of prostate cancer: a systematic review and meta-analysis. BJU Int. 2012;110(10):1414–23; discussion 1423.
29. Hong CW, Amalou H, Xu S, et al. Prostate biopsy for the interventional radiologist. J Vasc Interv Radiol. 2014;25(5):675–84.
30. Kurhanewicz J, Swanson MG, Nelson SJ, et al. Combined magnetic resonance imaging and spectroscopic imaging approach to molecular imaging of prostate cancer. J Magn Reson Imaging. 2002;16(4):451–63.
31. Ismail MT, Gomella LG. Transrectal prostate biopsy. Urol Clin North Am. 2013;40(4):457–72.
32. Pallwein L, Mitterberger M, Struve P, et al. Comparison of sonoelastography guided biopsy with systematic biopsy: impact on prostate cancer detection. Eur Radiol. 2007;17(9):2278–85.
33. Brock M, von Bodman C, Palisaar RJ, et al. The impact of real-time elastography guiding a systematic prostate biopsy to improve cancer detection rate: a prospective study of 353 patients. J Urol. 2012;187(6):2039–43.
34. Aigner F, Pallwein L, Schocke M, et al. Comparison of real-time sonoelastography with T2-weighted endorectal magnetic resonance imaging for prostate cancer detection. J Ultrasound Med. 2011;30(5):643–9.
35. Zhang Y, Tang J, Li YM, et al. Differentiation of prostate cancer from benign lesions using strain index of transrectal real-time tissue elastography. Eur J Radiol. 2012;81(5):857–62.
36. Ahmad S, Cao R, Varghese T, et al. Transrectal quantitative shear wave elastography in the detection and characterisation of prostate cancer. Surg Endosc. 2013;27(9):3280–7.
37. Woo S, Kim S, Cho J, et al. Shear wave elastography for detection of prostate cancer: a preliminary study. Korean J Radiol. 2014;15(3):346–55.
38. Trabulsi EJ, Sackett D, Gomella LG, et al. Enhanced transrectal ultrasound modalities in the diagnosis of prostate cancer. Urology. 2010;76(5):1025–33.
39. Burns PN, Wilson SR. Microbubble contrast for radiological imaging: 1. Principles. Ultrasound Q. 2006;22(1):5–13.
40. Lee HJ, Han JG. A study of parameters in spiral CT volumetry using balloon phantoms. J Korean Radiol Soc. 2001;45(2):221–8.
41. Choi JI, Kim SH, Seong CK, et al. Recurrent uterine cervical carcinoma: spectrum of imaging findings. Korean J Radiol. 2000;1(4):198–207.
42. Brawer MK, Deering RE, Brown M, et al. Predictors of pathologic stage in prostatic carcinoma. The role of neovascularity. Cancer. 1994;73(3):678–87.
43. Ismail M, Petersen RO, Alexander AA, et al. Color Doppler imaging in predicting the biologic behavior of prostate cancer: correlation with disease-free survival. Urology. 1997;50(6):906–12.
44. Furlow B. Contrast-enhanced ultrasound. Radiol Technol. 2009;80(6):547s–61.
45. Weidner N, Carroll PR, Flax J, et al. Tumor angiogenesis correlates with metastasis in invasive prostate carcinoma. Am J Pathol. 1993;143(2):401–9.
46. Lee HJ, Hwang SI, Chung JH, et al. Evaluation of tumor angiogenesis in a mouse PC-3 prostate cancer model using dynamic contrast-enhanced sonography. J Ultrasound Med. 2012;31(8):1223–31.
47. Sedelaar JP, van Leenders GJ, Hulsbergen-van de Kaa CA, et al. Microvessel density: correlation between contrast ultrasonography and histology of prostate cancer. Eur Urol. 2001;40(3):285–93.
48. Mitterberger M, Pinggera G, Horninger W, et al. Comparison of contrast enhanced color Doppler targeted biopsy to conventional systematic biopsy: impact on Gleason score. J Urol. 2007;178:464–8.
49. Jiang J, Chen Y, Zhu Y, et al. Contrast-enhanced ultrasonography for the detection and characterization of prostate cancer: correlation with microvessel density and Gleason score. Clin Radiol. 2011;66:732–7.
50. Li Y, Tang J, Fei X, et al. Diagnostic performance of contrast enhanced ultrasound in patients with prostate cancer: a meta-analysis. Acad Radiol. 2013;20(2):156–64.
51. Smeenge M, Mischi M, Laguna Pes MP, et al. Novel contrast-enhanced ultrasound imaging in prostate cancer. World J Urol. 2011;29(5):581–7.
52. Fischer T, Thomas A, Tardy I, et al. Vascular endothelial growth factor receptor 2-specific microbubbles for molecular ultrasound detection of prostate cancer in a rat model. Invest Radiol. 2010;45(10):675–84.
53. Perner S, Hofer MD, Kim R, et al. Prostate-specific membrane antigen expression as a predictor of prostate cancer progression. Hum Pathol. 2007;38(5):696–701.
54. Wang L, Li L, Guo Y, et al. Construction and in vitro/in vivo targeting of PSMA-targeted nanoscale microbubbles in prostate cancer. Prostate. 2013;73(11):1147–58.
55. Stroumbakis N, Cookson MS, Reuter VE, et al. Clinical significance of repeat sextant biopsies in prostate cancer patients. Urology. 1997;49(3A Suppl):113–8.
56. Halpern EJ, Strup SE. Using gray-scale and color and power Doppler sonography to detect prostatic cancer. AJR Am J Roentgenol. 2000;174(3):623–7.
57. Barentsz JO, Richenberg J, Clements R, et al. ESUR prostate MR guidelines 2012. Eur Radiol. 2012;22(4):746–57.
58. Hricak H, Choyke PL, Eberhardt SC, et al. Imaging prostate cancer: a multidisciplinary perspective. Radiology. 2007;243(1):28–53.
59. Dickinson L, Ahmed HU, Allen C, et al. Magnetic resonance imaging for the detection, localisation,

and characterisation of prostate cancer: recommendations from a European consensus meeting. Eur Urol. 2011;59(4):477–94.
60. Westphalen AC, Reed GD, Vinh PP, et al. Multiparametric 3T endorectal mri after external beam radiation therapy for prostate cancer. J Magn Reson Imaging. 2012;36(2):430–7.
61. Sonn GA, Natarajan S, Margolis DJ, et al. Targeted biopsy in the detection of prostate cancer using an office based magnetic resonance ultrasound fusion device. J Urol. 2013;189(1):86–91.
62. Labanaris AP, Engelhard K, Zugor V, et al. Prostate cancer detection using an extended prostate biopsy schema in combination with additional targeted cores from suspicious images in conventional and functional endorectal magnetic resonance imaging of the prostate. Prostate Cancer Prostatic Dis. 2010;13(1):65–70.
63. Kasivisvanathan V, Dufour R, Moore CM, et al. Transperineal magnetic resonance image targeted prostate biopsy versus transperineal template prostate biopsy in the detection of clinically significant prostate cancer. J Urol. 2013;189(3):860–6.
64. Stephenson SK, Chang EK, Marks LS. Screening and detection advances in magnetic resonance image-guided prostate biopsy. Urol Clin North Am. 2014;41(2):315–26.
65. Sonn GA, Chang E, Natarajan S, et al. Value of targeted prostate biopsy using magnetic resonance-ultrasound fusion in men with prior negative biopsy and elevated prostate-specific antigen. Eur Urol. 2014;65(4):809–15.
66. Ukimura O, Desai MM, Palmer S, et al. 3-Dimensional elastic registration system of prostate biopsy location by real-time 3-dimensional transrectal ultrasound guidance with magnetic resonance/transrectal ultrasound image fusion. J Urol. 2012;187(3):1080–6.
67. Rabbani F, Stroumbakis N, Kava BR, et al. Incidence and clinical significance of false-negative sextant prostate biopsies. J Urol. 1998;159(4):1247–50.
68. Kvale R, Moller B, Wahlqvist R, et al. Concordance between Gleason scores of needle biopsies and radical prostatectomy specimens: a population-based study. BJU Int. 2009;103(12):1647–54.
69. Park EA, Lee HJ, Kim KG, et al. Prediction of pathological stages before prostatectomy in prostate cancer patients: analysis of 12 systematic prostate needle biopsy specimens. Int J Urol. 2007;14(8):704–8.
70. D'Amico AV, Tempany CM, Cormack R, et al. Transperineal magnetic resonance image guided prostate biopsy. J Urol. 2000;164(2):385–7.
71. Epstein JI, Walsh PC, Carmichael M, et al. Pathologic and clinical findings to predict tumor extent of nonpalpable (stage T1c) prostate cancer. JAMA. 1994;271(5):368–74.
72. Punglia RS, D'Amico AV, Catalona WJ, et al. Effect of verification bias on screening for prostate cancer by measurement of prostate-specific antigen. N Engl J Med. 2003;349(4):335–42.
73. NCCN guidelines: prostate cancer early detection (v.2.2012). Comprehensive Cancer Network Website. Available at: http://www.nccn.org. Accessed 28 Apr 2013.
74. Bertaccini A, Fandella A, Prayer-Galetti T, et al. Systematic development of clinical practice guidelines for prostate biopsies: a 3-year Italian project. Anticancer Res. 2007;27(1b):659–66.
75. Presti Jr JC, Chang JJ, Bhargava V, et al. The optimal systematic prostate biopsy scheme should include 8 rather than 6 biopsies: results of a prospective clinical trial. J Urol. 2000;163(1):163–6; discussion 166–167.
76. Ozden E, Yaman O, Gogus C, et al. The optimum doses of and injection locations for periprostatic nerve blockade for transrectal ultrasound guided biopsy of the prostate: a prospective, randomized, placebo controlled study. J Urol. 2003;170(6 Pt 1):2319–22.
77. Seymour H, Perry MJ, Lee-Elliot C, et al. Pain after transrectal ultrasonography-guided prostate biopsy: the advantages of periprostatic local anaesthesia. BJU Int. 2001;88(6):540–4.
78. Schostak M, Christoph F, Muller M, et al. Optimizing local anesthesia during 10-core biopsy of the prostate. Urology. 2002;60(2):253–7.
79. Alavi AS, Soloway MS, Vaidya A, et al. Local anesthesia for ultrasound guided prostate biopsy: a prospective randomized trial comparing 2 methods. J Urol. 2001;166(4):1343–5.
80. Addla SK, Adeyoju AA, Wemyss-Holden GD, et al. Local anaesthetic for transrectal ultrasound-guided prostate biopsy: a prospective, randomized, double blind, placebo-controlled study. Eur Urol. 2003;43(5):441–3.
81. Cormio L, Lorusso F, Selvaggio O, et al. Noninfiltrative anesthesia for transrectal prostate biopsy: a randomized prospective study comparing lidocaine-prilocaine cream and lidocaine-ketorolac gel. Urol Oncol. 2013;31(1):68–73.
82. Leibovici D, Zisman A, Siegel YI, et al. Local anesthesia for prostate biopsy by periprostatic lidocaine injection: a double-blind placebo controlled study. J Urol. 2002;167(2 Pt 1):563–5.
83. Ismail T, Janane A, Dakkak Y. The contribution of periapical nerve block in transrectal ultrasound-guided prostate biopsy: results from a prospective randomized trial. Afr J Urol. 2012;18:78–81.
84. Lee HY, Lee HJ, Byun SS, et al. Effect of intraprostatic local anesthesia during transrectal ultrasound guided prostate biopsy: comparison of 3 methods in a randomized, double-blind, placebo controlled trial. J Urol. 2007;178(2):469–72; discussion 472.
85. Chun FK, Epstein JI, Ficarra V, et al. Optimizing performance and interpretation of prostate biopsy: a critical analysis of the literature. Eur Urol. 2010;58(6):851–64.
86. Delongchamps NB, de la Roza G, Jones R, et al. Saturation biopsies on autopsied prostates for detecting and characterizing prostate cancer. BJU Int. 2009;103(1):49–54.

87. Jones JS. Prostate cancer: are we over-diagnosing-or under-thinking? Eur Urol. 2008;53(1):10–2.
88. Campos-Fernandes JL, Bastien L, Nicolaiew N, et al. Prostate cancer detection rate in patients with repeated extended 21-sample needle biopsy. Eur Urol. 2009;55(3):600–6.
89. Zaytoun OM, Moussa AS, Gao T, et al. Office based transrectal saturation biopsy improves prostate cancer detection compared to extended biopsy in the repeat biopsy population. J Urol. 2011;186(3):850–4.
90. Desmond PM, Clark J, Thompson IM, et al. Morbidity with contemporary prostate biopsy. J Urol. 1993;150(5 Pt 1):1425–6.
91. Ajzen SA, Goldenberg SL, Allen GJ, et al. Palpable prostatic nodules: comparison of US and digital guidance for fine-needle aspiration biopsy. Radiology. 1989;171(2):521–3.
92. Berger AP, Gozzi C, Steiner H, et al. Complication rate of transrectal ultrasound guided prostate biopsy: a comparison among 3 protocols with 6, 10 and 15 cores. J Urol. 2004;171(4):1478–80; discussion 1480–1471.
93. Hegde JV, Mulkern RV, Panych LP, et al. Multiparametric MRI of prostate cancer: an update on state-of-the-art techniques and their performance in detecting and localizing prostate cancer. J Magn Reson Imaging. 2013;37(5):1035–54.
94. Hricak H, Dooms GC, McNeal JE, et al. MR imaging of the prostate gland: normal anatomy. AJR Am J Roentgenol. 1987;148(1):51–8.
95. Durmus T, Baur A, Hamm B. Multiparametric magnetic resonance imaging in the detection of prostate cancer. Rofo. 2014;186(3):238–46.
96. Nakashima J, Tanimoto A, Imai Y, et al. Endorectal MRI for prediction of tumor site, tumor size, and local extension of prostate cancer. Urology. 2004;64(1):101–5.
97. Beyersdorff D, Taupitz M, Winkelmann B, et al. Patients with a history of elevated prostate-specific antigen levels and negative transrectal US-guided quadrant or sextant biopsy results: value of MR imaging. Radiology. 2002;224(3):701–6.
98. Langer DL, van der Kwast TH, Evans AJ, et al. Prostate tissue composition and MR measurements: investigating the relationships between ADC, T2, K(trans), v(e), and corresponding histologic features. Radiology. 2010;255(2):485–94.
99. Bourne R, Kurniawan N, Cowin G, et al. 16 T diffusion microimaging of fixed prostate tissue: preliminary findings. Magn Reson Med. 2011;66(1):244–7.
100. Neto JA, Parente DB. Multiparametric magnetic resonance imaging of the prostate. Magn Reson Imaging Clin N Am. 2013;21(2):409–26.
101. Cruz M, Tsuda K, Narumi Y, et al. Characterization of low-intensity lesions in the peripheral zone of prostate on pre-biopsy endorectal coil MR imaging. Eur Radiol. 2002;12(2):357–65.
102. Ikonen S, Kivisaari L, Tervahartiala P, et al. Prostatic MR imaging. Accuracy in differentiating cancer from other prostatic disorders. Acta radiologica (Stockholm, Sweden: 1987). 2001;42(4):348–54.
103. Shukla-Dave A, Hricak H, Eberhardt SC, et al. Chronic prostatitis: MR imaging and 1H MR spectroscopic imaging findings – initial observations. Radiology. 2004;231(3):717–24.
104. Tamada T, Sone T, Toshimitsu S, et al. Age-related and zonal anatomical changes of apparent diffusion coefficient values in normal human prostatic tissues. J Magn Reson Imaging. 2008;27(3):552–6.
105. Akin O, Sala E, Moskowitz CS, et al. Transition zone prostate cancers: features, detection, localization, and staging at endorectal MR imaging. Radiology. 2006;239(3):784–92.
106. Purysko AS, Herts BR. Prostate MRI: the hemorrhage exclusion sign. J Urol. 2012;188(5):1946–7.
107. Turkbey B, Aras O, Karabulut N, et al. Diffusion-weighted MRI for detecting and monitoring cancer: a review of current applications in body imaging. Diagn Interv Radiol. 2012;18(1):46–59.
108. Koh DM, Collins DJ. Diffusion-weighted MRI in the body: applications and challenges in oncology. AJR Am J Roentgenol. 2007;188(6):1622–35.
109. Issa B. In vivo measurement of the apparent diffusion coefficient in normal and malignant prostatic tissues using echo-planar imaging. J Magn Reson Imaging. 2002;16(2):196–200.
110. Rosenkrantz AB, Kong X, Niver BE, et al. Prostate cancer: comparison of tumor visibility on trace diffusion-weighted images and the apparent diffusion coefficient map. AJR Am J Roentgenol. 2011;196(1):123–9.
111. Yagci AB, Ozari N, Aybek Z, et al. The value of diffusion-weighted MRI for prostate cancer detection and localization. Diagn Interv Radiol. 2011;17(2):130–4.
112. Haider MA, van der Kwast TH, Tanguay J, et al. Combined T2-weighted and diffusion-weighted MRI for localization of prostate cancer. AJR Am J Roentgenol. 2007;189(2):323–8.
113. Kim CK, Park BK, Lee HM, et al. Value of diffusion-weighted imaging for the prediction of prostate cancer location at 3T using a phased-array coil: preliminary results. Invest Radiol. 2007;42(12):842–7.
114. Kim CK, Park BK, Kim B. High-b-value diffusion-weighted imaging at 3 T to detect prostate cancer: comparisons between b values of 1,000 and 2,000 s/mm2. AJR Am J Roentgenol. 2010;194(1):W33–7.
115. Metens T, Miranda D, Absil J, et al. What is the optimal b value in diffusion-weighted MR imaging to depict prostate cancer at 3T? Eur Radiol. 2012;22(3):703–9.
116. Kim JH, Kim JK, Park BW, et al. Apparent diffusion coefficient: prostate cancer versus noncancerous tissue according to anatomical region. J Magn Reson Imaging. 2008;28(5):1173–9.
117. Hambrock T, Somford DM, Huisman HJ, et al. Relationship between apparent diffusion coefficients at 3.0-T MR imaging and Gleason grade in peripheral zone prostate cancer. Radiology. 2011;259(2):453–61.

118. Vargas HA, Akin O, Franiel T, et al. Diffusion-weighted endorectal MR imaging at 3 T for prostate cancer: tumor detection and assessment of aggressiveness. Radiology. 2011;259(3):775–84.
119. Oto A, Yang C, Kayhan A, et al. Diffusion-weighted and dynamic contrast-enhanced MRI of prostate cancer: correlation of quantitative MR parameters with Gleason score and tumor angiogenesis. AJR Am J Roentgenol. 2011;197(6):1382–90.
120. Turkbey B, Shah VP, Pang Y, et al. Is apparent diffusion coefficient associated with clinical risk scores for prostate cancers that are visible on 3-T MR images? Radiology. 2011;258(2):488–95.
121. Turkbey B, Bernardo M, Merino MJ, et al. MRI of localized prostate cancer: coming of age in the PSA era. Diagn Interv Radiol. 2012;18(1):34–45.
122. Durmus T, Vollnberg B, Schwenke C, et al. Dynamic contrast enhanced MRI of the prostate: comparison of gadobutrol and Gd-DTPA. Rofo. 2013;185(9): 862–8.
123. Tofts PS, Brix G, Buckley DL, et al. Estimating kinetic parameters from dynamic contrast-enhanced T(1)-weighted MRI of a diffusable tracer: standardized quantities and symbols. J Magn Reson Imaging. 1999;10(3):223–32.
124. Franiel T, Hamm B, Hricak H. Dynamic contrast-enhanced magnetic resonance imaging and pharmacokinetic models in prostate cancer. Eur Radiol. 2011;21(3):616–26.
125. Futterer JJ, Heijmink SW, Scheenen TW, et al. Prostate cancer localization with dynamic contrast-enhanced MR imaging and proton MR spectroscopic imaging. Radiology. 2006;241(2):449–58.
126. Hara N, Okuizumi M, Koike H, et al. Dynamic contrast-enhanced magnetic resonance imaging (DCE-MRI) is a useful modality for the precise detection and staging of early prostate cancer. Prostate. 2005;62(2):140–7.
127. Cirillo S, Petracchini M, Scotti L, et al. Endorectal magnetic resonance imaging at 1.5 Tesla to assess local recurrence following radical prostatectomy using T2-weighted and contrast-enhanced imaging. Eur Radiol. 2009;19(3):761–9.
128. Haider MA, Chung P, Sweet J, et al. Dynamic contrast-enhanced magnetic resonance imaging for localization of recurrent prostate cancer after external beam radiotherapy. Int J Radiat Oncol Biol Phys. 2008;70(2):425–30.
129. Ocak I, Bernardo M, Metzger G, et al. Dynamic contrast-enhanced MRI of prostate cancer at 3 T: a study of pharmacokinetic parameters. AJR Am J Roentgenol. 2007;189(4):849.
130. Kozlowski P, Chang SD, Jones EC, et al. Combined diffusion-weighted and dynamic contrast-enhanced MRI for prostate cancer diagnosis – correlation with biopsy and histopathology. J Magn Reson Imaging. 2006;24(1):108–13.
131. Delongchamps NB, Rouanne M, Flam T, et al. Multiparametric magnetic resonance imaging for the detection and localization of prostate cancer: combination of T2-weighted, dynamic contrast-enhanced and diffusion-weighted imaging. BJU Int. 2011; 107(9):1411–8.
132. Bloch BN, Furman-Haran E, Helbich TH, et al. Prostate cancer: accurate determination of extracapsular extension with high-spatial-resolution dynamic contrast-enhanced and T2-weighted MR imaging – initial results. Radiology. 2007;245(1): 176–85.
133. Kurhanewicz J, Vigneron DB. Advances in MR spectroscopy of the prostate. Magn Reson Imaging Clin N Am. 2008;16(4):697–710, ix–x.
134. Scheenen TW, Futterer J, Weiland E, et al. Discriminating cancer from noncancer tissue in the prostate by 3-dimensional proton magnetic resonance spectroscopic imaging: a prospective multicenter validation study. Invest Radiol. 2011;46(1):25–33.
135. Hoeks CM, Barentsz JO, Hambrock T, et al. Prostate cancer: multiparametric MR imaging for detection, localization, and staging. Radiology. 2011; 261(1):46–66.
136. Kaji Y, Kurhanewicz J, Hricak H, et al. Localizing prostate cancer in the presence of postbiopsy changes on MR images: role of proton MR spectroscopic imaging. Radiology. 1998;206(3):785–90.
137. Girouin N, Mege-Lechevallier F, Tonina Senes A, et al. Prostate dynamic contrast-enhanced MRI with simple visual diagnostic criteria: is it reasonable? Eur Radiol. 2007;17(6):1498–509.
138. Tanimoto A, Nakashima J, Kohno H, et al. Prostate cancer screening: the clinical value of diffusion-weighted imaging and dynamic MR imaging in combination with T2-weighted imaging. J Magn Reson Imaging. 2007;25(1):146–52.
139. Turkbey B, Pinto PA, Mani H, et al. Prostate cancer: value of multiparametric MR imaging at 3 T for detection – histopathologic correlation. Radiology. 2010;255(1):89–99.
140. Puech P, Betrouni N, Makni N, et al. Computer-assisted diagnosis of prostate cancer using DCE-MRI data: design, implementation and preliminary results. Int J Comput Assist Radiol Surg. 2009;4(1):1–10.
141. Vos PC, Hambrock T, Hulsbergen-van de Kaa CA, et al. Computerized analysis of prostate lesions in the peripheral zone using dynamic contrast enhanced MRI. Med Phys. 2008;35(3):888–99.
142. Vos P. Combining T2-weighted with dynamic MR images for computerized classification of prostate lesions. In: Editor A, Editor B, editors. Proceedings of SPIE: medical imaging 2008. Bellingham: SPIE-The International Society for Optical Engineering.
143. Ruprecht O, Weisser P, Bodelle B, et al. MRI of the prostate: interobserver agreement compared with histopathologic outcome after radical prostatectomy. Eur J Radiol. 2012;81(3):456–60.

144. Rothke M, Blondin D, Schlemmer HP, et al. PI-RADS classification: structured reporting for MRI of the prostate. Rofo. 2013;185(3):253–61.
145. Takeuchi M, Matsuzaki K, Nishitani H. Hyperintense uterine myometrial masses on T2-weighted magnetic resonance imaging: differentiation with diffusion-weighted magnetic resonance imaging. J Comput Assist Tomogr. 2009;33(6):834–7.
146. Rechichi G, Galimberti S, Signorelli M, et al. Myometrial invasion in endometrial cancer: diagnostic performance of diffusion-weighted MR imaging at 1.5-T. Eur Radiol. 2010;20(3):754–62.
147. Punwani S. Diffusion weighted imaging of female pelvic cancers: concepts and clinical applications. Eur J Radiol. 2011;78(1):21–9.
148. Haffner J, Lemaitre L, Puech P, et al. Role of magnetic resonance imaging before initial biopsy: comparison of magnetic resonance imaging-targeted and systematic biopsy for significant prostate cancer detection. BJU Int. 2011;108(8 Pt 2):E171–8.
149. Bott SR, Young MP, Kellett MJ, et al. Anterior prostate cancer: is it more difficult to diagnose? BJU Int. 2002;89(9):886–9.
150. Ouzzane A, Puech P, Lemaitre L, et al. Combined multiparametric MRI and targeted biopsies improve anterior prostate cancer detection, staging, and grading. Urology. 2011;78(6):1356–62.
151. Klotz L. Active surveillance for favorable-risk prostate cancer: background, patient selection, triggers for intervention, and outcomes. Curr Urol Rep. 2012;13(2):153–9.
152. Lees K, Durve M, Parker C. Active surveillance in prostate cancer: patient selection and triggers for intervention. Curr Opin Urol. 2012;22(3):210–5.
153. de la Rosette J, Ahmed H, Barentsz J, et al. Focal therapy in prostate cancer-report from a consensus panel. J Endourol. 2010;24(5):775–80.
154. Cooperberg MR, Lubeck DP, Meng MV, et al. The changing face of low-risk prostate cancer: trends in clinical presentation and primary management. J Clin Oncol. 2004;22(11):2141–9.
155. Sella T, Schwartz LH, Hricak H. Retained seminal vesicles after radical prostatectomy: frequency, MRI characteristics, and clinical relevance. AJR Am J Roentgenol. 2006;186(2):539–46.
156. Cooperberg MR, Broering JM, Carroll PR. Time trends and local variation in primary treatment of localized prostate cancer. J Clin Oncol. 2010;28(7):1117–23.
157. Fraass BA. The development of conformal radiation therapy. Med Phys. 1995;22(11 Pt 2):1911–21.
158. Vargas HA, Wassberg C, Akin O, Hricak H. MR imaging of treated prostate cancer. Radiology. 2012;262(1):26–42.
159. Sharifi N, Gulley JL, Dahut WL. Androgen deprivation therapy for prostate cancer. JAMA. 2005;294(2):238–44.
160. Yen YF, Nagasawa K, Nakada T. Promising application of dynamic nuclear polarization for in vivo (13) C MR imaging. Magn Reson Med Sci. 2011;10(4):211–7.
161. Franiel T, Ludemann L, Rudolph B, et al. Differentiation of prostate cancer from normal prostate tissue: role of hotspots in pharmacokinetic MRI and histologic evaluation. AJR Am J Roentgenol. 2010;194(3):675–81.
162. Delongchamps NB, Beuvon F, Eiss D, et al. Multiparametric MRI is helpful to predict tumor focality, stage, and size in patients diagnosed with unilateral low-risk prostate cancer. Prostate Cancer Prostatic Dis. 2011;14(3):232–7.
163. Arani A, Plewes D, Krieger A, et al. The feasibility of endorectal MR elastography for prostate cancer localization. Magn Reson Med. 2011;66(6):1649–57.
164. Li S, Chen M, Wang W, et al. A feasibility study of MR elastography in the diagnosis of prostate cancer at 3.0T. Acta Radiol. 2011;52(3):354–8.
165. Hanahan D, Weinberg RA. Hallmarks of cancer: the next generation. Cell. 2011;144:646–74.
166. Kem EE, Lee MC, Inoue T, Wong WH, editors. Clinical PET and PET/CT: principles and applications. New York: Springer; 2013.
167. Rahim MK, Kim SE, So H, et al. Recent trends in PET image interpretations using volumetric and texture-based quantification methods in nuclear oncology. Nucl Med Mol Imaging. 2014;48:1–15.
168. Jadvar H. Imaging evaluation of prostate cancer with 18F-fluorodeoxyglucose PET/CT: utility and limitations. Eur J Nucl Med Mol Imaging. 2013;40:5–10.
169. Liu IJ, Zafar MB, Lai YH, et al. Fluorodeoxyglucose positron emission tomography studies in diagnosis and staging of clinically organ-confined prostate cancer. Urology. 2001;57:108–11.
170. Oyama N, Akino H, Suzuki Y, et al. The increased accumulation of [18F]fluorodeoxyglucose in untreated prostate cancer. Jpn J Clin Oncol. 1999;29:623–9.
171. Hillner BE, Siegel BA, Shields AF, et al. Relationship between cancer type and impact of PET and PET/CT on intended management: findings of the national oncologic PET registry. J Nucl Med. 2008;49:1926–35.
172. Inoue T, Oriuchi N, Tomiyoshi K, et al. A shifting landscape: what will be next FDG in PET oncology. Ann Nucl Med. 2002;16:1–9.
173. Jadvar H. Molecular imaging of prostate cancer: PET radiotracers. AJR Am J Roentgenol. 2012;199:278–91.
174. Hong H, Zhang Y, Sun J, Cai W. Positron emission tomography imaging of prostate cancer. Amino Acids. 2010;39:11–27.
175. Umbehr MH, Muntener M, Hany T, et al. The role of choline and 18F-fluorocholine positron emission tomography (PET) and PET/CT in prostate cancer: a systematic review and meta-analysis. Eur Urol. 2013;64:106–17.

176. Jadvar H. Molecular imaging of prostate cancer with PET. J Nucl Med. 2013;54:1685–8.
177. Hara T, Kosaka N, Kishi H. PET imaging of prostate cancer using carbon-11-choline. J Nucl Med. 1998;39:990–5.
178. Okudaira H, Nakanishi T, Oka S, et al. Kinetic analyses of trans-1-amino-3-[18F]fluorocyclobutanecarboxylic acid transport in Xenopus laevis oocytes expressing human ASCT2 and SNAT2. Nucl Med Biol. 2013;40:670–5.
179. Castellucci P, Jadvar H. PET/CT in prostate cancer: non-choline radiopharmaceuticals. Q J Nucl Med Mol Imaging. 2012;56:367–74.
180. Mease RC, Foss CA, Pomper MG. PET imaging in prostate cancer: focus on prostate-specific membrane antigen. Curr Top Med Chem. 2013;13:951–62.
181. Sauter AW, Wehrl HF, Kolb A, Judenhofer MS, Pichler BJ. Combined PET/MRI: one step further in multimodality imaging. Trends Mol Med. 2010;16:508–15.
182. Kim YI, Cheon GJ, Paeng JC, et al. Usefulness of MTI-assisted metabolic volumetric parameters provided by simultaneous 18F-fluorocholine PET/MRI for primary prostate cancer characterization. Eur J Nucl Med Mol Imaging. 2015;42:1247–56.
183. Wetter A, Lipponer C, Nensa F, et al. Simultaneous 18F choline positron emission tomography/magnetic resonance imaging of the prostate: initial results. Invest Radiol. 2013;48:256–62.
184. Choi J, Park JC, Nah H, et al. A hybrid nanoparticle probe for dual-modality positron emission tomography and magnetic resonance imaging. Angew Chem Int Ed Engl. 2008;47:6259–62.
185. Andreoiu M, Cheng L. Multifocal prostate cancer: biologic, prognostic, and therapeutic implications. Hum Pathol. 2010;41(6):781–93.
186. Huang CC, Deng FM, Kong MX, et al. Re-evaluating the concept of "dominant/index tumor nodule" in multifocal prostate cancer. Virchows Arch Int J Pathol. 2014;464(5):589–94.
187. Noguchi M, Stamey TA, McNeal JE, et al. Prognostic factors for multifocal prostate cancer in radical prostatectomy specimens: lack of significance of secondary cancers. J Urol. 2003;170(2 Pt 1):459–63.
188. Parsons JK, Gage WR, Nelson WG, et al. p63 protein expression is rare in prostate adenocarcinoma: implications for cancer diagnosis and carcinogenesis. Urology. 2001;58(4):619–24.
189. Shah RB, Zhou M, LeBlanc M, et al. Comparison of the basal cell-specific markers, 34betaE12 and p63, in the diagnosis of prostate cancer. Am J Surg Pathol. 2002;26(9):1161–8.
190. Bailar 3rd JC, Mellinger GT, Gleason DF. Survival rates of patients with prostatic cancer, tumor stage, and differentiation – preliminary report. Cancer Chemother Rep 1. 1966;50(3):129–36.
191. Gleason DF. Classification of prostatic carcinomas. Cancer Chemother Rep 1. 1966;50(3):125–8.
192. Epstein JI, Allsbrook Jr WC, Amin MB, et al. The 2005 International Society of Urological Pathology (ISUP) consensus conference on Gleason grading of prostatic carcinoma. Am J Surg Pathol. 2005;29(9):1228–42.
193. Jung DC, Lee HJ, Kim SH, et al. Preoperative MR imaging in the evaluation of seminal vesicle invasion in prostate cancer: pattern analysis of seminal vesicle lesions. J Magn Reson Imaging. 2008;28(1):144–50.
194. Edge SB, Byrd DR, Carducci MA, Compton CC, editors. AJCC cancer staging manual. 7th ed. New York: Springer; 2010.
195. Welch HG, Albertsen PC. Prostate cancer diagnosis and treatment after the introduction of prostate-specific antigen screening: 1986–2005. J Natl Cancer Inst. 2009;101(19):1325–9.
196. Klotz L. Active surveillance for favorable-risk prostate cancer: who, how and why? Nat Clin Pract Oncol. 2007;4(12):692–8.
197. Choo R, Klotz L, Danjoux C, Morton GC, DeBoer G, Szumacher E, Fleshner N, Bunting P, Hruby G. Feasibility study: watchful waiting for localized low to intermediate grade prostate carcinoma with selective delayed intervention based on prostate specific antigen, histological and/or clinical progression. J Urol. 2002;167(4):1664–9.
198. Klotz L. Active surveillance for prostate cancer: for whom? J Clin Oncol. 2005;23(32):8165–9.
199. Bastian PJ, Mangold LA, Epstein JI, Partin AW. Characteristics of insignificant clinical T1c prostate tumors. Cancer. 2004;101(9):2001–5.
200. Jeldres C, Suardi N, Walz J, Hutterer GC, Ahyai S, Lattouf J-B, Haese A, Graefen M, Erbersdobler A, Heinzer H. Validation of the contemporary epstein criteria for insignificant prostate cancer in European men. Eur Urol. 2008;54(6):1306–13.
201. Mohler JL, Armstrong AJ, Bahnson RR, Boston B, Busby JE, D'Amico AV, Eastham JA, Enke CA, Farrington T, Higano CS. Prostate cancer, version 3.2012 featured updates to the NCCN guidelines. J Natl Compr Canc Netw. 2012;10(9):1081–7.
202. Lee SE, Kim DS, Lee WK, Park HZ, Lee CJ, Doo SH, Jeong SJ, Yoon CY, Byun SS, Choe G. Application of the Epstein criteria for prediction of clinically insignificant prostate cancer in Korean men. BJU Int. 2010;105(11):1526–30.
203. Boorjian SA, Karnes RJ, Rangel LJ, Bergstralh EJ, Blute ML. Mayo Clinic validation of the D'amico risk group classification for predicting survival following radical prostatectomy. J Urol. 2008;179(4):1354–61.
204. Hardie C, Parker C, Norman A, Eeles R, Horwich A, Huddart R, Dearnaley D. Early outcomes of active surveillance for localized prostate cancer. BJU Int. 2005;95(7):956–60.

205. Roemeling S, Roobol MJ, de Vries SH, Wolters T, Gosselaar C, van Leenders GJ, Schröder FH. Active surveillance for prostate cancers detected in three subsequent rounds of a screening trial: characteristics, PSA doubling times, and outcome. Eur Urol. 2007;51(5):1244–51.
206. Dall'Era MA, Konety BR, Cowan JE, Shinohara K, Stauf F, Cooperberg MR, Meng MV, Kane CJ, Perez N, Master VA. Active surveillance for the management of prostate cancer in a contemporary cohort. Cancer. 2008;112(12):2664–70.
207. Klotz L, Zhang L, Lam A, Nam R, Mamedov A, Loblaw A. Clinical results of long-term follow-up of a large, active surveillance cohort with localized prostate cancer. J Clin Oncol. 2010;28(1):126–31.
208. Tosoian JJ, Trock BJ, Landis P, Feng Z, Epstein JI, Partin AW, Walsh PC, Carter HB. Active surveillance program for prostate cancer: an update of the Johns Hopkins experience. J Clin Oncol. 2011;29(16):2185–90.
209. Carter HB, Kettermann A, Warlick C, Metter EJ, Landis P, Walsh PC, Epstein JI. Expectant management of prostate cancer with curative intent: an update of the Johns Hopkins experience. J Urol. 2007;178(6):2359–65.
210. van den Bergh RC, Roemeling S, Roobol MJ, Aus G, Hugosson J, Rannikko AS, Tammela TL, Bangma CH, Schröder FH. Outcomes of men with screen-detected prostate cancer eligible for active surveillance who were managed expectantly. Eur Urol. 2009;55(1):1–8.
211. Soloway MS, Soloway CT, Eldefrawy A, Acosta K, Kava B, Manoharan M. Careful selection and close monitoring of low-risk prostate cancer patients on active surveillance minimizes the need for treatment. Eur Urol. 2010;58(6):831–5.
212. Kakehi Y, Kamoto T, Shiraishi T, Ogawa O, Suzukamo Y, Fukuhara S, Saito Y, Tobisu K-i, Kakizoe T, Shibata T. Prospective evaluation of selection criteria for active surveillance in Japanese patients with stage T1cN0M0 prostate cancer. Jpn J Clin Oncol. 2008;38(2):122–8.
213. Hadway P, Barrett LK, Waghorn DJ, Hasan K, Bdesha A, Haldar N, Kelleher J. Urodepsis ams bacteraemia caused by antibiotic-resistant organisms after transrectal ultrasonography-guided prostate biopsy. BJU Int. 2009;104(11):1556–8.
214. Loeb S, Carter HB, Berndt SI, Ricker W, Schaeffer EM. Complications after prostate biopsy: data from SEER-Medicare. J Urol. 2011;186(5):1830–4.
215. Mouraviev V, Mayes JM, Polascik TJ. Pathologic basis of focal therapy for early-stage prostate cancer. Nat Rev Urol. 2009;6(4):205–15.
216. Cooperberg MR, Broering JM, Kantoff PW, Carroll PR. Contemporary trends in low risk prostate cancer: risk assessment and treatment. J Urol. 2007;178(3):S14–9.
217. Beerlage H, Thüroff S, Madersbacher S, Zlotta A, Aus G, de Reijke TM, de la Rosette J. Current status of minimally invasive treatment options for localized prostate carcinoma. Eur Urol. 2000;37(1):2–13.
218. Rees J, Patel B, MacDonagh R, Persad R. Cryosurgery for prostate cancer. BJU Int. 2004;93(6):710–4.
219. Han KR, Belldegrun AS. Third-generation cryosurgery for primary and recurrent prostate cancer. BJU Int. 2004;93(1):14–8.
220. Chaussy C, Thüroff S. The status of high-intensity focused ultrasound in the treatment of localized prostate cancer and the impact of a combined resection. Curr Urol Rep. 2003;4(3):248–52.
221. Long JP, Bahn D, Lee F, Shinohara K, Chinn DO, Macaluso Jr JN. Five-year retrospective, multi-institutional pooled analysis of cancer-related outcomes after cryosurgical ablation of the prostate. Urology. 2001;57(3):518–23.
222. Donnelly BJ, Saliken JC, Ernst DS, Ali-Ridha N, Brasher PM, Robinson JW, Rewcastle JC. Prospective trial of cryosurgical ablation of the prostate: five-year results. Urology. 2002;60(4): 645–9.
223. Han KR, Cohen JK, Miller RJ, Pantuck AJ, Freitas DG, et al. Treatment of organ confined prostate cancer with third generation cryosurgery: preliminary multicenter experience. J Urol. 2003;170(4 Pt 1):1126–30.
224. Bahn DK, Lee F, Badalament R, Kumar A, Greski J, Chernick M. Targeted cryoablation of the prostate: 7-year outcomes in the primary treatment of prostate cancer. Urology. 2002;60(2 Suppl 1):3–11.
225. Cohen JK, Miller RJ, Ahmed S, Lotz MJ, Baust J. Ten-year biochemical disease control for patients with prostate cancer treated with cryosurgery as primary therapy. Urology. 2008;71(3):515–8.
226. Levy DA, Pisters LL, Jones JS. Primary cryoablation nadir prostate specific antigen and biochemical failure. J Urol. 2009;182(3):931–7. 34. Madersbacher S, Marberger M. High-energy shockwaves and extracorporeal high-intensity focused ultrasound. J Endourol. 2003;17(8):667–72.
227. Foster RS, Bihrle R, Sanghvi N, Fry F, Kopecky K, Regan J, et al. Production of prostatic lesions in canines using transrectallky administrated high-intensity focused ultrasound. Eur Urol. 1993;23:330–6.
228. Uchida T, Nakano M, Hongo S, Shoji S, Nagata Y, Satoh T, Baba S, Usui Y, Terachi T. High-intensity focused ultrasound therapy for prostate cancer. Int J Urol. 2012;19(3):187–201.
229. Ahmed HU, Freeman A, Kirkham A, Sahu M, Scott R, Allen C, Van der Meulen J, Emberton M. Focal therapy for localized prostate cancer: a phase I/II trial. J Urol. 2011;185(4):1246–54.
230. Murat FJ, Poissonnier L, Rabilloud M, Belot A, Bouvier R, Rouviere O, Chapelon JY, Gelet A. Mid-term results demonstrate salvage high-intensity focused ultrasound (HIFU) as an effective and acceptably morbid salvage treatment option for

locally radiorecurrent prostate cancer. Eur Urol. 2009;55(3):640–9.

231. Zacharakis E, Ahmed HU, Ishaq A, Scott R, Illing R, Freeman A, Allen C, Emberton M. The feasibility and safety of high-intensity focused ultrasound as salvage therapy for recurrent prostate cancer following external beam radiotherapy. BJU Int. 2008;102(7):786–92.
232. Uchida T, Shoji S, Nakano M, Hongo S, Nitta M, Usui Y, Nagata Y. High-intensity focused ultrasound as salvage therapy for patients with recurrent prostate cancer after external beam radiation, brachytherapy or proton therapy. BJU Int. 2011;107(3):378–82.
233. Hayashi M, Shinmei S, Asano K. Transrectal high-intensity focused ultrasound for treatment for patients with biochemical failure after radical prostatectomy. Int J Urol. 2007;14(11):1048–50.
234. Murota-Kawano A, Nakano M, Hongo S, Shoji S, Nagata Y, Uchida T. Salvage high-intensity focused ultrasound for biopsy-confirmed local recurrence of prostate cancer after radical prostatectomy. BJU Int. 2010;105(12):1642–5.
235. Uchida T, Illing RO, Cathcart PJ, Emberton M. To what extent does the prostate-specific antigen nadir predict subsequent treatment failure after transrectal high-intensity focused ultrasound therapy for presumed localized adenocarcinoma of the prostate? BJU Int. 2006;98(3):537–9.
236. Ganzer R, Rogenhofer S, Walter B, Lunz JC, Schostak M, Wieland WF, Blana A. PSA nadir is a significant predictor of treatment failure after high-intensity focussed ultrasound (HIFU) treatment of localised prostate cancer. Eur Urol. 2008;53(3):547–53.
237. Crouzet S, Rebillard X, Chevallier D, Rischmann P, Pasticier G, Garcia G, Rouviere O, Chapelon JY, Gelet A. Multicentric oncologic outcomes of high-intensity focused ultrasound for localized prostate cancer in 803 patients. Eur Urol. 2010;58(4):559–66.
238. Blana A, Rogenhofer S, Ganzer R, Lunz JC, Schostak M, Wieland WF, Walter B. Eight years' experience with high-intensity focused ultrasonography for treatment of localized prostate cancer. Urology. 2008;72(6):1329–33.
239. Misrai V, Roupret M, Chartier-Kastler E, Comperat E, Renard-Penna R, Haertig A, Bitker MO, Richard F, Conort P. Oncologic control provided by HIFU therapy as single treatment in men with clinically localized prostate cancer. World J Urol. 2008;26(5):481–5.
240. Uchida T, Shoji S, Nakano M, Hongo S, Nitta M, Murota A, Nagata Y. Transrectal high-intensity focused ultrasound for the treatment of localized prostate cancer: eight-year experience. Int J Urol. 2009;16(11):881–6.
241. Inoue Y, Goto K, Hayashi T, Hayashi M. Transrectal high-intensity focused ultrasound for treatment of localized prostate cancer. Int J Urol. 2011;18(5):358–63.
242. Kupelian PA, Ciezki J, Reddy CA, Klein EA, Mahadevan A. Effect of increasing radiation doses on local and distant failures in patients with localized prostate cancer. Int J Radiat Oncol Biol Phys. 2008;71(1):16–22. doi:10.1016/j.ijrobp.2007.09.020.
243. Zelefsky MJ, Yamada Y, Fuks Z et al. Long-Term Results of Conformal Radiotherapy for Prostate Cancer: Impact of Dose Escalation on Biochemical Tumor Control and Distant Metastases-Free Survival Outcomes. Int J Radiat Oncol Biol Phys. 2008;71(4):1028–33. doi:10.1016/j.ijrobp.2007.11.066.
244. Bianco Jr FJ, Scardino PT, Eastham JA. Radical prostatectomy: long-term cancer control and recovery of sexual and urinary function ("trifecta"). Urology. 2005;66(5 Suppl):83–94.
245. Bill-Axelson A, Holmberg L, Filen F, Ruutu M, Garmo H, Busch C, Nordling S, Haggman M, Andersson SO, Bratell S, Spangberg A, Palmgren J, Adami HO, Johansson JE, Scandinavian Prostate Cancer Group Study N. Radical prostatectomy versus watchful waiting in localized prostate cancer: the Scandinavian prostate cancer group-4 randomized trial. J Natl Cancer Inst. 2008;100(16):1144–54.
246. Tewari A, Johnson CC, Divine G, Crawford ED, Gamito EJ, Demers R, Menon M. Long-term survival probability in men with clinically localized prostate cancer: a case–control, propensity modeling study stratified by race, age, treatment and comorbidities. J Urol. 2004;171(4):1513–9.
247. Augustin H, Hammerer P, Graefen M, Palisaar J, Noldus J, Fernandez S, Huland H. Intraoperative and perioperative morbidity of contemporary radical retropubic prostatectomy in a consecutive series of 1243 patients: results of a single center between 1999 and 2002. Eur Urol. 2003;43(2):113–8.
248. Lepor H, Nieder AM, Ferrandino MN. Intraoperative and postoperative complications of radical retropubic prostatectomy in a consecutive series of 1,000 cases. J Urol. 2001;166(5):1729–33.
249. Ficarra V, Novara G, Artibani W, Cestari A, Galfano A, Graefen M, Guazzoni G, Guillonneau B, Menon M, Montorsi F, Patel V, Rassweiler J, Van Poppel H. Retropubic, laparoscopic, and robot-assisted radical prostatectomy: a systematic review and cumulative analysis of comparative studies. Eur Urol. 2009;55(5):1037–63.
250. Parsons JK, Bennett JL. Outcomes of retropubic, laparoscopic, and robotic-assisted prostatectomy. Urology. 2008;72(2):412–6.
251. Hu JC, Wang Q, Pashos CL, Lipsitz SR, Keating NL. Utilization and outcomes of minimally invasive radical prostatectomy. J Clin Oncol Off J Am Soc Clin Oncol. 2008;26(14):2278–84.
252. Hu JC, Gu X, Lipsitz SR, Barry MJ, D'Amico AV, Weinberg AC, Keating NL. Comparative

effectiveness of minimally invasive vs open radical prostatectomy. JAMA. 2009;302(14):1557–64.
253. Walsh PC, Donker PJ. Impotence following radical prostatectomy: insight into etiology and prevention. J Urol. 1982;128(3):492–7.
254. Loughlin KR, Prasad MM. Post-prostatectomy urinary incontinence: a confluence of 3 factors. J Urol. 2010;183(3):871–7.
255. Tal R, Alphs HH, Krebs P, Nelson CJ, Mulhall JP. Erectile function recovery rate after radical prostatectomy: a meta-analysis. J Sex Med. 2009;6(9): 2538–46.
256. Briganti A, Chun FK, Salonia A, Gallina A, Farina E, Da Pozzo LF, Rigatti P, Montorsi F, Karakiewicz PI. Validation of a nomogram predicting the probability of lymph node invasion based on the extent of pelvic lymphadenectomy in patients with clinically localized prostate cancer. BJU Int. 2006;98(4): 788–93.
257. Cagiannos I, Karakiewicz P, Eastham JA, Ohori M, Rabbani F, Gerigk C, Reuter V, Graefen M, Hammerer PG, Erbersdobler A, Huland H, Kupelian P, Klein E, Quinn DI, Henshall SM, Grygiel JJ, Sutherland RL, Stricker PD, Morash CG, Scardino PT, Kattan MW. A preoperative nomogram identifying decreased risk of positive pelvic lymph nodes in patients with prostate cancer. J Urol. 2003;170(5): 1798–803.
258. Joslyn SA, Konety BR. Impact of extent of lymphadenectomy on survival after radical prostatectomy for prostate cancer. Urology. 2006;68(1):121–5.
259. Bader P, Burkhard FC, Markwalder R, Studer UE. Disease progression and survival of patients with positive lymph nodes after radical prostatectomy. Is there a chance of cure? J Urol. 2003;169(3):849–54.
260. Daneshmand S, Quek ML, Stein JP, Lieskovsky G, Cai J, Pinski J, Skinner EC, Skinner DG. Prognosis of patients with lymph node positive prostate cancer following radical prostatectomy: long-term results. J Urol. 2004;172(6 Pt 1):2252–5.
261. Wagner M, Sokoloff M, Daneshmand S. The role of pelvic lymphadenectomy for prostate cancer – therapeutic? J Urol. 2008;179(2):408–13.
262. Briganti A, Blute ML, Eastham JH, Graefen M, Heidenreich A, Karnes JR, Montorsi F, Studer UE. Pelvic lymph node dissection in prostate cancer. Eur Urol. 2009;55(6):1251–65.
263. Heidenreich A, Ohlmann CH, Polyakov S. Anatomical extent of pelvic lymphadenectomy in patients undergoing radical prostatectomy. Eur Urol. 2007;52(1):29–37.
264. Steiner MS. The puboprostatic ligament and the male urethral suspensory mechanism: an anatomic study. Urology. 1994;44(4):530–4.
265. Poore RE, McCullough DL, Jarow JP. Puboprostatic ligament sparing improves urinary continence after radical retropubic prostatectomy. Urology. 1998;51(1):67–72.
266. Deliveliotis C, Protogerou V, Alargof E, Varkarakis J. Radical prostatectomy: bladder neck preservation and puboprostatic ligament sparing – effects on continence and positive margins. Urology. 2002;60(5):855–8.
267. Costello AJ, Brooks M, Cole OJ. Anatomical studies of the neurovascular bundle and cavernosal nerves. BJU Int. 2004;94(7):1071–6.
268. Rogers CG, Trock BP, Walsh PC. Preservation of accessory pudendal arteries during radical retropubic prostatectomy: surgical technique and results. Urology. 2004;64(1):148–51.
269. Huggins C, Stevens R, Hodges CV. Studies on prostatic cancer: II. The effects of castration on advanced carcinoma of the prostate gland. Arch Surg. 1941;43(2):209–23.
270. Huggins C, Hodges CV. Studies on prostatic cancer: I. The effect of castration, of estrogen and of androgen injection on serum phosphatases in metastatic carcinoma of the prostate. J Urol. 2002;167(2): 948–51.
271. Mcleod DG. Hormonal therapy: historical perspective to future directions. Urology. 2003;61(2):3–7.
272. Menon M, Walsh PC. Hormonal therapy for prostatic cancer. Prostatic cancer. Littleton: PSG; 1979. p. 175.
273. Russell DW, Wilson JD. Steroid 5alpha-reductase: two genes/two enzymes. Annu Rev Biochem. 1994;63(1):25–61.
274. Desmond A, Arnold A, Hastie K. Subcapsular orchiectomy under local anaesthesia technique, results and implications. Br J Urol. 1988;61(2):143–5.
275. Oh WK. The evolving role of estrogen therapy in prostate cancer. Clin Prostate Cancer. 2002;1(2):81–9.
276. Jordan WP, Blackard CE, Byar DP. Reconsideration of orchiectomy in the treatment of advanced prostatic carcinoma. South Med J. 1977;70(12):1411.
277. Scherr DS, PITTS JRW. The nonsteroidal effects of diethylstilbestrol: the rationale for androgen deprivation therapy without estrogen deprivation in the treatment of prostate cancer. J Urol. 2003;170(5): 1703–8.
278. Oefelein MG, Resnick MI. Effective testosterone suppression for patients with prostate cancer: is there a best castration? Urology. 2003;62(2):207–13.
279. McLeod DG. Tolerability of nonsteroidal antiandrogens in the treatment of advanced prostate cancer. Oncologist. 1997;2(1):18–27.
280. Schally AV. Luteinizing hormone-releasing hormone analogs: their impact on the control of tumorigenesis. Peptides. 1999;20(10):1247–62.
281. Seidenfeld J, Samson DJ, Hasselblad V, Aronson N, Albertsen PC, Bennett CL, Wilt TJ. Single-therapy androgen suppression in men with advanced prostate cancera systematic review and meta-analysis. Ann Intern Med. 2000;132(7):566–77.
282. Bubley GJ. Is the flare phenomenon clinically significant? Urology. 2001;58(2):5–9.

283. McLeod D, Zinner N, Tomera K, Gleason D, Fotheringham N, Campion M, Garnick MB. A phase 3, multicenter, open-label, randomized study of abarelix versus leuprolide acetate in men with prostate cancer. Urology. 2001;58(5):756–61.
284. Trachtenberg J, Gittleman M, Steidle C, Barzell W, Friedel W, Pessis D, Fotheringham N, Campion M, Garnick MB, Group AS. A phase 3, multicenter, open label, randomized study of abarelix versus leuprolide plus daily antiandrogen in men with prostate cancer. J Urol. 2002;167(4):1670–4.
285. Van Poppel H, Tombal B, de la Rosette JJ, Persson B-E, Jensen J-K, Kold Olesen T. Degarelix: a novel gonadotropin-releasing hormone (GnRH) receptor blocker – results from a 1-yr, multicentre, randomised, phase 2 dosage-finding study in the treatment of prostate cancer. Eur Urol. 2008;54(4):805–15.
286. Anderson J. The role of antiandrogen monotherapy in the treatment of prostate cancer. BJU Int. 2003;91(5):455–61.
287. Iversen P. Antiandrogen monotherapy: indications and results. Urology. 2002;60(3):64–71.
288. Cabot RC, Harris NL, Rosenberg ES, Shepard J-AO, Cort AM, Ebeling SH, McDonald EK, Scher HI, Fizazi K, Saad F. Increased survival with enzalutamide in prostate cancer after chemotherapy. N Engl J Med. 2012;367(13):1187–97.
289. Ryan CJ, Smith MR, de Bono JS, Molina A, Logothetis CJ, de Souza P, Fizazi K, Mainwaring P, Piulats JM, Ng S. Abiraterone in metastatic prostate cancer without previous chemotherapy. N Engl J Med. 2013;368(2):138–48.
290. Crawford ED, Eisenberger MA, McLeod DG, Spaulding JT, Benson R, Dorr FA, Blumenstein BA, Davis MA, Goodman PJ. A controlled trial of leuprolide with and without flutamide in prostatic carcinoma. N Engl J Med. 1989;321(7):419–24.
291. Eisenberger MA, Blumenstein BA, Crawford ED, Miller G, McLeod DG, Loehrer PJ, Wilding G, Sears K, Culkin DJ, Thompson Jr IM. Bilateral orchiectomy with or without flutamide for metastatic prostate cancer. N Engl J Med. 1998;339(15):1036–42.
292. Samson DJ, Seidenfeld J, Schmitt B, Hasselblad V, Albertsen PC, Bennett CL, Wilt TJ, Aronson N. Systematic review and meta-analysis of monotherapy compared with combined androgen blockade for patients with advanced prostate carcinoma. Cancer. 2002;95(2):361–76.
293. Verhagen P, Wissenburg L, Wildhagen M, Bolle W, Verkerk A, Schröder F, Bangma C, Mickisch G. Quality of life effects of intermittent and continuous hormonal therapy by cyproterone acetate (CPA) for metastatic prostate cancer. Eur Urol Suppl. 2008;7(3):206.
294. Adib R, Anderson J, Ashken M, Baumber C, Bevis C, Beynon L, Blaxland J, Boag V, Bolger J, Boreham J. Immediate versus deferred treatment for advanced prostatic cancer: initial results of the Medical Research Council trial. Br J Urol. 1997;79(2):235–46.
295. Messing EM, Manola J, Sarosdy M, Wilding G, Crawford ED, Trump D. Immediate hormonal therapy compared with observation after radical prostatectomy and pelvic lymphadenectomy in men with node-positive prostate cancer. N Engl J Med. 1999;341(24):1781–8.
296. Wilt T, Nair B, MacDonald R, Rutks I. Early versus deferred androgen suppression in the treatment of advanced prostatic cancer. Cochrane Database Syst Rev. 2001;4.
297. Varghese SL, Grossfeld GD. The prostatic gland: malignancies other than adenocarcinomas. Radiol Clin North Am. 2000;38(1):179–202.
298. Hansel DE, Herawi M, Montgomery E, et al. Spindle cell lesions of the adult prostate. Mod Pathol Off J United States Can Acad Pathol. 2007;20(1):148–58.
299. Tavora F, Kryvenko ON, Epstein JI. Mesenchymal tumours of the bladder and prostate: an update. Pathology. 2013;45(2):104–15.
300. Bartolozzi C, Selli C, Olmastroni M, et al. Rhabdomyosarcoma of the prostate: MR findings. AJR Am J Roentgenol. 1988;150(6):1333–4.
301. Mott LJ. Squamous cell carcinoma of the prostate: report of 2 cases and review of the literature. J Urol. 1979;121(6):833–5.
302. Terris MK, Villers A, Freiha FS. Transrectal ultrasound appearance of transitional cell carcinoma involving the prostate. J Urol. 1990;143(5):952–6.
303. Eble J, Epstein J, Sesterhenn I, World Health Organization classification of tumours. Pathology and genetics of tumours of the urinary system and male genital organs. Lyon: IARC Press; 2004.
304. Schwartz LH, LaTrenta LR, Bonaccio E, et al. Small cell and anaplastic prostate cancer: correlation between CT findings and prostate-specific antigen level. Radiology. 1998;208(3):735–8.
305. Cho J. In: Kim SH, editor. Radiology illustrated: uroradiology. Philadelphia: Saunders; 2003. p. 571–606.
306. Agrons GA, Wagner BJ, Lonergan GJ, et al. From the archives of the AFIP. Genitourinary rhabdomyosarcoma in children: radiologic-pathologic correlation. Radiographics Rev Publ Radiol Soc North Am. 1997;17(4):919–37.
307. Chin W, Fay R, Ortega P. Malignant fibrous histiocytoma of prostate. Urology. 1986;27(4):363–5.
308. Shirakawa T, Fujisawa M, Gotoh A, et al. Complete resection of synovial sarcoma of prostatic fascia. Urology. 2003;61(3):644.
309. Arger PH, Malkowicz SB, VanArsdalen KN, et al. Color and power Doppler sonography in the diagnosis of prostate cancer: comparison between vascular density and total vascularity. J Ultrasound

Med Off J Am Inst Ultrasound Med. 2004;23(5): 623–30.
310. Barozzi L, Pavlica P, Menchi I, et al. Prostatic abscess: diagnosis and treatment. AJR Am J Roentgenol. 1998;170(3):753–7.
311. LaFontaine PD, Middleman BR, Graham Jr SD, et al. Incidence of granulomatous prostatitis and acid-fast bacilli after intravesical BCG therapy. Urology. 1997;49(3):363–6.
312. Rusch D, Moinzadeh A, Hamawy K, et al. Giant multilocular cystadenoma of the prostate. AJR Am J Roentgenol. 2002;179(6):1477–9.
313. Kaufman JJ, Berneike RR. Leiomyoma of the prostate. J Urol. 1951;65(2):297–310.
314. Imai S, Ayabe Y, Iiyama T, et al. Leiomyoma of the prostate: CT and MR findings. Abdom Imaging. 2002;27(6):674–6.

4 Tumors of the Male Genitalia

Min Hoan Moon, Kyung Chul Moon, Ja Hyeon Ku, Myong Kim, and Jin Ho Kim

4.1 Scrotal Tumor

4.1.1 Imaging Anatomy

On ultrasound, the testis appears as a structure of intermediate, homogenous echogenicity. Mediastinum testis is seen as echogenic band with craniocaudal extension just beneath the tunica albuginea. Cyst or tubular ectasia is often noted within the mediastinum testis. This cystic structure is normally not seen, and its presence suggests obstruction of the distal genital duct. The epididymis is the structure of an elongated shape around the testis. On ultrasound, the epididymis shows similar echogenicity with the testes, but the epididymal head is slightly higher in the echogenicity than the epididymal body and tail.

The testes appear as structures of homogenous signal intensity on MRI. The testes show high signal intensity on T2WI and iso signal intensity on T1WI compared with the muscle. The mediastinum testis and the epididymis show similar signal intensity to the testes on T1WI, but the mediastinum testis and the epididymis show low signal intensity distinguished from high signal intensity of the testis on T2WI. Therefore, T2WI is the standard imaging sequence that can assess the internal architecture of the testis (Fig. 4.1). The tunica albuginea appears as a membrane of low signal intensity on both T1WI and T2WI. Although MRI is an excellent imaging modality for assessment of testicular anatomy, MRI has yet to become a mainstay in the evaluation of testicular tumor because of its cost, prolonged scanning time, and relative unavailability. Furthermore, local staging of the testicular cancer is determined through surgical pathology.

M.H. Moon (✉)
Department of Radiology,
SMG-SNU Boramae Medical Center,
Seoul National University College of Medicine,
Seoul, Republic of Korea
e-mail: mmhoan@gmail.com

K.C. Moon
Department of Pathology,
Seoul National University Hospital,
Seoul National University College of Medicine,
Seoul, Republic of Korea

J.H. Ku
Department of Urology,
Seoul National University Hospital,
Seoul National University College of Medicine,
Seoul, Republic of Korea

M. Kim
Department of Urology,
Asan Medical Center, University of Ulsan College of Medicine, Seoul, Republic of Korea

J.H. Kim
Department of Radiation Oncology,
Seoul National University Hospital,
Seoul National University College of Medicine,
Seoul, Republic of Korea

S.H. Kim, J.Y. Cho (eds.), *Oncologic Imaging: Urology*, DOI 10.1007/978-3-662-45218-9_4

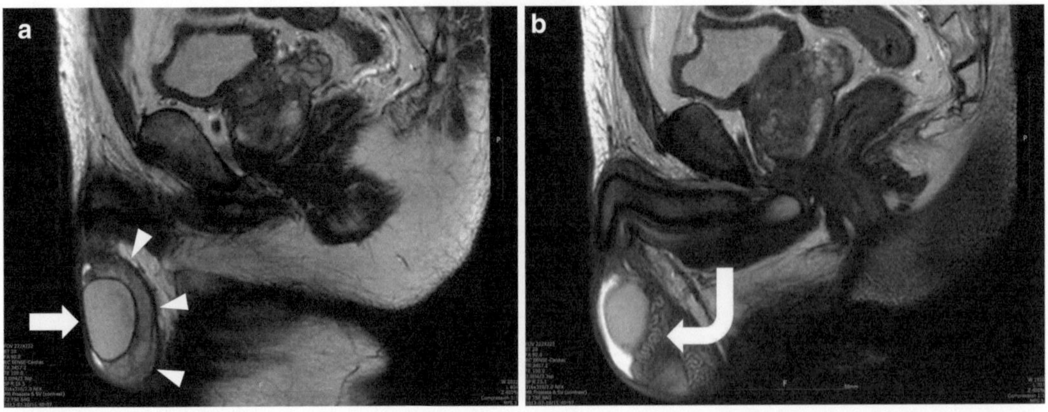

Fig. 4.1 Normal MR imaging of the scrotum. (**a**) On T2-weighted sagittal image through the right scrotum, the epididymis (*arrowheads*) shows low signal intensity compared to the high signal intensity of the testis (*arrow*). (**b**) On T2-weighted sagittal image obtained medial to (**a**), the vas deferens (*curved arrow*) appears as serpiginous tubular structure of relatively high signal intensity. Note that small hydrocele is present in the right scrotal sac

Table 4.1 Classification of testis tumor according to the origin

Germ cell tumor	Sex cord/stromal tumor	Mixed tumor	Nonprimary tumor
Seminoma	Leydig cell tumor	Gonadoblastoma	Lymphoma
Mixed GCT	Sertoli cell tumor		Leukemia
Embryonal cancer			Metastasis
Yolk sac tumor			
Teratoma			
Choriocarcinoma			

4.1.2 Tumor of the Testis

Testis tumor constitutes 1 % of male malignancies but is the most common malignant tumor in young men. The median age of diagnosis is 33 years. Testis tumor usually presents as a painless mass, and nearly one-fifth of patients will have metastatic disease at initial diagnosis. However, its prognosis is good with 5-year survival rate of above 90 %.

4.1.2.1 Tumor Subtypes

Testicular tumors are subdivided into four major categories: germ cell tumors, sex cord/stromal tumors, mixed tumors, and nonprimary tumors [1] (Table 4.1). Germ cell tumors account for most of testicular tumors (90–95 %) and further subdivided into seminoma and nonseminomatous germ cell tumors (NSGCT). Differentiation of seminoma from nonseminomatous germ cell tumor plays a critical role in the selection of appropriate treatment plan. Seminoma is extremely sensitive to radiation therapy, and its treatment is composed of radical orchiectomy followed by radiation therapy. On the contrary, nonseminomatous germ cell tumor is usually treated by radical orchiectomy with retroperitoneal lymph node dissection followed by chemotherapy. Most common histologic types of germ cell tumors include seminoma (35 %), embryonal carcinoma (20 %), and mixed germ cell tumor (40 %). The average age of onset of testicular cancer is slightly different according to the testicular tumor subtypes: yolk sac tumors (0–10 years), choriocarcinomas (20–30 years), embryonal carcinomas and teratomas (25–30 years), and seminomas (30–40 years) [2]. Tumor markers including AFP or hCG are helpful in the diagnosis, staging, and treatment response evaluation of testis tumors. The elevation of AFP

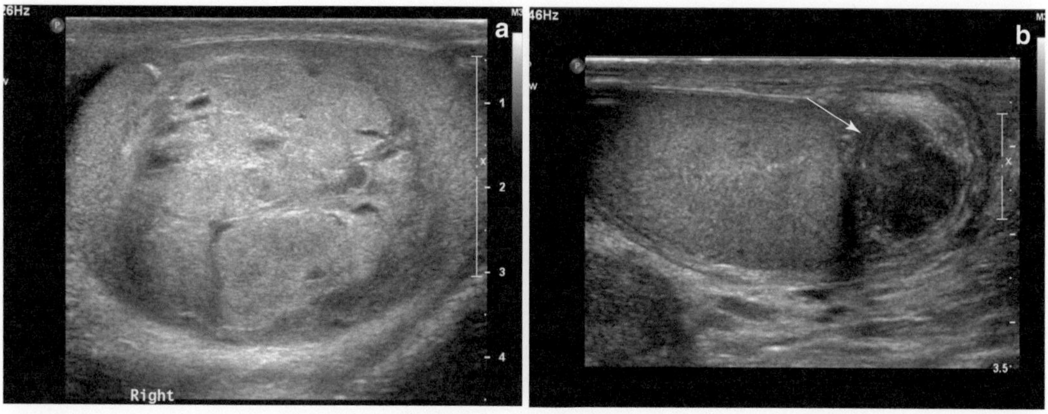

Fig. 4.2 Tumor versus non-tumor. The mass in (**a**) is regarded as testicular mass, and its final pathology was mixed germ cell tumor of the right testis. On the other hand, the mass (*arrow*) in (**b**) is deemed to be paratesticular mass, and its final clinical diagnosis was epididymitis

suggests yolk sac tumor and the elevation of hCG means seminoma or choriocarcinoma.

Sex cord–stromal tumors account for 4 % of all testicular tumors [1], and the majority of sex cord–stromal tumor is Leydig cell tumor or Sertoli cell tumor. Other sex cord–stromal tumors including granulosa cell tumors and fibroma–thecomas are very rare. Although sex cord–stromal tumors are usually benign, it is often difficult to determine the biologic behavior of sex cord–stromal tumors with histologic analysis. Sex cord–stromal tumors can produce estrogen or androgen so patients, especially with Leydig cell tumors, manifest as precocious virilization, gynecomastia, or decreased libido.

Nonprimary testicular tumor includes lymphoma, leukemia, and metastasis. Testicular lymphomas accounting for 5 % of all testicular tumors occur in a much older population and are the most common testicular neoplasm in men over 60 years of age. Primary testicular leukemia is very rare, but the testis is a common site of leukemia recurrence in children because the blood–testis barrier protects leukemic cells from chemotherapeutic agents.

4.1.2.2 Spread of Testicular Tumors

Testis tumor most commonly spreads via the lymphatic pathway, but choriocarcinoma can also spread hematogenously. The retroperitoneal lymph nodes are the most common site for metastatic disease, and evaluation of sentinel nodes is important in the assessment of testis tumor. Sentinel nodes of the right testicular cancers are located in the aortocaval area inferior to the renal hilar vessels, and those of the left testicular cancers are located in the para-aortic area bordering with left renal vein, ureter, aorta, and inferior mesenteric artery. As metastasis advances, metastasis in sentinel nodes spreads to adjacent retroperitoneum. Crossover drainage to the contralateral lymph nodes from the sentinel nodes is encountered in 15–20 %. Crossover drainage from aortocaval lymph nodes to the para-aortic lymph nodes is more common than vice versa [3, 4].

4.1.2.3 US Characterization of the Scrotal Mass

US is the first imaging modality in the evaluation of intrascrotal mass. US is a very sensitive imaging tool for identification of testis mass (almost 100 % in the sensitivity) and is helpful in the differentiation of testicular mass from paratesticular mass. The first step in the evaluation of the scrotal mass is to differentiate testicular mass from paratesticular mass. Testicular mass is usually malignant in its nature, but paratesticular mass is usually benign in its nature (Fig. 4.2). If the scrotal mass is regarded as testicular germ cell tumor, the next step is to differentiate seminomas from

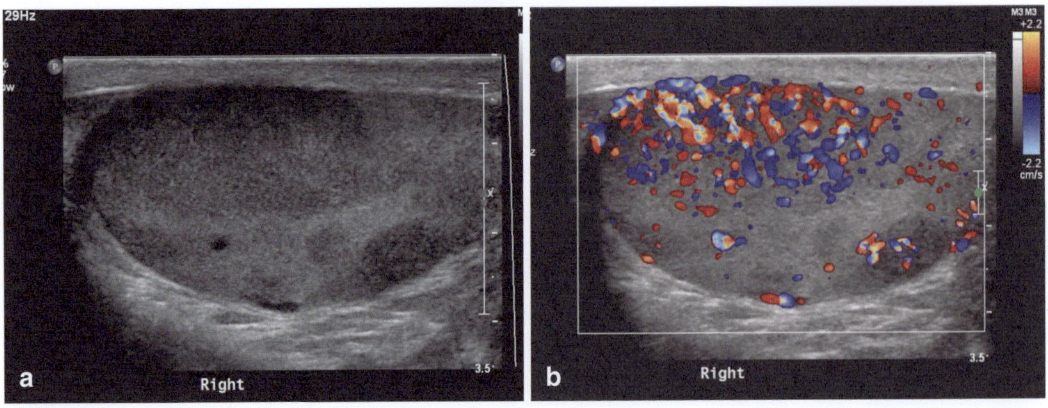

Fig. 4.3 US imaging findings of lymphoma. Gray scale US image (**a**) shows multiple homogenous hypoechoic masses in the right testis. On color Doppler US evaluation (**b**), the masses show markedly increased blood flow in those masses

nonseminomatous germ cell tumors. US imaging findings of the tumor reflect its histologic characteristics. Therefore, seminoma appears as homogenous low echoic mass due to its uniform internal architecture, whereas nonseminomatous germ cell tumor appears as a mixed echoic mass due to its necrosis or internal hemorrhage. If older men present with testis mass, the first impression of the testis mass is lymphoma or metastasis. On US, testicular lymphoma appears as homogenously hypoechoic lesions, and color Doppler evaluation shows markedly increased intralesional blood flow irrespective of lesion size (Fig. 4.3) [5]. Testicular metastasis is generally seen in the setting of widespread metastasis of primary cancers so the US diagnosis of testicular metastasis is not difficult although the US appearance of testicular metastasis is quite varied. Because the blood–testis barrier protects leukemic cells from chemotherapeutic agents, testicular leukemia should be considered in the differential diagnosis of testis mass in children with leukemia history. The US appearance of testicular leukemia is similar to the US appearance of testicular lymphoma that presents as homogenously hypoechoic lesions with markedly increased intralesional blood flow.

4.1.2.4 Rare Exception

Because most of intratesticular mass are malignant tumors and rare benign tumorous condition of the testis shows similar clinical and radiological manifestations to the malignant testicular tumors, intratesticular mass is usually treated by radical orchiectomy with tentative diagnosis of malignant testicular tumor. However, some of benign tumorous conditions like epidermoid cyst or testicular cyst show specific imaging findings and familiarity with those imaging features that can be helpful in the selection of testis-sparing enucleation in the treatment of intratesticular mass. The internal content of the epidermoid cyst is composed of cheesy laminated material. On US, the epidermoid cyst appears as onion-skin appearance due to its internal architecture. Preoperative diagnosis of epidermoid cyst makes urologists to select less invasive enucleation instead of more invasive radical orchiectomy. Testicular cyst is usually detected incidentally in men at least 40 years of age. On US, testicular cyst appears as a pure cyst without a perceptible wall or internal solid portion. These cysts are usually solitary but can also be multiple. Testicular cysts adjacent to or within the mediastinum testis are associated with extratesticular spermatoceles. Testicular cysts do not require treatment.

4.1.2.5 Staging

The staging system of the American Joint Committee on Cancer (AJCC) is commonly used. AJCC staging is a TNMS-based classification (T=tumor, N=node, M=metastases, S=serum markers) (Table 4.2) [6]. Because T staging is determined through surgical pathology, the role of

Table 4.2 TNM classification of testicular cancer [5]

Stage	Description
Tumor (T)	The extent of the primary tumor is usually classified after radical orchiectomy, and for this reason, a pathologic category is assigned
pTx	Primary tumor cannot be assessed
pT0	No evidence of primary tumor (e.g., histologic scar in testis)
pTis	Intratubular germ cell neoplasia (carcinoma in situ)
pT1	Tumor limited to the testis and epididymis without vascular or lymphatic invasion; tumor may invade into the tunica albuginea but not the tunica vaginalis
pT2	Tumor limited to the testis and epididymis with vascular or lymphatic invasion or tumor extending through the tunica albuginea with involvement of the tunica vaginalis
pT3	Tumor invades the spermatic cord with or without vascular or lymphatic invasion
pT4	Tumor invades scrotum with or without vascular or lymphatic invasion
Lymph node (N)	Clinical category
Nx	Regional lymph node cannot be assessed
N0	No regional lymph node metastasis
N1	Metastasis with a lymph node mass 2 cm or less in greatest dimension or multiple lymph nodes, none more than 2 cm in greatest dimension
N2	Metastasis with a lymph node mass more than 2 cm but not more than 5 cm in greatest dimension or multiple lymph nodes, any one mass greater than 2 cm but not more than 5 cm in greatest dimension
N3	Metastasis with a lymph node mass more than 5 cm in greatest dimension
Lymph node (N)	Pathologic category
pNx	Regional lymph node cannot be assessed
pN0	No regional lymph node metastasis
pN1	Metastasis with a lymph node mass 2 cm or less in greatest dimension and five or fewer nodes positive, none more than 2 cm in greatest dimension
pN2	Metastasis with a lymph node mass more than 2 cm but not more than 5 cm in greatest dimension; more than five nodes positive, none more than 5 cm; or evidence of extranodal extension of tumor
pN3	Metastasis with a lymph node mass more than 5 cm in greatest dimension
Metastasis (M)	
M0	No evidence of distant metastasis
M1	Distant metastasis
M1a	Nonregional nodal or pulmonary metastasis
M1b	Distant metastasis other than to nonregional nodes and lungs
Serum tumor markers (S)	S category is determined using the nadir value of the postorchiectomy tumor markers
Sx	Tumor marker studies not available or not performed
S0	Tumor marker levels within normal limits
S1	Lactate dehydrogenase (LDH) <1.5 times normal and hCG <5000 mIU/mL and α-fetoprotein (AFP) <1000 g/mL
S2	LDH 1.5–10 times normal or hCG 5000–50,000 mIU/mL or AFP 1000–10,000 g/mL
S3	LDH >10 times normal or hCG >50,000 mIU/mL or AFP >10,000 g/mL

imaging is focused on the assessment of N and M staging. Abdominopelvic CT is the reference standard for the assessment of N and M staging of testis tumors (Fig. 4.4). Testicular cancer has a high propensity for nodal micrometastasis [7]. Because the identification of metastatic lymph nodes is based on size criteria, abdominopelvic CT provides sensitivity of about 70–80 %. Chest CT is performed if metastatic adenopathy is noted in the abdominopelvic CT and additional imaging like brain imaging is warranted if clinical suspicions are present. Testicular cancers can be grouped into three major categories according to the TNMS-based classification: tumors limited to the testis are stage I, those with retroperitoneal nodal involvement are stage II, and those with distant disease are stage III [6].

4.1.3 Special Consideration in Testis Tumor

4.1.3.1 Testicular Microlithiasis

Testicular microlithiasis is defined as five or more microliths on US image (Fig. 4.5) [1]. Microcalcifications within the lumen of the seminiferous tubules are responsible for testicular microlithiasis, and defect of the phagocytic activity of Sertoli cells is regarded as being responsible for testicular microlithiasis [8]. The prevalence of testicular microlithiasis is reported as being between 0.6 and 9 % of symptomatic men [9]. Although the risk of testicular cancer is increased up to 21.6 times [10], it is doubtful whether US follow-up would substantially change the outcome [11].

4.1.3.2 Burned-Out Germ Cell Tumor

Burned-out germ cell tumor is defined as a germ cell tumor with spontaneous regression.

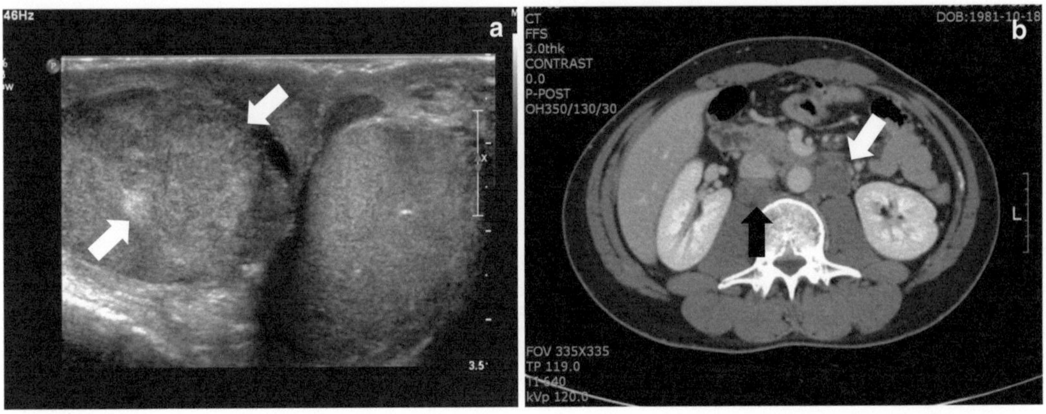

Fig. 4.4 Seminoma with lymph node metastasis. (**a**) US image through the scrota shows ill-defined, slightly hypoechoic mass (*arrow*) in the right testis. (**b**) Abdominopelvic CT scan shows metastatic lymph nodes in the retrocaval and para-aortic area (*arrow*)

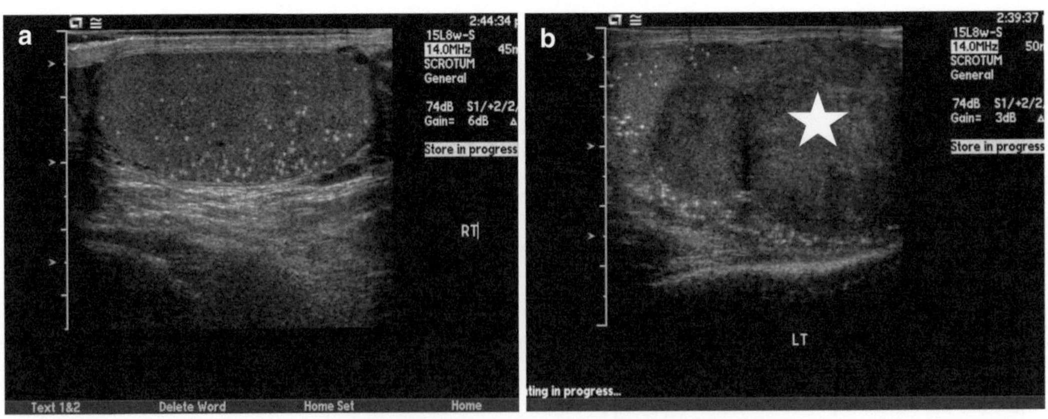

Fig. 4.5 US imaging finding of testicular microlithiasis. US image through the right testis (**a**) shows multiple echogenic spots in the testicular parenchyma, suggestive of microlithiasis. On the longitudinal scan of the left testis (**b**), hypoechoic mass (*asterisk*) is noted in the left testis with microlithiasis

The pathogenesis of burned-out germ cell tumor is uncertain but is presumed to be due to rapid outgrowth beyond the blood supply [1]. Because burned-out germ cell tumor presents with metastasis in the form of extragonadal germ cell tumor, we should consider two possibilities when faced with extragonadal germ cell tumors. One is a primary germ cell tumor originated from the extragonadal germ cells that is aberrantly migrated from the yolk sac, and the other is an extragonadal metastasis of burned-out germ cell tumor. Primary extragonadal germ cell tumors occur commonly in the pineal gland, mediastinum, retroperitoneum, or sacrum [12]. Because retroperitoneal germ cell tumors are more likely to be a metastasis from a primary testicular tumor, the testis should be thoroughly interrogated to rule out the possibility of an occult testicular primary lesion.

4.1.3.3 Germ Cell Tumor in Undescended Testis

There is a strong association between undescended testis and testicular carcinoma, especially seminoma. Therefore, the possibility of testicular cancer should be considered in the evaluation of undescended testis. The pathophysiology of malignant transformation in undescended testes is uncertain, and orchiopexy, performed even at an early age, does not decrease the risk of testicular carcinoma. Furthermore, the risk of testicular cancer is not limited to the undescended testis, and the risk extends to the contralateral normal testis [1]. MR is the most helpful imaging modality in the detection of associated testicular carcinoma in men with undescended testis. US or CT is not good due to its poor tissue contrast. Undescended testis of over 2 cm in US or CT should consider the possibility of associated testicular carcinoma. The majority of the cases present as homogenous mass developed in the abdominally located testis. The demonstration of ipsilateral spermatic cord absence makes specific diagnosis of testicular tumor associated with undescended testis.

4.1.4 Tumor of the Epididymis and Spermatic Cord

4.1.4.1 Epididymal Tumor

Tumorous conditions of the epididymis and spermatic cord are rarely encountered in the clinical practice, and most of them are benign in their nature. The adenomatoid tumor is the most common benign tumor of the epididymis. Leiomyoma or papillary cystadenoma is the next common benign tumor of the epididymis. Adenomatoid tumor is a benign neoplasm of uncertain origin. Adenomatoid tumor occurs frequently in the epididymal tail and appears as a well-defined round mass on US evaluation. The internal echogenicity of the adenomatoid tumor seems to be homogenous and slightly hyperechoic compared with the epididymis. Papillary cystadenoma is frequently associated with von Hippel–Lindau disease. On US evaluation, papillary cystadenoma shows nonspecific imaging features indistinguishable from adenomatoid tumor or leiomyoma, but papillary cystadenoma has the tendency to be more cystic compared with adenomatoid tumor or leiomyoma. Sperm granuloma is a nontumorous condition mimicking epididymal tumor. Most of epididymal tumor needs enucleation, but sperm granuloma is treated conservatively or by epididymectomy for relief of postvasectomy pain syndrome. Therefore, differentiation of sperm granuloma from epididymal tumor is clinically important. Sperm granuloma itself shows imaging feature indistinguishable from epididymal tumor, but previous vasectomy-related findings including dilated epididymal system can be helpful in the differential diagnosis.

4.1.4.2 Spermatic Cord Tumor

Lipoma is the most common extratesticular neoplasm and can occur anywhere within the scrotal sac. Lipoma accounts for more than half of the neoplasms that developed in the spermatic cord. Lipoma appears as echogenic mass on US evaluation (Fig. 4.6). However, this US imaging feature is a nonspecific finding that can be also seen in other disease entities such as inguinal hernia or sarcoma. Cross-sectional imaging like CT or MR might be helpful for specific diagnosis of lipoma by demonstrating internal fat content. When the mass of the spermatic cord is not lipoma, the possibility of malignant spermatic cord mass is increased. A report says that spermatic cord mass other than lipoma is a malignant mass in about 56 % [13]. Rhabdomyosarcoma is the most common malignant tumor of the spermatic cord in children, and liposarcoma is the most common malignant tumor of the spermatic cord in adults. Because the malignant mass of the spermatic cord is usually large and the relationship with adjacent structure can be helpful in the assessment of its origin, MR with large FOV and good tissue contrast is helpful in the evaluation of malignant spermatic cord tumor.

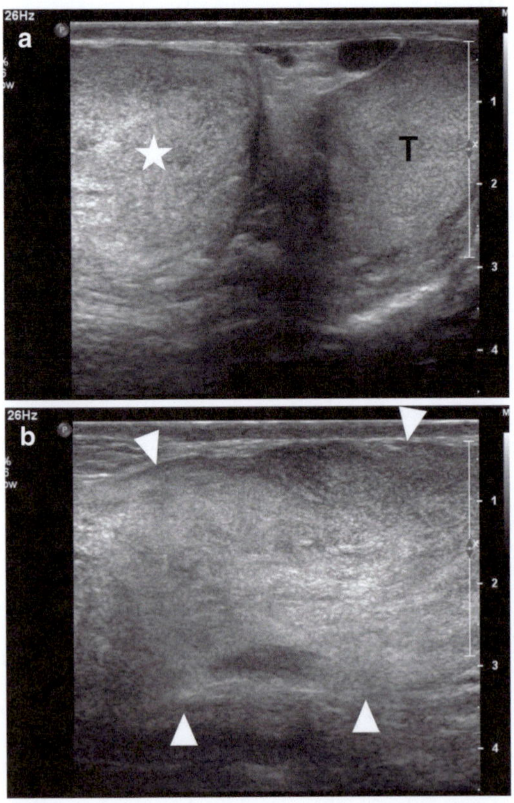

Fig. 4.6 Lipoma of the spermatic cord in a 62-year-old man. (**a**) Longitudinal scan of the left scrotum shows echogenic mass (*asterisk*), separated from the left testis (*T*). (**b**) The mass appears as heterogeneously high echoic mass (*arrowheads*) along the spermatic cord

4.1.5 Pathologic Consideration of Scrotal Tumors

4.1.5.1 Pathology of Germ Cell Tumor

Seminoma

Grossly seminoma is well-circumscribed, frequently lobulated mass with homogenous gray-white cut surface (Fig. 4.7a). Hemorrhage and

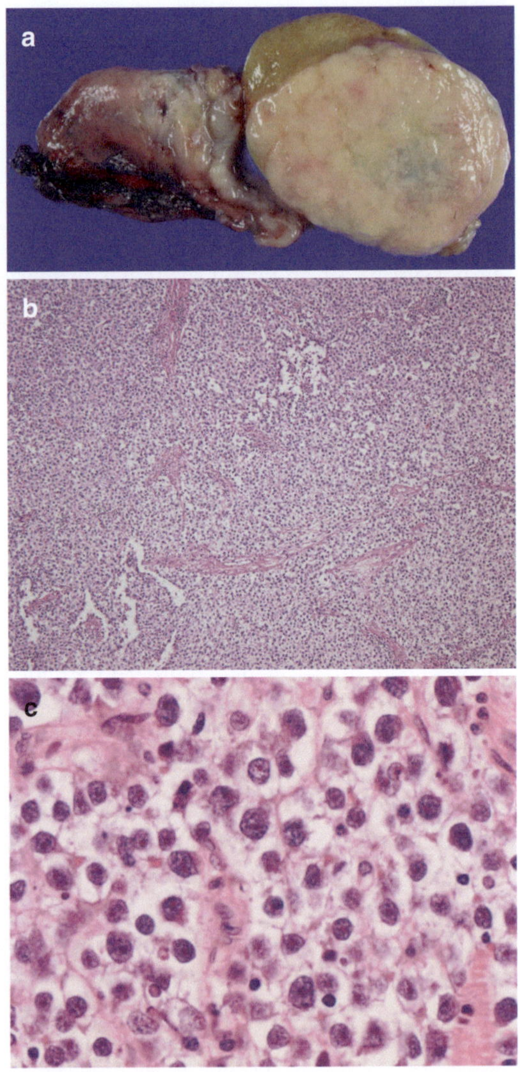

Fig. 4.7 Pathologic findings of seminoma. (**a**) Grossly seminoma is well-circumscribed and lobulated mass with homogenous whitish cut surface. (**b**) Microscopically tumor cells are arranged in solid pattern. (**c**) Tumor cells have round uniform nuclei, prominent nucleoli, and abundant clear cytoplasm

necrosis usually are not found. The presence of hemorrhage and necrosis may suggest mixed germ cell tumor with other nonseminomatous component. Microscopically, main architectural pattern is solid sheets or nests (Fig. 4.7b). Tubular, alveolar structures can be admixed. Tumor cells are round, uniform cells with abundant cytoplasm and distinct cell membrane (Fig. 4.7c). Nuclei are centrally located, round and uniform with prominent nucleoli. Fibrous septa between tumor cell sheets or nests are often prominent. Lymphocytes and plasma cell infiltration are frequently found. Granulomatous reaction and syncytiotrophoblastic giant cells can be seen.

Embryonal Carcinoma

Grossly embryonal carcinoma is poorly demarcated mass with variegated cut surface. Hemorrhage and necrosis are common (Fig. 4.8a). Microscopically embryonal carcinoma shows variable growth patterns such as solid growth, papillary, or glandular pattern (Fig. 4.8b, c). Tumor cells are large and highly pleomorphic with amphophilic cytoplasm. Mitotic figures, hemorrhage, and necrosis are common (Fig. 4.8d).

Yolk Sac Tumor

Grossly yolk sac tumor is solid, gray-white to yellowish mass with myxoid or gelatinous cut surface (Fig. 4.9a). Microscopically, yolk sac tumor reveals variable growth patterns such as microcystic or reticular pattern, macrocystic pattern, solid pattern, glandular–alveolar pattern, endodermal sinus pattern, papillary pattern, myxomatous pattern, polyvascular vitelline pattern, hepatoid pattern, and enteric pattern (Fig. 4.9b, c). Microcystic or reticular pattern is the most common pattern. This pattern is

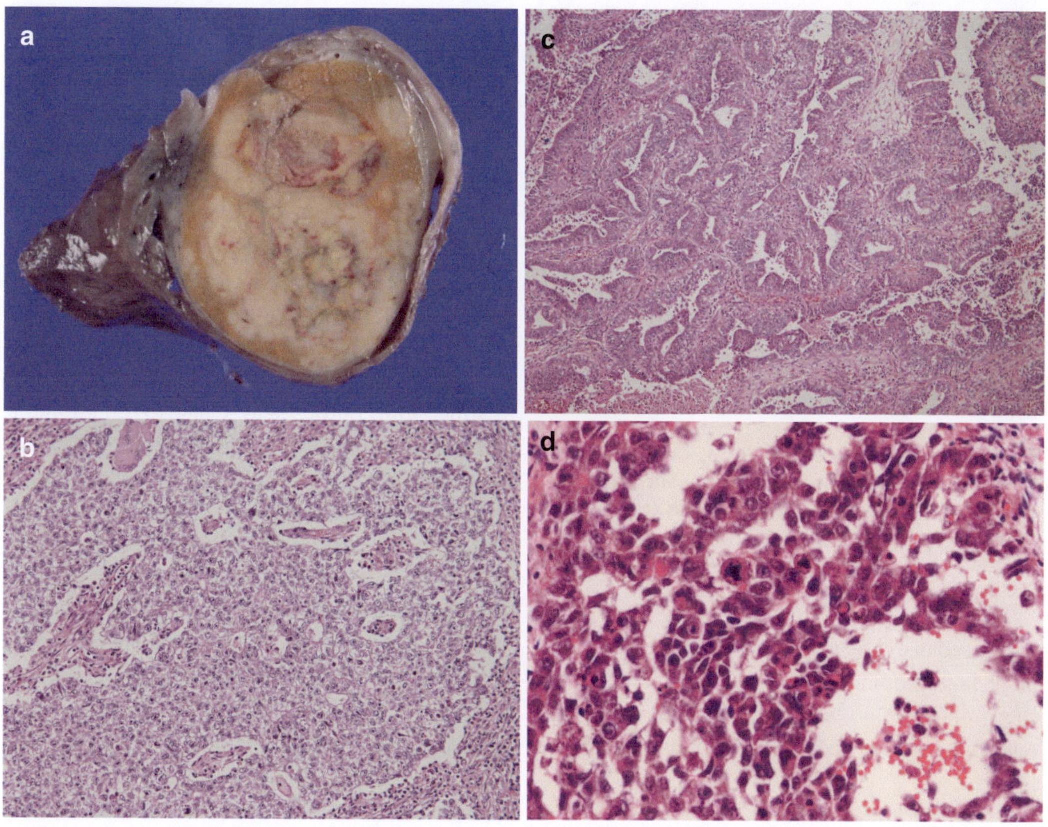

Fig. 4.8 (**a**) Cut surface of embryonal carcinoma shows poorly demarcated whitish mass with focal hemorrhage and necrosis. Microscopically embryonal carcinoma shows variable growth pattern including solid growth (**b**) and glandular pattern (**c**). Nuclear pleomorphism and mitosis are common (**d**)

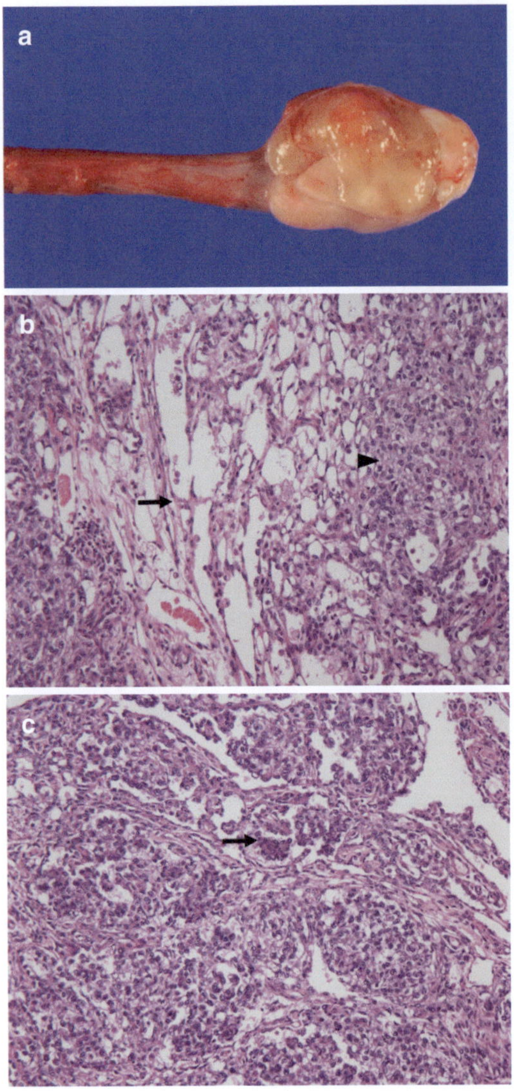

Fig. 4.9 (**a**) Cut surface of yolk sac tumor is grayish homogenous and somewhat myxoid. Microscopically yolk sac tumor shows variable patterns including microcystic pattern (**b**, *center*, *arrow*), solid pattern (**b**, *right side*, *arrow head*), and endodermal sinus pattern (**c**) with Schiller–Duval body (*arrow*)

composed of aggregates of vacuolated cells resembling honeycomb appearance. Each tumor often shows multiple growth patterns. Tumor cells are relatively uniform and somewhat bland looking.

Choriocarcinoma

Choriocarcinoma generally is mixed with other germ cell tumor component, and pure choriocarcinoma in testis is very rare [14].

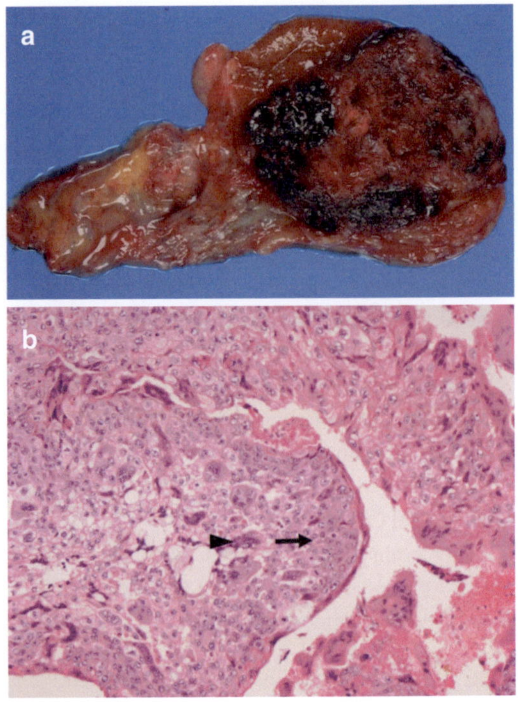

Fig. 4.10 (**a**) Grossly choriocarcinoma is hemorrhagic mass with frequent necrosis. (**b**) Microscopically choriocarcinoma is composed of mononuclear cytotrophoblasts (*arrow*) and multinucleated syncytiotrophoblasts (*arrowhead*)

Grossly this tumor usually shows hemorrhage and necrosis (Fig. 4.10a). Microscopically, choriocarcinoma is composed of cytotrophoblasts and syncytiotrophoblasts (Fig. 4.10b). Cytotrophoblast is round mononuclear cells with distinct cell border and clear to amphophilic cytoplasm. Syncytiotrophoblast is multinucleated cells with smudged nuclei and abundant eosinophilic cytoplasm. Syncytiotrophoblasts frequently cover the nest of cytotrophoblasts.

Teratoma

Teratoma is defined as germ cell tumor composed of more than one type of tissue of different germinal layers (endoderm, mesoderm, and ectoderm). Grossly teratoma shows variegated cut surface with partly solid and cystic areas. Hair, cartilage, or bone can be found (Fig. 4.11a). Microscopically teratoma consists of mixture of tissues of three germ layers (Fig. 4.11b). Well-differentiated mature elements consist of squamous epithelium,

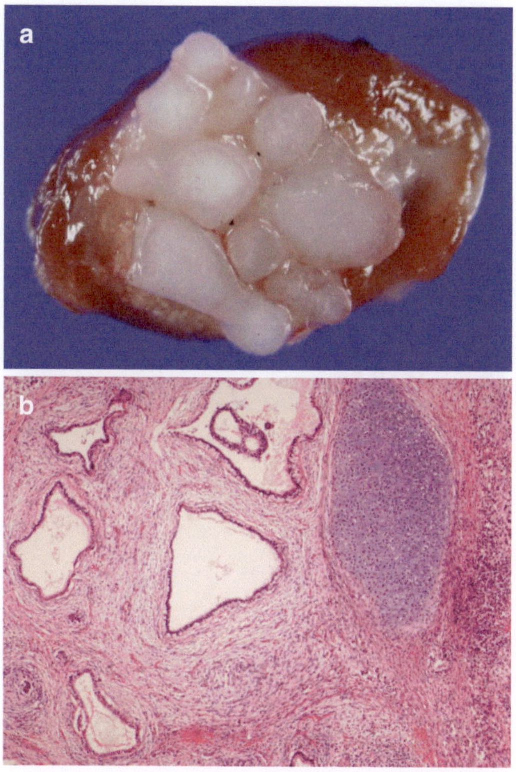

Fig. 4.11 (**a**) This gross photograph of teratoma mainly shows cartilaginous component. (**b**) Microscopically this tumor has cartilage and glandular components

neural tissue, glandular elements, or muscular tissues. Fetal-type immature elements such as undifferentiated mesenchyme, fetal-type glands, or primitive neuroepithelium can be admixed.

Dermoid Cyst and Epidermoid Cyst

Dermoid cyst means monodermal teratoma composed of cysts lined by keratinizing squamous epithelium with skin appendages [15]. Epidermoid cyst does not contain skin appendages (Fig. 4.12).

Mixed Germ Cell Tumor

Mixed germ cell tumor is defined as germ cell tumor composed of more than one histologic type. Grossly mixed germ cell tumor shows heterogeneous cut surface with frequent hemorrhage and necrosis (Fig. 4.13a). Microscopically various germ cell tumor components can be admixed (Fig. 4.13b). Mixed germ cell tumors account for 35–54 % of all testicular germ cell tumors [14].

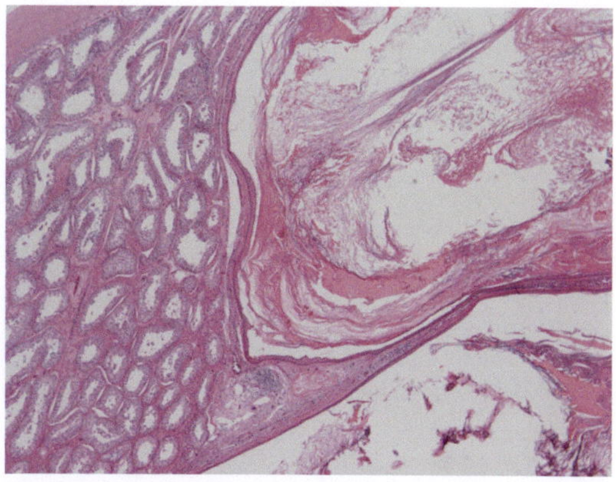

Fig. 4.12 Epidermal cyst of testis is composed of cyst lined by squamous epithelium and filled with keratin materials

4.1.5.2 Pathology of Sex Cord Stromal Tumor

Leydig Cell Tumor

Grossly Leydig cell tumor is well-demarcated yellow to gray mass with homogenous cut surface (Fig. 4.14a). Microscopically Leydig cell tumor is composed of round to polygonal tumor cells with abundant eosinophilic cytoplasm resembling Leydig cells (Fig. 4.14b). Leydig cell tumor shows solid or nodular growth pattern.

Sertoli Cell Tumor

Sertoli cell tumor is grossly well-circumscribed mass with tan to yellow color. Microscopically tumor cells are uniform round, oval, or columnar cells with clear to eosinophilic cytoplasm. Tumor cells frequently show tubular arrangement. Solid, cord, microcyst, or nest formations can be found [16, 17].

4.1.5.3 Tumors of Paratesticular Structures

Adenomatoid Tumor

Adenomatoid tumor is a benign mesothelial origin tumor. Grossly adenomatoid tumor is small well-demarcated tumor. Microscopically this tumor is mainly composed of vacuolated mesothelial cells. Tumor cell arrangement is cord, nest, or tubule formation (Fig. 4.15).

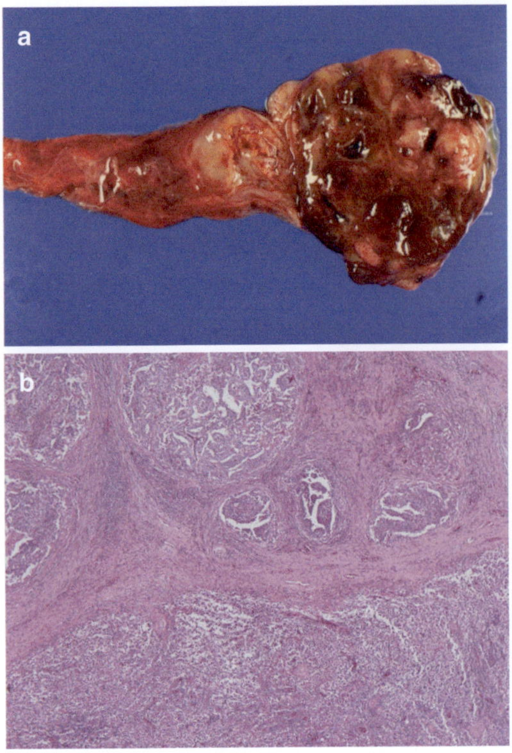

Fig. 4.13 (**a**) Grossly mixed germ cell tumor shows variable morphology depending on the proportion of germ cell tumor components. Hemorrhage and necrosis are common findings. (**b**) This photograph shows embryonal carcinoma (*upper part*) and seminoma (*lower part*)

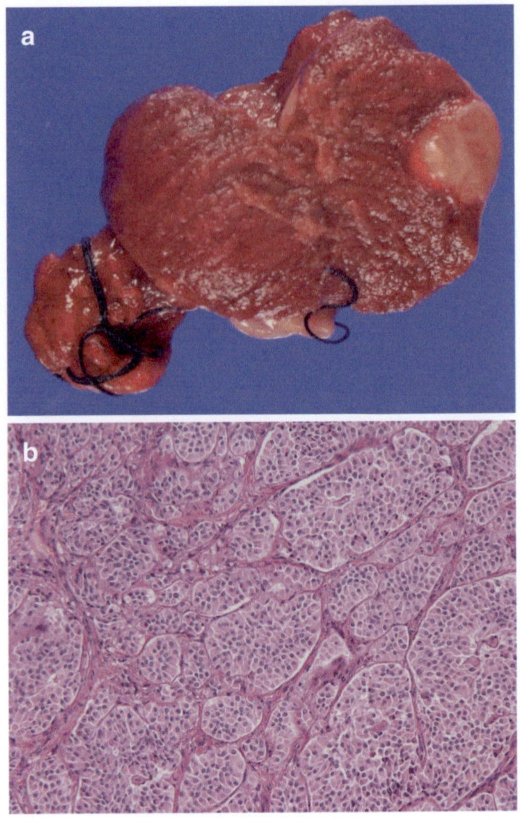

Fig. 4.14 (**a**) This photograph reveals small Leydig cell tumor showing grayish homogenous cut surface. (**b**) Microscopically tumor cells resemble Leydig cells having abundant eosinophilic cytoplasm and round uniform nuclei

Papillary Cystadenoma of Epididymis

This tumor is a benign epithelial tumor showing papillary arrangement and frequently associated with von Hippel–Lindau disease [18]. Grossly this tumor is well circumscribed and variably cystic [18]. Tumor cells are cuboidal to columnar epithelial cells with clear cytoplasm, and these cells are arranged in tubular, cystic, and papillary architecture (Fig. 4.16).

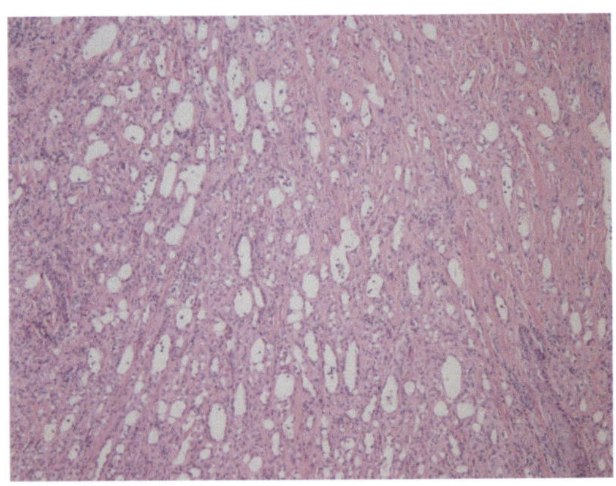

Fig. 4.15 Microscopic findings of adenomatoid tumor of testis showing variable-sized tubule formation

4.1.6 Therapeutic Consideration of Scrotal Tumors

Testis tumor can be broadly categorized as seminoma and nonseminomatous germ cell tumor (NSGCT) due to difference in their natural history and treatment. The multidisciplinary treatment approach including surgical management to testis tumor enables the dramatic improvements of cancer-specific survival rate around 60 % in the 1960s to over than 90 % in the 1990s [19].

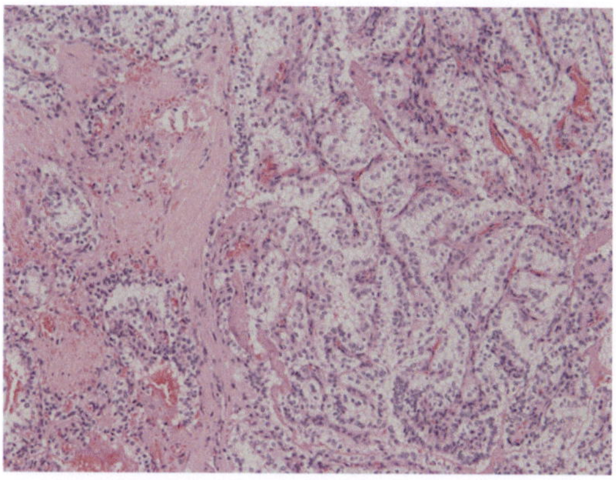

Fig. 4.16 Papillary cystadenoma is composed of clear cells with tubulopapillary architecture

The management decisions are directly related to the clinical stage (CS) and histologic subtype of the primary tumor. The American Joint Committee on Cancer (AJCC) and Union Internationale Contre le Cancer (UICC) developed the international consensus classification for testis tumor in 1997 and lastly updated in 2002 [20, 21]. The CSs are broadly categorized as follows: CS I, disease confined to testis; CS II, presence of regional (or retroperitoneal) lymph node metastasis; and CS III, cases with nonregional lymph node or visceral metastasis [20, 21].

4.1.6.1 Surgical Management

In the treatment of testis tumor, surgery remains as a core part of the management. However, the advance in chemotherapy and improvement in clinical staging due to the exquisite imaging modality and serum tumor markers reduced their role in the past few decades [22].

Because testis tumors are rapidly growing, surgery should be performed immediately without delays longer than 1–2 weeks. However, unfortunately, delays in the diagnosis and treatment of testis tumors are very frequent [23]. Bosl et al. reported that there are significant differences in delayed intervals for diagnosis between the early (CS I) and advanced (CS II and III) stage testis tumor. Painless scrotal mass is often ignored up to 18 % [24]. Careful history taking and physical examination, as well as imaging modality and serum tumor markers, are important for correct diagnosis.

Radical Orchiectomy

Patients who are suspected the testis tumor should undergo orchiectomy. Approximately 80–85 % of CS I seminoma and 70–80 % of CS I NSGCT can be curative by the radical orchiectomy itself. Moreover, radial orchiectomy can provide the information regarding histologic subtype and their primary T stage. Those reviews of primary testis tumor specimens are important for decision-making for further treatments [25].

Radical orchiectomy with removal of testis and their spermatic cord to the level of internal inguinal ring is the choice of the first treatment. A simple orchiectomy via trans-scrotal incision is not generally recommended, because this procedure leaves the inguinal spermatic cord.

This leaved cord enables the lymphatic drainage from the testis; therefore, the risks for local recurrence and lymph node metastasis are increasing. Open or trans-scrotal aspiration biopsies were also prohibited due to the increasing chance of tumor spillage.

The procedure is routinely performed under general or spinal anesthesia. Patient was placed to supine position and aseptically draped the lower abdomen including the genitalia. An oblique incision is made in the inguinal area. About 5–7 cm sized incision is made above 2 cm and parallel to the inguinal ligament. The incision can be extended to the upper scrotum in cases of large tumors. Transverse incision along the Langerhans skin line can be made for cosmetic advantage, but delivery of testis from scrotum can be more difficult.

The external inguinal ring should be identified for orientation. From there, external oblique muscle fascia (Camper and Scarpa's fascia) is incised sharply with awareness not to injure the ilioinguinal nerve running just beneath it. The spermatic cord including the cremaster muscle is bluntly dissected using the peanut dissectors inferiorly and then isolated. Isolated cord is tagged with a 0.5 in. Penrose or a 14 Fr Nelaton tourniquet. The cord is lifted by the tourniquet and dissected cephalad as far as the internal ring.

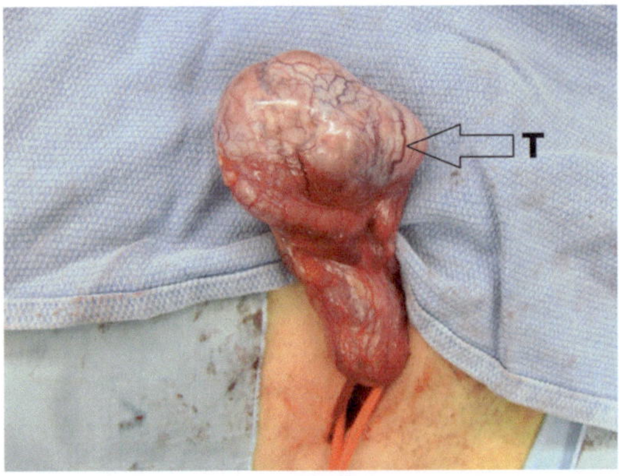

Fig. 4.17 Delivery of the testis (*T*)

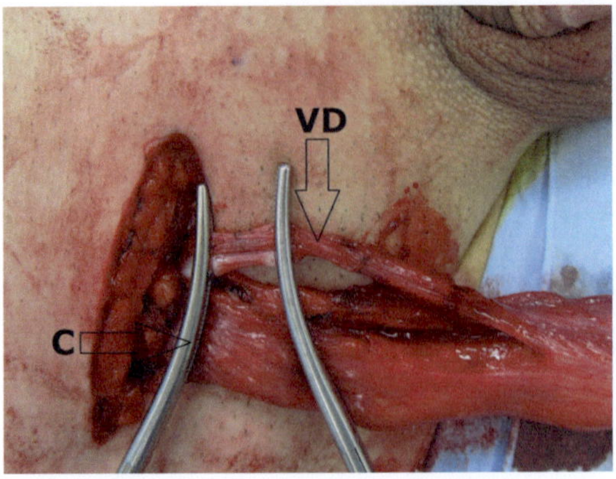

Fig. 4.18 Division of spermatic cord into the vas deferens (*VD*) and cord vessels (*C*)

At the level of internal ring, the cord is clamped using a tourniquet or Kelly preventing the upward spreading of the tumor.

After that, the testis is delivered onto the field via skin incision. The neck of the scrotum was stretched to be in a straight line; thereafter, the scrotum is gently pushed to deliver the testis (Fig. 4.17). Further dissection of Scarpa's fascia or division of gubernacular attachment may be needed for delivery. The delivered testis should be draped off from the field using a sterile towel to prevent the spillage. At this point, if there is any suspicion about the diagnosis, the biopsy of the testis can be considered without risk of spread. If the results of the intraoperative frozen biopsy are implying the cancer, the orchiectomy can be gone ahead.

After mobilizing the spermatic cord 1–2 cm inside the internal ring, the vas deferens and the cord vessels should be dissected and clamped separately (Fig. 4.18). The ligations also should be performed individually. After the double clamps of divided cords, at the proximal of the clamping, double ligations for each cord using 2-0 or 3-0 nonabsorbable ligatures should be performed. The cord is transected at the proximal of the double ligation.

After the orchiectomy, meticulous bleeding control of operative bed should be done. Irrigation with sterile distilled water also should be performed. Thereafter, conjoined tendon is sutured to the leaved edge of the inguinal ligament. External oblique muscle fascia is imbricated with interrupt or continuous 3-0 absorbable sutures. Subcutaneous tissue is closed using 3-0 or 4-0 absorbable sutures. Skin is sutured with metallic stapler or nonabsorbable interrupt sutures. Drain is not necessary to place. Concomitant placement of testicular prosthesis is not generally recommended. In cases of spinal anesthesia, transient placement of Foley urethral catheter or intermittent catheterization for urinary drainage may be needed.

Testis-Sparing Surgery

Testis-sparing surgery such as partial orchiectomy has no role in patients with normal contralateral testis. However, it can be considerable for small-sized organ-confined tumor in patients with bilateral testis tumor or with solitary testis. Patients with suspected benign tumor also can consider this surgical procedure. Partial orchiectomy is not feasible when the testis tumors are not small (>2 cm), because the leaved normal parenchyma is often insufficient after all [25]. In the cases of testis-sparing surgery, adjuvant radiotherapy using dose of >20 Gy is recommended by some groups. Heidenreich et al. reported that there had been no recurrence during 91 months follow-up in 46 patients with small organ-confined testis tumor, who underwent adjuvant radiotherapy after the partial orchiectomy [26].

When partial orchiectomy is performed, biopsy for adjacent normal parenchyma should be done to rule out the accompanying intratubular germ cell neoplasia (ITGCN). The ITGCN has a 50 % risk of testis tumor in a 5-year follow-up therefore that is well known to be a prodromal lesion of testis tumor [27].

The procedure is routinely performed under general or spinal anesthesia. From the positioning to the delivery of the testis, whole procedures are similar with radical orchiectomy. After the delivery, delivered testis is placed on a folded sterile towel to prevent the spillage. If there are doubts about the diagnosis, intraoperative testis biopsy can be done without risk of spread because the testis is draped out of field. After exposure of the testis, the tunica albuginea is incised along the whole length of the testis. The edge of tunica albuginea is grasped with mosquito clamps. The testicular tubules are bluntly dissected from the inner layer of tunica albuginea using 4×4 in. gauze wrapped around the index finger. After blunt dissection, remained stalk which supplies testis tubule tissues is ligated with 2-0 absorbable ligatures and resected. Remained stump and entire inner surface of tunica albuginea should be fulgurated using an electrocautery to ablate potential residual tumor cells. Tunica albuginea is closed with 3-0 absorbable continuous sutures. Skin repair procedure is similar to that of radical orchiectomy.

Simple Orchiectomy

Simple orchiectomy is not recommended for the treatment of testis tumor, because this procedure leaves the inguinal spermatic cord. Leaved cord enables the lymphatic drainage; therefore, the risks for local recurrence and lymph node metastasis are increasing. A recent meta-analysis reported that local recurrence rate was 2.9 % of 206 patients with scrotal violation compared to 0.4 % of patients who underwent radical orchiectomy [28]. It has been reported that suboptimal approaches for testis tumors occurred up to 17 % of tumors [29, 30].

Simple orchiectomy is generally performed for the purpose of androgen axis blockage in advanced prostate cancer. Bilateral simple orchiectomy reduces circulating testosterone levels <50 ng/dL, which is considered the castration level within 24 h of the surgery [30]. A series of large clinical trials established the effectiveness of this procedure in advanced prostate cancer [31, 32].

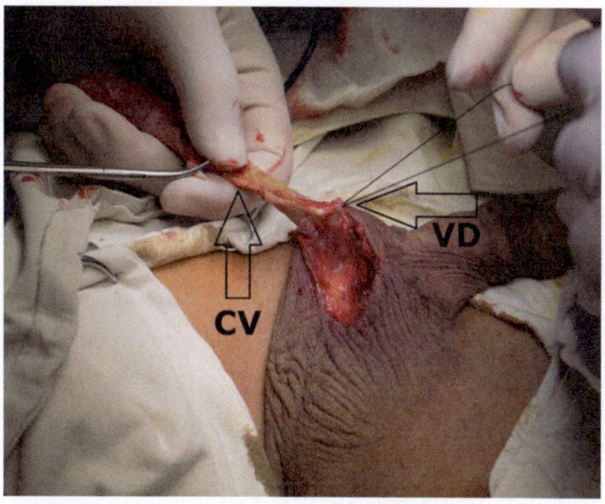

Fig. 4.19 Resection and ligation of isolated vas deferens (*VD*) from cord vessels (*CV*)

The procedure is routinely performed under general, spinal, or local anesthesia. Position of patients is similar to that of radical orchiectomy. Initially, a vertical 3 to 5 cm incision on the scrotal median raphe is made.

After initial incision, electrocautery is recommended to utilize for transection of inner layers including dartos muscle and cremasteric layers that can reduce the risk of scrotal hematoma formation. Transection is made until the bluish tunica vaginalis is presenting. Within the tunica vaginalis the testis is pushed and delivered into the wound. If the delivery is interfered by the tunica vaginalis, that layer can be alternatively opened for mobilizing the testis. Mobilized testis is drawn until the epididymis and cord are exposed.

The cord is dissected to divide into the vas deferens and cord vessels. Divided vas deferens is ligated separately using 3-0 synthetic absorbable suture (Fig. 4.19). The cord vessels are resected at the level lower than internal inguinal ring. To ensure the cord is not slippery, proximal double clamping is mandatory. Remained stump of the cord should be doubly ligated. Using more than one suture ligation with 2-0 synthetic absorbable suture is recommended, because remained cord vessels tend to retract into the internal inguinal ring after division. If the ligature is lost, the uncontrolled major bleeding may occur at scrotal or inguinal area.

Before closing, awareness for bleeding is needed because a scrotal hematoma can be dramatically large. Any bleeders in the dartos and subcutaneous tissue should be electrocauterized meticulously to avoid a distressing scrotal hematoma. Drains are rarely placed. The transected dartos layer and skin are individually repaired using 4-0 or 5-0 synthetic absorbable sutures. In spinal anesthesia, transient placement of the Foley urethral catheter can be considered.

Retroperitoneal Lymph Node Dissection (RPLND)

Postorchiectomy levels of serum tumor markers (AFP, hCG, and LDH) are important for staging and the selection of further treatment. Therefore, all patients are recommended to assess for appropriate decline in those markers after the orchiectomy. Further management decisions should be referred to the levels of serum tumor markers measured within 4 weeks after the orchiectomy. The presence or new elevation of serum tumor marker levels after orchiectomy implies metastatic diseases; thus, those patients should be considered to receive the induction chemotherapy.

Except for choriocarcinoma, almost all testis tumors are spreading via lymphatic channels from the testis to the retroperitoneal lymph nodes (RPLNs). On the other hand, choriocarcinoma tends to disseminate hematogenously. Therefore, retroperitoneum is the most common initial metastatic site of the testis tumor accounting up to 70–80 % of total cases. Detailed mapping studies using RPLND series identified that the primary "lending zone" of right testis tumors is the interaortocaval lymph nodes, after which lymphatics are drained to paracaval or para-aortic lymph nodes. For left testis tumors the primary drained site is the para-aortic lymph nodes followed by the interaortocaval nodes [3]. Because the direction of lymphatic drainage in the retroperitoneum is from right to left, contralateral lymph node spread from right-sided testis tumors is common, but contralateral retroperitoneal spread from left-sided tumor is rare. Therefore, extents of templates for RPLND are different between the right- and left-sided testis tumors.

Conventionally RPNLD should be considered in all NSGCT patients with stage IIB or lower [33, 34]. However, improved accuracy of clinical staging by imaging work-up and the extended application of cisplatin-based chemotherapy cut back the conventional role of RPLND [4, 35]. The possible infertility resulting from retrograde ejaculation also limits the clinical use of RPLND. In patients with stage 1A and 1B (T2 only), the surveillance instead of RPLND can be considered [34]. The suitable clinical indications for preferred RPLND in NSGCT are as follows: (1) clinical stage IB (≥T3) with negative marker; (2) stage IIA with negative marker; (3) stage IIB with unifocal tumors size <3 cm, with ipsilateral nodes restricted to the primary lending zone with negative marker; and (4) all stage II treated with primary chemotherapy with residual mass (≥1 cm) on CT scan. Chemotherapy should be considered as a first-line treatment in persistent tumor marker (≥S1) or advanced stage (≥III) NSGCT [33, 34].

For standard RPLND, the nodal area to be resected for right-sided tumors stops over the aorta and includes interaortocaval, right paracaval, and right iliac nodes. For left-sided tumors, dissection stops medially over the vena cava and includes the interaortocaval, left para-aortic, and left iliac nodes. A modified nerve-sparing RPLND can be also considered in low-stage tumors (stage ≤1B) to prevent the retrograde ejaculation [33, 34]. A modified dissection template is unilateral below the inferior mesenteric artery and bilateral above.

4.1.6.2 Radiation Therapy

Radiation therapy has its role in seminoma. Approximately 80 % of seminoma patients are clinical stage I. In those patients surveillance, single-agent carboplatin, and radiation therapy are accepted as treatment options [33, 34]. The long-term cancer control with those modalities approached nearly 100 %. Seminoma patients with stage IIA or IIB with non-bulky disease also can consider the radiation therapy [34].

Generally, the radiation therapy is recommended to start after the orchiectomy wound has fully healed. Patients are routinely treated 5 days a week. Linear accelerators with >6 MV protons should be utilized when possible. A non-contrast CT scan simulation should be performed in the treatment position. In stage IA, IB, and IS of seminoma, a total dose of 20 Gy in ten fractions is recommended. Irradiated field may be determined by bony anatomy. The superior and inferior borders are recommended as the bottom of vertebral body T11 and L5. The width of lateral borders is generally 10 cm wide (strip fields). In stage IIA and IIB, two consecutive phase radiation therapies are recommended. First phase is performed in modified dog-leg fields [36] with 20 Gy in ten fractions. Second phase is performed in nodal mass contoured fields with daily 2 Gy fractions to a total cumulative dose of 30 Gy (stage IIA) and 36 Gy (stage IIB) [34].

4.1.6.3 Chemotherapy

One of the most important features of testis tumor is their sensitivity to cisplatin-based chemotherapy. This characteristic of testis tumor enables cure in most of the patients even though with extensive metastasis. With the establishment of cisplatin-based chemotherapy on testis tumor, cancer-specific survival has been dramatically improved [19]. Before the cisplatin-based chemotherapy was introduced, cure chance for patients with advanced testis tumor was lower than 10 %. However, the long-term survival for patients with metastatic testis tumor has been higher than 80 % [18].

Chemotherapy has its important roles in all histologic subtypes of testis tumor. In seminoma, one or two cycles of single-agent carboplatin (regimen, 700 mg/m^2 IV) can be considered as a treatment option in stage IA and IB. In stage II and III seminoma, four cycles of EP (regimen: etoposide 100 mg/m^2 IV on days 1–5, cisplatin 20 mg/m^2 IV on days 1–5, repeat every 3 weeks) or three cycles of BEP (regimen: etoposide 100 mg/m^2 IV on days 1–5, cisplatin 20 mg/m^2 IV on days 1–5, bleomycin 30 units IV weekly on days 1, 8, and 15, repeat every 3 weeks) should be considered [33, 34].

In NSGCT, one or two cycles of BEP can be considered in stage IB. In NSGCT stages IS, II, and IIIA, four cycles of EP or three cycles of BEP are recommended. Only four cycles of BEP can be applied in stage IIIB; four cycles of BEP or four cycles of VIP (regimen: etoposide 75 mg/m^2 IV on days 1–5, mesna 120 mg/m^2 slow IV push before ifosfamide on day 1, 1200 mg/m^2 IV on days 1–5, ifosfamide 1200 mg/m^2 on days 1–5, cisplatin 20 g/m^2 IV on days 1–5, repeat every 3 weeks) are recommended as treatment options. In stages IIA and IIB, if there are residual masses (≥1 cm) after the chemotherapy, consolidative bilateral RPLND should be performed [33, 34].

4.2 Penile Tumor

4.2.1 Imaging Anatomy

The penis is divided into a penile root, a penile shaft, and a penile glans. The penile shaft consists of the paired dorsolateral corpora cavernosa and the single ventral corpus spongiosum. In the penile root, the corpora cavernosa is attached to the symphysis pubis, and the corpus spongiosum is attached to the urogenital diaphragm (Fig. 4.20). The glans of the penis is an anterior extension of the corpus spongiosum which contains the urethra. Three fascial layers (the Colles fascia, the Buck's fascia, and the tunica albuginea) surround the corpora cavernosa and the corpus spongiosum. The innermost fascia is the tunica albuginea and it surrounds each corpus individually. The Buck's fascia surrounds the corpora cavernosa and the corpus spongiosum while separating the corpora cavernosa from the corpus spongiosum. The Buck's fascia acts as a barrier to corporal invasion and hematogenous spread of the penile cancer [37]. The outermost Colles fascia is located between the subcutaneous connective tissue and the overlying skin. The lymphatic drainage from the skin of the penis and prepuce is toward the superficial inguinal nodes, and the lymphatic drainage from the glans penis is toward the deep

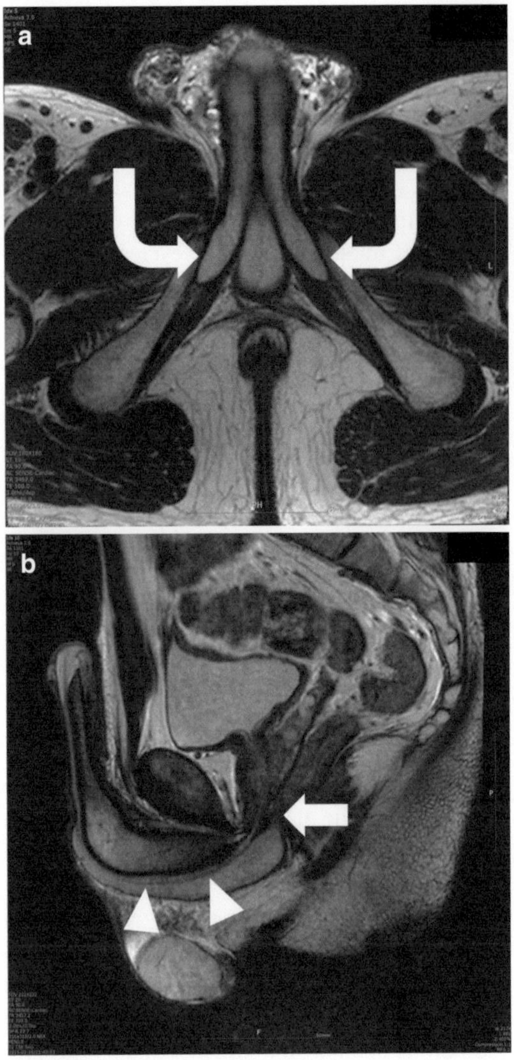

Fig. 4.20 Normal MR imaging of the penile root. (**a**) On T2-weighted axial scan of the penile root, both corpora cavernosa (*curved arrows*) are attached to the inferior ramus of the symphysis pubis. (**b**) On T2-weighted sagittal scan, the corpus spongiosum containing the urethra (*arrowheads*) is attached to the urogenital diaphragm (*arrow*)

inguinal lymph nodes. The lymphatic drainage from the erectile tissue and penile urethra is toward the internal iliac nodes [38].

US is the primary imaging modality for assessment of the penis because of its widespread availability and low cost. On US evaluation, the corpora cavernosa and corpus spongiosum appear as a tubular structure of a homogenous echotexture (Fig. 4.21). The surrounding tunica albuginea and

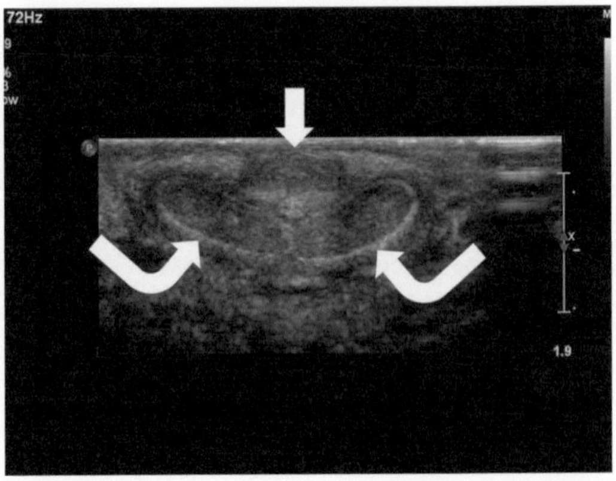

Fig. 4.21 US performed with the penis in the anatomic position. Corpora cavernosa (*curved arrow*) and a corpus spongiosum (*arrow*) appear as tubular structures of homogenous echogenicity

Buck's fascia could not be clearly defined on US evaluation. MR imaging is the most accurate imaging modality in the assessment of the penile anatomy. For appropriate patient positioning, a towel is placed between the patient's legs to elevate the scrotum and penis with the patient in supine position. The penis is then dorsiflexed against the lower abdomen along the midline and taped in position to reduce the motion of the penis during the examination. The corpora cavernosa and corpus spongiosum show intermediate signal intensity on T1-weighted MR imaging and high signal intensity on T2-weighted imaging. Both the tunica albuginea and the Buck's fascia are hypointense on T1- and T2-weighted imaging and could not be separated from each other (Fig. 4.22). The outermost Colles fascia is also hypointense on T1- and T2-weighted imaging. T2-weighted imaging is the preferred imaging sequence for depicting the penile anatomy due to its superior tissue contrast between the corpora and overlying fascia. CT is unable to depict the penile anatomy due to its poor tissue contrast. The role of CT is limited to the evaluation of pelvic lymph nodes that are inaccessible by clinical methods.

4.2.2 Penile Cancer

Penile cancer is an uncommon neoplasm in the developed countries with an incidence of 0.4 % of all male malignancies [39], but it accounts for

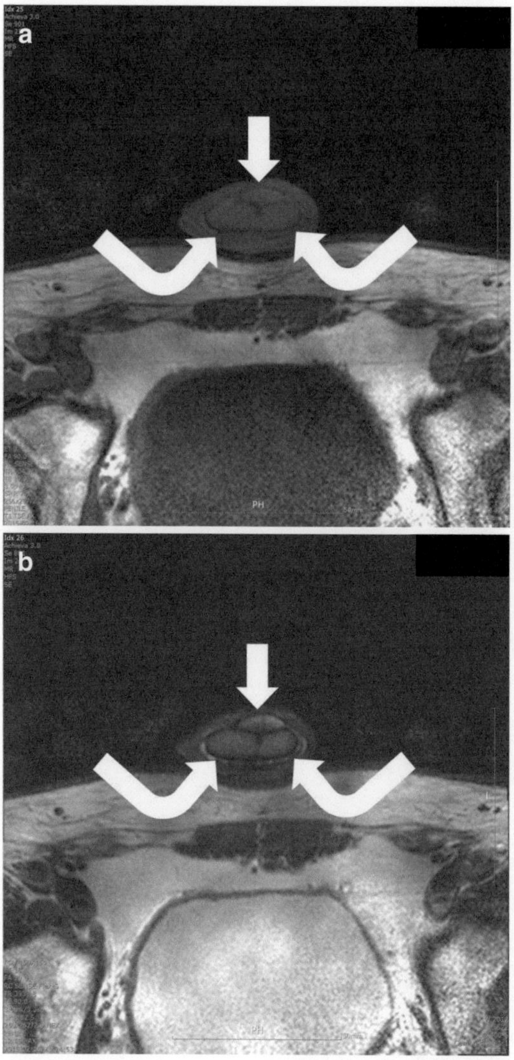

Fig. 4.22 MRI performed with the penis in the anatomic position. The corpora cavernosa (*curved arrow*) and corpus spongiosum (*arrow*) show intermediate signal intensity on T1-weighted imaging (**a**) and high signal intensity on T2-weighted imaging (**b**). Both the tunica albuginea and Buck's fascia are hypointense on T1- and T2-weighted imaging and could not be separated from each other

10–20 % of all male malignancies in some areas such as Africa and South America [40]. The most frequent penile neoplasm is squamous cell carcinoma accounting for 95 % of penile neoplasms [40]. Penile neoplasms other than squamous cell carcinoma are very rare. These include primary nonsquamous malignancies like sarcoma, melanoma, basal-cell carcinoma, and lymphoma and secondary penile cancer like metastasis. Clinically, penile cancer presents as erythema, induration, bleeding, or enlarging ulcer. The most common site of penile cancer involvement is the penile glans (48 %), followed by the prepuce (21 %), coronal sulcus (6 %), and penile shaft [41, 42].

4.2.2.1 Staging of Penile Cancer

The lymphatic spread is the major pathway of the metastasis of the penile cancer. The skin of the penis and prepuce drains into the superficial inguinal lymph nodes, the glans penis drains in the deep inguinal lymph node, and the corpora drain into the internal iliac lymph nodes (Fig. 4.23). Two staging systems are used to determine the optimal therapeutic approach in men with penile cancer: the Jackson classification system (Table 4.3) and the TNM classification system (Table 4.4). The presence and extent of nodal metastasis is the most significant predictor of survival in men with penile cancer and is related to the stage of primary lesion. The incidence of lymph node metastases increases from 20 % of T1 tumors to 47–66 % of T2–T4 penile cancers [43]. Other factors that influence the lymphatic spread of penile cancer are the histologic grade, the vertical growth of the tumor, and the presence of vascular or lymphatic invasion [44].

4.2.2.2 Treatment

Treatment of penile cancer varies depending on the site and extent of the primary penile mass. Ablation, excision, partial penectomy, or total penectomy can be given for the treatment of primary penile cancer, according to the clinical stage. Controversy regarding inguinal lymphadenectomy exists and practices vary considerably [45]. Some surgeons favor reevaluation of palpable inguinal lymph nodes after 4–6 weeks of antibiotic treatment and perform inguinal lymphadenectomy for the continued presence of lymph nodes in the inguinal lesion. This approach is based on the theoretical backgrounds that reactive lymphadenopathy will resolve following antibiotic treatment, whereas metastatic lymphadenopathy will persist [38]. Others favor prophylactic inguinal lymphadenectomy at the time of the penile surgery, and prophylactic inguinal lymphadenectomy has been shown to improve long-term survival rates [46, 47]. However, inguinal lymphadenectomy is

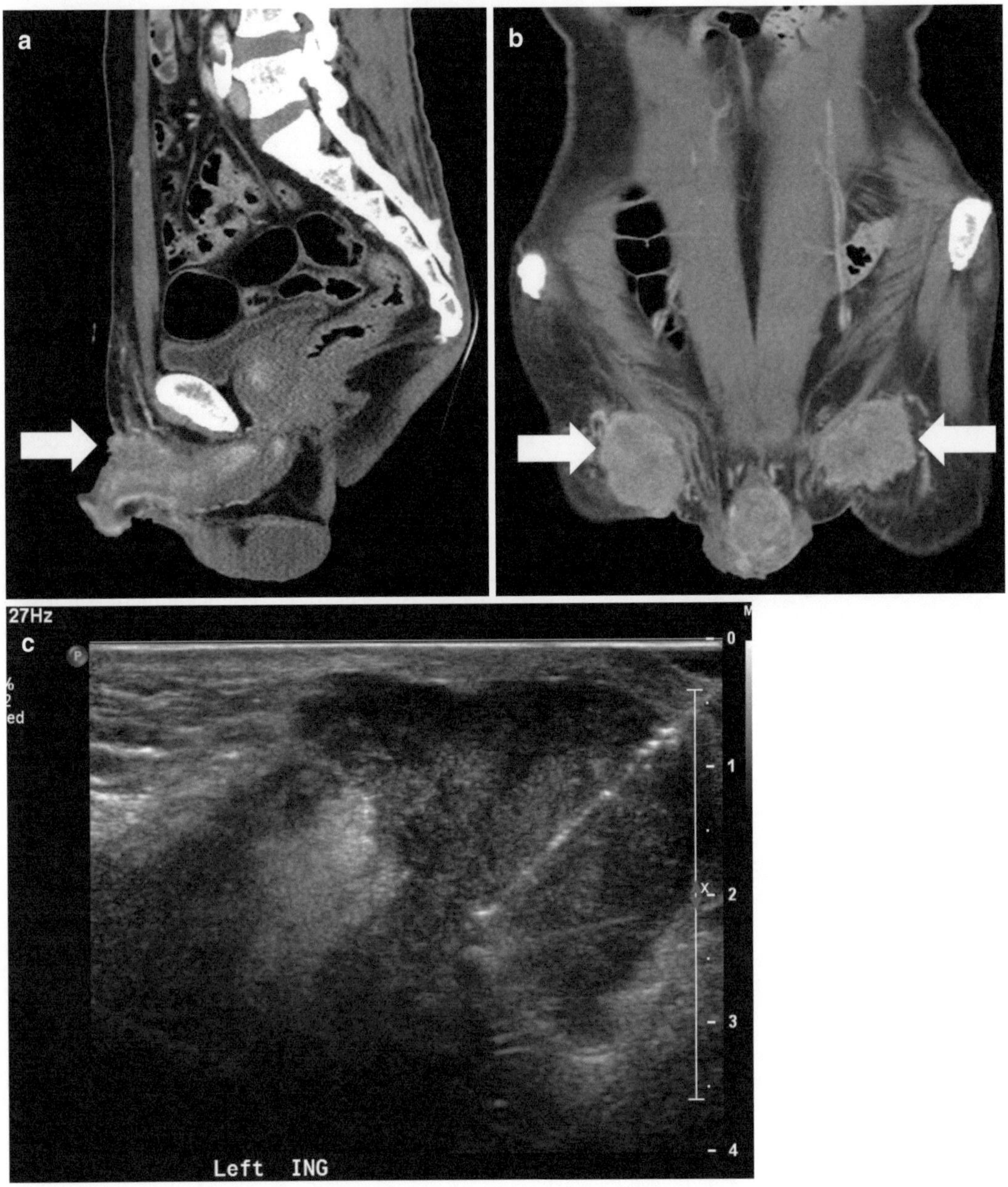

Fig. 4.23 Penile cancer with lymph node metastasis in a 52-year-old man. Contrast-enhanced sagittal CT scan (**a**) shows infiltrative mass in the penile shaft (*arrow*). On the coronal reformatted image (**b**), metastatic lymph nodes (*arrow*) are noted in both inguinal areas. US-guided biopsy (**c**) of the metastatic lymph node revealed squamous cell carcinoma

Table 4.3 Jackson classification of penile cancer

Stage	Involvement
1	Confined to the glans penis
2	Invasion of the shaft or corpora
3	Operable inguinal lymph node metastasis
4	Invasion of adjacent structures, inoperable inguinal lymph node metastasis

associated with a high incidence of major morbidity like severe lymphedema and skin flap necrosis. Bevan-Thomas et al. reported minor morbidity of 68 % and major morbidity of 32 % associated with inguinal lymphadenectomy [48]. Therefore, an effort should be made to identify the patients who will benefit from the inguinal lymphadenectomy.

4.2.2.3 Role of Imaging

Traditionally, the evaluation of the penile cancer is performed clinically by palpation of the penile tumor and the inguinal lymph nodes. However, the clinical approach is often inaccurate in the assessment of local invasion of the penile cancer and its inguinal node metastases [49, 50]. Ultrasound is a useful imaging modality in the assessment of local invasion of penile cancer. On ultrasound, interruption of the thin echogenic line surrounding corpora suggests infiltration of the tunica albuginea by penile cancer. MRI can be also used to stage penile cancers. T2-weighted imaging and contrast-enhanced T1-weighted imaging are the most commonly used imaging sequences in defining the local extent of a penile neoplasm. Squamous cell carcinomas appear as ill-defined infiltrating tumors of low intensity on both T2-weighted imaging and contrast-enhanced T1-weighted imaging (Fig. 4.24) [38]. Although MR imaging can be useful in the detection of pelvic or retroperitoneal lymph node metastasis, the capacity of MR imaging to detect lymph node metastases is limited because the diagnosis is based on lymph node size. MR imaging cannot detect microscopic metastases in normal-sized lymph nodes and is unable to distinguish inflammatory lymphadenopathy from metastatic lymphadenopathy. CT plays a limited role in the evaluation of the extent of the primary tumor, but it is useful in the evaluation of lymph node or distant metastasis. However, same limitation is present in the evaluation of metastatic lymph nodes.

Table 4.4 TNM classification of penile cancer

Stage	Description
Tumor (T)	
Tx	Primary tumor cannot be assessed
T0	No evidence of primary tumor
Tis	Carcinoma in situ
T1	Invasion of subepithelial connective tissue
T2	Invasion of one or more corpora
T3	Invasion of urethra or prostate gland
T4	Invasion of other adjacent structures
Lymph node (N)	
Nx	Regional lymph node cannot be assessed
N0	No regional lymph node metastasis
N1	Metastasis in a single superficial inguinal lymph node
N2	Metastases in multiple or bilateral superficial inguinal lymph nodes
N3	Unilateral or bilateral metastases in deep inguinal or pelvic lymph nodes
Metastasis (M)	
Mx	Distant metastasis cannot be assessed
M0	No evidence of distant metastasis
M1	Distant metastasis

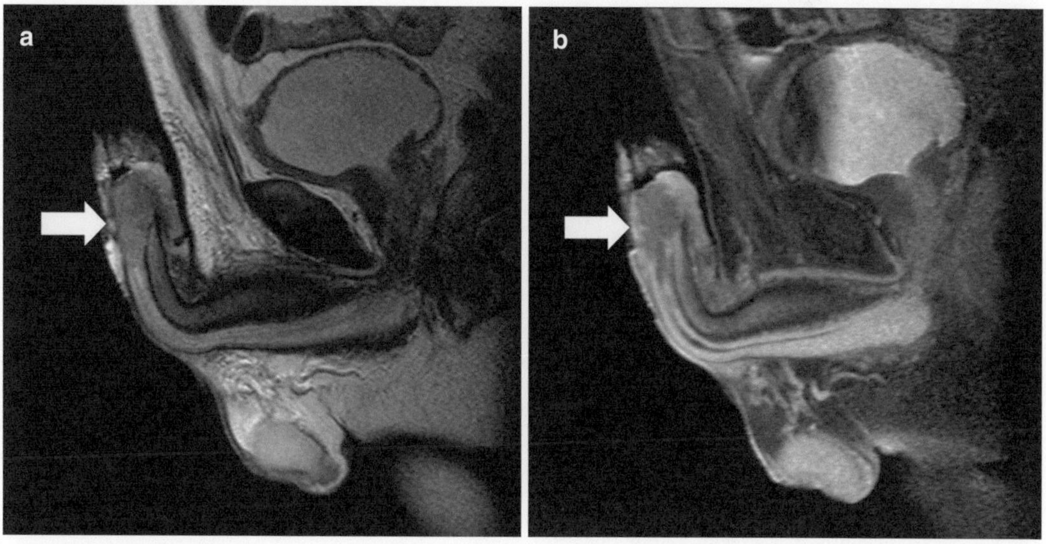

Fig. 4.24 Penile cancer in a 67-year-old man. T2-weighted sagittal image (**a**) shows infiltrative mass of low signal intensity (*arrow*) of the penile glans. The mass appears as less enhancing infiltrative lesion (*arrow*) on the contrast-enhanced T1-weighted imaging (**b**)

4.2.3 Pathologic Consideration of Penile Tumors

4.2.3.1 Squamous Cell Carcinoma

Squamous cell carcinoma of the penis is often large tumor with white granular surface (Fig. 4.25a, b). Growth pattern of penile squamous cell carcinoma can be classified as three patterns: superficial spreading, vertical growth, and multicentric. Microscopically penile squamous cell carcinoma mainly shows well or moderate differentiation frequently having keratinization (Fig. 4.25c). Some variants of squamous cell carcinoma such as basaloid carcinoma, warty carcinoma, verrucous carcinoma, or pseudohyperplastic carcinoma are present [14, 51].

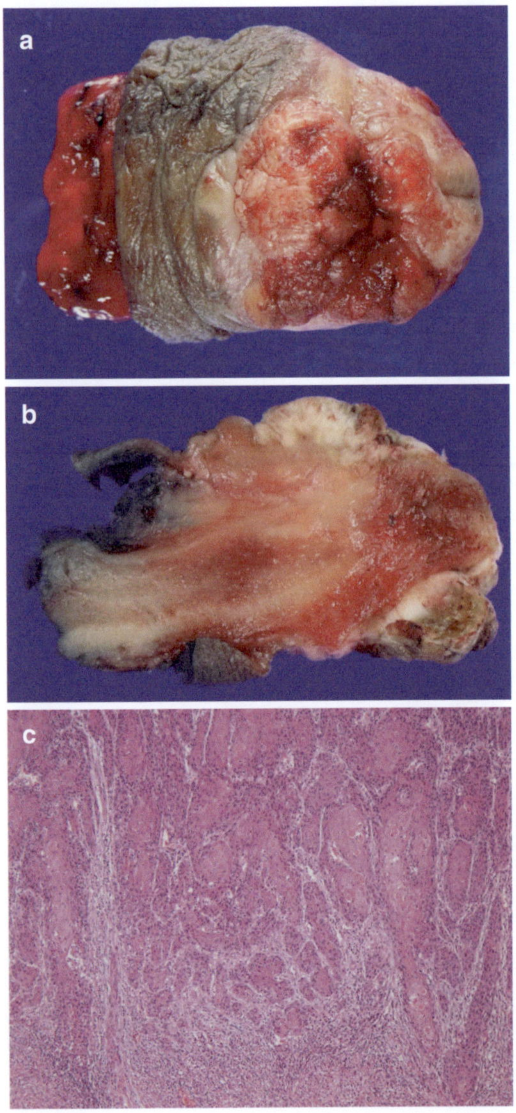

Fig. 4.25 (**a**) Gross photograph of squamous cell carcinoma of penis shows ulcerative whitish lesion. (**b**) Cut surface shows whitish mass with infiltration. (**c**) Microscopically well-differentiated squamous cell carcinoma is found

4.2.3.2 Other Carcinomas

Small cell carcinoma, Merkel cell carcinoma, and clear cell carcinoma are rarely reported in the penis [14].

4.2.3.3 Other Tumors

Mesenchymal tumors of the penis are very rare. Kaposi sarcomas and leiomyosarcomas are the most common sarcomas in the penis [52].

4.2.4 Therapeutic Consideration of Penile Cancer

Penile cancer is extremely uncommon tumor which accounts for 0.4–0.6 % of all male malignancy in the United States [53]. Previous reports have been implied that not only the pathological features of primary tumor but also the nodal status is important for determining their prognosis and further treatment planning of penile cancer [46, 54]. The development of imaging staging and accumulation of knowledge regarding nodal spreading behavior have enabled modification of surgical strategy to lessen potential morbidities. The selection of patients who are suitable for organ-preserving surgery also became possible.

4.2.4.1 Surgical Management

Despite accumulating knowledge, the surgery remains as a primary treatment. Only the early sufficient surgical resection with close follow-up can ensure the best chance for cure. It is also well known that effective control of nodal disease is critical for survival outcomes.

Circumcision

The preventive role of neonatal routine circumcision in penile cancer is still a controversy.

Although circumcision can improve the personal hygiene status and therefore enable the avoidance of risk factors such as HPV infections, however this may be less effective in countries with good hygiene status. Frisch et al. reported decreased incidence of penile cancer in an uncircumcised Danish population from 1940s to 1990s and concluded that this is due to the dissemination of in-house bath [55]. Although circumcision can lessen the phimosis-related infections, other modifiable behaviors such as condom use, avoidance of ultraviolet exposure, smoking, and improvement of general hygiene status also should be considered for prevention of malignant transformation. Moreover, HPV vaccination is expected to play an important role in penile cancer prevention. However, the efficacy is not yet confirmed [56, 57].

Laser Therapy

Laser therapy has been proposed as a conservative treatment modality in penile squamous cell carcinoma. Laser has the advantage of sharp ablation of primary tumor with preservation of surrounding tissues. The carbon dioxide (CO_2), potassium titanyl phosphate (KTP), and neodymium-doped yttrium aluminum garnet (Nd:YAG) lasers are commonly used for this purpose. Because the CO_2 has an extremely narrow penetration depth (0.01 mm), it has been often used for treatment of precancerous lesion or carcinoma in situ (CIS) [58–60]. However, local recurrence rate is reported up to 30 % [60].

In international recommendations, the laser treatment can be considered in Tis, Ta, and T1 low grade ($\leq$2) as a treatment option for penile squamous cell carcinoma [61, 62]. In that procedure, it is recommended to secure safety margins of 3–5 mm from the lesions. Approximately 20 min before that procedure, the skin is prepared with 5 % acetic acid, because HPV-induced area is whitened by the acetic acid [59]. After that the laser ablation can be performed completely. Disadvantages of laser therapy lie in difficulty in determining the proper depth and latency of healing in obese or immunocompromised patients [59].

Mohs Micrographic Surgery

Mohs micrographic surgery enables excision of penile cancer tissue in thin layers [63]. This was originally devised as a fixed tissue technique; however, the application has been extended to the fresh tissues for the treatment of smaller lesions [64, 65]. Mohs micrographic surgery is ideally suitable for Tis or small Ta lesions, and their treatment outcomes are comparable to that of partial penectomy. However, the outcome may be dependent on technical skills and experience of surgeon [65, 66].

Prior to the surgical procedure, color coding with tissue dyes should be performed. That enables the accurate orientation and tissue mapping during the surgery. Under surface of removed tissue is horizontally cut for intraoperative frozen biopsy. Lateral margins are also cut vertically. In frozen examination, whole deep and lateral margins are thoughtfully evaluated. If the presence of tumor is identified, further resection is performed until the whole tumor is removed. Mohs et al. reported that the long-term local control rate is 94 % [66].

Partial Penectomy

Penile amputation remains the oncologic gold standard for definitive treatment for primary tumor. Local recurrence rates after partial or total penectomy are reported as 0–8 % [67–69]. Among them, partial penectomy is the most frequently performed surgery for the treatment of penile squamous cell carcinoma. General indication for partial penectomy is T1 with high grade ($\geq$3) and $\geq$T2 [61, 62]. This procedure has two major goals. One is a successful local control to ensure $\geq$2 cm safety margin from primary lesion. The other is preservation of the penis to enable to void in standing and to perform intercourse.

The patient is placed in a supine position under general or spinal anesthesia. To prevent the spillage, the lesion is initially draped out from the fields using sterile towel or surgical glove. For the same purpose, tourniquet clamping of penile roots is also recommendable (Fig. 4.26). Proposed line for incision is drawn on the skin. Along this line, the skin and dartos fascia are incised circumferentially. Buck's fascia is

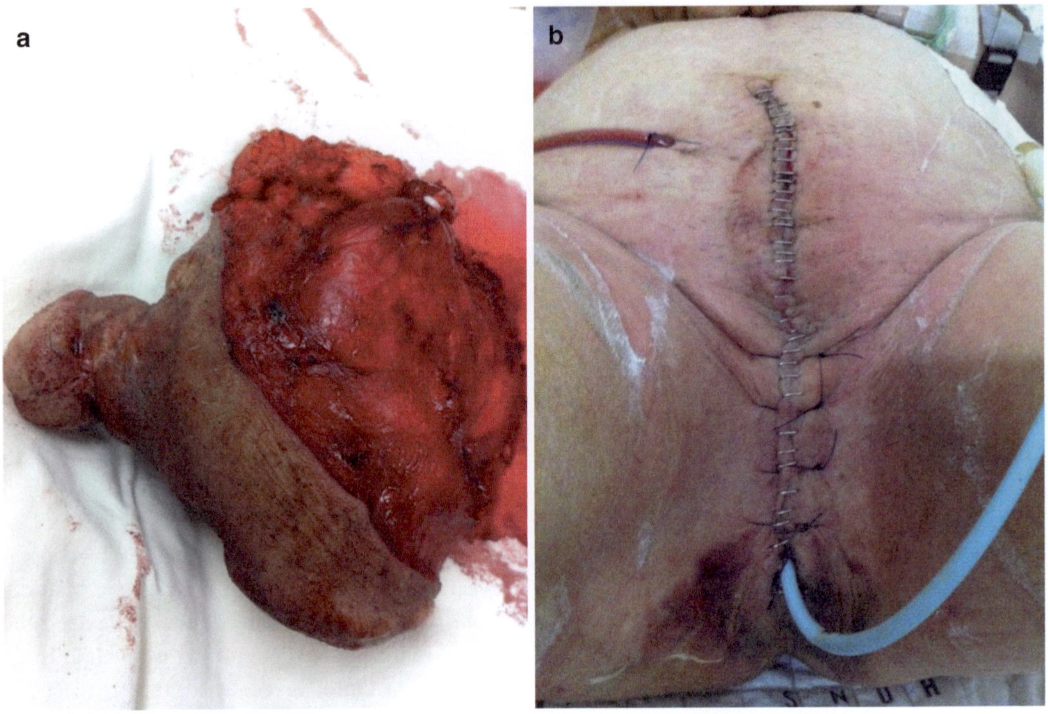

Fig. 4.26 Surgical specimen (**a**) and postoperative wound (**b**) after radical penectomy with scrotectomy

transected laterally, and neurovascular bundle at laterodorsal side of penis was dissected from tunica albuginea. Penile dorsal vein is also isolated. Dissected vessels are ligated and divided.

Resection points are marked; ≥2 cm safety margin from tumor should be ensured at that time. The urethra is resected 1–1.5 cm longer than the remained corpus cavernosum. Corpus spongiosum including urethra is also dissected from the bilateral corpus cavernosum. Dissected urethra and corpus cavernosum are transected at marked point separately (Fig. 4.26).

The remained and opened stumps of corpus cavernosum are closed with 2-0 nonabsorbable interrupt sutures. Using the redundant urethral mucosa, urethrostomy is matured using 4-0 absorbable suture. The penile skin is repaired at the midline from the dorsal side of penis with 3-0 or 4-0 absorbable interrupt sutures. Foley urethral catheter is place for 3–5 days postoperatively.

Total Penectomy

Total penectomy is a procedure that amputates the total penis at the level of the suspensory ligament. Recommended indications for total penectomy are similar to that of partial penectomy (T1 with high grade (≥3) and ≥T2) [61]. The choice of two surgical procedures is mainly determined by the tumor location and size. If the size or location of tumor does not allow the sufficient remained penile urethral length for voiding on standing, total penectomy can be considered.

The resection procedures of tumor with sufficient resection margin are similar to those of partial penetomy. Only different point is that the resection is made more proximally at the level of suspension ligament. At total penectomy, opening of urethrostomy is formed at perineal area to facilitate the voiding in sitting position.

Radical Penectomy

Patients who should consider radical penectomy are extremely rare. We experienced one case of radical penectomy with scrotectomy (Fig. 4.27). Generally, the patient is placed in a lithotomy position under general or spinal anesthesia. Initially, perineal incision is made for radical penectomy. The corpus cavernosum is mobilized

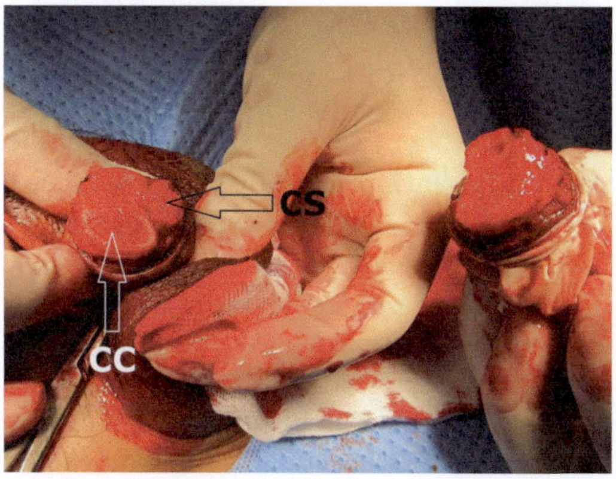

Fig. 4.27 Transection of dissected corpus spongiosum (*CS*) and corpus cavernosum (*CC*)

from the ishiopubic rami. Thereafter corpus is ligated and divided, and dorsal vein may be seen coursing under the pubis at that point. A perineal incision is made, and the mobilized penis is delivered via this wound. Dissection of the corpus cavernosum continues to the crura (proximal end). After the penis is completely excised, dorsal vein is ligated using 1-0 or 2-0 suture ligature and divided. Using the remained proximal urethra, urethrostomy is matured at perineum.

Inguinal Lymph Node Dissection

Conventionally, bilateral inguinal lymph node dissection (ILND) is recommended, because the cure rate with ILND when nodes are positive for malignancy is as high as 80%. This feature of penile cancer contrasts with other genitourinary malignancies such as bladder, prostate, or kidney cancers which are generally surgically incurable when nodal metastasis is present. However, the reluctance of routine application of the bilateral ILND is originated from the relatively high rates of the procedure-related morbidities. Complications such as pulmonary embolism, wound infection, severe lymphedema of lower extremity, or scrotum have been reported as ILND-related morbidities [48, 70]. Generally, the false-negative (malignancy positive) rate of routine administration of ILND in clinically negative nodal disease is known to be approximately 30% [71]. That means 70% of patients are at risk of major morbidity after the routine ILND with no survival benefit.

Decision of ILND is made mainly based on the palpation of inguinal area and the pathologic stage of the primary lesion [61, 62]. Patients with non-palpable inguinal lymph node with low risk (Tis, Ta, T1a) of primary penile lesion are not generally recommended to undergo surveillance or dynamic sentinel node biopsy (DSNB) [61, 62]. DSNB is the procedure to define the location of sentinel nodes using the vital blue dyes or gamma-ray emission-detecting techniques in the surgical fields. However, even though inguinal nodes are non-palpable, ILND or DSNB is recommended in patients with intermediate- (T1b) or high-risk (any T2 or G3–4) tumors [61, 62].

When nodes are palpable, clinical decisions for ILND are based on the laterality and size of the nodes. If the palpable node is unilateral or bilateral with smaller than 4 cm, ILND is generally recommended. In this situation, lymph node biopsy also can be considered prior to ILND in patients with primary low-risk penile lesions [61]. However, if the size of the palpable node is larger than 4 cm, the decision for further treatment can be more complicated according to their number, location, and movability of the nodes. If the large palpable node is unilateral and movable, ILND alone or neoadjuvant chemotherapy followed by ILND should be considered. If the positive nodes of ILND are two or more, pelvic lymph node dissection (PLND) should be followed. Patients with multiple and/or bilateral large nodes are needed to consider the neoadjuvant chemotherapy followed with ILND and PLND as the further treatment regardless of their movability. In cases of positive pelvic nodes, the possibility of resectability is important for clinical decision. If the nodes are potentially resectable, neoadjuvant chemotherapy with consolidation surgery can be the option. However, if the patient is a nonsurgical candidate, radiotherapy with concurrent chemotherapy should be considered [61, 62].

Modified Inguinal Lymph Node Dissection

The therapeutic benefit of modified ILND is known to be similar to that of standard ILND with lower morbidity [72]. This procedure can be considered in patients with clinically non-palpable nodes but with intermediate- (T1b) or high-risk (any T2 or G3–4) primary tumors [73]. The extent of modified ILND is confined to medial to the femoral artery and cephalad to the fossa ovalis (Fig. 4.11). This procedure has the advantage of smaller skin incision, saphenous vein preservation, and lower risk for the injury of sartorius muscle.

For this procedure, patient is placed on a frog-legged position under general or spinal anesthesia. Approximately 10 cm length of incision is made below 1 fingerbreadth under the inguinal ligament. Undermining beneath the skin was made sufficiently 6–8 cm superiorly and inferiorly from the initial incision. Fatty tissue including nodes located within the aforementioned boundaries is cautiously dissected and ligated. The upper and medial borders of dissection are determined by the fascia of the external oblique muscle and the adductor longus muscle. As previously described, the saphenous vein is preserved during the procedure, which is expected to be helpful for the prevention of lymphedema of lower extremities. After the dissection is completed, closed vacuum drain is placed and the incision is closed. Postoperative compression of wound may be helpful to prevent the formation of the dead space.

Standard Inguinal Lymph Node Dissection

The standard ILND is generally indicated when the extent of metastasis is limited to the inguinal nodes, and those are expected to be surgically resectable [61, 62]. This procedure is commonly performed at 4–6 weeks after the surgery of the primary tumor. The boundary of dissection is wider than that of the modified ILND. Nodes located at lateral to the femoral artery and caudal to the fossa ovalis are also dissected in the standard ILND. Because the saphenous vein is sacrificed during the procedure, the risk for lymphedema is higher than that of the modified ILND. Position for this procedure is similar with modified ILND. Approximately 10 cm length of incision is made below 1 fingerbreadth under the inguinal ligament. Undermining beneath the skin was made sufficiently 6 cm superiorly and 15 cm inferiorly from the initial incision. The lateral and lower borders of dissection are wider than those of modified ILND which are reaching the anterior superior iliac spine (ASIS) and approximately 20 cm below the ASIS.

4.2.4.2 Radiation Therapy

In penile cancer, primary radiation therapy can be considered as curative treatment option in T1 and T2 (penile preservation protocol) [61, 62]. Primary radiation therapy has their advantage to permit relative preservation of penile function. If local control can be archived, salvage surgery still can be considered as curative modality. Therefore aforementioned subset of patient with early stage penile cancer can consider the radiation therapy as a reasonable initial treatment strategy. Both external beam radiation therapy (EBRT) and brachytherapy can be utilized for treatment of penile cancer. The circumcision is necessary before the commencement of radiation therapy. The purpose of the circumcision is to expose the lesion properly, to prevent the skin infection, and to prevent the skin edema. Radiotherapy with concurrent chemotherapy can also be considered in advanced cases (≥T3, non-resectable N3, or M1; surgically unresectable protocol).

In the penile preservation protocol, recommended regimen is different by the primary tumor size. If the tumor is <4 cm, brachytherapy alone or EBRT with or without chemotherapy using total dose of 65–70 Gy covering penile lesion with 2 cm margins is recommended [61]. If the tumor is ≥4 cm, EBRT with chemotherapy is preferred. Recommended regimen is the 45–50.4 Gy to the whole penile shaft and boost primary lesion with 2 cm margins (total dose, 60–70 Gy) [61]. In the surgically unresectable protocol, recommended regimen is EBRT with chemotherapy with the 45–50.4 Gy covering the whole penile shaft, pelvic lymph nodes, and bilateral inguinal lymph nodes and boost primary lesion with 2 cm margins (total dose, 60–70 Gy) [61].

4.2.4.3 Chemotherapy

In penile cancer, the role of chemotherapy is very limited [61]. In case of multiple or bilateral positive inguinal lymph nodes (N2) or potentially resectable positive pelvic lymph node (N3), neoadjuvant chemotherapy can be considered prior to ILND and PLND as previously described in the ILND session [61, 62]. In nonsurgical candidate of N3 and metastatic penile cancer (M1), systemic chemotherapy alone or radiotherapy with concurrent chemotherapy should be considered [61]. In those cases, recommended regimen is four cycles of TIP (paclitaxel, ifosfamide, and cisplatin). However, the effectiveness is not confirmed by the randomized controlled trial.

References

1. Woodward PJ, Sohaey R, O'Donoghue MJ, Green DE. From the archives of the AFIP: tumors and tumorlike lesions of the testis: radiologic-pathologic correlation. Radiographics Rev Publ Radiol Soc N Am Inc. 2002;22(1):189–216.
2. Kreydin EI, Barrisford GW, Feldman AS, Preston MA. Testicular cancer: what the radiologist needs to know. AJR Am J Roentgenol. 2013;200(6):1215–25.
3. Donohue JP, Zachary JM, Maynard BR. Distribution of nodal metastases in nonseminomatous testis cancer. J Urol. 1982;128(2):315–20.
4. Sheinfeld J. Nonseminomatous germ cell tumors of the testis: current concepts and controversies. Urology. 1994;44(1):2–14.
5. Mazzu D, Jeffrey Jr RB, Ralls PW. Lymphoma and leukemia involving the testicles: findings on gray-scale and color Doppler sonography. AJR Am J Roentgenol. 1995;164(3):645–7.
6. Edge SB, Byrd DR, Compton CC, Fritz AG, Greene FL, Trotti A. American Joint Committee on Cancer (AJCC) staging handbook. New York: Springer; 2010.
7. Hilton S, Herr HW, Teitcher JB, Begg CB, Castellino RA. CT detection of retroperitoneal lymph node metastases in patients with clinical stage I testicular nonseminomatous germ cell cancer: assessment of size and distribution criteria. AJR Am J Roentgenol. 1997;169(2):521–5.
8. Vegni-Talluri M, Bigliardi E, Vanni MG, Tota G. Testicular microliths: their origin and structure. J Urol. 1980;124(1):105–7.
9. Kim B, Winter 3rd TC, Ryu JA. Testicular microlithiasis: clinical significance and review of the literature. Eur Radiol. 2003;13(12):2567–76.
10. Cast JE, Nelson WM, Early AS, et al. Testicular microlithiasis: prevalence and tumor risk in a population referred for scrotal sonography. AJR Am J Roentgenol. 2000;175(6):1703–6.
11. Richenberg J, Brejt N. Testicular microlithiasis: is there a need for surveillance in the absence of other risk factors? Eur Radiol. 2012;22(11):2540–6.
12. Parada D, Pena KB, Moreira O, Cohen I, Parada AM, Mejias LD. Extragonadal retroperitoneal germ cell tumor: primary versus metastases? Arch Esp Urol. 2007;60(6):713–9.
13. Beccia D, Krane R, Olsson C. Clinical management of non-testicular intrascrotal tumors. J Urol. 1976; 116(4):476–9.
14. Eble JN, Sauter G, Epstein JI, et al. Pathology and genetics of tumours of the urinary system and male genital organs. Lyon: IARC Press; 2004.
15. Ulbright TM, Srigley JR. Dermoid cyst of the testis: a study of five postpubertal cases, including a pilomatrixoma-like variant, with evidence supporting its separate classification from mature testicular teratoma. Am J Surg Pathol. 2001;25(6):788–93.
16. Young RH, Talerman A. Testicular tumors other than germ cell tumors. Semin Diagn Pathol. 1987;4(4): 342–60.
17. Young RH, Koelliker DD, Scully RE. Sertoli cell tumors of the testis, not otherwise specified: a clinicopathologic analysis of 60 cases. Am J Surg Pathol. 1998;22(6):709–21.
18. Odrzywolski KJ, Mukhopadhyay S. Papillary cystadenoma of the epididymis. Arch Pathol Lab Med. 2010;134(4):630–3.
19. Brown LM, Pottern LM, Hoover RN, Devesa SS, Aselton P, Flannery JT. Testicular cancer in the United States: trends in incidence and mortality. Int J Epidemiol. 1986;15:164–70.
20. Wilkinson PM, Read G. International Germ Cell Consensus Classification: a prognostic factor-based staging system for metastatic germ cell cancers. International Germ Cell Cancer Collaborative Group. J Clin Oncol. 1997;15:594–603.
21. Greene FL, editor. AJCC cancer staging manual. Springer; New York: 2002.
22. Sheinfeld J, Herr HW. Role of surgery in management of germ cell tumor. Semin Oncol. 1998;25: 203–9.
23. Huyghe E, Muller A, Mieusset R, Bujan L, Bachaud J-M, Chevreau C, et al. Impact of diagnostic delay in testis cancer: results of a large population-based study. Eur Urol. 2007;52:1710–6.
24. Bosl GJ, Goldman A, Lange PH, Vogelzang NJ, Fraley EE, Levitt SH, et al. Impact of delay in diagnosis on clinical stage of testicular cancer. Lancet. 1981;318:970–3.
25. Krege S, Beyer J, Souchon R, Albers P, Albrecht W, Algaba F, et al. European consensus conference on diagnosis and treatment of germ cell cancer: a report of the second meeting of the European Germ Cell Cancer Consensus group (EGCCCG): part I. Eur Urol. 2008;53:478–96.
26. Heidenreich A, Weißbach L, Höltl W, Albers P, Kliesch S, Köhrmann KU. Organ sparing surgery for malignant germ cell tumor of the testis. J Urol. 2001;166:2161–5.
27. Montironi R. Intratubular germ cell neoplasia of the testis: testicular intraepithelial neoplasia. Eur Urol. 2002;41:651–4.
28. Capelouto CC, Clark PE, Ransil BJ, Loughlin KR. Original articles: testis cancer: a review of scrotal

violation in testicular cancer: is adjuvant local therapy necessary? J Urol. 1995;153:981–5.
29. Leibovitch I, Baniel J, Foster RS, Donohue JP. The clinical implications of procedural deviations during orchiectomy for nonseminomatous testis cancer. J Urol. 1995;154:935–9.
30. Maatman TJ, Gupta MK, Montie JE. Effectiveness of castration versus intravenous estrogen therapy in producing rapid endocrine control of metastatic cancer of the prostate. J Urol. 1985;133:620–1.
31. Byar DP. The veterans administration cooperative urological research group's studies of cancer of the prostate. Cancer. 1973;32:1126–30.
32. Byar DP, Corle DK. Hormone therapy for prostate cancer: results of the Veterans Administration Cooperative Urological Research Group studies. NCI Monogr. 1988;7:165–70.
33. Albers P, Albrecht W, Algaba F, Bokemeyer C, Cohn-Cedermark G, Fizazi K, et al. EAU guidelines on testicular cancer: 2011 update. Eur Urol. 2011;60:304–19.
34. Motzer RJ, Agarwal N, Beard C, Bolger GB, Boston B, Carducci MA, et al. Testicular cancer. J Natl Compr Canc Netw. 2009;7:672–93.
35. Francis R, Bower M, Brunström G, Holden L, Newlands ES, Rustin GJS, et al. Surveillance for stage I testicular germ cell tumours: results and cost benefit analysis of management options. Eur J Cancer. 2000;36:1925–32.
36. Classen J, Schmidberger H, Meisner C, Souchon R, Sautter-Bihl M-L, Sauer R, et al. Radiotherapy for stages IIA/B testicular seminoma: final report of a prospective multicenter clinical trial. J Clin Oncol. 2003;21:1101–6.
37. Vossough A, Pretorius ES, Siegelman ES, Ramchandani P, Banner MP. Magnetic resonance imaging of the penis. Abdom Imaging. 2002;27(6):640–59.
38. Singh AK, Saokar A, Hahn PF, Harisinghani MG. Imaging of penile neoplasms. Radiographics Rev Publ Radiol Soc N Am Inc. 2005;25(6):1629–38.
39. Culkin DJ, Beer TM. Advanced penile carcinoma. J Urol. 2003;170(2 Pt 1):359–65.
40. Lucia MS, Miller GJ. Histopathology of malignant lesions of the penis. Urol Clin North Am. 1992; 19(2):227–46.
41. Algaba F, Horenblas S, Pizzocaro-Luigi Piva G, Solsona E, Windahl T, European Association of Urology. EAU guidelines on penile cancer. Eur Urol. 2002;42(3):199–203.
42. Burgers JK, Badalament RA, Drago JR. Penile cancer. Clinical presentation, diagnosis, and staging. Urol Clin North Am. 1992;19(2):247–56.
43. Ornellas AA, Seixas AL, Marota A, Wisnescky A, Campos F, de Moraes JR. Surgical treatment of invasive squamous cell carcinoma of the penis: retrospective analysis of 350 cases. J Urol. 1994;151(5):1244–9.
44. Slaton JW, Morgenstern N, Levy DA, et al. Tumor stage, vascular invasion and the percentage of poorly differentiated cancer: independent prognosticators for inguinal lymph node metastasis in penile squamous cancer. J Urol. 2001;165(4):1138–42.
45. Singh AK, Gonzalez-Torrez P, Kaewlai R, Tabatabaei S, Harisinghani MG. Imaging of penile neoplasm. Semin Ultrasound CT MR. 2007;28(4):287–96.
46. McDougal WS. Carcinoma of the penis: improved survival by early regional lymphadenectomy based on the histological grade and depth of invasion of the primary lesion. J Urol. 1995;154(4):1364–6.
47. Theodorescu D, Russo P, Zhang ZF, Morash C, Fair WR. Outcomes of initial surveillance of invasive squamous cell carcinoma of the penis and negative nodes. J Urol. 1996;155(5):1626–31.
48. Bevan-Thomas R, Slaton JW, Pettaway CA. Contemporary morbidity from lymphadenectomy for penile squamous cell carcinoma: the M.D. Anderson Cancer Center Experience. J Urol. 2002;167(4): 1638–42.
49. Vapnek JM, Hricak H, Carroll PR. Recent advances in imaging studies for staging of penile and urethral carcinoma. Urol Clin North Am. 1992;19(2):257–66.
50. Horenblas S. Lymphadenectomy for squamous cell carcinoma of the penis. Part 2: the role and technique of lymph node dissection. BJU Int. 2001;88(5): 473–83.
51. Chaux A, Velazquez EF, Barreto JE, et al. New pathologic entities in penile carcinomas: an update of the 2004 world health organization classification. Semin Diagn Pathol. 2012;29(2):59–66.
52. Katona TM, Lopez-Beltran A, MacLennan GT, et al. Soft tissue tumors of the penis: a review. Anal Quant Cytol Histol Int Acad Cytol Am Soc Cytol. 2006;28(4):193–206.
53. Percy CL, Miller BA, Ries LAG. Effect of changes in cancer classification and the accuracy of cancer death certificates on trends in cancer mortality. Ann N Y Acad Sci. 1990;609:87–97.
54. Ravi R. Correlation between the extent of nodal involvement and survival following groin dissection for carcinoma of the penis. Br J Urol. 1993;72: 817–9.
55. Frisch M, Friis S, Kjaer SK, Melbye M. Falling incidence of penis cancer in an uncircumcised population (Denmark 1943–90). BMJ. 1995;311:1471.
56. Bleeker MCG, Heideman DAM, Snijders PJF, Horenblas S, Dillner J, Meijer CJLM. Penile cancer: epidemiology, pathogenesis and prevention. World J Urol. 2009;27:141–50.
57. Block SL, Nolan T, Sattler C, Barr E, Giacoletti KED, Marchant CD, et al. Comparison of the immunogenicity and reactogenicity of a prophylactic quadrivalent human papillomavirus (types 6, 11, 16, and 18) L1 virus-like particle vaccine in male and female adolescents and young adult women. Pediatrics. 2006;118: 2135–45.
58. Greenbaum SS, Glogau R, Stegman SJ, Tromovitch TA. Carbon dioxide laser treatment of erythroplasia of Queyrat. J Dermatol Surg Oncol. 1989;15:747–50.

59. Tietjen DN, Malek RS. Laser therapy of squamous cell dysplasia and carcinoma of the penis. Urology. 1998;52:559–65.
60. van Bezooijen BPJ, Horenblas S, Meinhardt W, Newling DWW. Laser therapy for carcinoma in situ of the penis. J Urol. 2001;166:1670–1.
61. Clark PE, Spiess PE, Agarwal N, Biagioli MC, Eisenberger MA, Greenberg RE, et al. Penile cancer. J Natl Compr Canc Netw. 2013;11:594–615.
62. Pizzocaro G, Algaba F, Horenblas S, Solsona E, Tana S, Van Der Poel H, et al. EAU penile cancer guidelines 2009. Eur Urol. 2010;57:1002–12.
63. Mohs FE, Snow SN, Messing EM, Kuglitsch ME. Microscopically controlled surgery in the treatment of carcinoma of the penis. J Urol. 1985;133:961–6.
64. Brown MD, Zachary CB, Grekin RC, Swanson NA. Penile tumors: their management by Mohs micrographic surgery. J Dermatol Surg Oncol. 1987;13:1163–7.
65. Shindel AW, Mann MW, Lev RY, Sengelmann R, Petersen J, Hruza GJ, et al. Mohs micrographic surgery for penile cancer: management and long-term follow up. J Urol. 2007;178:1980–5.
66. Mohs FE, Snow SN, Larson PO. Mohs micrographic surgery for penile tumors. Urol Clin North Am. 1992;19:291–304.
67. DeKernion J, Tynberg P, Persky L, Fegen J. Carcinoma of the penis. Cancer. 1973;32:1256–62.
68. McDougal WS, Kirchner Jr FK, Edwards RH, Killion LT. Treatment of carcinoma of the penis: the case for primary lymphadenectomy. J Urol. 1986;136:38–41.
69. Horenblas S, van Tinteren H, Delemarre JF, Boon TA, Moonen LM, Lustig V. Squamous cell carcinoma of the penis. II. Treatment of the primary tumor. J Urol. 1992;147:1533–8.
70. Nelson BA, Cookson MS, Smith Jr JA, Chang SS. Complication of inguinal and pelvic lymphadenectomy for squamous cell carcinoma of the penis: a contemporary series. J Urol. 2004;172:494–7.
71. Pettaway CA, Lance RS, Davis JW. Tumors of the penis. In: Wein AJ, Kavoussi LR, Novick AC, Partin AW, Peters CA, editors. Campbell-Walsh urology. 10th ed. Philadelphia: Elsevier; 2012. p. 901–33.
72. Colberg JW, Andriole GL, Catalona WJ. Long-term follow-up of men undergoing modified inguinal lymphadenectomy for carcinoma of the penis. Br J Urol. 1997;79:54–7.
73. Sharp DS, Angermeier KW. Surgery of penile and urethral carcinoma. In: Wein AJ, Kavoussi LR, Novick AC, Partin AW, Peters CA, editors. Campbell-Walsh urology. 10th ed. Philadelphia: Elsevier; 2012. p. 934–55.

Adrenal Tumors

5

Byung Kwan Park, Kyung Chul Moon,
Ja Hyeon Ku, Minyong Kang, and Jin Ho Kim

5.1 Introduction

The adrenal glands are routinely scanned on every computed tomography (CT) scan or magnetic resonance imaging (MRI) of the abdomen and the chest. Incidental adrenal masses are increasingly being detected because of increasing number of imaging studies that are routinely performed; these lesions are encountered in approximately 5 % of imaged patients with no known adrenal disease [1]. Although the adrenal gland is involved by various diseases, almost all adrenal lesions detected are benign in patients without a history of malignancy. Therefore, diagnostic approach to adrenal lesions in these patients should not be as aggressive as those in oncologic patients.

In contrast, the possibility that adrenal masses are metastatic lesions is higher in patients with a known extra-adrenal malignancy. For the last decade, adrenal CT protocols had been introduced and currently help to differentiate adenoma and non-adenoma in patients with a history of malignancy. Adrenal metastasis characterization in oncologic patients is critical to stage and manage the primary disease. Adrenal mass biopsy is the confirmative examination for diagnosing a metastasis, but this invasive procedure should be limited to oncologic patients with adrenal metastasis in whom the cancer treatment or prognosis will be altered by means of the biopsy.

Most of functioning adrenal masses are already identified by clinician before CT or MRI is performed. The main role of radiologic studies is to detect or localize an adrenal mass for surgical excision. Hence, our description will focus on how to differentiate adenoma and non-adenoma and on imaging features of various non-adenomas as well.

B.K. Park (✉)
Department of Radiology, Samsung Medical Center,
Sungkyunkwan University School of Medicine,
Seoul, Republic of Korea
e-mail: bk1436.park@samsung.com

K.C. Moon
Department of Pathology,
Seoul National University Hospital,
Seoul National University College of Medicine,
Seoul, Republic of Korea

J.H. Ku
Department of Urology,
Seoul National University Hospital,
Seoul National University College of Medicine,
Seoul, Republic of Korea

M. Kang
Department of Urology,
Seoul National University Hospital,
Seoul, Republic of Korea

J.H. Kim
Department of Radiation Oncology,
Seoul National University Hospital,
Seoul National University College of Medicine,
Seoul, Republic of Korea

S.H. Kim, J.Y. Cho (eds.), *Oncologic Imaging: Urology*, DOI 10.1007/978-3-662-45218-9_5

5.2 Anatomy

The adrenal glands are paired endocrine organs which are located at anterosuperior and medial to the upper pole of each kidney. Adrenal glands histologically consist of cortex and medulla. The cortex is made up of three layers in which different corticosteroids are produced. The outer layer is zona glomerulosa producing mineralocorticoids. The middle layer is zona fasiculata producing glucocorticoids. The inner layer is zona reticularis producing sex steroids or gonadocorticoids.

The medulla is composed of chromaffin cells producing catecholamines including epinephrine and norepinephrine. Chromaffin cells are arranged in nest or sheet and typically concentrated in the body.

Adrenal gland is supplied by the superior, middle, and inferior suprarenal arteries. These arteries can originate from the inferior phrenic arteries, abdominal aorta, and renal arteries, respectively. Each adrenal vein is single in contrast to multiple adrenal arteries. Right adrenal vein directly drains into the inferior vena cava, and left adrenal vein drains into the left renal vein or inferior phrenic vein.

5.3 Detection

Most of adrenal masses are incidentally detected. Only a small number of adrenal tumors are functional, and an even smaller number are malignant [2]. Most incidentally discovered adrenal tumors are nonfunctional and benign, with fewer than 10 % having detectable endocrine functionality and fewer than 5 % being malignant [3]. Some functional adrenal lesions may not require imaging for initial clinical recognition, but imaging almost always plays an important role for determining surgical plan because it can show well the location, size, number, invasion, and metastasis of adrenal tumors.

5.3.1 Conn Syndrome

Aldosterone-secreting adrenal cortical adenoma (aldosteronoma) accounts for up to 2 % of all unanticipated adrenal masses [2]. Conn syndrome, or primary aldosteronism due to an adrenal cortical adenoma, has classically been characterized clinically by hypertension and hypokalemia. However, it has become increasingly recognized that most patients with primary aldosteronism do not have hypokalemia [4]. The more common causes of primary aldosteronism include bilateral idiopathic adrenal cortical hyperplasia (~60 % of cases) and an aldosterone-secreting adenoma (~35 %). Unilateral adrenal hyperplasia and other rarer causes account for the remainder of cases [4]. Plasma aldosterone-to-renin ratio is the diagnostic test of choice.

5.3.2 Cushing Syndrome

Cortisol is produced by between 2 and 15 % of adenomas [2]. Hypercortisolism can result in Cushing syndrome, which is clinically manifested with weight gain and fat deposition, hypertension, easy bruisability, amenorrhea, hirsutism, acne, muscle weakness, diabetes, and mood changes. Non-iatrogenic hypercortisolism results from pituitary dependence (Cushing disease) approximately 60–70 % of cases in adults, and the remaining cases are pituitary independent [5]. Pituitary-independent causes include ectopic adrenocorticotropic hormone (ACTH) production, rarely ectopic corticotropic-releasing factor secretion, primary pigmented nodular adrenocortical disease, and macronodular hyperplasia with marked adrenal enlargement. Cushing syndrome caused by an adrenal adenoma is one of ACTH-independent hypercortisolisms. Cortisol-producing adenomas are often >2 cm in size and easily detected with CT or MR imaging [6].

5.3.3 Catecholamines

Reportedly, the frequency of pheochromocytoma among adrenal masses is variable with prevalence likely being near 3–6 % [7]. Pheochromocytoma is increasingly detected due to the widespread use of CT and magnetic resonance (MR) imaging before the patient presumably becomes symptomatic. Increasing numbers of unanticipated pheochromocytomas are detected at CT or MR imaging that is performed for unrelated symptoms [8]. Clinically, pheochromocytomas may lead to a classic triad of palpitation, sweating, and hypertension due to excretion of catecholamine. The diagnosis is usually established with increased level of catecholamines in the 24-h urine.

5.4 Characterization

5.4.1 Benign Adrenal Tumors and Tumorlike Conditions

5.4.1.1 Cortical Adenoma

Adenoma is the most common tumor in the adrenal gland. The estimated prevalence ranges from 1.4 to 8.9 % based on autopsy series, and it increases with age [9].

Histologically, adenoma is typically a well-circumscribed encapsulated solid mass arising from the adrenal cortex. The cut surface of the specimen is yellow due to abundant neutral lipid content. At microscopic examination, tumor cells have abundant pale-staining lipid-rich cytoplasm, which is often arranged in short cords or nests. A relatively rich and delicate vascular supply is present. These findings of lipid-rich cells and an abundant vascular network is related with CT or MR imaging features.

Ultrasonography is not the first-line imaging modality to characterize an adrenal mass because most of adrenal adenomas are less than 3 cm. This imaging technique can guide a biopsy of a large adrenal mass which usually is inoperable. At ultrasonography, an adenoma appears as a round or oval mass that is well demarcated, slightly heterogeneous, and hypoechoic [10].

At CT, a small adenoma (<3 cm) is usually a well-demarcated mass with homogeneous attenuation. The CT attenuation values of adenomas depend predominantly on the amount of intracytoplasmic lipid. Studies have shown that using a cutoff value of 10 HU or less at unenhanced CT has high sensitivity (71 %) and specificity (98 %) for adenoma, which is so-called lipid-rich

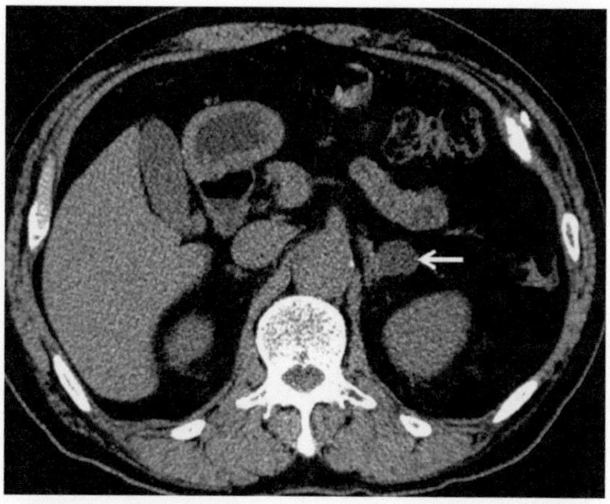

Fig. 5.1 Lipid-rich adenoma in a 69-year-old man. Unenhanced CT image shows a left adrenal mass (*arrow*) which is measured 1 HU, consistent with a lipid-rich adenoma

adenoma (Fig. 5.1) [11]. Therefore, the majority of adenomas has enough lipid content to be accurately characterized; the remaining about 30 % of adenomas, so-called "lipid-poor" adenoma, will have higher attenuation values (>10 HU) at unenhanced CT so that chemical shift MRI or washout CT is required to differentiate adenoma and non-adenoma.

Subsequent studies have shown that percentage loss of iodine contrast material is useful characterizing a lipid-poor adenoma at early and delayed contrast-enhanced CT examinations (Fig. 5.2). This concept is based on that adenoma shows early wash-in and washout of contrast material. This is why adenoma is histologically hypervascular and why adenoma does not retain contrast material for delayed time periods, as opposed to most of non-adenoma. Washout values can be calculated using a few different methods, with most institutes adopting non-contrast images, early contrast-enhanced images (usually 1 min after contrast material injection), and delayed contrast-enhanced images (at 15 min). Absolute percentage washout (APW) and relative percentage washout (RPW) are calculated using the attenuation values that are measured to place a region of interest (ROI) on the lesion at the different phases of contrast enhancement.

Generally, formulas for calculating APW or RPW are as follows: APW = [early contrast-enhanced

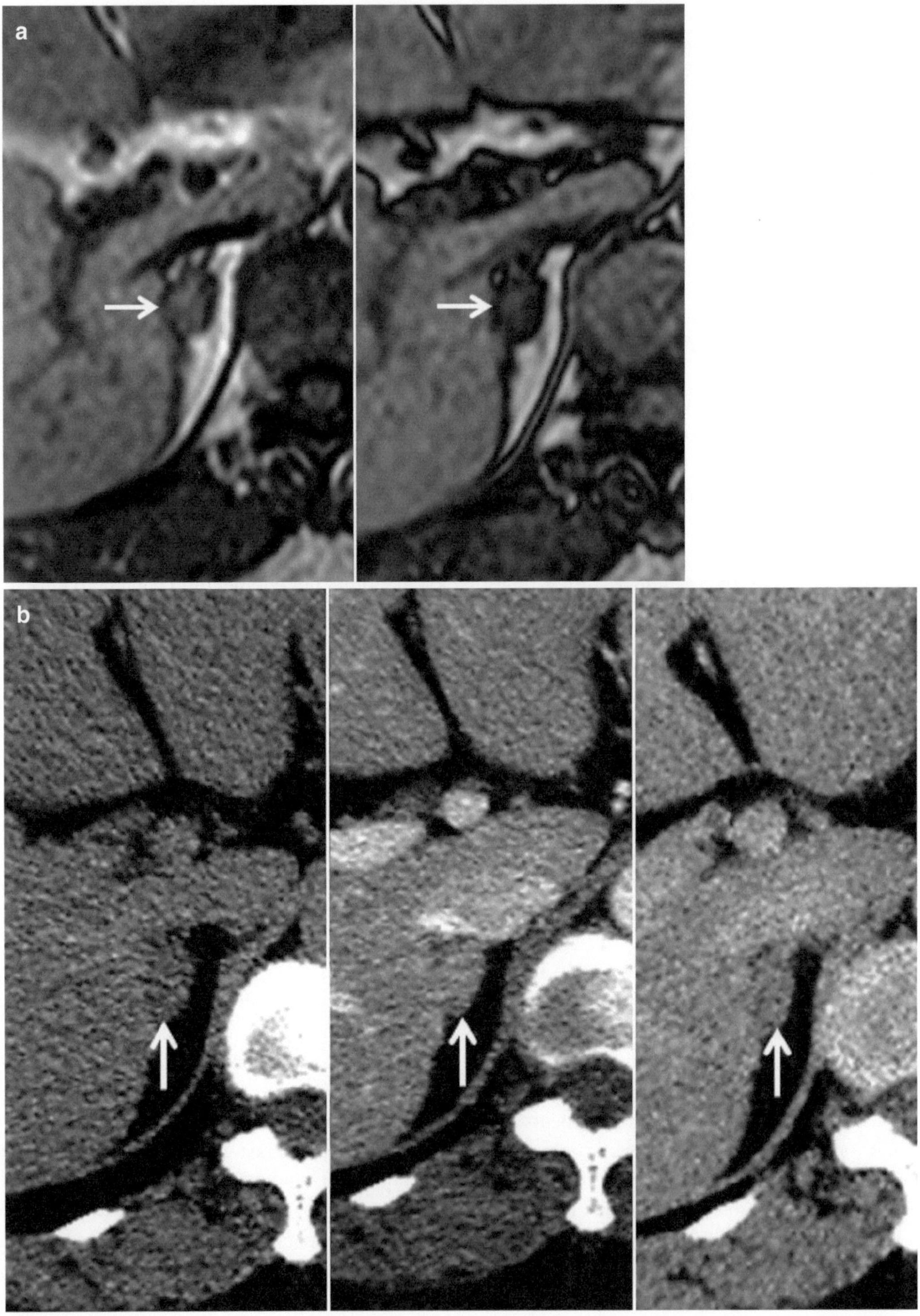

Fig. 5.2 Lipid-poor adenoma in a 57-year-old woman. (**a**) The signal intensity of a right adrenal mass (*arrow*) does not show any difference between in-phase (*left*-side) and opposed-phase (*right*-side) MR images. Adrenal-to-spleen ratio is 1.2 and signal intensity index is 4.2 %. Accordingly, MR diagnosis of the lesion is non-adenoma. (**b**) The right adrenal mass (*arrow*) is measured 35 HU, 129 HU, and 62 HU on unenhanced (*right-side* image), early enhanced (*middle*), and delayed (*left-side* image) enhanced CT images, respectively. Absolute and relative washout values are calculated 71 % and 52 %, respectively. Accordingly, CT diagnosis of the lesion is adenoma

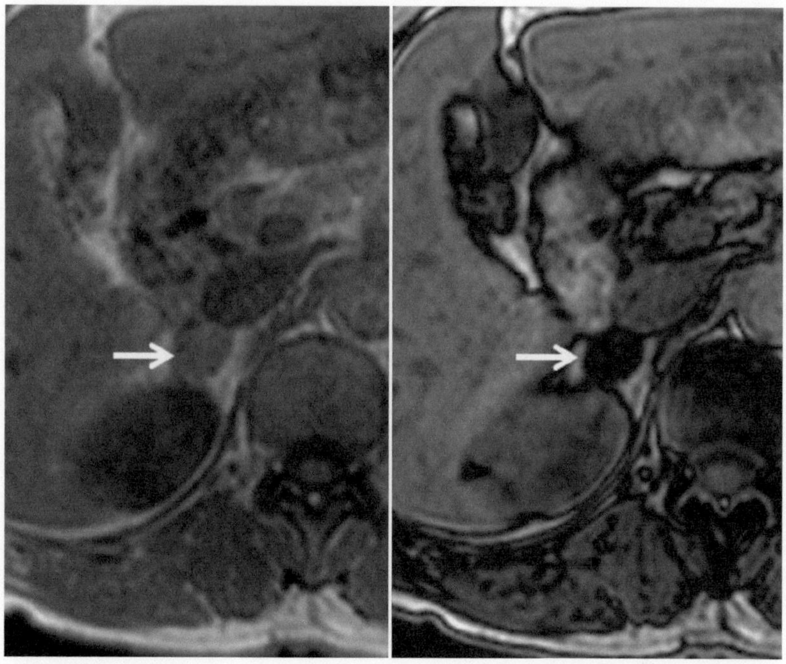

Fig. 5.3 Lipid-rich adenoma in a 62-year-old man. A right adrenal mass (*arrow*) is hyperintense on in-phase MR image (*left-side* image), while the lesion shows signal void on opposed-phase MR image (*right-side* image)

CT (HU)−delayed contrast-enhanced CT (HU)] x 100/[early contrast-enhanced CT (HU)−unenhanced CT (HU)]. RPW=[early contrast-enhanced CT (HU)−delayed contrast-enhanced CT (HU)] x 100/[early contrast-enhanced CT (HU)]. APW of 60% or more or RPW of 40% or more offers confident diagnosis of adenoma, with sensitivity ranging from 88 to 96% and specificity ranging from 96 to 100%.

Chemical shift MR imaging uses the different precession frequencies of protons in both water fat within the same voxel and creates in-phase and opposed-phase images in which signal from the protons is either additive or subtractive from one another (Fig. 5.3). This MR technique is useful in detecting abundant intracytoplasmic lipid found. Regarding detection of adenoma, chemical shift MR imaging is better than unenhanced CT because this MR technique detects more adenomas that are measured more than 10 HU at unenhanced CT. Visual MR assessment provides a confident diagnosis of adenoma that is measured 10 HU or less at unenhanced CT (Fig. 5.3). However, quantitative MR assessment should be performed for characterizing adenoma that is measured between 10 and 20 HU at unenhanced CT (Fig. 5.4) [12–14]. For quantitative analysis, adrenal-to-spleen ratio (ASR) and signal intensity index (SII) are frequently used. SII is more sensitive for adenoma than ASR (Fig. 5.4) [12, 15]. ASR and SII are calculated as follows:

$$\mathrm{ASR} = \left(\mathrm{SI_{OP}}\ \text{of adrenal mass} / \mathrm{SI_{OP}}\ \text{of spleen}\right) / \left(\mathrm{SI_{IP}}\ \text{of adrenal mass} / \mathrm{SI_{IP}}\ \text{of spleen}\right)$$

$$\mathrm{SII} = \left(\mathrm{SI_{IP}}\ \text{of adrenal mass} - \mathrm{SI_{OP}}\ \text{of adrenal mass}\right) \times 100 / \mathrm{SI_{IP}}\ \text{of adrenal mass}$$

SI_{OP} and SI_{IP} indicate signal intensity on opposed-phase image and in-phase image, respectively.

Adenoma can be diagnosed if ASR is less than 0.71 or if SII is more than 16.5%. However, if adenoma is measured more than 20 HU on unenhanced CT, the sensitivity begins to be lower (Fig. 5.2). Adenoma that is measured more than 40 HU at unenhanced CT hardly is diagnosed on

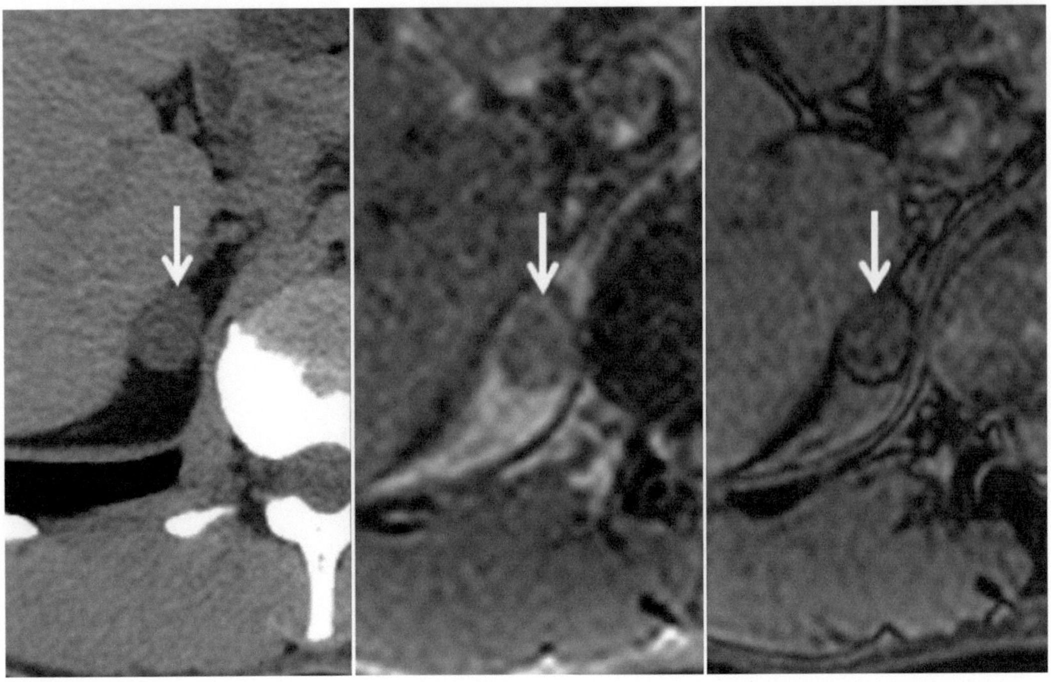

Fig. 5.4 Lipid-rich adenoma in a 43-year-old man. Unenhanced CT image (*left-side* image) shows a right adrenal mass (*arrow*) which is measured 12 HU. CT diagnosis is not consistent with a lipid-rich adenoma. The lesion is slightly hyperintense on in-phase MR image (*middle* image) and slightly hypointense on opposed-phase MR image (*right-side* image). The adrenal-to-spleen ratio is 0.92, but the signal intensity index is 24 %. MR diagnosis is lipid-rich adenoma

chemical shift MR imaging [12, 15]. Therefore, adrenal masses that is measured more than 20 HU on unenhanced CT should be evaluated using early and delayed contrast-enhanced CT imaging rather than chemical shift MR imaging [12].

Imaging features of adenoma may overlap with those of other benign and malignant lesions, including pheochromocytomas, metastases, and cortical carcinomas [16–19]. While small size (<3 cm) of adrenal mass can suggest a benign lesion, the size criterion is not a reliable finding. Adrenal lesion's lipid or fat which is detected on CT or MR imaging is not totally specific for adenoma because adrenal hyperplasia, adenoma with a carcinoma or metastasis focus or metastases from renal cell carcinoma, hepatocellular carcinoma, and liposarcoma have potential to contain intracytoplasmic lipid or adipose tissue [16–18, 20]. Furthermore, hypervascular pheochromocytomas, adrenal hyperplasia, and hypervascular metastasis from renal cell carcinoma or hepatocellular carcinoma may meet washout criteria of adenoma.

Adenoma may include cystic degeneration, hemorrhage, and calcification, which are frequent when adenoma grows 3 cm or more (Fig. 5.5) [16, 19]. These unusual features make it difficult to differentiate adenoma from cortical carcinoma. Right adrenal adenoma may arise from the adrenohepatic tissue and subsequently can manifest as a primary or metastatic hepatic tumor (Fig. 5.6) [21].

5.4.1.2 Hyperplasia

The prevalence of adrenal hyperplasia is estimated to be 0.51 % in the autopsy series of approximately 3500 subjects [22]. Hyperplasia manifests as either a diffuse or focal enlargement of adrenal gland. Hyperplasia involves adrenal gland multifocally and bilaterally. A series of 113 consecutive adult necropsies reported that 35 % appear normal, 50 % mildly nodular, and 15 % distinctly nodular [23]. The mean age of patients with distinctly nodular hyperplasia was 65 years while that of normal adrenal group was 50 years.

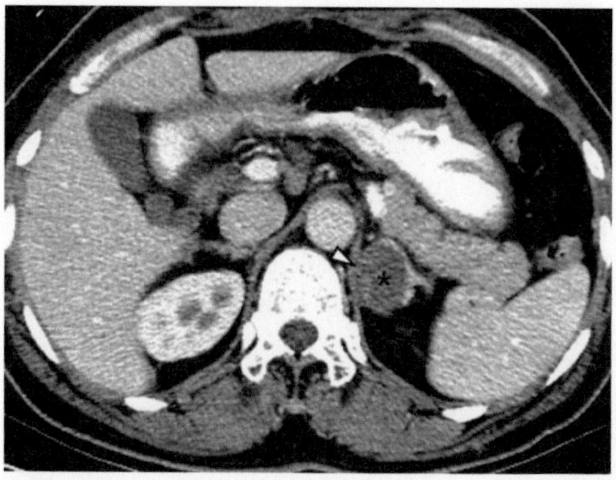

Fig. 5.5 Degenerated adenoma in a 47-year-old woman. Contrast-enhanced CT image shows a left adrenal mass (*arrow*) which is measured 3.3 cm. The central area (*asterisk*) of the lesion is not enhanced, but the medial aspect (*arrowhead*) shows crescent-like marginal enhancement. She underwent left adrenalectomy, and histologic diagnosis was adenoma with cystic degeneration and hemorrhage

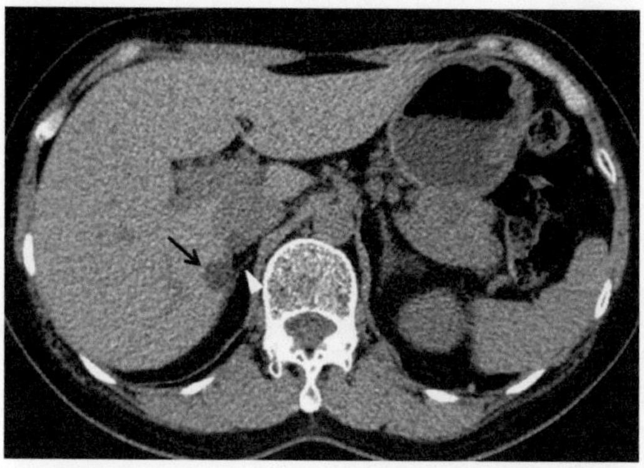

Fig. 5.6 Adrenohepatic fusion adenoma in a 59-year-old woman. Unenhanced CT shows a hypoattenuating hepatic mass (*arrow*) which is measured 0 HU. Right adrenal limb (*arrowhead*) is attached to the medial aspect of the lesion. The lesion shows adenoma-like enhancement (early wash-in and washout) on early and delayed enhanced CT images (not shown). Clinically, the diagnosis is considered adenoma arising adrenohepatic fusion

With age increasing, adrenal gland becomes nodular [23].

Hyperplasia is histologically composed of mainly lipid-rich cortical cells which form variable-sized nodules due to overgrowth. Hyperplastic nodules appear micronodular or macronodular in appearance, depending on whether or not the nodules are visible with at gross examination.

Clinically, hyperplasia often is similar to hyperfunctioning adenoma. Actively hormone-producing hyperplasia can cause pituitary- or ACTH-independent Cushing syndrome or hyperaldosteronism [5].

Hyperplasia is detected at CT or MR imaging if the hyperplastic nodules are apparently large. At unenhanced CT, hyperplasia appears frequently hypodense nodules which are measured 10 HU or less because of lipid-rich cells as it were adenoma [16] (Fig. 5.7). Less frequently, hyperplasia appears isodense compared to adjacent normal adrenal tissue, which tends to be atrophic due to decreased ACTH. Accordingly, it is not unusual that hyperplasia shows signal drops on opposed-phase MR imaging (Fig. 5.7). In addition, hyperplastic nodules may show high washout which meets criteria for adenoma (Fig. 5.7) [16]. For these reasons, hyperplasia is not easy to differentiate from multiple adenomas clinically, radiologically, and histologically.

5.4.1.3 Hemorrhage

Adrenal hemorrhage may result from various conditions including trauma, burn, sepsis, surgery, hypotension, and anticoagulant therapy [5, 24]. Trauma is the most common cause to adrenal hemorrhage [24, 25]. Adrenal hemorrhage involves unilateral or bilateral adrenal glands.

Adrenal hemorrhage may occur in adenoma, myelolipoma, pheochromocytoma, metastasis, and cortical carcinoma, which may be spontaneously ruptured due to excessive bleeding [26].

Usually, adrenal hemorrhage is not symptomatic and is mostly an incidental finding at CT or MR imaging. Symptom is flank or back pain that ranges from mild to severe pain. It depends on the degree of hemorrhage. However, adrenal insufficiency is rare even if adrenal hemorrhage is bilateral [25, 27].

On CT images, adrenal hemorrhage appears a round or oval mass in which the attenuation value depends on the stage of hemorrhage (Fig. 5.8). Less commonly, adrenal hemorrhage may manifest as extensive suprarenal hematoma that obliterates the gland entirely [5, 28]. More recent hemorrhage appears relatively hyperdense. Over time, the size and attenuation value of adrenal hemorrhage decreases. In most cases, adrenal hemorrhage spontaneously disappears. Calcification may develop in the late stage of adrenal hemorrhage (Fig. 5.9).

On MR imaging, the signal intensity of adrenal hemorrhage also depends on the stage of hemorrhage. Early hemorrhage tends to be isointense on T1-weighted images and hypointense on T2-weighted images. Intermediate hemorrhage tends to be hyperintense on both T1- and T2-weighted images due to the paramagnetic effects of methemoglobin. Finally, adrenal hemorrhage shows a T1- and T2-hypointense rim due to formation of fibrous capsule and deposition of hemosiderin, resulting in a variable degree of susceptibility artifact on gradient-echo images [24, 25, 29].

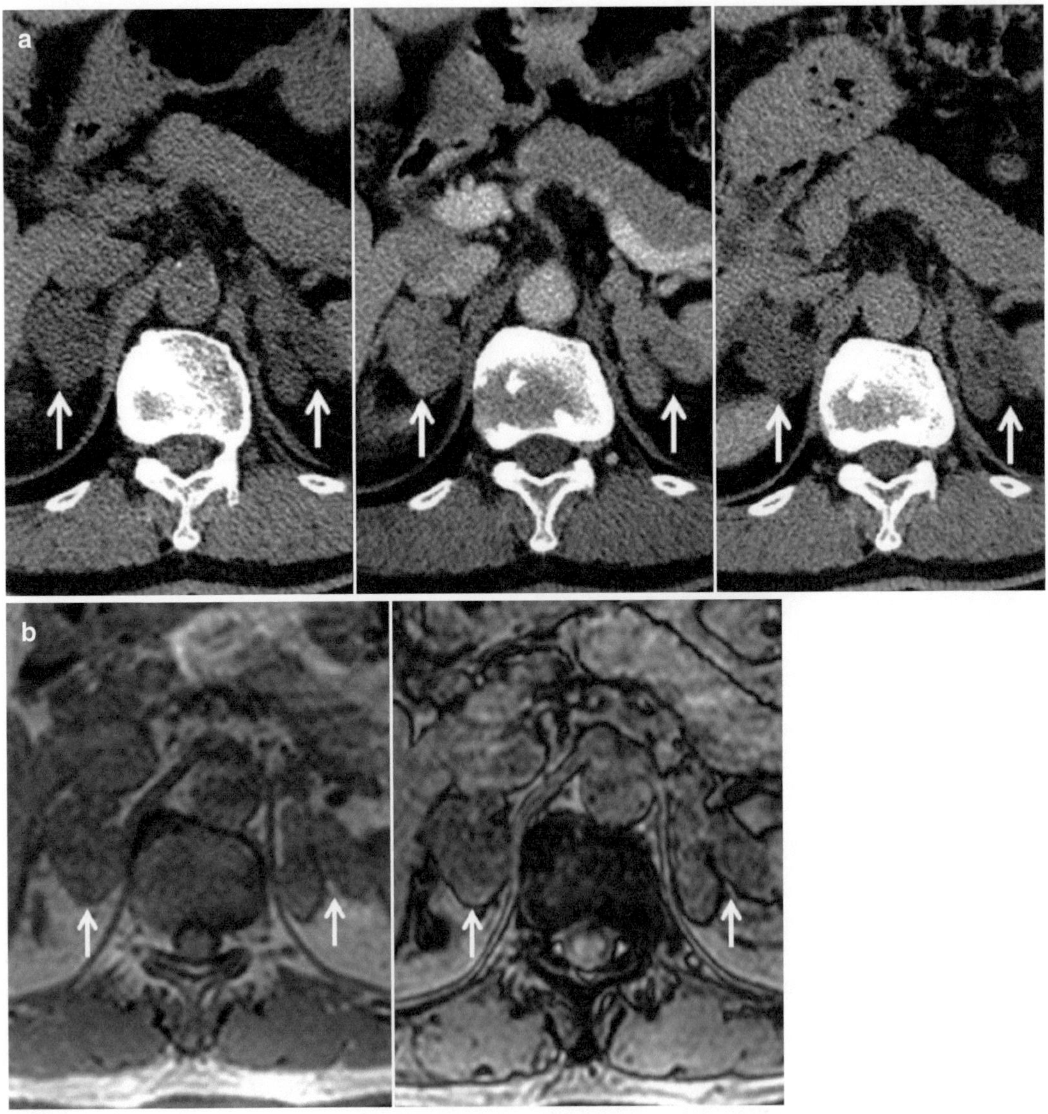

Fig. 5.7 Macronodular hyperplasia in a 53-year-old man. (**a**) Unenhanced CT image (*right-side* image) shows bilateral adrenal hypodense masses (*arrows*) which are measured less than 10 HU. Early (*middle* image) and delayed (*left-side* image) enhanced images show adenoma-like enhancement with APW ≥ 60 % and RPW ≥ 60 %. (**b**) Bilateral adrenal masses are hyperintense on in-phase MR image and hypointense on opposed-phase MR image with ASR < 0.71 and SII > 16.5 %. Histologic diagnosis was macronodular hyperplasia after percutaneous biopsy

5.4.1.4 Cyst

Most of adrenal cysts are incidentally detected at CT or MR imaging that is performed for unrelated reason. Usually, these lesions are asymptomatic but infrequently cause discomfort or mild pain because of mass effect to adjacent organs. Pathologically, adrenal cysts consist of endothelial cyst, epithelial cyst, pseudocyst, and parasitic cyst [30]. Almost all adrenal cysts appear a unilocular cyst with fine wall and simple fluid [31]. However, pseudocysts may have a minimally thick cyst wall and complicated fluid resulting from internal hemorrhage or fluid-fluid level [31, 32].

At CT, adrenal cyst usually shows a well-demarcated, non-enhancing, hypoattenuating lesion with simple water attenuation (<20 HU) and a thin wall (Fig. 5.10) [31]. Sometimes, internal hemorrhage or calcification can be detected. Wall calcification is seen more often in the pseudocysts and parasitic cysts, while septum calcification is present in endothelial cysts [31].

At MR imaging, adrenal cysts show a well-demarcated, non-enhancing, thin-walled lesion which is uniformly hypointense on T1-weighted images and hyperintense on T2-weighted images similar to those of simple cyst [29]. Hemorrhagic fluid within an adrenal cyst may show T1 hyperintense signal [29]. The imaging appearances of

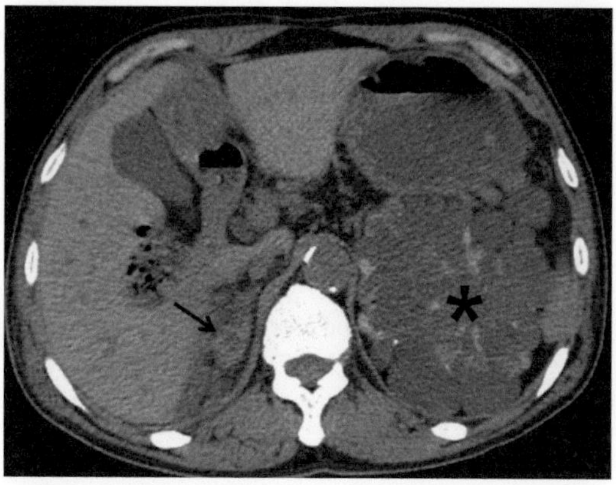

Fig. 5.8 Adrenal hematoma in a 28-year-old man. Unenhanced CT image shows a hyperdense right adrenal mass which is measured 62 HU. He underwent right nephrectomy due to autosomal dominant polycystic kidney disease (*asterisk*)

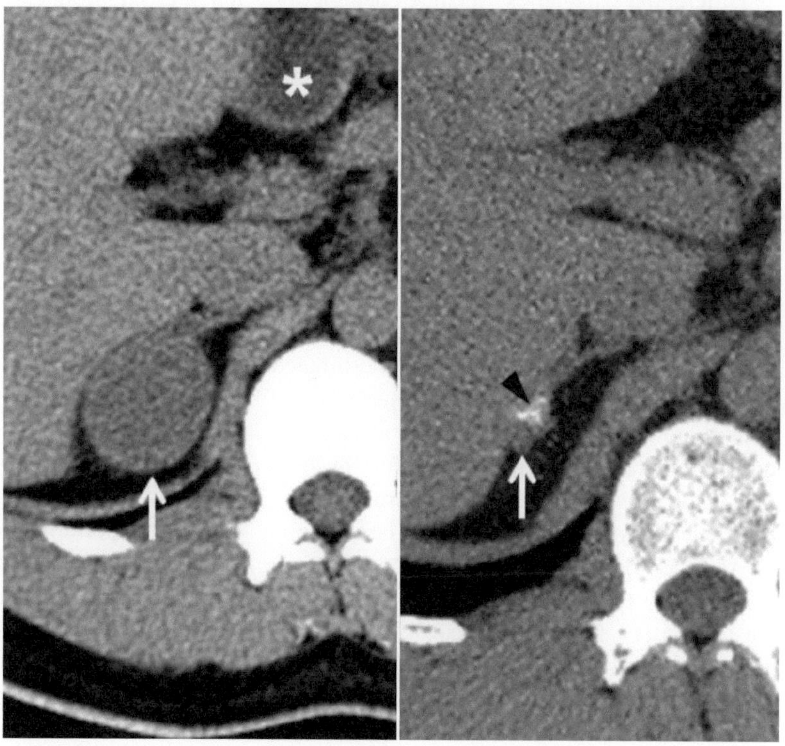

Fig. 5.9 Adrenal hematoma in a 29-year-old man. Unenhanced CT image (*right-side* image) shows subacute hematoma (*arrow*) in the right adrenal gland. The lesion (22 HU) is more hyperdense than stomach fluid (*asterisk*). The adrenal hematoma (*arrow*) is decreased and calcified (*arrowhead*) on 2 years later CT image (*left-side* image)

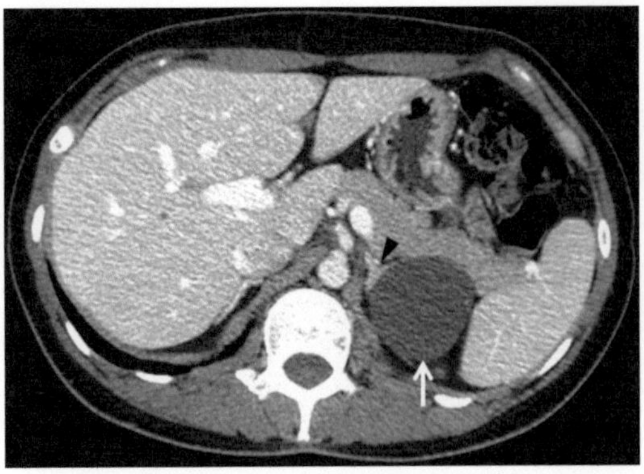

Fig. 5.10 Adrenal cyst in a 35-year-old woman. Contrast-enhanced CT image shows a left adrenal cyst (*arrow*) with thin wall and simple fluid. An *arrowhead* indicates the other left adrenal tissue

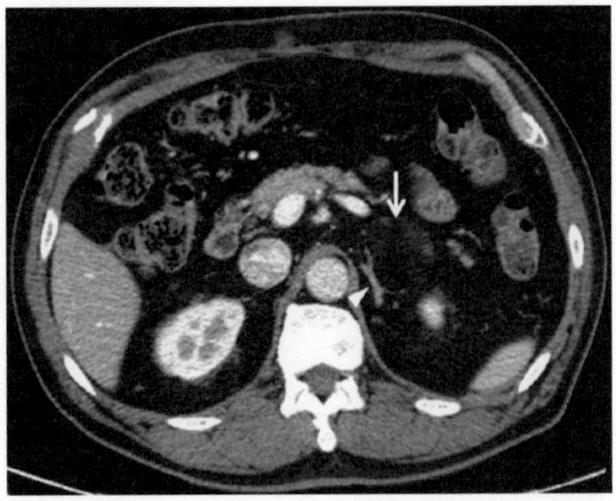

Fig. 5.11 Myelolipoma in a 67-year-old man. Contrast-enhanced CT image shows a left adrenal myelolipoma (*arrow*) in which attenuation value is measured as low as −54 HU. An *arrowhead* indicates the other left adrenal tissue

an echinococcal adrenal cyst may include a simple cyst, a multilocular cyst with septa, daughter vesicles, the "water lily" sign, and calcifications depending on the stage of infection [31, 33]. Detecting extra-adrenal Echinococcus is useful in making a confident diagnosis of echinococcal cysts, since isolated adrenal involvement is rare [33].

Differential diagnoses include benign or malignant adrenal masses with cystic degeneration. Adenoma, hemangioma, pheochromocytoma, cortical carcinoma, and metastasis may have varying degrees of a cystic appearance, but the wall is much thicker or more irregular than a usual adrenal cyst [31, 34].

5.4.1.5 Myelolipoma

Adrenal myelolipoma is a benign tumor histologically composed of adipose and myeloid tissues. The prevalence of myelolipoma is estimated 0.08–0.2 % in autopsy series [35]. Usually, these tumors are hormonally inactive and are asymptomatic. In rare incidence, discomfort or pain may occur due to mass effect or internal hemorrhage when myelolipoma grows to a large size.

At CT, myelolipoma is easily diagnosed because gross fat (less than −30 HU) is almost always visible (Fig. 5.11). Calcification can be detected in approximately 24 % [36]. At MR imaging, myelolipomas show hyperintense foci on T1-weighted images due to gross fat. These T1 hyperintense signals are suppressed on fat-saturated MR images [1, 5, 6, 29]. However, internal hemorrhage may obliterate adipose tissue so that hemorrhagic myelolipoma is not easy to diagnose.

5.4.1.6 Pheochromocytoma

Pheochromocytoma is a catecholamine-producing tumor arising from chromaffin cells in the adrenal medulla. This tumor is closely related to extra-adrenal sympathetic and parasympathetic paraganglia, so-called as extra-adrenal pheochromocytoma. Pheochromocytomas typically produce and secrete both norepinephrine and epinephrine. Norepinephrine is usually the predominant catecholamine. The prevalence of pheochromocytoma is still unknown.

Widespread use of CT or MRI increases detection of asymptomatic pheochromocytoma. Therefore, the number of small or asymptomatic pheochromocytoma appears greater than that of large or symptomatic pheochromocytoma [5]. The number of pheochromocytoma with classical triad symptoms becomes fewer. Biochemical test should be performed to detect subclinical or asymptomatic pheochromocytoma or other hormone-producing adrenal tumors.

Pheochromocytomas are a typically firm and gray-white tumor that may have areas of central degenerative changes including fibrosis, hemorrhage, and cystic change.

CT is the first-line modality for detecting, localizing, and characterizing pheochromocytoma. These tumors are round or oval masses of similar attenuation to the back muscles at unenhanced CT [37]. Scattered or punctate calcifications can be detected in approximately 10% [17, 38]. The size of pheochromocytoma becomes smaller because of early detection. These tumors usually are measured 3–5 cm in diameter when they are detected but can grow to 10 cm or more mostly in symptomatic cases [5, 17, 26]. Degenerated pheochromocytoma may show hyperdense texture on unenhanced CT due to hemorrhage or poor enhancement due to cystic or necrotic change on contrast-enhanced CT. When the lesion is small, it can show adenoma-like enhancement due to strong enhancement on early enhanced CT (Fig. 5.12).

At MR imaging, the classic sign "light bulb" on T2-weighted image is not so frequently encountered because it can be seen in case of a pheochromocytoma that contains at least more than one half of cystic or necrotic change [17, 39]. Majority of pheochromocytomas show slightly high signal intensity compared to adjacent adrenal tissue on T2-weighted images [5]. Also, hyperintense foci due to cystic or necrotic changes can be encountered within the tumor on T2-weighted images. These masses are homogeneous or heterogeneous depending on internal components of calcification, fibrosis, necrosis, hemorrhage, and cyst degeneration [39].

CT or MR imaging features of pheochromocytoma are overlapped with adenoma and cortical carcinoma. Pheochromocytoma is usually so hypervascular that this tumor cannot be easily differentiated with adenoma regarding washout of contrast material [16, 17, 40]. When the size of pheochromocytoma is less than 3 cm, this tumor is a homogeneous solid mass because of rare cystic or necrotic changes. From this point of view, small pheochromocytoma may meet the criteria for washout of adenoma. When pheochromocytoma becomes larger, this tumor contains frequently hemorrhage, calcification, cystic or necrotic change, and fibrosis. These imaging appearances often overlap with those of large adenoma (≥3 cm) and cortical carcinoma [17, 19, 41, 42].

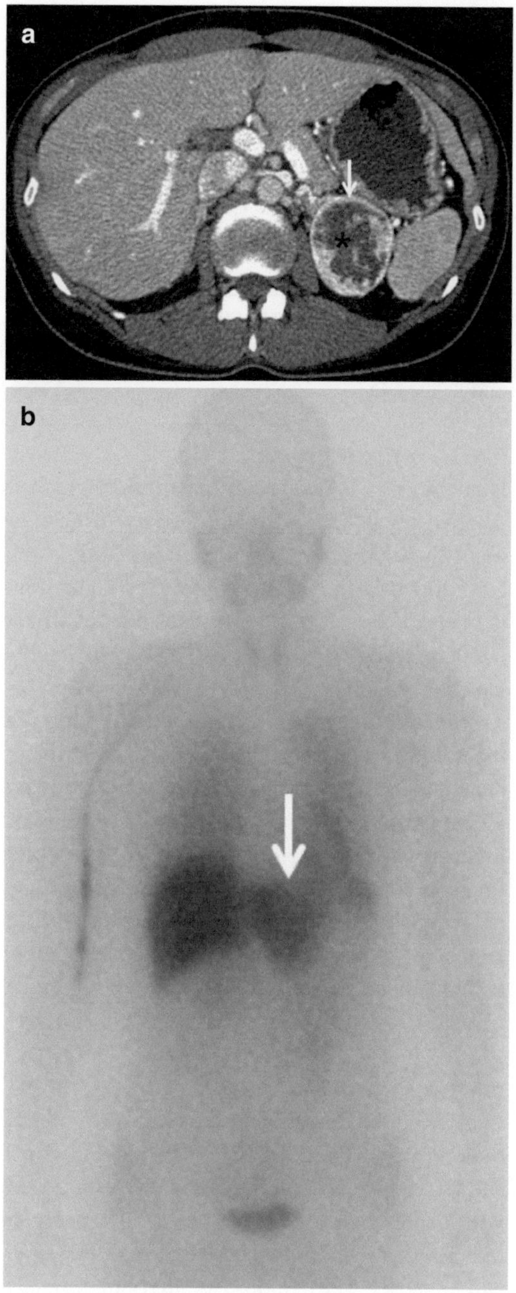

Fig. 5.12 Pheochromocytoma in a 49-year-old woman. (**a**) Contrast-enhanced CT image shows a left pheochromocytoma (*arrow*) with non-enhancing degeneration area (*asterisk*). (**b**) I123 MIBG scan shows a hypermetabolic mass (*arrow*) which is well correlated with CT findings

Pheochromocytoma shows a wide range of imaging features, which is so-called an imaging chameleon [43]. Radiologists are kept in mind that pheochromocytoma should be included for the differential diagnosis of masses with high washout lesions or dominant cystic change, depending on the clinical and laboratory findings.

No imaging feature can reliably distinguish benign and malignant pheochromocytomas unless there is evidence of distant metastasis or invasion to the surrounding structures [43]. Regional lymph nodes are the most frequent metastatic location, followed by the bone, liver, lung, and kidney [5].

5.4.1.7 Hemangioma

Hemangioma is a rare adrenal tumor which is discovered incidentally on CT or MRI. The main histologic types of this tumor are capillary and cavernous hemangiomas. Cavernous hemangioma is more frequent than capillary hemangioma. These tumors tend to be highly vascular. Unenhanced CT shows these tumors are seen well-demarcated hypoattenuating solid masses [44]. Phleboliths or calcification is characteristic imaging features for diagnosis. Hemangioma is hypointense on T1-weighted images and hyperintense on T2-weighted images. Hemorrhage or necrosis increases signal intensity on T1-weighted image. Contrast-enhanced CT or MRI shows peripheral nodular enhancement with or without delayed central filling.

5.4.1.8 Lymphangioma

Lymphangioma is an exceedingly rare adrenal tumor which is discovered incidentally. CT shows a thin-walled non-enhancing cystic lesion with near-water attenuation. Mild enhancement can be identified in the cyst wall or thin septa. MRI shows the tumor is hypointense on T1-weighted images and hyperintense on T2-weighted images [29]. A multilocular cyst with thin septa and water-like fluid is most suggestive of a lymphangioma.

5.4.1.9 Schwannoma

Schwannoma is a benign nerve sheath tumor which is rarely discovered in the adrenal gland [45]. This tumor appears as a heterogeneously enhancing hypoattenuating mass at CT (Fig. 5.13). Adrenal schwannoma is isointense on T1-weighted images and hyperintense on T2-weighted images compared to muscle. However, these MR imaging features are nonspecific, as lesion signal intensity depends on the degree of degenerative change [45]. Accordingly, the differential diagnoses include pheochromocytoma and malignant tumors.

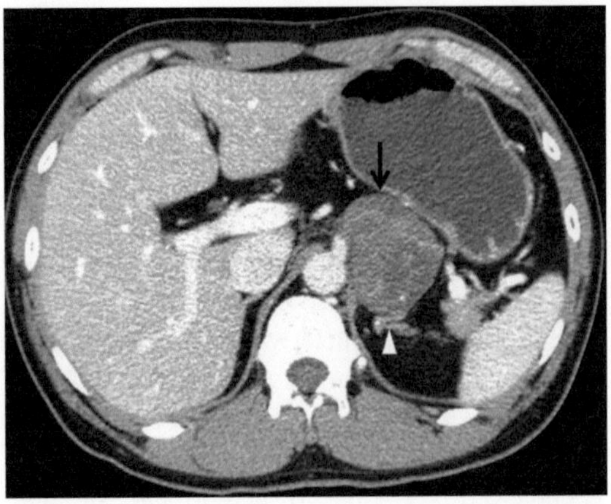

Fig. 5.13 Schwannoma in a 36-year-old man. Contrast-enhanced CT image shows a left adrenal schwannoma (*arrow*) which is heterogeneously enhanced. An *arrowhead* indicates the residual left adrenal tissue

5.4.1.10 Ganglioneuroma

Ganglioneuroma is a benign neurogenic tumor arising along the sympathetic nerve or adrenal gland. This lesion is more frequent in the mediastinum or retroperitoneum than in the adrenal medulla. Adrenal ganglioneuroma accounts for 20–30 % of all cases [46].

Unenhanced CT shows the lesion is so hypoattenuating that the attenuation value is measured <40 HU [47]. Punctate or discrete calcifications can be seen. Early enhanced CT shows a hypoattenuating mass while delayed enhanced CT shows that the lesion is hyperattenuating as compared to muscle due to persistent enhancement (Fig. 5.14a) [48]. Characteristically, the lesion grows by wrapping vessels without obstruction [49]. MRI shows the lesion is hypointense on T1-weighted images, hyperintense on T2-weighted images (Fig. 5.14b), and gradual or persistent enhancement on contrast-enhanced images.

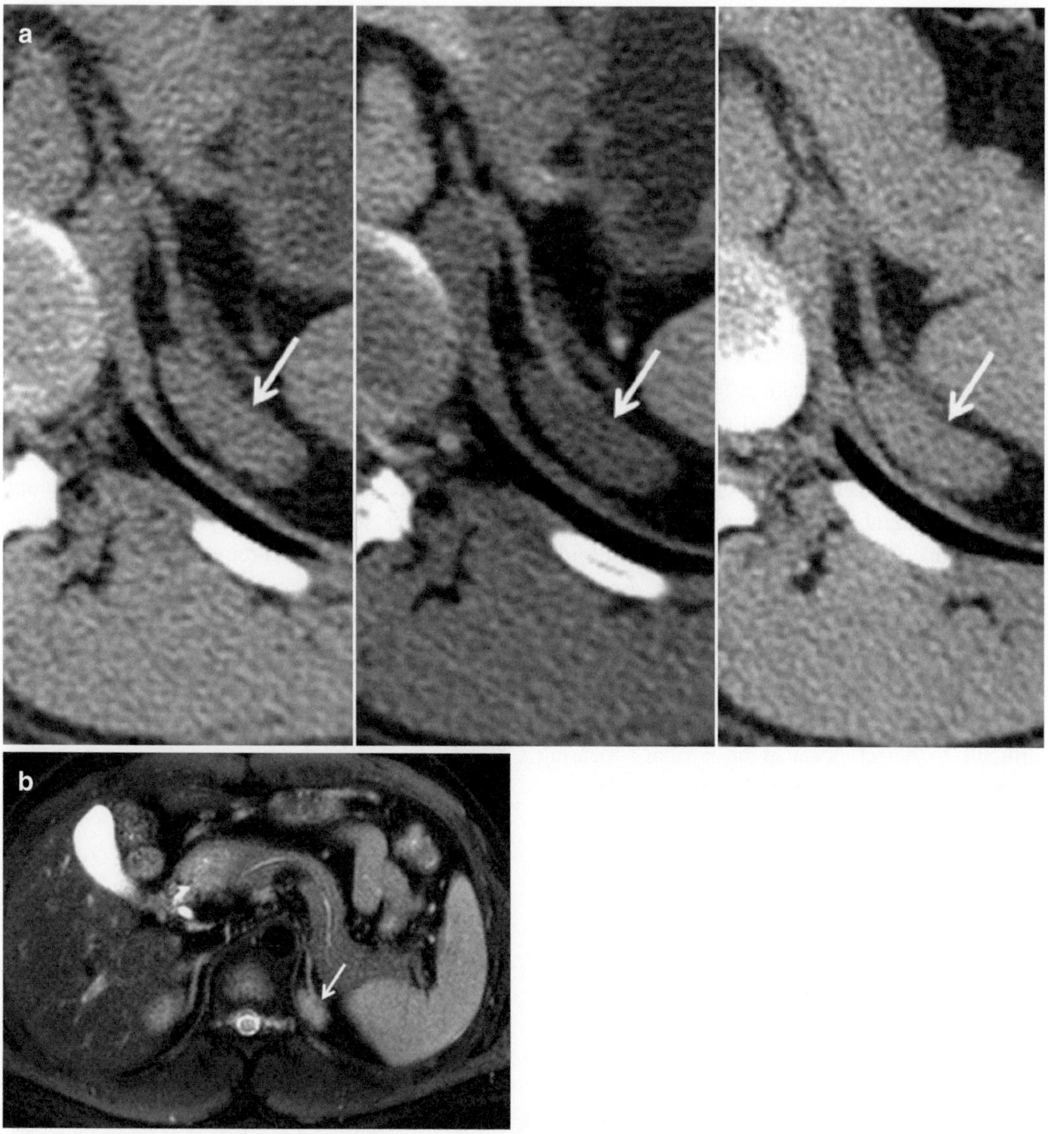

Fig. 5.14 Ganglioneuroma in a 30-year-old man. (**a**) A left ganglioneuroma (*arrow*) is measured 12 HU, 21 HU, and 34 HU on unenhanced (*right-side*), early enhanced (*middle*), and delayed enhanced (*left-side*) CT images. The lesion shows gradual and persistent enhancement. (**b**) T2-weighted MR image shows that the lesion (*arrow*) is hyperintense

5.4.1.11 Adenomatoid Tumor

Adenomatoid tumor is a rare benign adrenal lesion of mesothelial origin. Contrast-enhanced CT shows the lesion is well-circumscribed and heterogeneously hypoattenuating. Calcification may be present. MRI shows lesion signal intensity is variable on T1-weighted, T2-weighted, and contrast-enhanced images. Differential diagnoses include pheochromocytoma and adrenocortical carcinoma [50].

5.4.1.12 Oncocytoma

Oncocytoma is a rare adrenal tumor which is histologically benign but clinically malignant in some cases [51, 52]. CT or MRI shows the lesion is a well-demarcated mass with heterogeneous enhancement [52]. Differential diagnoses include adrenocortical carcinoma, lymphoma, or lipid-poor myelolipoma. Generally, the lack of vascular invasion or lymphadenopathy argues against the former diagnoses.

5.4.1.13 Adrenal Infection

Adrenal infection is caused by fungus, bacteria, mycobacteria, parasite, and virus. Hydatid involvement shows the classic appearance of a primary cyst with daughter cysts internally. Histoplasmosis and paracoccidioidomycosis are the most common fungal infections [3]. Less common infections are blastomycosis, coccidioidomycosis, and cryptococcosis. Typically, bilateral adrenal enlargement is a common feature [53]. Lung infection can precede detection of adrenal involvement.

Tuberculosis also can affect both adrenal glands. CT shows decreased central attenuation due to necrosis and calcifications.

Adrenal abscess formation occurs rarely and is usually unilateral. Bacteria such as *Escherichia coli*, group B streptococcus, and Bacteroides spread hematogenously and may be associated with hemorrhage. So, this infection appears as adrenal tumor [7]. Immunocompromised patients can have cytomegalovirus (CMV) infection affecting the adrenals [54]. However, CMV infection is difficult to detect because of normal-appearing adrenal gland at cross-sectional imaging [55].

5.5 Malignant Adrenal Tumors

5.5.1 Cortical Carcinoma

Cortical carcinoma is an uncommon malignant adrenal tumor [56, 57]. This lesion shows a biphasic two peak incidences in early childhood and middle ages [57]. It is sporadic or associated with hereditary syndromes including Li-Fraumeni syndrome, Beckwith-Wiedemann syndrome, Carney complex, congenital adrenal hyperplasia, and multiple endocrine neoplasia (MEN) type 1 [58].

Clinically, cortical carcinoma may show abdominal pain, back pain, weight loss, or early satiety depending on cancer stage. This lesion may result in Cushing syndrome, hyperaldosteronism, or virilization or feminization due to overproduction of steroids [56, 57].

Usually, cortical carcinoma is detected as a large tumor which is superior to the kidney. Necrosis, hemorrhage, or calcification is frequent. This lesion shows typically unilateral involvement. Large cortical carcinoma tends to locally spread into adjacent organs, regional lymph nodes, and the renal vein or IVC [56, 57].

At US, a small cortical carcinoma shows homogeneous echotexture, while a large cortical carcinoma shows heterogeneous echotexture due to hemorrhage and necrosis. Both hyperechoic and hypoechoic regions may be present. US is good to determine whether or not adjacent organs are invaded because of real-time imaging.

Unenhanced CT shows cortical carcinoma is measured greater than 10 HU [19]. Contrast-enhanced CT show heterogeneous lesion enhancement due to necrosis, hemorrhage, or calcification (Fig. 5.15a) [19]. Generally, a large

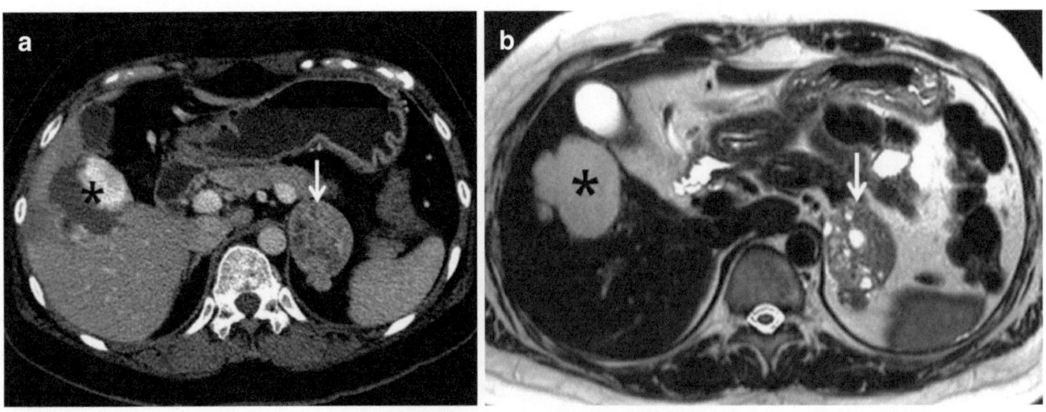

Fig. 5.15 Cortical carcinoma in a 47-year-old woman. (**a**) Contrast-enhanced CT shows a left cortical carcinoma (*arrow*) which is heterogeneously enhanced due to multifocal necrosis. An *asterisk* indicates a hepatic hemangioma. (**b**) T2-weighted MR image shows the lesion (*arrow*) contains multifocal hyperintense foci due to necrosis. An *asterisk* indicates a hepatic hemangioma

cortical carcinoma shows lower relative (<40 %) and absolute (<60 %) percentage washouts than adenoma [19]. However, small cortical carcinoma may show high relative percentage washout (≥40 %) [19]. Tumor thrombus within the renal vein or IVC is not uncommon. Local invasion, regional and para-aortic lymphadenopathy, and distant metastases to the lungs, liver, and bones are common initial presentations of large cortical carcinoma [59].

MRI shows cortical carcinoma is hypointense on T1-weighted images and hyperintense on T2-weighted images (Fig. 5.15b). Areas of hemorrhage appear hyperintense foci on T1-weighted images [59]. Occasionally, this lesion may contain small areas that lose signal on out-of-phase images [60]. Therefore, this feature alone cannot completely exclude the diagnosis of cortical carcinoma. Cortical carcinoma shows a heterogeneous enhancement and slow washout at contrast-enhanced MRI.

A heterogeneously enhancing large adrenal mass is one of important features for identifying cortical carcinoma. However, the high likelihood of cortical carcinoma is only 70 % although adrenal tumor is measured more than 6 cm [59, 61]. This is why there is some overlap between large adenoma (≥3 cm) and cortical carcinoma in terms of lesion size [19]. Therefore, CT or MRI features can provide more confident differentiation of adenoma from cortical carcinoma than lesion size.

5.5.2 Lymphoma

Primary adrenal lymphoma is extremely rare. Almost all cases of adrenal lymphoma are secondary [62]. Adrenal lymphoma manifests as nodular or diffuse enlargement. The diffuse type of adrenal lymphoma reflects uniform organ infiltration often leading to adrenal thickening or enlargement [62]. The nodular type of adrenal lymphoma appears a well-demarcated round solid mass [62]. Characteristically, adrenal lymphoma shows homogeneous texture irrespective of nodular or diffuse pattern because necrosis, hemorrhage, and calcification are uncommon unless there has been prior treatment [63]. Bilateral adrenal involvement is seen in approximately 50 % of cases [64]. For nodular type of adrenal lymphoma, differential diagnoses include adenoma, hyperplasia, and metastasis. For diffuse type of adrenal lymphoma, differential diagnoses include hyperplasia, hemorrhage, and metastasis.

Sonographically, adrenal lymphoma manifests homogeneously hypoechoic masses or adrenal enlargement. Sometimes, the lesion appears an anechoic mass or enlargement with or without posterior sonic enhancement as if it were a cyst mass.

At CT images, adrenal lymphoma mostly manifests a hypoattenuating mass with slight to moderate enhancement (Fig. 5.16) [65, 66]. Extensive extra-adrenal involvement is not

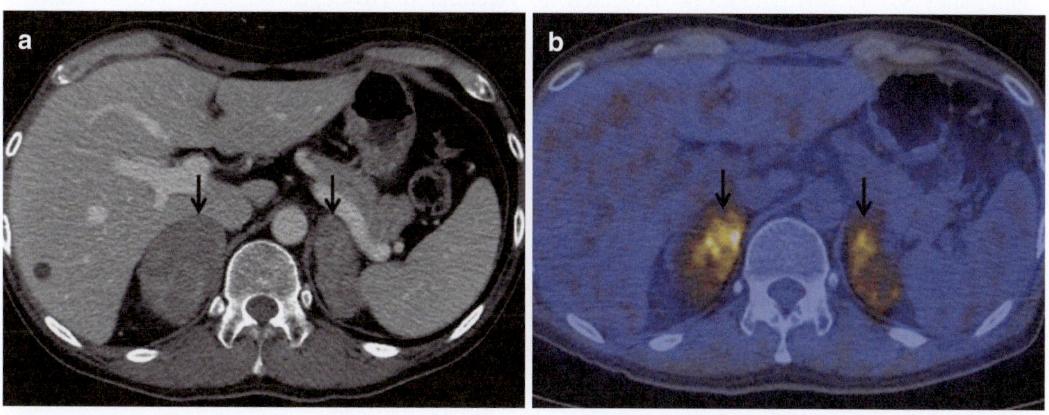

Fig. 5.16 Adrenal lymphoma in a 52-year-old man. (**a**) Contrast-enhanced CT shows bilateral lymphomas (*arrow*) which are homogeneously enhancing solid masses. (**b**) FDG-PETCT shows FDG uptake of adrenal lymphoma (*arrow*) that is higher than that of liver

uncommon in the lymph node, liver, spleen, testis, and retroperitoneal space.

At MRI, adrenal lymphoma is hypointense to isointense on T1-weighted images and slightly hyperintense on T2-weighted images when compared with the liver [66]. Contrast-enhanced MR images show mild to moderate enhancement in the adrenal lymphoma [100]. Adrenal lymphoma shows mild diffusion restriction at diffusion-weighted images [65].

Because adrenal lymphoma is not a surgical disease, percutaneous biopsy is often needed for definitive diagnosis.

5.5.3 Metastases

Adrenal incidentalomas in patients without a history of extra-adrenal malignancy are benign in almost all cases. However, the possibility that adrenal masses are metastatic lesions is higher in patients with a known extra-adrenal malignancy than non-oncologic patients with adrenal incidentaloma. Adrenal metastases are reported in 27 % of an autopsy series of patients with extra-adrenal malignant tumors [67]. The most common metastatic tumor is lung cancer and followed by breast cancer, colon cancer, and malignant melanoma [68].

Bilateral metastasis is more common than unilateral metastasis. However, any new adrenal mass should be considered a potential metastatic lesion in a patient with a known extra-adrenal malignancy. CT or MRI should be dedicated to detect intracytoplasmic lipid or to assess percentage washout for the purpose of excluding possibility of adenoma (Fig. 5.17). If an adrenal mass is not adenoma on imaging studies, PETCT or percutaneous biopsy is necessary to exclude the diagnoses of non-metastatic non-adenomas [20]. PETCT is superior to CT or MRI for detecting adrenal metastasis, while the former is inferior to the latter for characterizing adenoma [20]. However, it should be kept in mind that extra-adrenal malignant tumor can metastasize to a preexisting adrenal lesion [20].

5.6 Pathology of Adrenal Tumors

5.6.1 Adrenal Cortical Adenoma

Grossly adrenal cortical adenoma is well-demarcated intra-adrenal mass with yellow to yellow-brown color and is frequently encapsulated (Fig. 5.18a). Cut surface is solid and homogeneous. Microscopically cortical adenoma is composed of clear to eosinophilic cells with small, relatively uniform nuclei (Fig. 5.18b). Mild nuclear pleomorphism can be found. Architectural pattern is solid sheets, nest, or cord. Mitosis is usually absent.

5.6.2 Adrenal Cortical Carcinoma

Adrenal cortical carcinoma is generally large tumor with invasive border. Tumor cut surface is often variegated frequently containing necrosis and hemorrhage (Fig. 5.19a). Microscopically, carcinoma is often composed of tumor cells with atypical bizarre nuclei (Fig. 5.19b). High mitotic figures and atypical mitosis are frequent in carcinomas. Carcinomas often show patternless sheets. Invasion into capsule, vascular invasion, broad fibrous bands, and necrosis are another features of carcinoma. Several scoring systems have been used to evaluate malignant potential of adrenal cortical neoplasm, and the Weiss scoring system is commonly used [69–71]. Weiss scoring system includes nuclear grade, mitotic rate, presence of atypical mitosis, clear cells, diffuse architecture, microscopic necrosis, and invasion of venous, sinusoidal and capsular structures [72].

5.6.3 Pheochromocytoma

Pheochromocytomas are variable-sized tumor with yellow to reddish color. This tumor is frequently encapsulated and often shows hemorrhage and necrosis (Fig. 5.20a). Microscopically pheochromocytoma reveals well-defined tumor cell clusters mainly showing alveolar pattern with abundant vascular network (Fig. 5.20b). Tumor cells have

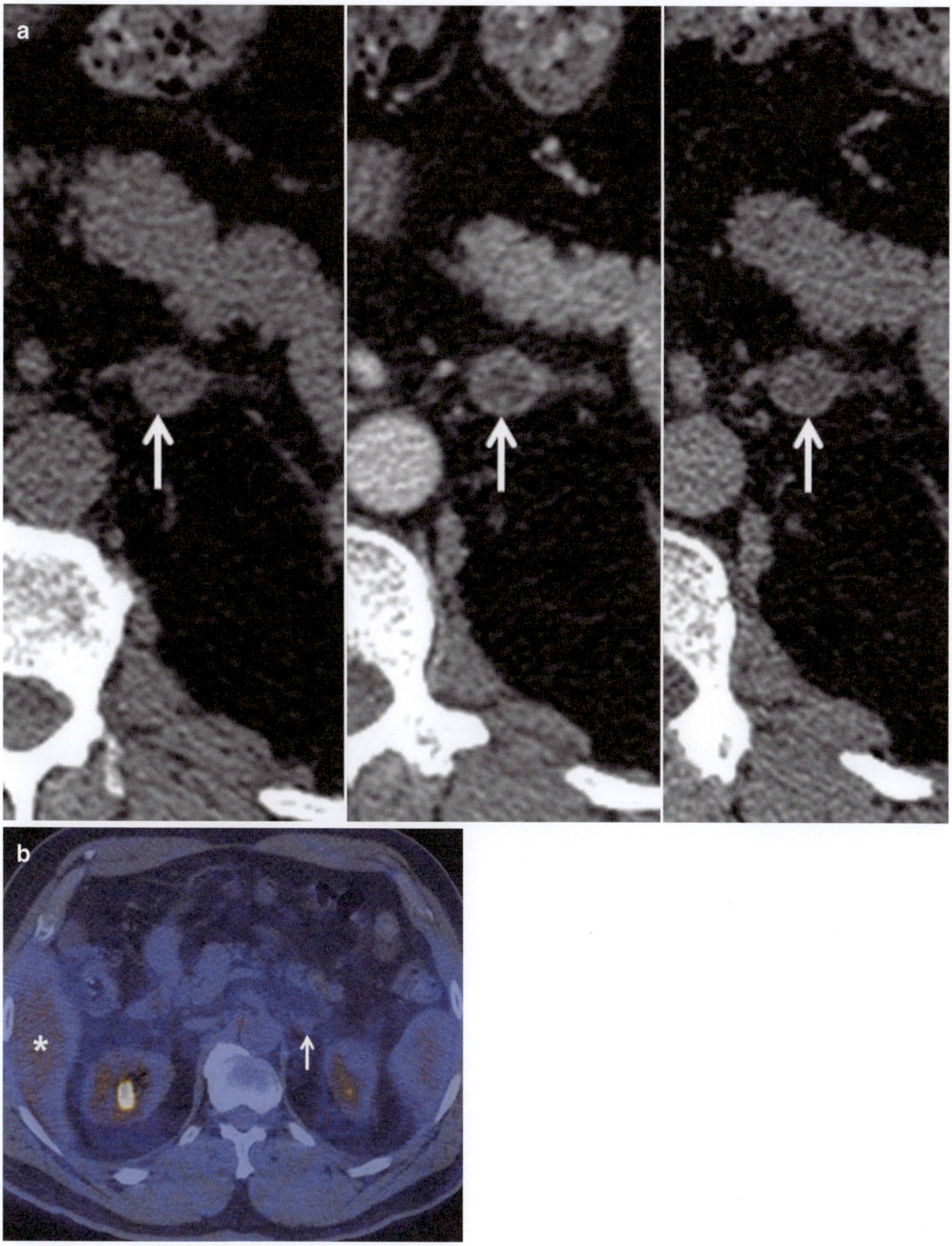

Fig. 5.17 Adrenal metastasis in a 66-year-old man. (**a**) Contrast-enhanced CT shows a left adrenal metastatic nodule (*arrow*) in which absolute and relative percentage washouts are calculated less than 60 % and less than 40 %, respectively. He underwent surgery of sigmoid colon cancer previously. These CT findings are suggestive of metastasis. Follow-up CT shows increased size of the lesion, consistent with metastasis. (**b**) PETCT shows a small left adrenal nodule (*arrow*) in which FDG uptake is less than that (*asterisk*) of the liver, suggesting a benign lesion. However, a small or necrotic metastatic nodule may manifests as a false-negative lesion

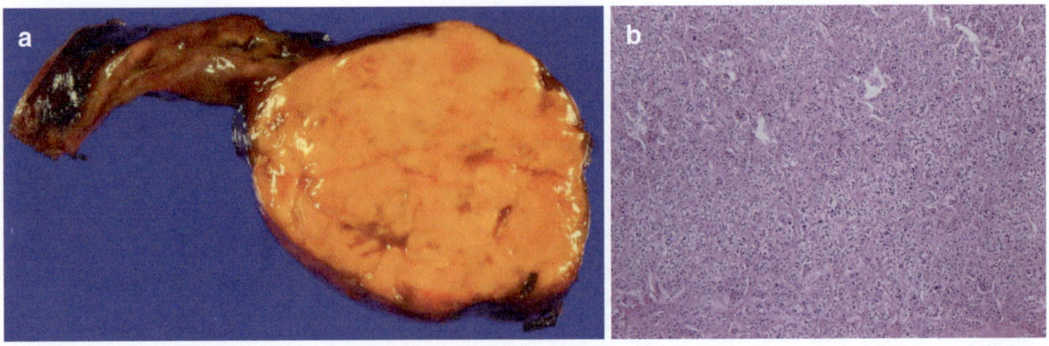

Fig. 5.18 (**a**) Gross photograph of adrenal cortical adenoma shows well-demarcated mass surrounded by normal adrenal tissue with yellow color. (**b**) Microscopically this adrenal cortical adenoma shows small tumor cell nests, and tumor cells have small round uniform nuclei and eosinophilic cytoplasm

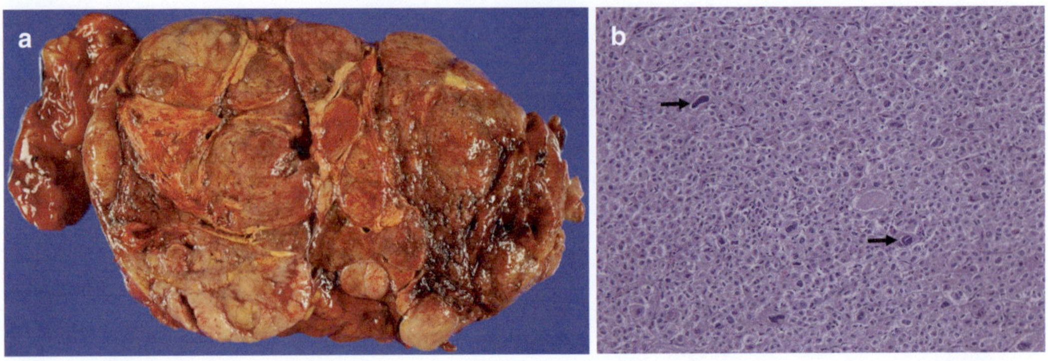

Fig. 5.19 (**a**) Adrenal cortical carcinoma is large mass with frequent hemorrhage and necrosis. (**b**) Bizarre nuclei (*arrows*) are found

granular eosinophilic, basophilic, or amphophilic cytoplasm with round nuclei and prominent nucleoli. Nuclear pleomorphisms are sometimes found. Morphologic markers of malignant pheochromocytoma are not reliable [73]. But malignant pheochromocytomas are generally larger tumor than benign pheochromocytoma with more necrosis (Fig. 5.20c). Pheochromocytoma of the adrenal gland scaled score (PASS) can be applied to separate benign from malignant pheochromocytoma [74, 75]. PASS includes capsular invasion, vascular invasion, extension into periadrenal adipose tissue, presence of large nests or diffuse growth pattern, central tumor necrosis or confluent necrosis, high cellularity, tumor cell spindling, cellular monotony, mitosis more than 3 per ten high-power fields, atypical mitosis, nuclear pleomorphism, and nuclear hyperchromasia (Fig. 5.20d, e).

5.6.4 Neuroblastic Tumors

Neuroblastomas are large well-demarcated soft, gray-tan-colored mass often showing hemorrhage, necrosis, and cystic change (Fig. 5.21a). Microscopically this tumor is composed of small primitive round cells (neuroblast) with little cytoplasm in fibrillary background (Fig. 5.21b). Architectural pattern is mainly solid sheet. Homer-Wright rosettes are often found.

Ganglioneuroblastoma is a tumor showing some degree of differentiation that lies between neuroblastoma and ganglioneuroma. Ganglioneuroblastoma contains varying proportion of larger ganglion cells admixed with primitive neuroblasts (Fig. 5.21c, d) [76]. Ganglioneuroma has little or no neuroblasts.

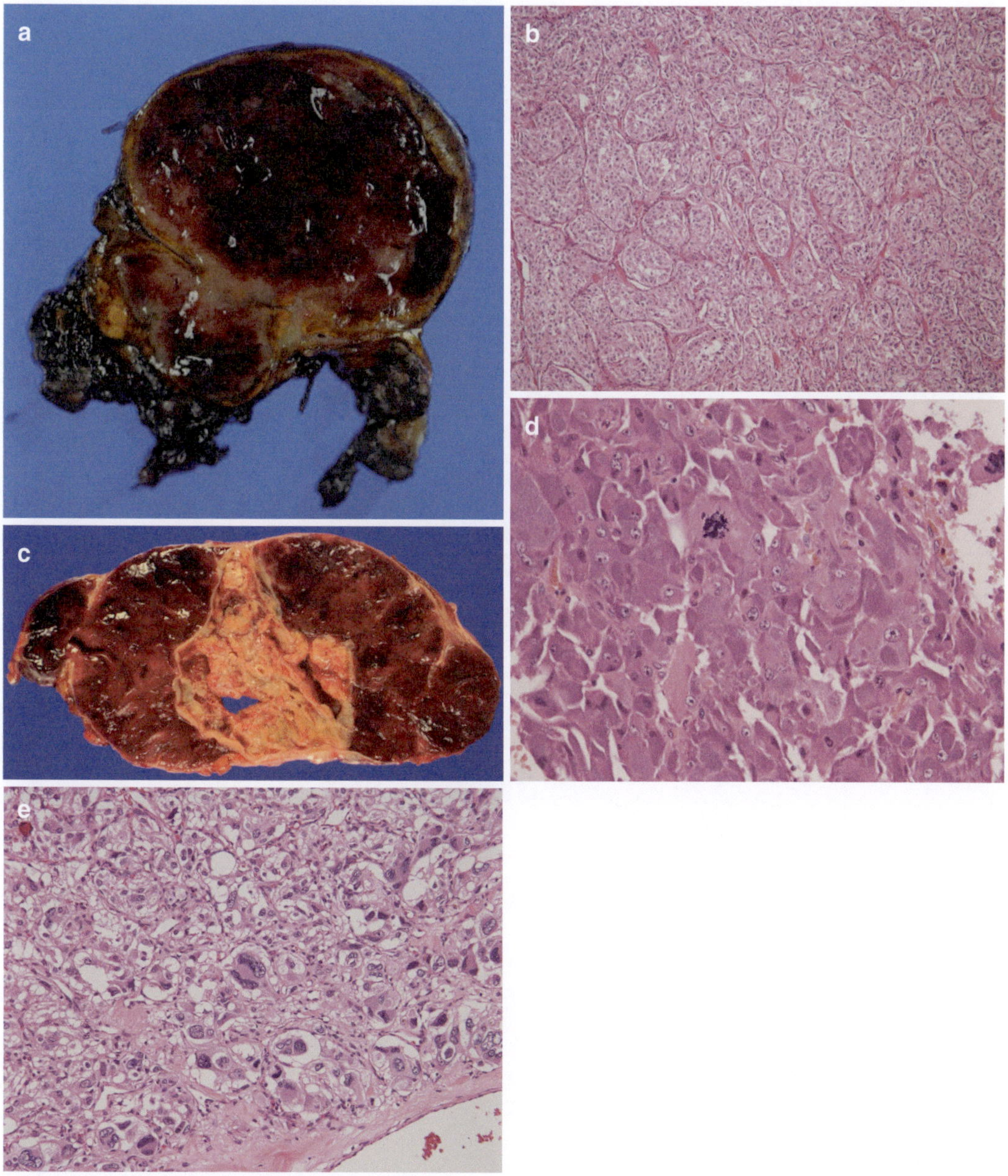

Fig. 5.20 (**a**) Cut surface of pheochromocytoma shows whitish to reddish color with hemorrhage. Normal adrenal tissue is noted around pheochromocytoma. (**b**) Microscopically pheochromocytoma reveals alveolar pattern with granular eosinophilic cytoplasm. (**c**) Grossly malignant pheochromocytoma is large tumor with frequent hemorrhage and necrosis. Microscopically malignant pheochromocytoma can show atypical mitosis (**d**) or nuclear pleomorphism (**e**)

5.6.5 Other Tumors

5.6.5.1 Adrenal Cyst

Adrenal cyst can be classified into endothelial (simple) cyst, pseudocyst, and true epithelial cyst [77]. Endothelial cyst shows flat endothelial lining (Fig. 5.22a). Pseudocyst has fibrous wall without lining cells and contains serous or bloody fluid (Fig. 5.22b). True epithelial-lined adrenal cyst is rare [78].

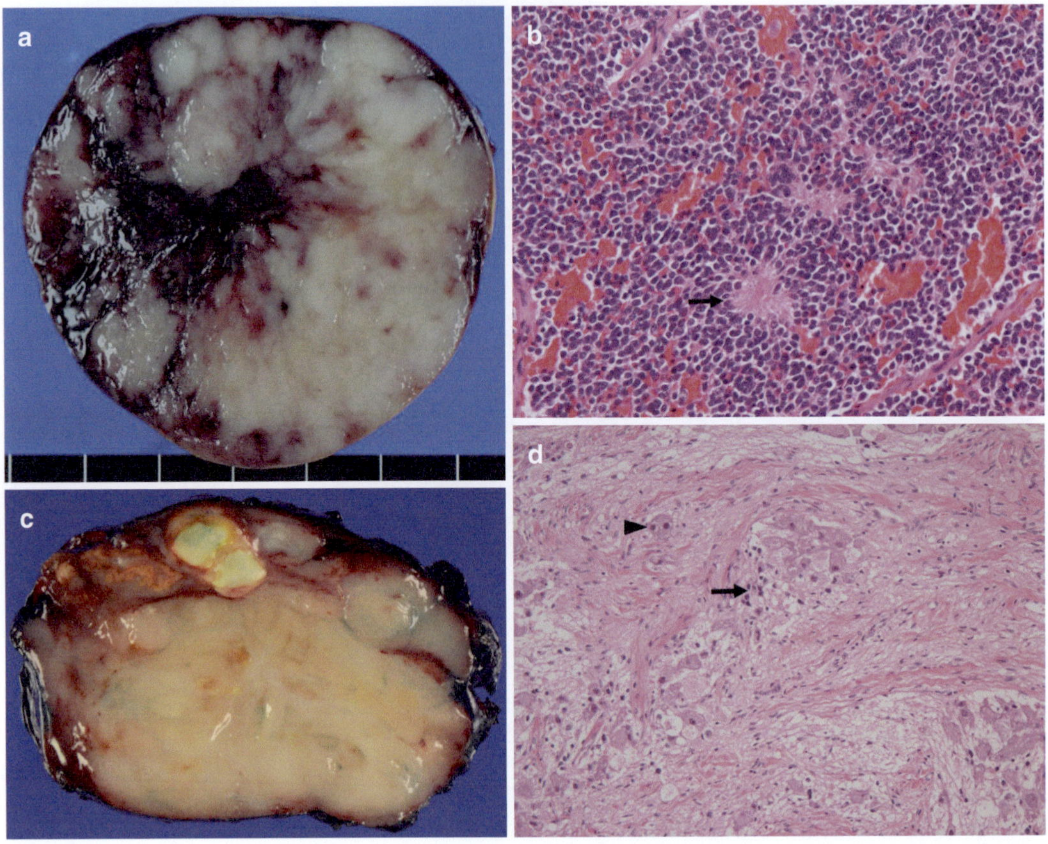

Fig. 5.21 (**a**) Grossly neuroblastoma is large well-demarcated mass with hemorrhage. (**b**) Microscopically neuroblastoma is composed of uniform small round cells with occasional Homer-Wright rosette (*arrow*). (**c**) Ganglioneuroblastoma is whitish, relatively homogeneous mass. (**d**) Microscopically ganglioneuroblastoma contains variable amounts of neuroblasts (*arrow*), ganglion cells (*arrow head*), and schwannian stroma

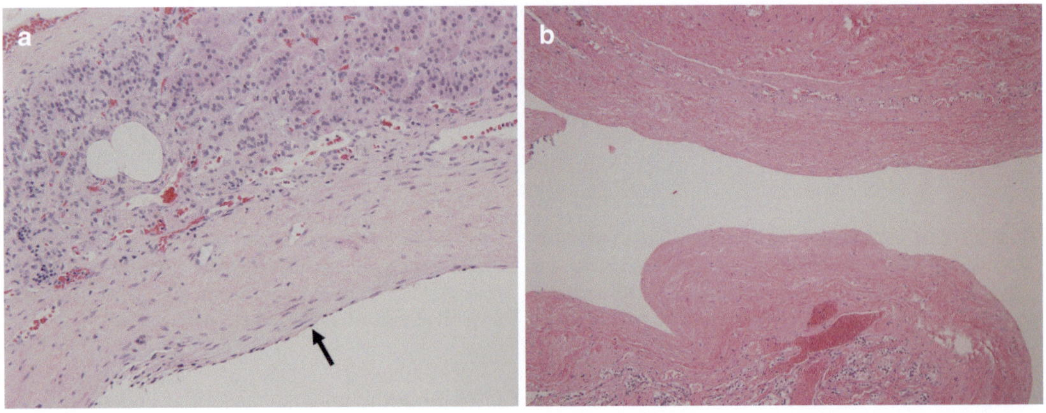

Fig. 5.22 Adrenal cysts. (**a**) Endothelial cyst shows endothelial lining (*arrow*) on cyst wall. (**b**) Pseudocyst shows no lining cells on cyst wall

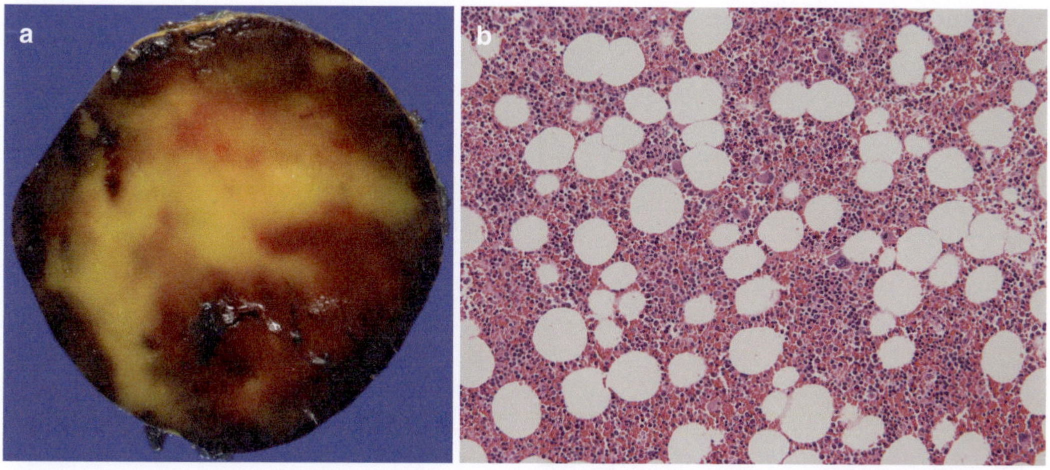

Fig. 5.23 (**a**) Myelolipoma is yellowish mass with hemorrhage. (**b**) Microscopically myelolipoma is composed of mature fat and hematopoietic elements

5.6.5.2 Myelolipoma

Grossly myelolipoma shows yellow-colored cut surface with hemorrhagic area (Fig. 5.23a). Microscopically this tumor is composed of adipose tissue and hematopoietic (Fig. 5.23b).

5.7 Percutaneous Thermal Ablation

Imaging-guided thermal ablation is indicated as an alternative treatment for patients who are not eligible for surgery because of coexisting morbidities and for patients who do not want to undergo surgery [79]. This minimally invasive treatment requires a multidisciplinary team approach from interventional radiologist, oncologist, urologist, surgeon, and endocrinologist. They should thoroughly evaluate physical examination, sign, and symptoms.

Pre-ablation CT or MR images are reviewed for tumor size, location, and potential difficulties in approach to the tumor. The international normalized ratio should be less than 1.5–1.8 and the platelet count $5 \times 10^3/\mu L$ or greater. Biochemical serum or urine assays for cortisol, aldosterone, and catecholamines should be performed before ablation to measure interval change after treatment.

A pre-ablation biopsy is recommended to confirm the pathologic diagnosis because no tissue is removed during percutaneous ablative therapy. A hypertensive crisis may occur during a biopsy, particularly if a pheochromocytoma is suspected. A biopsy should be obviated if catecholamine is positive in the urine or serum.

Endocrinologic consultation is necessary in the management of functioning adrenal tumors and helps in preprocedure preparation for a hypertensive crisis [79]. An endocrinologist may initiate premedication with α- and β-blockers. A typical pretreatment protocol can include 10–60 mg of oral phenoxybenzamine with titration of β-blockers for 10–14 days before ablation.

Although most renal and hepatic tumors are ablated with conscious sedation, adrenal tumor ablations should be performed under general anesthesia to preempt hypertensive crisis and to prepare for treatment.

Radiofrequency ablation [80–82] is the most common ablation therapy for adrenal tumor and followed by cryoablation [83, 84] and microwave ablation [85, 86].

CT is the most common guiding modality for adrenal tumor ablation to visualize ablation area during the course of treatment (Fig. 5.24). MRI can depict ablation area well because of excellent soft tissue contrast but also can avoid radiation exposure to both patients and radiologists.

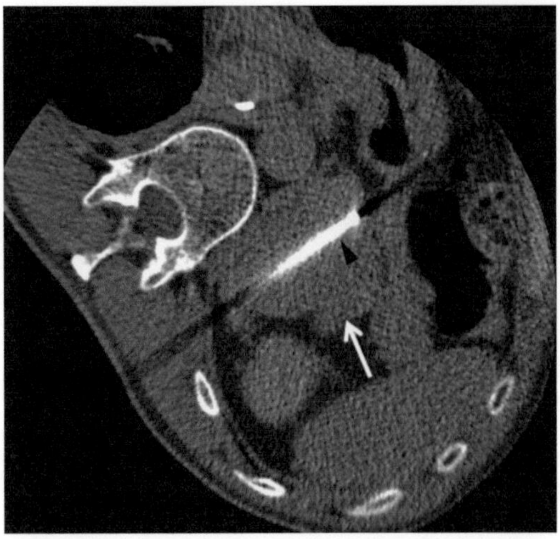

Fig. 5.24 Radiofrequency ablation of an adrenal metastatic mass in a 57-year-old man. Unenhanced CT shows a left adrenal metastatic mass (*arrow*) in which a radiofrequency electrode (*arrowhead*) is placed. Left-side down of the patient collapses the ipsilateral lung so that no lung tissue is intervened in the pathway of the electrode

Complications of adrenal tumor ablation include hypertensive crisis, bowel injury, pneumothorax, hemorrhage, adrenal insufficiency, infection, and pain. Hypertensive crisis results from excessively released catecholamines. This complication requires intravenous administration of α- and β-blockers. Bowel injury is a result of thermal damage to small bowel. This complication can be avoided by hydrodissection displacing bowel. Ipsilateral side down of patients helps to avoid pneumothorax by means of collapsing the ipsilateral lung (Fig. 5.24). Subsequently, lung tissue does not exist in the pathway of ablation applicators. Transhepatic approach may avoid pneumothorax by means of providing another route for accessing right adrenal tumor [87]. Hemorrhage may result from mechanical injury to critical structures including the inferior vena cava, aorta, renal arteries, and lumbar collateral vessels. Ablation applicators should be meticulously manipulated during the tumor targeting. Adrenal insufficiency is a rare complication of thermal ablation because normal adrenal tissue is more likely to be preserved with thermal ablation compared to surgery.

Long-term outcome after imaging-guided ablation depends on the type of tumor treated and size of the tumor. Technical success can be achieved for tumors smaller than 5 cm. For functioning adrenal tumors, technical success requires non-enhancing adrenal tumors and normalizing biochemical abnormalities. For adrenal metastatic tumors, the eventual outcome depends on the prognosis of the primary tumor although local control is achieved [80].

5.8 Surgery for Adrenal Tumors

The indications for adrenalectomy are various, including primary aldosteronism, Cushing syndrome, pheochromocytoma, adrenal adenoma, adrenocortical adenoma, neuroblastoma, adrenal cyst, myelolipoma, metastatic adrenal tumor, and incidentaloma [88]. Among various approaches, laparoscopic adrenalectomy is generally considered as the surgical treatment of choice [89]. However, open adrenalectomy is better in the cases of adrenocortical carcinoma, large size of pheochromocytoma, severe obesity, and previous history of multiple abdominal surgeries [90].

5.8.1 Open Surgical Approach to Adrenal Gland

For open adrenalectomy, several approaches are available, including flank, lumbodorsal posterior, thoracoabdominal, and subcostal incision [88]. Particularly, thoracoabdominal approach is useful for large tumor or invasive adrenocortical carcinoma due to good surgical field. Conversely, lumbodorsal posterior approach for adrenalectomy should not be recommended for large-sized tumor or adrenocortical carcinoma due to the small operative filed. Subcostal approach can be useful for larger adrenal tumors with better surgical exposure of great vessels.

Initial step of adrenalectomy is to identify the surgical plane between the Gerota fascia and the visceral peritoneum. The peritoneum is freed and mobilized from the Gerota fascia. On the right side, inferior vena cava (IVC) and duodenum are seen, and the adrenal gland can be visualized following cephalad dissection toward the lower border of the

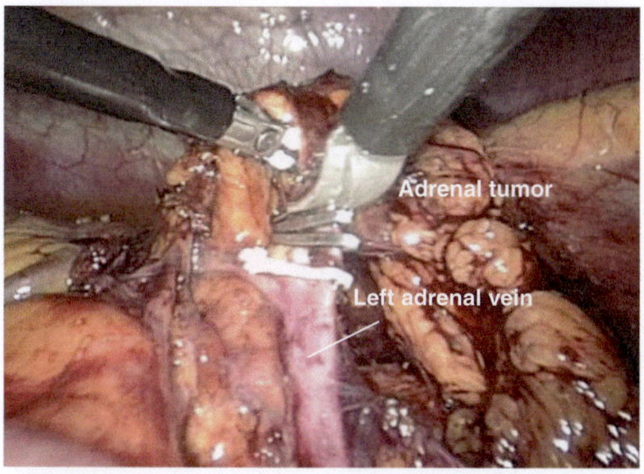

Fig. 5.25 Control of left adrenal vein; the identification and handling of adrenal vein are important steps in adrenalectomy. In left adrenalectomy, the left adrenal vein can be ligated and transected using clipping material, such as metal clip and Hem-o-lok

liver. The adrenal gland is dissected along the plane between medial aspect of adrenal gland and lateral boarder of IVC. The adrenal vein can be identified during dissection of this plane, and it is ligated by either surgical ties or metal clips. Arterial control of the adrenal gland is typically performed with harmonic scalpel for effective hemostasis. Attachment to the kidney of inferomedial surface of the adrenal gland is divided by using harmonic scalpel or electrocautery hook. For the resection of left adrenal gland, same surgical process is used; otherwise aorta is identified medially as well as the spleen and pancreas are visualized superiorly. Left adrenal vein draining into renal vein is identified and ligated. After meticulous control of arterial branch with harmonic scalpel, the adrenal gland is mobilized and finally resected.

5.8.2 Laparoscopic Approach to Adrenal Gland

Laparoscopic surgery to remove the adrenal tumors has several advantages, such as less pain and shorter hospital day, compared to open adrenalectomy. Particularly, laparoscopic resection is preferred in tumors with its diameter less than 6 cm and in benign tumors [91]. Transperitoneal and retroperitoneal approaches are available in laparoscopic adrenalectomy.

In transperitoneal technique, patient is generally placed in a semilateral position at 70 degree. Anterior supine position is recommended in the case of bilateral adrenal tumors for a better accessibility and surgical view. For left-side adrenal tumor with lateral approach, four ports are placed. First of all, white line of Toldt is incised off the parietal peritoneum, and the descending colon is mobilized toward medial side. The lienorenal ligament is divided to detach the spleen from kidney upper pole, which makes to facilitate the exposure of adrenal gland. The left renal vein is identified at the medial side of the renal vein. After control with Hem-o-lok and metal clips, the adrenal vein is divided (Fig. 5.25).

Then, the adrenal gland bearing tumors is dissected from the kidney upper pole and detached from perivascular connective tissues. In this procedure, adrenal arteries are mostly not visible, and dissection with harmonic scalpel is useful for effective bleeding control. Finally, remaining periadrenal attachment is further dissected, and then, absorbable hemostat (Surgicel®; Ethicon Endo-Surgery Inc, Blue Ash, OH, USA) is placed on tumor resection bed. The tumor specimen is extracted from the abdomen cavity by using LAPSAC®, Cook Medical, Bloomington, IN, USA.

For right-side tumor, the whole step of surgery is similar to left-side tumor; otherwise one more assist-trocar is needed for liver traction. Initially, attachment between the liver and Gerota's fascia is dissected, and then IVC is exposed beside the duodenum. Adrenal tumor can be identified between the liver and IVC at the upper pole side of the kidney. After detection of the right adrenal vein draining into IVC, it is clamped with metal clip and resected. Upper aspect of the adrenal gland, where unvisible adrenal arteries can be existed, is dissected (Fig. 5.26).

In this step, harmonic scalpel is recommended for efficient bleeding control. Lower aspect of adrenal gland is dissected from kidney upper pole. Then, adrenal tumor is fully resected, and specimen is removed from tumor bed by using LAPSAC®. Representative images of adrenal tumors specimens are shown.

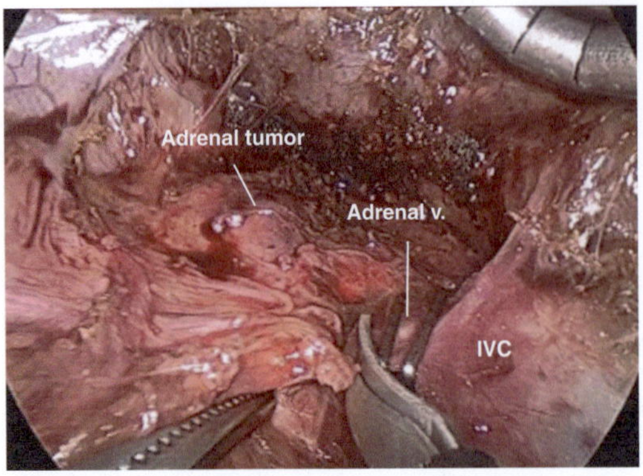

Fig. 5.26 Dissecting the superior border of tumor; the upper part of adrenal tumor is separated from the inferior border of the liver

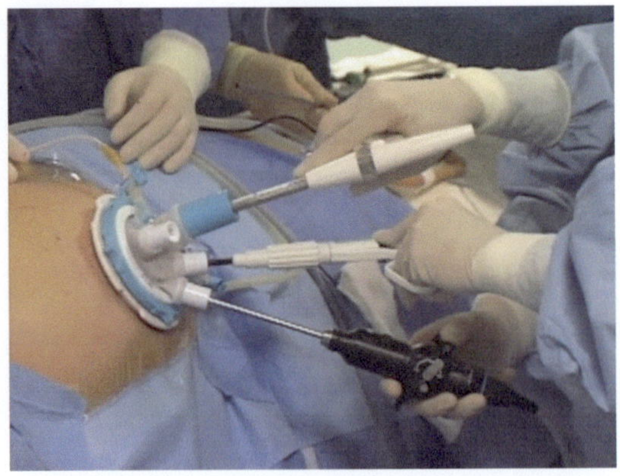

Fig. 5.27 Insertion of surgical instruments in OCTO™PORT system; laparoendoscopic single-site surgery (LESS) for renal or adrenal mass removal can be performed using commercialized port device, such as OCTO™PORT

Whittle et al. reported the first case of laparoscopic retroperitoneal adrenalectomy 20 years ago [92]; this surgical technique is not widely used due to several difficulties such as small working space and paucity of anatomic landmark during surgery [93]. Therefore, some surgeons perform retroperitoneal adrenalectomy in selected indications, for example, small tumors and nonobese patients.

5.8.3 Approach to Adrenal Gland with Laparoendoscopic Single-Site Surgery (LESS)

In 2009, LESS-nephrectomy in children was reported in Korea [94]. After then, various indications of LESS techniques were tried, and several studies of LESS-adrenalectomy were reported [95, 96]. Patient is placed in semilateral position. About 2.5 cm-sized incision is made at the umbilicus (contralateral side of the tumor). In our department, homemade single-port system was initially applied for LESS.

The retractor of Lap-disc is inserted through the incision. Surgical glove is docked with retractor of Lap-disc. After cutting three tips of glove, 5 mm trocar is inserted and stayed with rubber band as working channels. Recently, commercial single-port system, OCTO™PORT (DalimsurgNET, Seoul, Korea), can be used for LESS in Korea. Flexible instruments for LESS-adrenalectomy are entered into OCTO™PORT system (Fig. 5.27).

After completion of tumor resection, specimen is extracted via the retractor of single port. Only small single incision site remains after surgery with good cosmetic result.

For LESS-right adrenalectomy, hepatorenal ligament is initially detached from the kidney upper pole side like laparoscopic surgery. Then, IVC and duodenum are identified followed by adrenal mass detection.

Adrenal vein is exposed and controlled by harmonic scalpel (Fig. 5.28). Remained attachment of adrenal tumor is resected from the kidney upper pole and lower margin of the liver. After complete resection of the adrenal gland, specimen is extracted by using LAPSAC®. Finally, surgical glue (Tissel®) and surgical are applied on tumor resection bed for effective bleeding control. The surgical step for left LESS-adrenalectomy is similar to laparoscopic surgery, and key procedures are presented as following figures. Port placement and detailed skill for single-port surgery are described above.

5.8.4 Robot-Assisted Laparoscopic Approach to Adrenal Gland

Robot-assisted laparoscopic surgery has become mainstay of urologic surgery, such as radical prostatectomy and partial nephrectomy [97]. Although it remains open question whether robotic adrenalectomy is superior to conventional

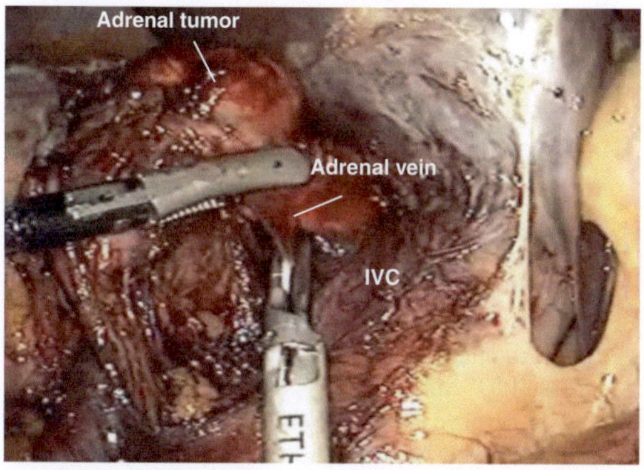

Fig. 5.28 Identification and control of right adrenal vein; right adrenal vein directly originates from inferior vena cava (IVC), and the length of right adrenal vein is generally shorter than that of left adrenal vein. Therefore, adequate dissection of medial and posterior side of IVC is necessary to identify and control of right adrenal vein. Right adrenal vein can be sacrificed using energy device, such as Harmonic scalpel™

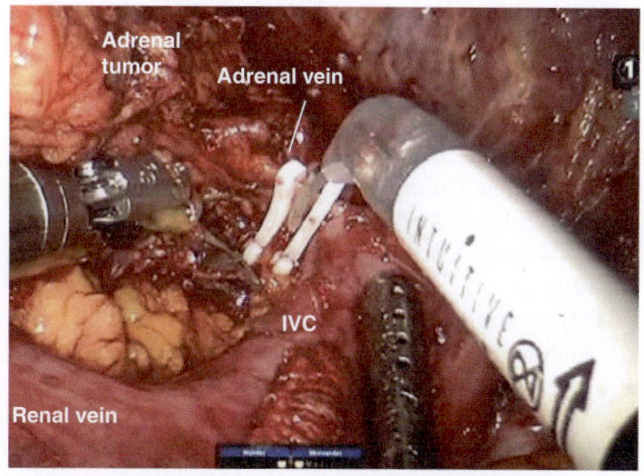

Fig. 5.29 Completion of right adrenal tumor resection; complete removal of adrenal mass can be made after processing adrenal vein

laparoscopic surgery, the interest in robot-assisted laparoscopic surgery for adrenal mass has also been increased [98]. Three-dimensional vision and handlike movement are the technical benefits of robot-assisted surgery.

Typically, transperitoneal approach is used, and thus, patient is prepared in flank position and draped. Four to five trocars are inserted as following the surgeon's preference, and the robot should be docked at an angle at the upper side of operative table for great accessibility of adrenal gland. Detailed procedures of the operative technique for robot-assisted adrenalectomy are nearly identical to conventional laparoscopic surgery as described previously. Briefly, for right-side tumor, detachment of hepatorenal ligament is initially done. IVC and adrenal vein are identified at the medial side of duodenum. Then, adrenal vein is clamped and resected (Fig. 5.29). Remained connective tissues of adrenal gland are dissected and then fully detached from tumor bed.

5.9 Radiotherapy

Primary adrenal tumors are rarely indications for definitive or adjuvant RT. Adrenal gland is prone to metastatic involvement from certain malignancies. In selected oligometastatic cases, stereotactic body ablative radiotherapy (SBRT) may be used to ablate metastatic lesions in adrenal gland. To accurately define target volume for SBRT of adrenal metastases, contrast-enhanced CT scanning is useful to differentiate uninvolved adrenal parenchyma from metastatic lesions.

Conclusion

Radiologists should focus on characterizing adrenal adenoma when an adrenal mass is incidentally detected because adenoma is the most common adrenal lesion. Unenhanced CT, MRI, and contrast-enhanced CT provide excellent accuracy for lipid-rich or lipid-poor adenoma and myelolipoma. The other benign and malignant non-adenomas are evaluated by team approach involving radiologists, endocrinologists, and surgeons based on clinical findings and biochemical tests in addition to imaging features. Therefore, they need to be familiar with imaging protocols and various imaging features for differential diagnoses.

References

1. Blake MA, Cronin CG, Boland GW. Adrenal imaging. AJR Am J Roentgenol. 2010;194(6):1450–60.
2. Arnold DT, Reed JB, Burt K. Evaluation and management of the incidental adrenal mass. Proc (Bayl Univ Med Cent). 2003;16(1):7–12.
3. Cawood TJ, Hunt PJ, O'Shea D, Cole D, Soule S. Recommended evaluation of adrenal incidentalomas is costly, has high false-positive rates and confers a risk of fatal cancer that is similar to the risk of the adrenal

lesion becoming malignant; time for a rethink? Eur J Endocrinol. 2009;161(4):513–27.

4. Young WF. Primary aldosteronism: renaissance of a syndrome. Clin Endocrinol (Oxf). 2007;66(5):607–18.
5. Lattin Jr GE, Sturgill ED, Tujo CA, et al. From the Radiologic Pathology Archives: Adrenal Tumors and Tumor-like Conditions in the Adult: Radiologic-Pathologic Correlation. Radiographics. 2014;34(3):805–29.
6. Mayo-Smith WW, Boland GW, Noto RB, Lee MJ. State-of-the-art adrenal imaging. Radiographics. 2001;21(4):995–1012.
7. Terzolo M, Stigliano A, Chiodini I, et al. AME position statement on adrenal incidentaloma. Eur J Endocrinol. 2011;164(6):851–70.
8. Motta-Ramirez GA, Remer EM, Herts BR, Gill IS, Hamrahian AH. Comparison of CT findings in symptomatic and incidentally discovered pheochromocytomas. AJR Am J Roentgenol. 2005;185(3):684–8.
9. Kloos RT, Gross MD, Francis IR, Korobkin M, Shapiro B. Incidentally discovered adrenal masses. Endocr Rev. 1995;16(4):460–84.
10. Abrams HL, Siegelman SS, Adams DF, et al. Computed tomography versus ultrasound of the adrenal gland: a prospective study. Radiology. 1982;143(1):121–8.
11. Boland GW, Lee MJ, Gazelle GS, Halpern EF, McNicholas MM, Mueller PR. Characterization of adrenal masses using unenhanced CT: an analysis of the CT literature. AJR Am J Roentgenol. 1998;171(1):201–4.
12. Seo JM, Park BK, Park SY, Kim CK. Characterization of lipid-poor adrenal adenoma: chemical-shift MRI and washout CT. AJR Am J Roentgenol. 2014;202(5):1043–50.
13. Haider MA, Ghai S, Jhaveri K, Lockwood G. Chemical shift MR imaging of hyperattenuating (>10 HU) adrenal masses: does it still have a role? Radiology. 2004;231(3):711–6.
14. Israel GM, Korobkin M, Wang C, Hecht EN, Krinsky GA. Comparison of unenhanced CT and chemical shift MRI in evaluating lipid-rich adrenal adenomas. AJR Am J Roentgenol. 2004;183(1):215–9.
15. Park BK, Kim CK, Kim B, Lee JH. Comparison of delayed enhanced CT and chemical shift MR for evaluating hyperattenuating incidental adrenal masses. Radiology. 2007;243(3):760–5.
16. Park BK, Kim B, Ko K, Jeong SY, Kwon GY. Adrenal masses falsely diagnosed as adenomas on unenhanced and delayed contrast-enhanced computed tomography: pathological correlation. Eur Radiol. 2006;16(3):642–7.
17. Park BK, Kim CK, Kwon GY, Kim JH. Re-evaluation of pheochromocytomas on delayed contrast-enhanced CT: washout enhancement and other imaging features. Eur Radiol. 2007;17(11):2804–9.
18. Choi YA, Kim CK, Park BK, Kim B. Evaluation of adrenal metastases from renal cell carcinoma and hepatocellular carcinoma: use of delayed contrast-enhanced CT. Radiology. 2013;266(2):514–20.
19. Park SY, Park BK, Park JJ, Kim CK. CT sensitivities for large (≥3 cm) adrenal adenoma and cortical carcinoma. Abdom Imaging. 2014;40:310–7.
20. Park SY, Park BK, Kim CK. The value of adding (18) F-FDG PET/CT to adrenal protocol CT for characterizing adrenal metastasis (>/= 10 mm) in oncologic patients. AJR Am J Roentgenol. 2014;202(2):W153–60.
21. Park BK, Kim CK, Jung BC, Suh YL. Cortical adenoma in adrenohepatic fusion tissue: clue to making a correct diagnosis at preoperative computed tomography examination. Eur Urol. 2009;56(6):1082–5.
22. Russell RP, Masi AT. The prevalence of adrenal cortical hyperplasia at autopsy and its association with hypertension. Ann Intern Med. 1970;73(2):195–205.
23. Dobbie JW. Adrenocortical nodular hyperplasia: the ageing adrenal. J Pathol. 1969;99(1):1–18.
24. Rana AI, Kenney PJ, Lockhart ME, et al. Adrenal gland hematomas in trauma patients. Radiology. 2004;230(3):669–75.
25. Kawashima A, Sandler CM, Ernst RD, et al. Imaging of nontraumatic hemorrhage of the adrenal gland. Radiographics. 1999;19(4):949–63.
26. Park BK, Kim CK, Kwon GY. Spontaneous rupture of pheochromocytoma: computed tomography-pathologic features and correlation. Acta Radiol. 2008;49(2):230–2.
27. Xarli VP, Steele AA, Davis PJ, Buescher ES, Rios CN, Garcia-Bunuel R. Adrenal hemorrhage in the adult. Medicine (Baltimore). 1978;57(3):211–21.
28. Burks DW, Mirvis SE, Shanmuganathan K. Acute adrenal injury after blunt abdominal trauma: CT findings. AJR Am J Roentgenol. 1992;158(3):503–7.
29. Elsayes KM, Mukundan G, Narra VR, et al. Adrenal masses: mr imaging features with pathologic correlation. Radiographics. 2004;24 Suppl 1:S73–86.
30. Incze JS, Lui PS, Merriam JC, Austen G, Widrich WC, Gerzof SG. Morphology and pathogenesis of adrenal cysts. Am J Pathol. 1979;95(2):423–32.
31. Sanal HT, Kocaoglu M, Yildirim D, et al. Imaging features of benign adrenal cysts. Eur J Radiol. 2006;60(3):465–9.
32. Carvounis E, Marinis A, Arkadopoulos N, Theodosopoulos T, Smyrniotis V. Vascular adrenal cysts: a brief review of the literature. Arch Pathol Lab Med. 2006;130(11):1722–4.
33. Polat P, Kantarci M, Alper F, Suma S, Koruyucu MB, Okur A. Hydatid disease from head to toe. Radiographics. 2003;23(2):475–94; quiz 536–477.
34. Otal P, Escourrou G, Mazerolles C, et al. Imaging features of uncommon adrenal masses with histopathologic correlation. Radiographics. 1999;19(3):569–81.
35. Olsson CA, Krane RJ, Klugo RC, Selikowitz SM. Adrenal myelolipoma. Surgery. 1973;73(5):665–70.
36. Kenney PJ, Wagner BJ, Rao P, Heffess CS. Myelolipoma: CT and pathologic features. Radiology. 1998;208(1):87–95.
37. Miyake H, Maeda H, Tashiro M, et al. CT of adrenal tumors: frequency and clinical significance of low-attenuation lesions. AJR Am J Roentgenol. 1989;152(5):1005–7.

38. Brink I, Hoegerle S, Klisch J, Bley TA. Imaging of pheochromocytoma and paraganglioma. Fam Cancer. 2005;4(1):61–8.
39. Jacques AE, Sahdev A, Sandrasagara M, et al. Adrenal phaeochromocytoma: correlation of MRI appearances with histology and function. Eur Radiol. 2008;18(12): 2885–92.
40. Patel J, Davenport MS, Cohan RH, Caoili EM. Can established CT attenuation and washout criteria for adrenal adenoma accurately exclude pheochromocytoma? AJR Am J Roentgenol. 2013;201(1):122–7.
41. Newhouse JH, Heffess CS, Wagner BJ, Imray TJ, Adair CF, Davidson AJ. Large degenerated adrenal adenomas: radiologic-pathologic correlation. Radiology. 1999; 210(2):385–91.
42. Colby GW, Banks KP, Torres E. AJR teaching file: Incidental adrenal mass and hypertension. AJR Am J Roentgenol. 2006;187(3 Suppl):S470–2.
43. Blake MA, Kalra MK, Maher MM, et al. Pheochromocytoma: an imaging chameleon. Radiographics. 2004;24 Suppl 1:S87–99.
44. Kawashima A, Sandler CM, Fishman EK, et al. Spectrum of CT findings in nonmalignant disease of the adrenal gland. Radiographics. 1998;18(2):393–412.
45. Inokuchi T, Takiuchi H, Moriwaki Y, et al. Retroperitoneal ancient schwannoma presenting as an adrenal incidentaloma: CT and MR findings. Magn Reson Imaging. 2006;24(10):1389–93.
46. Guo YK, Yang ZG, Li Y, et al. Uncommon adrenal masses: CT and MRI features with histopathologic correlation. Eur J Radiol. 2007;62(3):359–70.
47. Maweja S, Materne R, Detrembleur N, et al. Adrenal ganglioneuroma. Am J Surg. 2007;194(5):683–4.
48. Park BK, Kim CK, Kim B, Kwon GY. Adrenal tumors with late enhancement on CT and MRI. Abdom Imaging. 2007;32(4):515–8.
49. Radin R, David CL, Goldfarb H, Francis IR. Adrenal and extra-adrenal retroperitoneal ganglioneuroma: imaging findings in 13 adults. Radiology. 1997;202(3):703–7.
50. Liu YQ, Zhang HX, Wang GL, Ma LL, Huang Y. A giant cystic adenomatoid tumor of the adrenal gland: a case report. Chin Med J (Engl). 2010;123(3):372–4.
51. de Krijger RR, van Nederveen FH, Korpershoek E, Dinjens WN. New developments in the detection of the clinical behavior of pheochromocytomas and paragangliomas. Endocr Pathol. 2006;17(2):137–41.
52. Juliano JJ, Cody RL, Suh JH. Metastatic adrenocortical oncocytoma: a case report. Urol Oncol. 2008;26(2):198–201.
53. Kumar N, Singh S, Govil S. Adrenal histoplasmosis: clinical presentation and imaging features in nine cases. Abdom Imaging. 2003;28(5):703–8.
54. Pulakhandam U, Dincsoy HP. Cytomegaloviral adrenalitis and adrenal insufficiency in AIDS. Am J Clin Pathol. 1990;93(5):651–6.
55. Freda PU, Wardlaw SL, Brudney K, Goland RS. Primary adrenal insufficiency in patients with the acquired immunodeficiency syndrome: a report of five cases. J Clin Endocrinol Metab. 1994;79(6):1540–5.
56. Allolio B, Fassnacht M. Clinical review: Adrenocortical carcinoma: clinical update. J Clin Endocrinol Metab. 2006;91(6):2027–37.
57. Wooten MD, King DK. Adrenal cortical carcinoma. Epidemiology and treatment with mitotane and a review of the literature. Cancer. 1993;72(11):3145–55.
58. Soon PS, McDonald KL, Robinson BG, Sidhu SB. Molecular markers and the pathogenesis of adrenocortical cancer. Oncologist. 2008;13(5):548–61.
59. Bharwani N, Rockall AG, Sahdev A, et al. Adrenocortical carcinoma: the range of appearances on CT and MRI. AJR Am J Roentgenol. 2011;196(6):W706–14.
60. Ferrozzi F, Bova D. CT and MR demonstration of fat within an adrenal cortical carcinoma. Abdom Imaging. 1995;20(3):272–4.
61. Hussain S, Belldegrun A, Seltzer SE, Richie JP, Gittes RF, Abrams HL. Differentiation of malignant from benign adrenal masses: predictive indices on computed tomography. AJR Am J Roentgenol. 1985;144(1):61–5.
62. Leite NP, Kased N, Hanna RF, et al. Cross-sectional imaging of extranodal involvement in abdominopelvic lymphoproliferative malignancies. Radiographics. 2007;27(6):1613–34.
63. Sohaib SA, Reznek RH. Adrenal imaging. BJU Int. 2000;86 Suppl 1:95–110.
64. Anis M, Irshad A. Imaging of abdominal lymphoma. Radiol Clin North Am. 2008;46(2):265–85, viii-ix.
65. Rashidi A, Fisher SI. Primary adrenal lymphoma: a systematic review. Ann Hematol. 2013;92(12):1583–93.
66. Hussain HK, Korobkin M. MR imaging of the adrenal glands. Magn Reson Imaging Clin N Am. 2004; 12(3):515–44, vii.
67. Abrams HL, Spiro R, Goldstein N. Metastases in carcinoma; analysis of 1000 autopsied cases. Cancer. 1950;3(1):74–85.
68. Boland GW, Blake MA, Hahn PF, Mayo-Smith WW. Incidental adrenal lesions: principles, techniques, and algorithms for imaging characterization. Radiology. 2008;249(3):756–75.
69. de Krijger RR, Papathomas TG. Adrenocortical neoplasia: evolving concepts in tumorigenesis with an emphasis on adrenal cortical carcinoma variants. Virchows Arch. 2012;460(1):9–18.
70. Tissier F. Classification of adrenal cortical tumors: what limits for the pathological approach? Best Pract Res Clin Endocrinol Metab. 2010;24(6):877–85.
71. McNicol AM. A diagnostic approach to adrenal cortical lesions. Endocr Pathol. 2008;19(4):241–51.
72. Weiss LM. Comparative histologic study of 43 metastasizing and nonmetastasizing adrenocortical tumors. Am J Surg Pathol. 1984;8(3):163–9.
73. Tischler AS. Pheochromocytoma and extra-adrenal paraganglioma: updates. Arch Pathol Lab Med. 2008;132(8):1272–84.
74. Thompson LD. Pheochromocytoma of the Adrenal gland Scaled Score (PASS) to separate benign from malignant neoplasms: a clinicopathologic and immunophenotypic study of 100 cases. Am J Surg Pathol. 2002;26(5):551–66.

75. Strong VE, Kennedy T, Al-Ahmadie H, et al. Prognostic indicators of malignancy in adrenal pheochromocytomas: clinical, histopathologic, and cell cycle/apoptosis gene expression analysis. Surgery. 2008;143(6):759–68.
76. Lonergan GJ, Schwab CM, Suarez ES, et al. Neuroblastoma, ganglioneuroblastoma, and ganglioneuroma: radiologic-pathologic correlation. Radiographics. 2002;22(4):911–34.
77. Wedmid A, Palese M. Diagnosis and treatment of the adrenal cyst. Curr Urol Rep. 2010;11(1):44–50.
78. Chien HP, Chang YS, Hsu PS, et al. Adrenal cystic lesions: a clinicopathological analysis of 25 cases with proposed histogenesis and review of the literature. Endocr Pathol. 2008;19(4):274–81.
79. Uppot RN, Gervais DA. Imaging-guided adrenal tumor ablation. AJR Am J Roentgenol. 2013;200(6):1226–33.
80. Mayo-Smith WW, Dupuy DE. Adrenal neoplasms: CT-guided radiofrequency ablation--preliminary results. Radiology. 2004;231(1):225–30.
81. Xiao YY, Tian JL, Li JK, Yang L, Zhang JS. CT-guided percutaneous chemical ablation of adrenal neoplasms. AJR Am J Roentgenol. 2008;190(1):105–10.
82. Lo WK, vansonnenberg E, Shankar S, et al. Percutaneous CT-guided radiofrequency ablation of symptomatic bilateral adrenal metastases in a single session. J Vasc Interv Radiol. 2006;17(1):175–9.
83. Atwell TD, Wass CT, Charboneau JW, Callstrom MR, Farrell MA, Sengupta S. Malignant hypertension during cryoablation of an adrenal gland tumor. J Vasc Interv Radiol. 2006;17(3):573–5.
84. Welch BT, Atwell TD, Nichols DA, et al. Percutaneous image-guided adrenal cryoablation: procedural considerations and technical success. Radiology. 2011; 258(1):301–7.
85. Wang Y, Liang P, Yu X, Cheng Z, Yu J, Dong J. Ultrasound-guided percutaneous microwave ablation of adrenal metastasis: preliminary results. Int J Hyperthermia. 2009;25(6):455–61.
86. Li X, Fan W, Zhang L, et al. CT-guided percutaneous microwave ablation of adrenal malignant carcinoma: preliminary results. Cancer. 2011;117(22):5182–8.
87. Park SY, Park BK, Kim CK. Sonographically guided transhepatic core biopsies of right renal and adrenal masses: safety and short-term follow-up. J Ultrasound Med. 2013;32(11):2013–21.
88. Miller BS, Doherty GM. Surgical management of adrenocortical tumours. Nat Rev Endocrinol. 2014; 10(5):282–92.
89. Micali S, Peluso G, De Stefani S, Celia A, Sighinolfi MC, Grande M, Bianchi G. Laparoscopic adrenal surgery: new frontiers. J Endourol. 2005;19(3):272–8.
90. Kuruba R, Gallagher SF. Current management of adrenal tumors. Curr Opin Oncol. 2008;20(1): 34–46.
91. Elfenbein DM, Scarborough JE, Speicher PJ, Scheri RP. Comparison of laparoscopic versus open adrenalectomy: results from American College of Surgeons-National Surgery Quality Improvement Project. J Surg Res. 2013;184(1):216–20.
92. Whittle DE, Schroeder D, Purchas SH, Sivakumaran P, Conaglen JV. Laparoscopic retroperitoneal left adrenalectomy in a patient with Cushing's syndrome. Aust N Z J Surg. 1994;64(5):375–6.
93. Shonkwiler RJ, Lee JA. Laparoscopic retroperitoneal adrenalectomy. Surg Laparosc Endosc Percutan Tech. 2011;21(4):243–7.
94. Park YH, Kang MY, Jeong MS, Choi H, Kim HH. Laparoendoscopic single-site nephrectomy using a homemade single-port device for single-system ectopic ureter in a child: initial case report. J Endourol. 2009;23(5):833–5.
95. Jeong CW, Park YH, Shin CS, Kim HH. Synchronous bilateral laparoendoscopic single-site adrenalectomy. J Endourol. 2010;24(8):1301–5.
96. Jeong BC, Park YH, Han DH, Kim HH. Laparoendoscopic single-site and conventional laparoscopic adrenalectomy: a matched case-control study. J Endourol. 2009;23(12):1957–60.
97. Lin CY, Yang CR, Cheng CL, Ho HC, Chiu KY, Su CK, Chen WM, Wang SS, Chen CS, Li JR, Yang CK, Ou YC. Application in robotic urologic surgery. J Chin Med Assoc. 2014;77(5):242–5.
98. Brandao LF, Autorino R, Zargar H, Krishnan J, Laydner H, Akca O, Mir MC, Samarasekera D, Stein R, Kaouk J. Robot-assisted Laparoscopic Adrenalectomy: Step-by-Step Technique and Comparative Outcomes. Eur Urol. 2014;66:898–905.

Retroperitoneal Tumors

6

Chang Kyu Sung, Bohyun Kim, Kyung Chul Moon, Ja Hyeon Ku, and Seung Beom Ha

6.1 Introduction

The retroperitoneum is a large compartmentalized space bounded anteriorly by the posterior parietal peritoneum and posteriorly by the transversalis fascia (Fig. 6.1). The abdominal retroperitoneum is divided by the fascial planes into three distinct compartments: the anterior pararenal, the perirenal, and the posterior pararenal spaces. The anterior and posterior pararenal spaces merge inferior to the level of the kidneys, which communicates inferiorly with the prevesical space and extraperitoneal compartments of the pelvis [1]. Retroperitoneal tumors represent a broad, diverse group of benign and malignant lesions, which may be primary or secondary in origin [2]. Primary tumors of the retroperitoneum develop independently from cells distinct from the major retroperitoneal organs such as the kidneys, adrenal glands, pancreas, colon and duodenum, and major blood vessels. The majority of retroperitoneal tumors arise from retroperitoneal organs and are therefore not considered primary retroperitoneal tumors [3].

Primary retroperitoneal tumors present a broad spectrum of pathologic entities and arise from actual tissues in the same space or from embryonic rests found therein [4]. Diagnosis of these tumors begins with affirmation of their retroperitoneal location and then determination of whether the lesion is primarily retroperitoneal or is arising secondarily from a retroperitoneal organ [5]. Primary retroperitoneal tumors can be further categorized into four main groups: mesodermal neoplasms; neurogenic tumors; germ cell, sex cord, and stromal tumors; and lymphoid neoplasms [5] (Table 6.1). When lymph nodes are regarded as a retroperitoneal organ, lymphoma is not considered a primary retroperitoneal tumor. Because of high incidence of retroperitoneal lymphadenopathy including metastases and lymphoma, the term primary retroperitoneal tumors should be considered after exclusion of lymphadenopathy and anatomic connection to any retroperitoneal organs.

Malignant retroperitoneal tumors account for approximately 0.1 % of all malignancies and are more common than benign tumors in

C.K. Sung (✉)
Department of Radiology, SMG-SNU Boramae Medical Center, Seoul National University College of Medicine, Seoul, Republic of Korea
e-mail: sckmd@daum.net

B. Kim (✉)
Department of Radiology, Mayo Clinic, Rochester, MN, USA
e-mail: kim.bohyun@mayo.edu

K.C. Moon
Department of Pathology, Seoul National University Hospital, Seoul National University College of Medicine, Seoul, Republic of Korea

J.H. Ku
Department of Urology, Seoul National University Hospital, Seoul National University College of Medicine, Seoul, Republic of Korea

S.B. Ha
Seoul Urology Group, Seoul, Republic of Korea

S.H. Kim, J.Y. Cho (eds.), *Oncologic Imaging: Urology*, DOI 10.1007/978-3-662-45218-9_6

the retroperitoneal space [6, 7]. Retroperitoneal sarcomas account for 90 % of mesodermal primary retroperitoneal malignancies, with liposarcoma, leiomyosarcoma, and malignant fibrous histiocytoma making up more than 80 % of these tumors [1, 8]. Retroperitoneal sarcomas have a peak incidence in the fifth and sixth decades of life and occur with equal frequency in males and females [8].

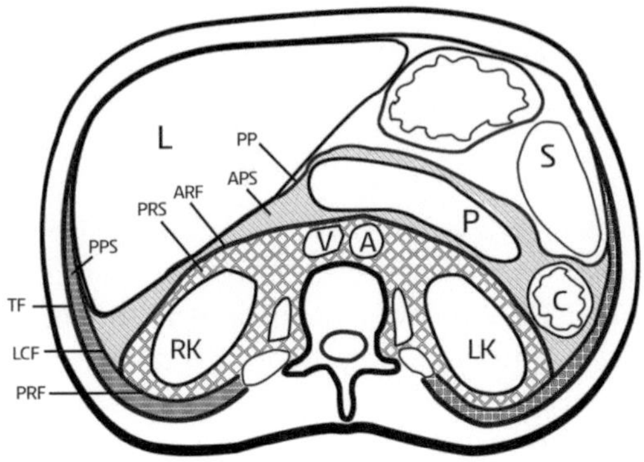

Fig. 6.1 Schematic diagram of retroperitoneal anatomy at the level of the kidneys. The retroperitoneum is subdivided into the three distinct compartments: the anterior pararenal (AP*S*), the perirenal (PRS), and the posterior pararenal (PPS) spaces. *A* aorta, *V* inferior vena cava, *P* pancreas, *S* spleen, *L* liver, *C* colon, *RK* right kidney, *LK* left kidney, *PP* parietal peritoneum, *ARF* anterior renal fascia, *LCF* lateroconal fascia, *PRF* posterior renal fascia, *TF* transversalis fascia

They usually reach a large size without producing symptoms. Therefore, they can present later in life with nonspecific symptoms such as abdominal pain and fullness and usually have poor prognosis. The 5-year survival rate of the patients including those with sarcoma was reportedly 22–50 % [9]. Therefore, it is important to diagnose retroperitoneal tumors as early as possible and discriminate the malignant from the benign tumors precisely in order to properly treat and to avoid unnecessary aggressive treatment for benign tumors. However, since the diagnostic imaging findings of these tumors are not specific for the histological diagnosis and even imaging-guided biopsy of large retroperitoneal tumors may not be conclusive, prediction of the definitive histological diagnosis remains a challenge [7, 10].

6.2 Diagnostic Evaluation

Cross-sectional imaging plays an important role in the characterization of these masses and in the evaluation of their extent, direct involvement of adjacent structures, and detection of distant metastases and therefore in treatment planning. It is also useful in guiding biopsy, planning surgery, evaluating response to treatment, restaging, and in the

Table 6.1 Classification of primary retroperitoneal tumors

Tissue of origin	Benign	Malignant
Mesodermal origin		
Adipocytic	Lipoma	Liposarcoma
Smooth muscle	Leiomyoma	Leiomyosarcoma
Skeletal muscle	Rhabdomyoma	Rhabdomyosarcoma
Fibroblastic	Fibroma	Fibrosarcoma
Vascular	Hemangioma Lymphangioma	Hemangioendothelioma
Nervous origin		
Nerve sheath	Schwannoma	Malignant peripheral nerve sheath tumor
Sympathetic nervous system	Neurofibroma	Ganglioneuroblastoma
Chromaffin/paraganglionic cells	Ganglioneuroma	Neuroblastoma
	Paraganglioma	Malignant paraganglioma
Germ cell, sex cord, and stromal cell origin		
Embryonic rests	Benign teratoma	Malignant teratoma
Notochord	Chordoma	
Embryonic hindgut	Tailgut cyst (retrorectal cystic hamartoma)	
Lymphoid origin		Lymphoma
Miscellaneous	Erdheim–Chester disease Castleman's disease	

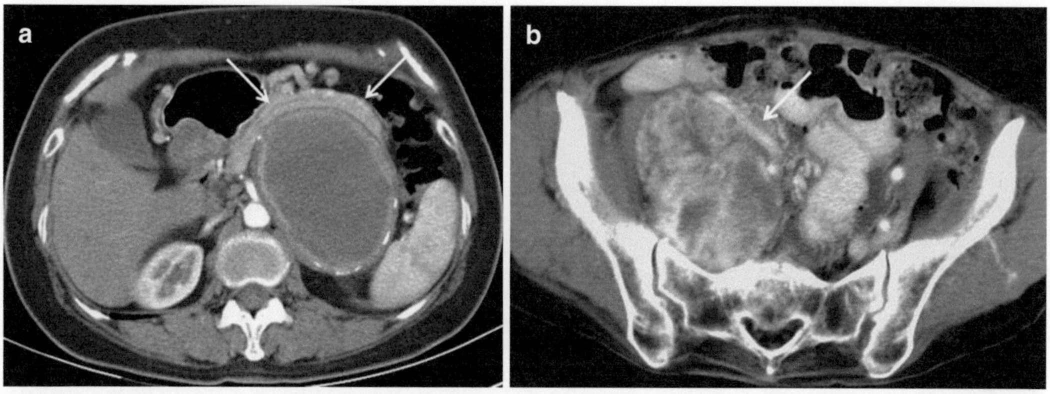

Fig. 6.2 Determining tumor location within the retroperitoneal space. (**a**) Anterior displacement of retroperitoneal structures such as pancreas (*arrows*) in this case of schwannoma suggests that the mass arises in the retroperitoneum. (**b**) Anteromedial displacement of right iliac vessels (*arrow*) by the mass (leiomyosarcoma) suggests that the mass arises in the retroperitoneum

long-term follow-up for local recurrence. An abdominopelvic computed tomography (CT) scan is the most commonly used modality for evaluating retroperitoneal disease, whereas magnetic resonance imaging (MRI) is more often used as a problem-solving tool. In most cases, CT is less sensitive to motion artifact than MRI, and it better defines the anatomic relationship of the tumor to other abdominal organs. CT provides superior spatial resolution and detection of calcification, while MRI has superior soft tissue contrast and capabilities in the detection of fat within a lesion. MRI has advantage in assessing fat or hemorrhage and is particularly useful in differentiating solid from nonenhancing cystic or necrotic lesions and in evaluating the extent of disease and the presence and nature of vascular thrombosis or encasement [11].

In order to classify a mass as primary retroperitoneal, the location should be determined as within the retroperitoneal space and an organ of origin is excluded. Displacement of normal retroperitoneal organs or large vessels in the space strongly suggests that a mass is retroperitoneal in location (Fig. 6.2) [3]. Several radiological signs have been described to assist in determining the organ of origin. They include claw or beak sign, invisible or phantom organ sign, and embedded organ sign (Fig. 6.3) [3, 12, 13]. The claw or beak sign is positive when a mass causes the edge of an adjacent organ into a beak shape, meaning that the mass originates from that organ. Conversely, if a mass originates from a structure adjacent to the organ, it will form obtuse angles to abut and compress the organ. The invisible or phantom organ sign is positive when a large mass arises from a small organ that then becomes undetectable. The embedded organ sign is positive when a mass that arises from a given organ often appears embedded within it and the interface between the two may be difficult to appreciate [3]. Conversely, a mass that abuts but does not originate from a hollow structure compresses it and produces a crescentic deformity. Rounded rather than beaked edges of an adjacent organ (negative beak sign) with a crescentic deformation (negative embedded organ sign) by the tumor suggest a primary retroperitoneal tumor [3].

Location, size, and anatomical changes secondary to tumor growth are easily visualized, and tumor invasion of adjacent organs can be demonstrated or suggested on cross-sectional imaging. Although there are significant overlaps in the imaging characteristics of retroperitoneal tumors, the radiographic appearances can offer clues as to the histologic subtype and grade, which may guide decisions. Some lesions have distinctive characteristics and can be diagnosed with some accuracy on imaging. It is also possible to narrow the differential diagnosis of a retroperitoneal mass based on certain imaging characteristics in combination with the pattern of involvement and demographics [5].

If fatty components are obvious, a diagnosis of liposarcoma is possible, but differentiation

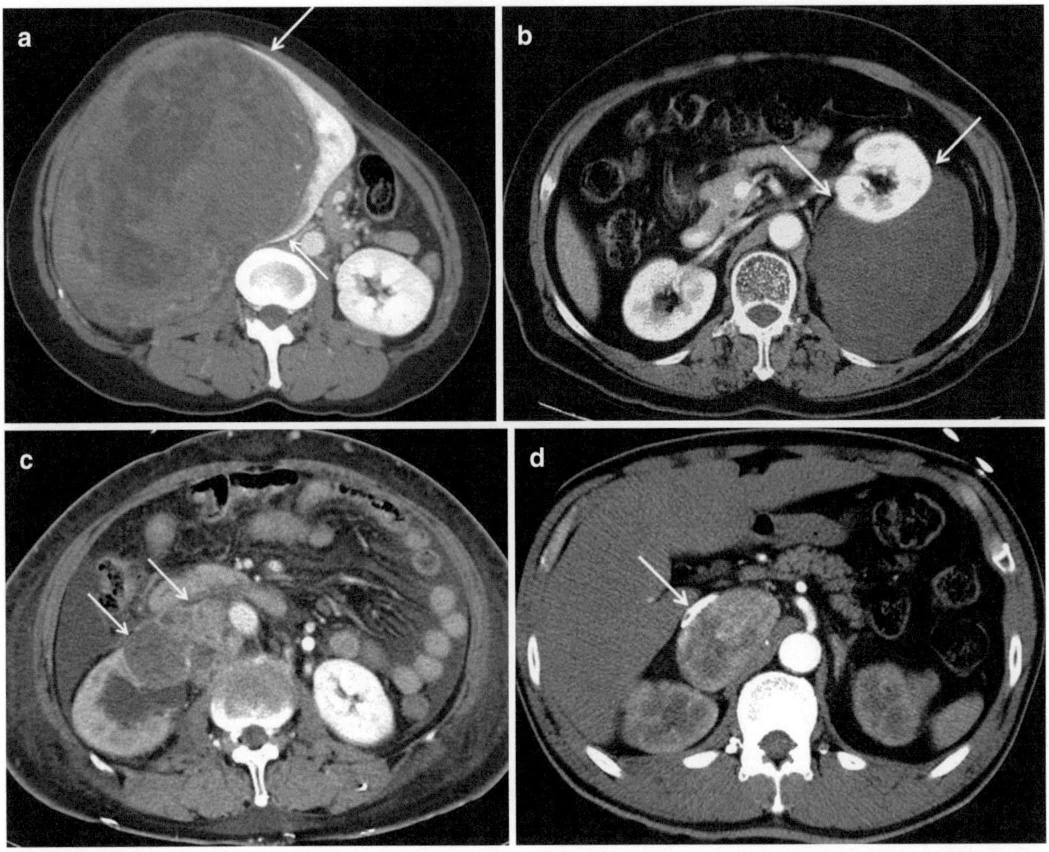

Fig. 6.3 Determining origin of the mass. (**a**) Positive beak sign: a large mass causes the edge of the kidney to become beak shaped (*arrows*), meaning that the lesion originates from the kidney and is not primary retroperitoneal tumor. The mass was confirmed as renal cell carcinoma. (**b**) Negative beak sign: a large low-density mass abuts left kidney with dull edge (*arrows*), meaning that the mass originates from adjacent to left kidney. The mass was confirmed as leiomyosarcoma. (**c**) Positive invisible or phantom organ sign: a heterogeneous mass (*arrows*) that was confirmed as leiomyosarcoma is located between the right kidney and abdominal aorta. The tumor's originating organ (inferior vena cava) appears totally incorporated by the tumor at this level and is no longer recognizable. (**d**) Negative embedded organ sign: the wall of inferior vena cava is compressed extrinsically from the tumor creating a crescent shape (*arrow*), meaning that the lesion does not originate from the IVC. The mass was confirmed as right adrenal pheochromocytoma

from a benign lipoma can be difficult. Cross-sectional imaging cannot reliably distinguish between retroperitoneal lymphomas and sarcomas: although lymphomas tend to be homogeneous on imaging and often envelope the inferior vena cava and aorta, while sarcomas are usually heterogeneous, these findings are unreliable. Imaging evidence of tumor necrosis suggests a high-grade component and portends a poor prognosis [14]. In general, extensive vascular involvement, peritoneal implants, and distant metastatic disease suggest unresectability.

Histological confirmation is required for diagnosis in many cases of primary retroperitoneal sarcomas because of overlap of imaging features and for tumor grading. However, when the diagnosis seems straightforward, preoperative tissue diagnosis is not necessary if surgery is planned to be the primary therapeutic intervention. Percutaneous biopsy can be a safe method in providing a tissue diagnosis for a locally advanced or unresectable lesion. Retroperitoneal biopsies can be safely performed under CT or US guidance. Imaging helps to identify and to guide specific targeted biopsy from the enhancing or soft tissue component of the mass, which is more likely to be the more aggressive component of the mass.

6.3 Tumors of Mesodermal Origin

Most of the primary retroperitoneal tumors are of mesodermal origin with liposarcoma, leiomyosarcoma, and malignant fibrous histiocytoma together, making up more than 80 % of primary retroperitoneal sarcomas [1, 15]. Historically, undifferentiated/unclassified soft tissue sarcomas are new terminology that replace or include the older term "malignant fibrous histiocytoma (MFH)" [16, 17]. The remaining primary retroperitoneal masses arise predominantly from the nervous system. Among children, the most common histologic types of retroperitoneal sarcomas are rhabdomyosarcoma and fibrosarcoma [18].

Retroperitoneal sarcomas typically present in the sixth and seventh decades of life and are often large at the time of clinical presentation because the loose connective tissue in the retroperitoneum provides little resistance to their growth [1]. Surgical resection is the only potentially curative treatment for a localized retroperitoneal sarcoma. The ability to perform a complete surgical resection at the time of initial presentation is the most important independent prognostic factor for survival followed only by histologic grade [5, 19–21]. The usual reasons for unresectability are extensive vascular involvement or the presence of multiple peritoneal implants. Overall, regional lymphadenopathy is uncommon in soft tissue sarcomas, with a frequency of less than 4 % at presentation, and less than one-third of patients have metastases at presentation [21]. The recurrence rates are high, and metastases to the liver, lung, bones, and brain may be seen [8, 22].

6.3.1 Liposarcoma

Liposarcoma is the most common (33 %) sarcoma to occur in the retroperitoneum [22]. Retroperitoneal liposarcomas account for 10–15 % of all liposarcomas, and they are more common in the 50–70-year age group, with no sex predilection [1, 22]. They are classified histologically into four main subtypes: atypical lipomatous tumor/well differentiated, dedifferentiated, myxoid, and pleomorphic (Fig. 6.4) [15, 23]. Different histological subtypes may coexist in the same lesion. Such histological subtypes are usually classified on the basis of the most aggressive cellular component. The fourth edition of the World Health Organization (WHO) Classification of Tumors of Soft Tissue and Bone was published in February 2013 [16]. The changes for adipocytic tumors in the fourth edition were the removal of the terms "round cell liposarcoma" and "mixed-type liposarcoma" [16, 17]. While the section heading lists only "atypical lipomatous tumor" on the recent WHO classification, the authors point out that retention of "well-differentiated liposarcoma" is still appropriate for tumors in sites at which margin-negative resection is often impossible (e.g., retroperitoneum, mediastinum), since such tumors are associated with substantial mortality [17]. The terminology "atypical lipomatous tumor" and "well-differentiated liposarcoma" continues to need clarification [17].

Liposarcoma is usually large (average diameter, >20 cm) and is a slow-growing tumor [1]. In general, liposarcomas may be distinguished based on the presence of fat, which varies depending on the subtype [1, 24]. The well-differentiated subtype is low-grade tumor and the most common type of retroperitoneal liposarcoma [1, 22]. The fact that well-differentiated liposarcoma shows no potential for metastasis unless it undergoes dedifferentiation led, in the late 1970s, to the introduction of terms such as atypical lipoma or atypical lipomatous tumor, particularly for lesions arising at surgically amenable locations in the limbs and on the trunk since, at these sites, wide excision should usually be curative, and hence the designation "sarcoma" is not warranted [25]. However, in sites such as the retroperitoneum and mediastinum, it is commonly impossible to obtain a wide surgical excision margin, and, in such cases, local recurrence is almost inevitable and often leads to death, even in the absence of dedifferentiation and metastasis – hence, at these sites, retention of the

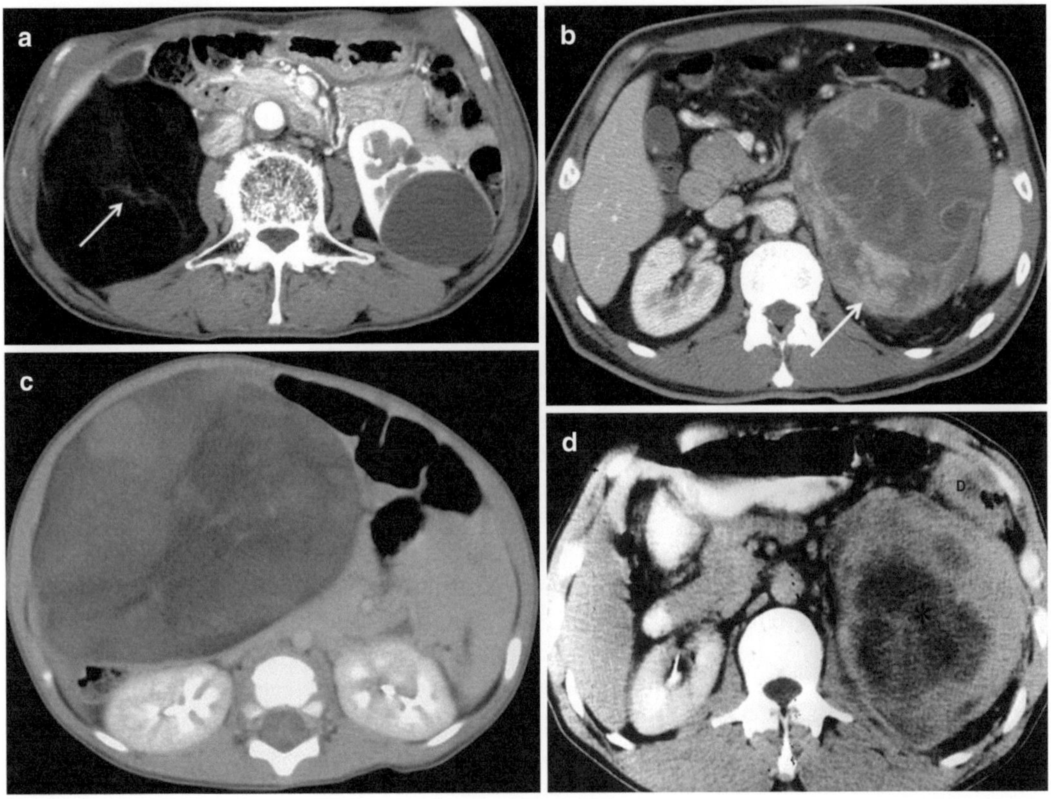

Fig. 6.4 Liposarcoma with four histologic types on postcontrast CT images. (**a**) Well-differentiated liposarcoma in a 79-year-old man is shown as a large homogeneous fat-containing mass with thick septa (*arrow*) in right perirenal space with superior displacement of the right kidney (not shown). (**b**) Dedifferentiated liposarcoma in a 58-year-old man is shown as a large well-marginated mass with heterogeneous attenuation and enhancing septa and soft tissue components (*arrow*). (**c**) Myxoid liposarcoma in a 1-year-old man is shown as a heterogeneous hypoattenuating mass with ground-glass appearance. (**d**) Pleomorphic liposarcoma in a 58-year-old man is shown as a large solid soft tissue mass with internal necrosis and no fatty component

term well-differentiated liposarcoma can readily be justified [17, 26].

Well-differentiated liposarcomas are predominantly hypoattenuating lesion with fat attenuation on CT images and typically round or lobulated with smooth margin and may displace or surround local structures (Fig. 6.4a). The fat content in the mass demonstrates high signal intensity on T1-weighted images and intermediate signal intensity on T2-weighted images, with loss of signal on fat-suppressed images. The macroscopic fat content may be greater than 75 %, and these lesions must be distinguished from other fat-containing neoplasms which may occur in the retroperitoneum, such as lipoma, adrenal myelolipoma, renal angiomyolipoma, and teratoma [27]. Retroperitoneal lipomas are fat-containing lesions that do not have any associated soft tissue component or nodularity. Although the appearance of well-differentiated liposarcoma may be similar to that of a lipoma, this subtype frequently has thicker, irregular, and nodular septa that show enhancement after contrast material administration [28]. Calcification or ossification is rare and considered a poor prognostic feature, which often indicates dedifferentiation [3]. Well-differentiated tumors can recur but do not metastasize [1].

Dedifferentiated liposarcomas are high-grade tumors with poor prognosis [29]. This subtype is defined by the presence of sharply demarcated regions of non-lipogenic sarcomatous tissue within

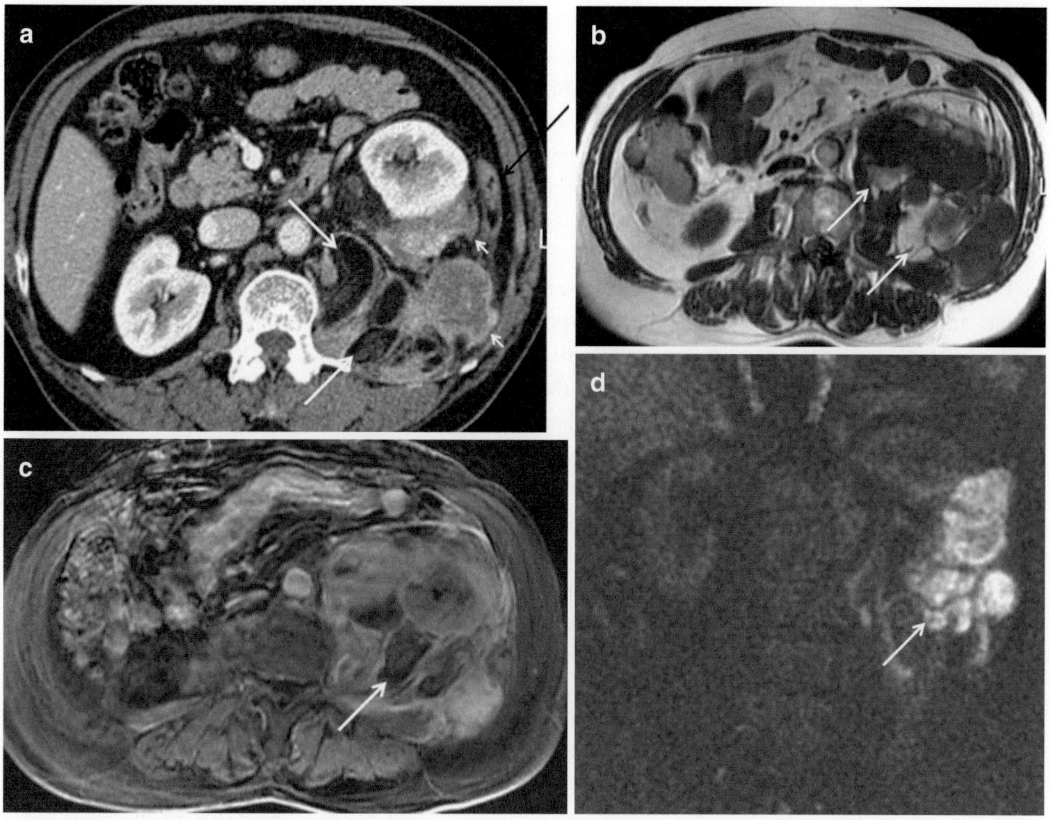

Fig. 6.5 Dedifferentiated liposarcoma in a 63-year-old man. (**a**) Contrast-enhanced axial CT demonstrates a poorly marginated and markedly heterogeneous mass with fatty component (*arrows*) and enhancing nonadipose solid-appearing regions (*small arrows*) in left retroperitoneal space. The tumor invades into left psoas and quadratus lumborum muscles medially and displaces the left kidney and descending colon (*black arrow*) anteriorly. (**b**) T1-weighted axial image shows fat component (*arrows*) with hyperintensity in the mass. (**c**) T1-weighted fat-suppressed gadolinium-enhanced MRI demonstrates reduction of the signal intensity at the fat component (*arrow*) and significant enhancement at the nonadipose solid component of the mass. (**d**) Diffusion-weighted imaging shows hyperintense signal (*arrow*) within the solid component of the mass

a well-differentiated tumor [16]. At CT and MR imaging, these dedifferentiated tumors appear as more heterogeneous tumors with both fat and solid components (Figs. 6.4b and 6.5) [1]. There may be no evidence of fat in up to 20 %, which makes the diagnosis difficult based on imaging alone [28]. Calcification is seen in as many as 30 % of these tumors and is an important sign of dedifferentiation [1, 30]. Variable signal intensity and enhancement of the solid portion may be seen [30].

Myxoid liposarcoma is of intermediate-grade malignancy and the second most common subtype of liposarcoma, accounting for more than one-third of liposarcomas and representing about 10 % of all adult soft tissue sarcomas. The lesions formerly known as round cell liposarcoma are interpreted as histologic continuum with myxoid subtype and are included in this category. This subtype shows a heterogeneous hypoattenuating mass, with attenuation less than that of muscle at CT (Fig. 6.4c). Homogeneous distribution of fat and soft tissue within the mass may result in a "pseudocystic" appearance, near fluid density, on non-contrast scan [15]. They characteristically show gradual, heterogeneous enhancement [15]. There is no macroscopic fat in over 50 % and calcifications are uncommon [28]. At MR imaging, there is low signal intensity on T1-weighted images and high signal intensity on T2-weighted images because of the mucopolysaccharide contents in the myxoid matrix [1]. Lacy, linear, or amorphous areas of high signal intensity on T1-weighted images and intermediate signal intensity on T2-weighted images may be seen because of the intratumoral fat content [1]. They demonstrate slowly progressive, reticular contrast enhancement due to solid components, which enables differentiation from a cyst [31].

Pleomorphic liposarcomas are high-grade sarcomas and the least common histologic subtype. This subtype tends to occur in the extremities (lower > upper limbs), whereas the trunk and the retroperitoneum are less frequently affected. They are seen as heterogeneous soft tissue masses with little or no fat within and may contain areas of necrosis that are indistinguishable from other solid tumors (Fig. 6.4d) [1]. Calcifications are rare.

Local recurrence after resection is the most common cause of relapse and is usually seen within 2 years. Recurrent liposarcomas may be difficult to differentiate from retroperitoneal fat, but recurrent tumors frequently have a slightly higher attenuation than the surrounding fat [13]. Recurrent liposarcomas often have a different appearance from the primary tumor and in many cases may not contain any visible fat.

6.3.2 Leiomyosarcoma

Leiomyosarcomas are the second most common primary retroperitoneal sarcoma, accounting for 28 % of all cases [22]. They arise from smooth muscle elements within the retroperitoneal muscle tissue, blood vessels, or Wolffian duct remnants [1, 19]. Leiomyosarcoma is more common in women, in the fifth to sixth decades of life [32]. They can grow to a large size (>10 cm) before compromising adjacent organs and precipitating clinical symptoms such as venous thrombosis [1]. Histopathologically, this tumor has large areas of necrosis and cystic degeneration, but calcification is uncommon [1]. They are large, well-circumscribed masses, which is isoattenuating to muscle on CT scan (Fig. 6.6). Contrast enhancement is often heterogeneous and predominantly peripheral. Small tumors may be homogeneously solid, but large tumors have extensive areas of low attenuation and represent necrosis and cystic degeneration. Rarely, leiomyosarcoma may appear as mostly cystic. At MR imaging, these tumors have intermediate to low signal intensity on T1-weighted images and intermediate to high signal intensity on T2-weighted images, depending on the amount of necrosis [1]. Mixed signal intensity and a fluid–debris level can be seen in hemorrhagic lesions [1]. The presence of extensive necrosis in a retroperitoneal mass, with contiguous involvement of a vessel, is highly suggestive of leiomyosarcoma [1]. Metastasis to the liver, lungs, or lymph nodes occurs late in the course of the disease [22, 32].

6.3.3 Undifferentiated/Unclassified Sarcoma

This new category in the 2013 WHO classification, which may comprise up to 20 % of all pleomorphic soft tissue sarcomas [33], encompasses tumors in which all recognizable lines of differentiation have been excluded. Many of these tumors would have been called MFH in the past. Since MFH was first described as a distinct histologic type of soft tissue sarcomas in 1964, large series of cases were reported [34, 35]. However, MFH has been plagued by controversy in terms of both its histogenesis and its validity as a clinicopathologic entity. Many pathologists recognized that most so-called MFH located in the retroperitoneum were dedifferentiated liposarcomas and only a few cases may be classified as undifferentiated pleomorphic sarcoma [35]. The latest WHO classification no longer includes MFH as a distinct diagnostic category but rather as subtypes of an undifferentiated/unclassified sarcoma [16, 17]. These tumors are typically high grade, show a wide range of morphological features, and are often associated with a poor prognosis. These tumors can be subclassified according to predominant morphological patterns: round cell, spindle cell, pleomorphic, and epithelioid. Undifferentiated sarcoma, formerly known as MFH, is the third most common sarcoma in the retroperitoneal space and has been regarded as the most common soft tissue sarcoma in the whole body [1].

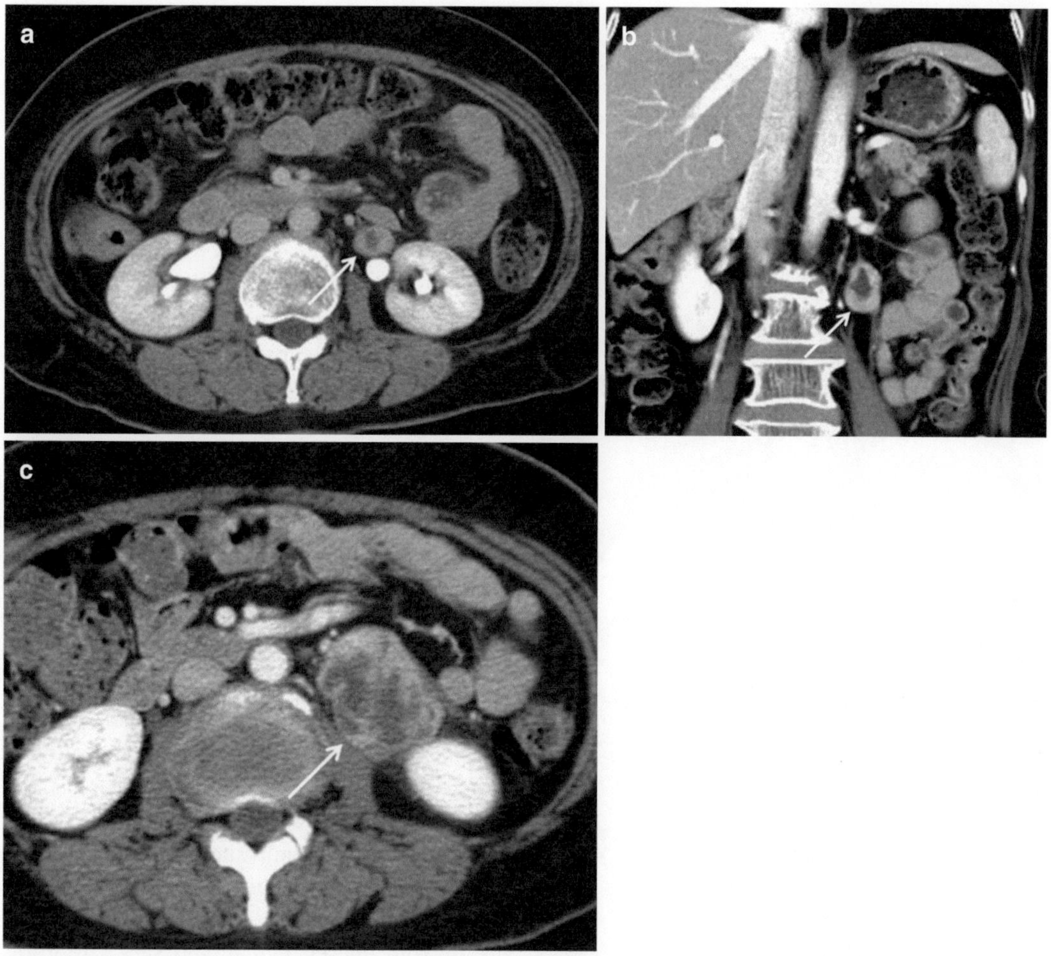

Fig. 6.6 Leiomyosarcoma in a 55-year-old woman. (**a**, **b**) Axial and coronal reformatted contrast-enhanced CT images incidentally discovered a solid-enhancing mass (*arrows*) containing internal cystic portion in left perirenal space. At that time, neurogenic tumor including neurilemmoma or paraganglioma was proposed as a radiological diagnosis. (**c**) After 7 months, the follow-up CT shows marked interval increase in size of the mass (*arrow*) with more heterogeneous enhancement and internal nonenhancing areas. Pathological examination after surgical resection confirmed leiomyosarcoma

CT and MRI findings of the MFH were nonspecific and demonstrated a large, infiltrating, and heterogeneously enhancing soft tissue mass with areas of necrosis and hemorrhage and with possible invasion of adjacent organs (Fig. 6.7). Variable patterns of calcification can be seen (7–20 % of cases) in the peripheral portions of these tumors [1]. The presence of calcification may help to distinguish MFH from leiomyosarcoma [22]. The changes or controversial application in terminology and classification has represented a source of potential diagnostic confusion. Imaging interpretation should be updated with the latest pathological classification to reach the more specific diagnosis in predicting the histological type or grade of retroperitoneal tumors.

6.3.4 Solitary Fibrous Tumor

Visceral pleura is the most common site of solitary fibrous tumor occurrence, but it can occur outside of the thoracic cavity. Retroperitoneal solitary fibrous tumors are rare, and their clinical manifestations depend on the location and size of the tumor. They grow slowly in an expansive way

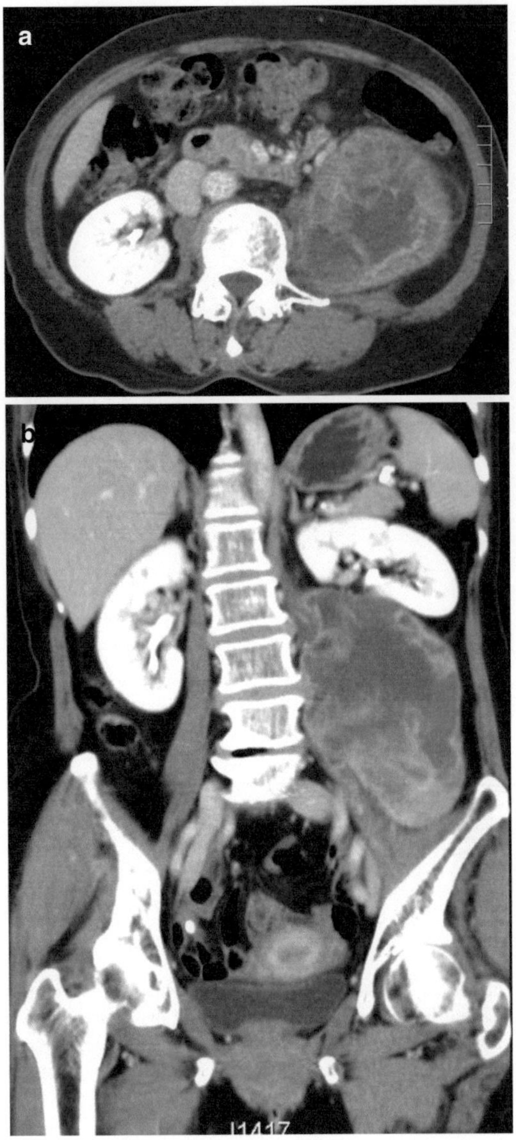

Fig. 6.7 Undifferentiated pleomorphic sarcoma in a 36-year-old woman. Contrast-enhanced CT ((**a**), axial; (**b**), coronal reformatted) shows a large well-circumscribed heterogeneous mass with internal necrotic areas at left retroperitoneal space. Direct tumor invasion of adjacent muscles, including the psoas and quadratus lumborum muscles, is shown, and the left kidney is displaced superiorly

and displace adjacent structures by compression. For extrapleural solitary fibrous tumor, there is now complete omission of the prior synonym "hemangiopericytoma" according to the WHO classification of soft tissue tumors [16, 17].

The retroperitoneal solitary fibrous tumors were mostly lobulated and large, in round or oval shape (Fig. 6.8). Myxoid degeneration, hemorrhage, and necrosis may be visible, especially in huge masses; the tumor density or signal intensity became more heterogeneous on imaging. Rarely, some may have calcification. Most retroperitoneal solitary fibrous tumors show moderate or intense enhancement. Complete surgical resection is the standard therapy for solitary fibrous tumor, and pathologically negative resection margins are important to achieve a good prognosis.

6.3.5 Less Common Sarcomas

Rhabdomyosarcoma is the most common soft tissue sarcoma in children. The tumor is believed to arise from primitive muscle cells, but tumors can occur anywhere in the body. The retroperitoneum is involved in 7 % of cases diagnosed with rhabdomyosarcoma [36]. Cross-sectional imaging shows a mass with heterogeneous attenuation or signal intensity, focal calcifications, necrosis, and significant contrast enhancement.

Extraskeletal chondrosarcoma in retroperitoneum is very rare. The histologic types of lesions that account for extraskeletal chondrosarcoma are myxoid, mesenchymal, and very rarely low grade [37]. On CT and MR images, both myxoid and mesenchymal chondrosarcomas have features similar to those described for tumors of these histologic types located in bone [37]. Imaging of these lesions demonstrates a nonspecific soft tissue mass with areas of chondroid matrix mineralization, which may be seen as ring- and arc-like, stippled, and highly opaque calcifications (Fig. 6.9).

Extraskeletal osteosarcoma is a rare malignant mesenchymal tumor characterized by the direct production of osteoid or bone by tumor cells without primary bone or periosteal involvement. The most common location of these tumors is the lower extremity, especially the thigh, followed by the upper extremity and the retroperitoneum [38]. Imaging shows a large soft tissue with areas of amorphous calcifications, necrosis, or old hemorrhage (Fig. 6.10). The imaging findings of

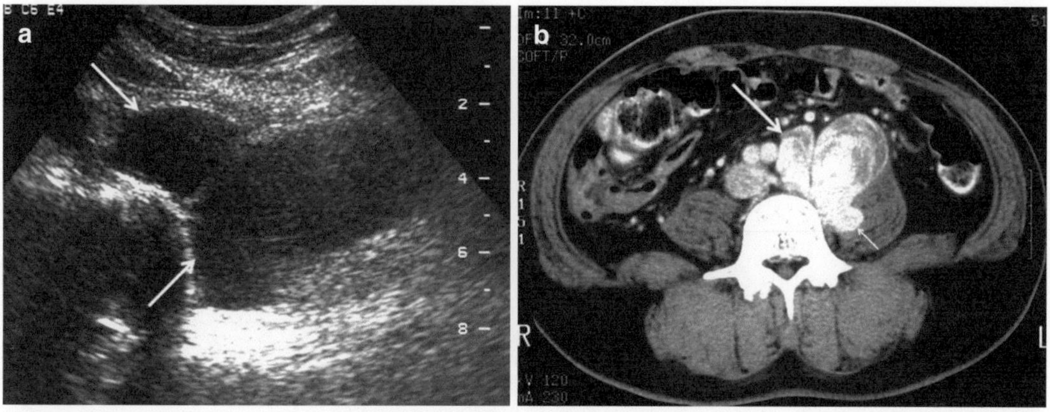

Fig. 6.8 Solitary fibrous tumor in a 46-year-old man. (**a**) Transabdominal sonogram shows a large, lobulated mass (*arrows*) at left paravertebral region. (**b**) Contrast-enhanced axial CT at aortic bifurcation level demonstrates a large, lobulated mass (*arrow*) with intense enhancement at left anterior paravertebral region. Note direct tumor invasion into the adjacent left psoas muscle (*small arrow*)

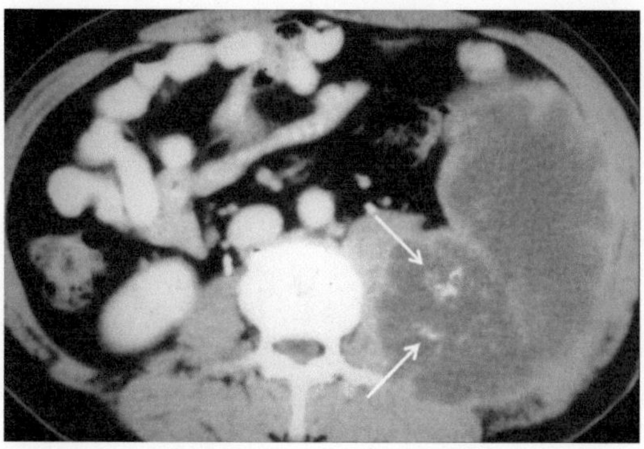

Fig. 6.9 Extraskeletal chondrosarcoma in retroperitoneum in a 51-year-old man. Contrast-enhanced CT scan of the abdomen shows a large soft tissue mass in the left retroperitoneum with invasion of the left psoas muscle. Note punctate or stippled calcifications (*arrows*) in the mass

extraskeletal osteosarcoma are nonspecific, with considerable overlap with other retroperitoneal masses. A wide range of differential diagnoses include several benign and malignant conditions that show mineralization, which include nontumoral benign conditions such as calcified hematoma or myositis ossificans and numerous benign and malignant retroperitoneal tumors.

6.4 Tumors of Neurogenic Origin

Neurogenic tumors constitute 10–20 % of primary retroperitoneal tumors in adult [1]. Compared with the tumors of mesodermal origin, they are generally benign, occur in a younger population, and have a better prognosis [1]. They are classified according to their cells of origin. They can originate from the nerve sheaths (schwannoma, neurofibroma, neurofibromatosis, malignant nerve sheath tumors), sympathetic nerves/ganglionic cells (ganglioneuroma, ganglioneuroblastoma, neuroblastoma), or chromaffin/paraganglionic cells (paraganglioma, pheochromocytoma). They are seen commonly along the sympathetic ganglia, which are located in the paraspinal region, and in the adrenal medulla or the organs of Zuckerkandl (para-aortic bodies) [1]. Less commonly, they occur in other sites, such as the urinary bladder, abdominal wall, bowel wall, or gallbladder [1, 39]. Neuroblastoma and ganglioneuroblastoma are malignancies of childhood and are very rare in adults [15].

6.4.1 Schwannoma

Schwannoma, also known as neurilemmoma, is the most common retroperitoneal neurogenic tumor and accounts for 4 % of all retroperitoneal tumors [5]. It is a solitary, slow-growing benign tumor that arises from peripheral nerve sheath and is usually located in the paravertebral or presacral region. Pathologically, it appears as a rounded or

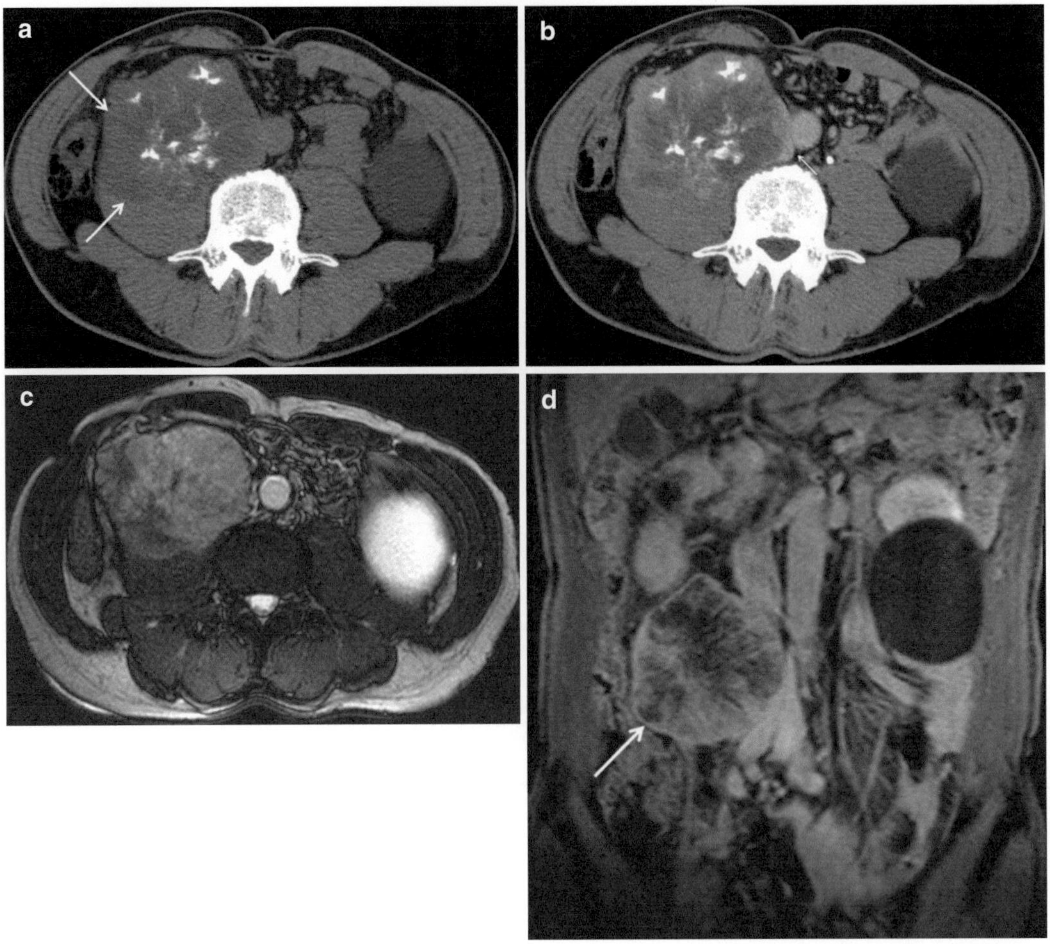

Fig. 6.10 Extraskeletal osteosarcoma in a 64-year-old man. (**a**, **b**) Precontrast (**a**) and post-contrast (**b**) axial CT images show a well-defined soft tissue mass (*arrow*) at right retroperitoneum with abutting the right psoas muscle and ICV (*arrowheads*). Multiple amorphous calcifications are seen in the mass. (**c**) Axial T2-weighted MR images show heterogeneously hyperintense mass. (**d**) Coronal T1-weighted fat-suppressed MR images after administration of contrast material shows avid contrast enhancement with radiating pattern in the mass (*arrow*). The mass compresses infrarenal IVC without invasion. Right ureter was also compressed by the mass, with resultant obstructive hydronephrosis

oval mass and is well encapsulated and extends along the course of a nerve, with the nerve of origin flattened against the periphery of the tumor [1]. Microscopically, it consists of two different components (Antoni A and Antoni B). Antoni A area is highly cellular, while Antoni B area is less cellular, with cystic and edematous area. At MR imaging, highly cellular areas are hypointense on T1- and T2-weighted images, while cystic and edematous areas appear hyperintense on T2-weighted images. Small schwannomas may be seen as round, well-circumscribed, and homogeneous masses, but large schwannomas have a heterogeneous appearance and are more likely to undergo degenerative changes (hemorrhage, necrosis or cystic changes, calcification, and hyalinization) (Fig. 6.11). Contrast enhancement is heterogeneous, with nonenhancing cystic components and enhancing solid components [1]. Malignant transformation rarely occurs [1, 40].

6.4.2 Neurofibroma

Neurofibroma is a benign nerve sheath tumor that can occur as an isolated tumor (90 %) or as part of

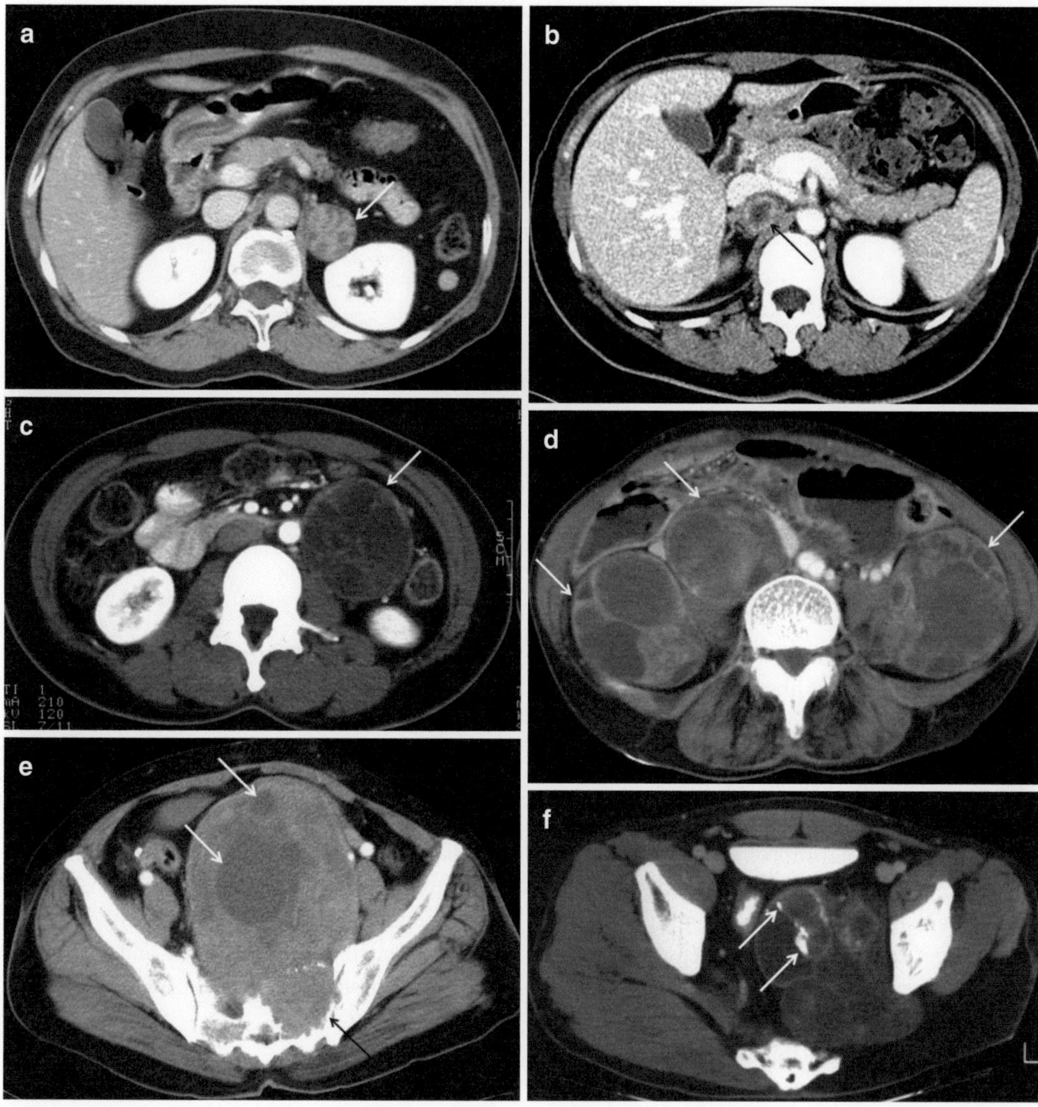

Fig. 6.11 Schwannoma: various patterns on axial contrast-enhanced CT images. (**a**) A small schwannoma in a 58-year-old woman is seen as a round, well-circumscribed solid mass (*arrow*) with slightly inhomogeneous enhancement at left retroperitoneal space of the periadrenal region. (**b**) Another case of small schwannoma in a 31-year-old woman is seen as an oval, well-circumscribed solid mass (*arrow*) with internal nonenhancing portion at retrocaval region. (**c**) A schwannoma in a 34-year-old woman is shown as a well-defined round mass (*arrow*) at left para-aortic region. The mass is seen to be predominantly cystic with septations. (**d**) Multiple schwannomas in a 6x-year-old woman are seen as bilateral retroperitoneal soft tissue masses (*arrows*) with prominent cystic degeneration. (**e**) A large schwannoma in a 54-year-old woman is seen as a heterogeneous presacral mass with internal cystic or necrotic changes (*arrows*) and neural foraminal widening and bone destruction (*black arrows*). (**f**) A benign schwannoma in a 48-year-old man demonstrates a multiloculated cystic mass with several septal calcifications (*arrows*) and extending into the left gluteal region through the greater sciatic foramen

type 1 neurofibromatosis [1]. Approximately one-third of patients with a solitary neurofibroma are associated with type 1 neurofibromatosis, and almost every patient with multiple tumors or plexiform neurofibromas has type 1 neurofibromatosis [39]. Neurofibroma is more common in men, particularly in the 20–40-year age group [39]. Histopathologically, neurofibroma is an unencapsulated solid tumor that is composed of nerve sheath cells and collagen bundles with variable

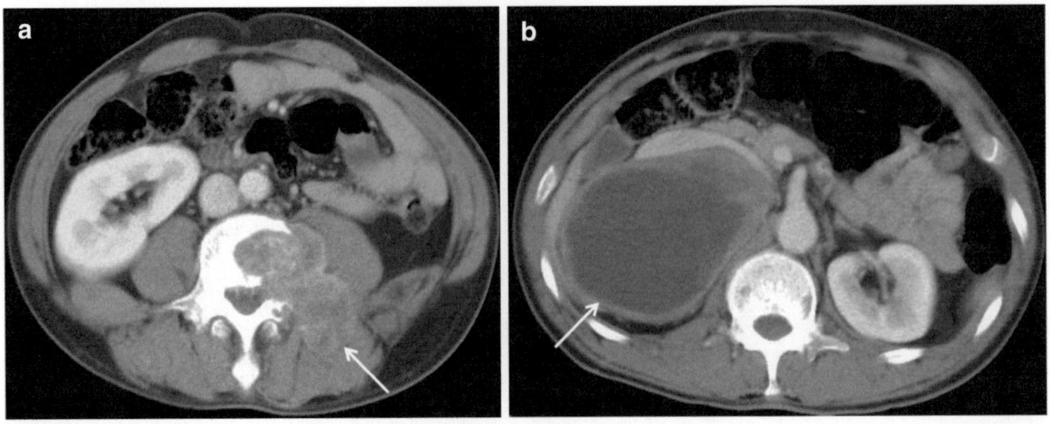

Fig. 6.12 Malignant peripheral nerve sheath tumor in a 44-year-old man. (**a**) Axial contrast-enhanced CT image shows a heterogeneously enhancing soft tissue mass (*arrow*) destroying left side of the vertebral body, pedicle, and transverse process with invasion of the neighboring paraspinal muscle. (**b**) Another mass (*arrow*) with predominantly cystic appearance is seen at right retroperitoneal space with anterior displacement of the inferior vena cava by the mass

myxoid degeneration and causes expansion of the entire nerve, with nerve fibers traversing the tumor [1]. Cystic degeneration is rare. Plexiform neurofibroma is seen as a large extensive infiltrating mass and is commonly located in the lumbosacral plexus.

On imaging, neurofibroma is depicted as a well-defined, rounded mass with homogeneous contrast enhancement. Occasionally, it demonstrate target-like enhancement representing the center of nerve tissue and the periphery of myxoid degeneration. On T1-weighted images, the central portion of the tumor has higher signal intensity that is due to neural tissue, and on T2-weighted images, the periphery has higher signal intensity that is due to myxoid degeneration [1]. Tumors involving the neural foramina may show a "dumbbell" shape with widening of the bony foramina or vertebral body scalloping.

6.4.3 Malignant Peripheral Nerve Sheath Tumor

Malignant peripheral nerve sheath tumors include malignant schwannoma, neurogenic sarcoma, and neurofibrosarcoma [1]. Fifty percent of these tumors originate de novo, and the rest of them are derived from neurofibroma or ganglioneuroma or occur after exposure to radiation [39]. These are highly aggressive and infiltrative tumors, may present with distant metastases, and demonstrate high recurrence rate. They may be clinically asymptomatic, but progressive enlargement and pain can be suggestive of malignancy, especially when associated with type 1 neurofibromatosis. Although imaging is not reliable in differentiating between benign and malignant tumors, a heterogeneous nature, irregular or infiltrative borders with invasion into adjacent tissues and destruction of adjacent bones can be helpful for detecting malignancy (Fig. 6.12).

6.4.4 Ganglioneuroma

Ganglioneuroma is a rare benign tumor that arises from the sympathetic ganglia. It is usually asymptomatic; however, approximately 57 % of ganglioneuromas may be functional and produce catecholamines or androgenic hormones [41]. In the retroperitoneum, the tumor is commonly seen along the paravertebral sympathetic ganglia (59 % of cases) or, less commonly, in the adrenal medulla [1].

This tumor appears as a well-circumscribed, longitudinally oriented, paravertebral soft tissue mass that may surround major blood vessels without compressing their lumen, usually do not result in osseous changes, and only infrequently extend

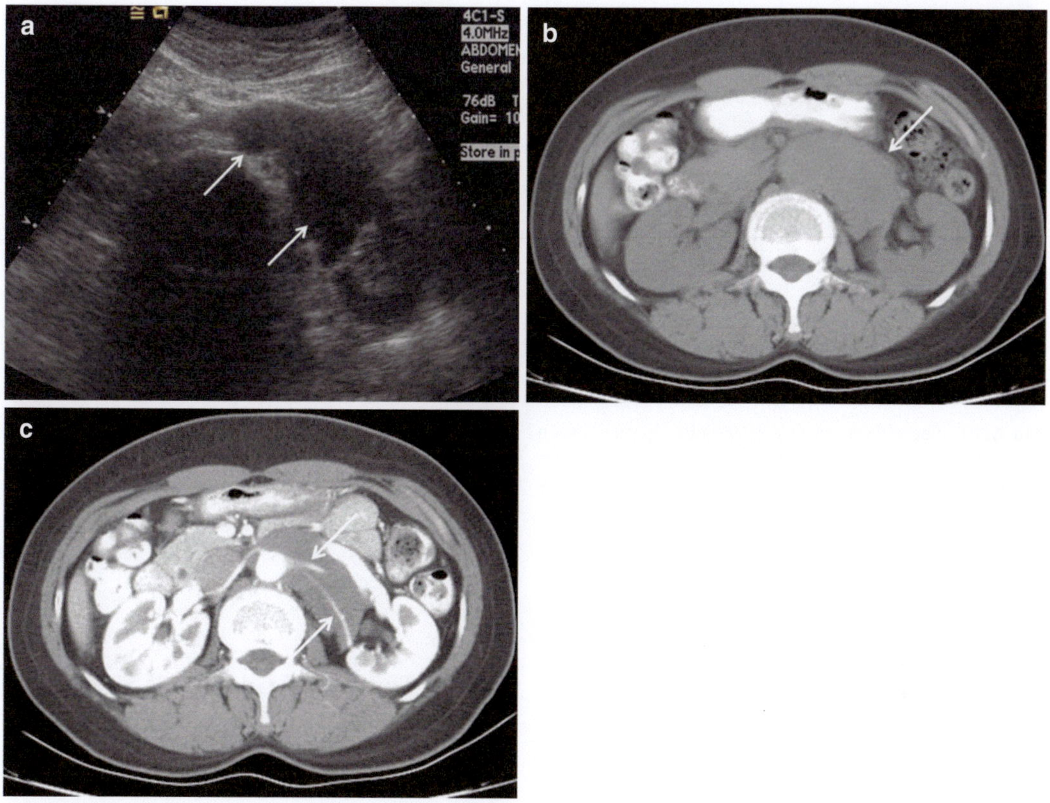

Fig. 6.13 Ganglioneuroma in a 48-year-old woman. (**a**) Transabdominal sonogram demonstrates a low echoic mass (*arrows*) in left retroperitoneum. (**b**) Precontrast axial CT image shows a soft tissue mass (*arrow*) at left para-aortic region that has homogeneous attenuation similar to that of the renal parenchyma. (**c**) Contrast-enhanced axial CT image shows a well-circumscribed, minimally enhancing, soft tissue mass that encase the left renal arteries (*arrows*) without causing significant luminal narrowing

into the neural foramina (Fig. 6.13) [1]. Discrete punctate calcifications are seen in 20–30 % of ganglioneuromas, unlike the coarse amorphous calcification of neuroblastomas [42]. Necrosis and hemorrhage are uncommon, and contrast enhancement is variable. On MRI, this tumor has homogeneously low signal intensity on T1-weighted images, with varying signal intensity on T2-weighted images, depending on the myxoid, cellular, and collagen components [1].

6.4.5 Ganglioneuroblastoma and Neuroblastoma

Ganglioneuroblastoma is an intermediate-grade tumor comprised of mixture of neuroblasts and ganglion cells in varying proportions. It is a pediatric tumor occurring in the 2–4-year age group, with no sex predilection, and is rare in adults. Imaging appearances vary, and the tumor could be solid or cystic with solid components [1].

Neuroblastoma is a rare malignant tumor in adults, while it is one of the most common malignant tumors in children. The most common locations are the adrenal gland and paravertebral region of the retroperitoneum since the tumor originates along the sympathetic ganglion chain, the Zuckerkandl organ, and the adrenal medulla. On imaging, neuroblastoma is seen as an irregular, lobulated, and heterogeneous mass with coarse amorphous calcifications and variable contrast enhancement (Fig. 6.14). It may invade into adjacent organs and surround blood vessels with luminal compression. As many as 70 % of patients have metastatic disease at the time of diagnosis [39].

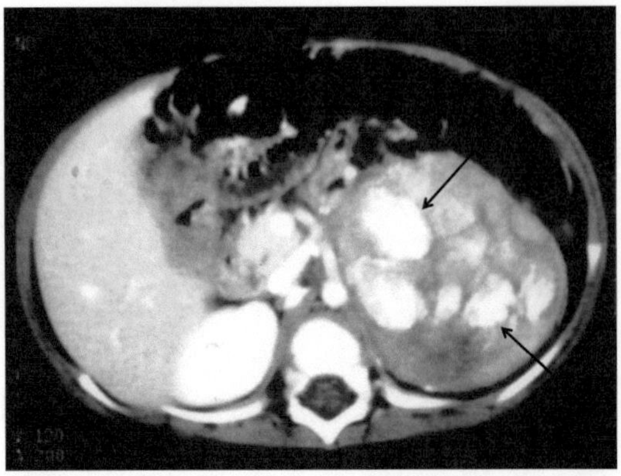

Fig. 6.14 Neuroblastoma in a 10-month-old girl is seen as a well-circumscribed, soft tissue mass in left upper retroperitoneum that contains multiple calcifications (*arrows*)

6.4.6 Paraganglioma (Extra-adrenal Pheochromocytoma)

A paraganglion is a group of non-neuronal cells derived of the neural crest. They are essentially of two types (chromaffin or sympathetic paraganglia made of chromaffin cells and nonchromaffin or parasympathetic ganglia made of glomus cells). Tumors that arise from the chromaffin cells of the adrenal medulla are called pheochromocytomas, and those that arise in an extra-adrenal location (10 %) are referred to as paragangliomas. In the retroperitoneum, the most common site for a paraganglioma is the organs of Zuckerkandl, which are located at the origin of the inferior mesenteric artery or at the bifurcation of the aorta. Up to 40 % of retroperitoneal paragangliomas are malignant, compared with 10 % of adrenal pheochromocytomas [43]. Malignancy is recognized by locally aggressive behavior or metastatic spread to other sites, as the histopathologic criteria do not distinguish the benign forms from the malignant ones [44]. Paragangliomas may be functional in up to 60 % of patients and produce symptoms caused by catecholamine secretion [5].

They usually appear as sharply circumscribed polypoid masses and are highly vascular tumors represented by intense contrast enhancement (Figs. 6.15, 6.16, and 6.17). They may have areas of intratumoral hemorrhage, necrosis, or punctate calcification. In general, the malignant paragangliomas are larger and heterogeneous with poorly defined margins and internal necrosis, while the benign ones are smaller and homogeneous with clear margins. Radiological imaging is helpful in giving information on resectability and detecting the benign or malignant character of the lesion. On MR imaging, they show low to intermediate T1 signal intensity and moderately high T2 signal intensity with marked and early enhancement after contrast material administration. They may show fluid–fluid levels representing the presence of hemorrhagic necrosis inside the lesion. Radionuclide imaging performed after administration of m-iodobenzylguanidine (MIBG) shows high uptake in paragangliomas and is a sensitive technique for localizing these lesions (Fig. 6.16) [39].

6.5 Tumors of Germ Cell, Sex Cord, and Stromal Cell Origin

6.5.1 Primary Extragonadal Germ Cell Tumors

Germ cell tumors arise predominantly from within the testis or ovaries, but approximately 5–10 % of all malignant germ cell tumors are of extragonadal origin, particularly in the mediastinum and retroperitoneum. Primary extragonadal germ cell tumor is more common in men. Extragonadal retroperitoneal germ cell tumors may have a pathological testis showing either viable tumor or lesions compatible with a "burned-out" or "autoinfarcted" primary testicular tumor [12, 45]. They should be considered to be metastases of a viable or burned-out testicular cancer until proven otherwise.

Germ cell tumors can be classified into two broad categories: seminomatous and nonseminomatous germ cell tumors, which include embryonal cell carcinoma, choriocarcinoma, yolk sac tumor, teratoma, and mixed germ cell tumors. The imaging appearances of primary extragonadal germ cell tumors are nonspecific

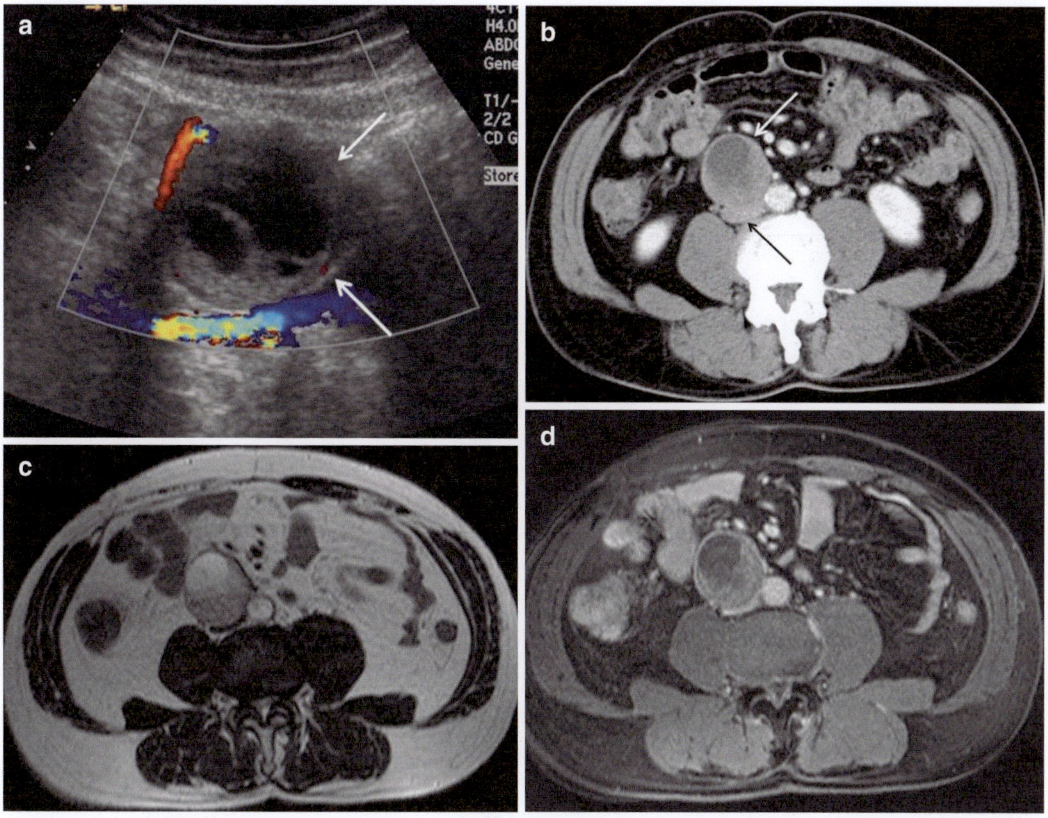

Fig. 6.15 Paraganglioma in a 65-year-old man. (**a**) Transabdominal sonogram demonstrates a round cystic mass (*arrows*) with solid portion. (**b**) Post-contrast axial CT image shows a well-defined mass (*arrow*) with internal cystic portion and moderately enhancing solid portion. The mass is located anterior to the inferior vena cava (*black arrow*). (**c**, **d**) Axial T2-weighted MR image (**c**) and post-contrast axial T1-weighted fat-suppressed MR image (**d**) show a precaval mass that contains both solid and cystic components

and are similar to those of their gonadal counterparts. Nonseminomatous germ cell tumors tend to be more heterogeneous tumors with areas of hemorrhage, necrosis, and heterogeneous enhancement.

Teratomas represent the most common form of all germ cell tumors. Teratomas contain multiple parenchymal tissues that are derived from more than one germ cell layer (ectoderm, mesoderm, and endoderm). Teratomas can be benign or malignant, and benign teratomas can be either mature or immature. Mature teratomas (dermoid cysts) are predominantly cystic and may have calcification, fat with or without fat–fluid level, and a villiform solid component known as a Rokitansky protuberance (Fig. 6.18). Malignant teratomas may be associated with irregular margins, wall thickening, and invasion of adjacent structures and vascular invasion.

6.5.2 Primary Sex Cord–Stromal Tumors

Extragonadal sex cord–stromal tumors are exceedingly rare, while extragonadal germ cell tumors are not infrequently encountered. Most of these tumors are granulosa cell tumors. Other histopathologic types (thecomas, Sertoli–Leydig cell tumors, and other unclassified sex cord tumors) are exceedingly rare. An elevated estrogen level may be seen in granulosa cell tumors and

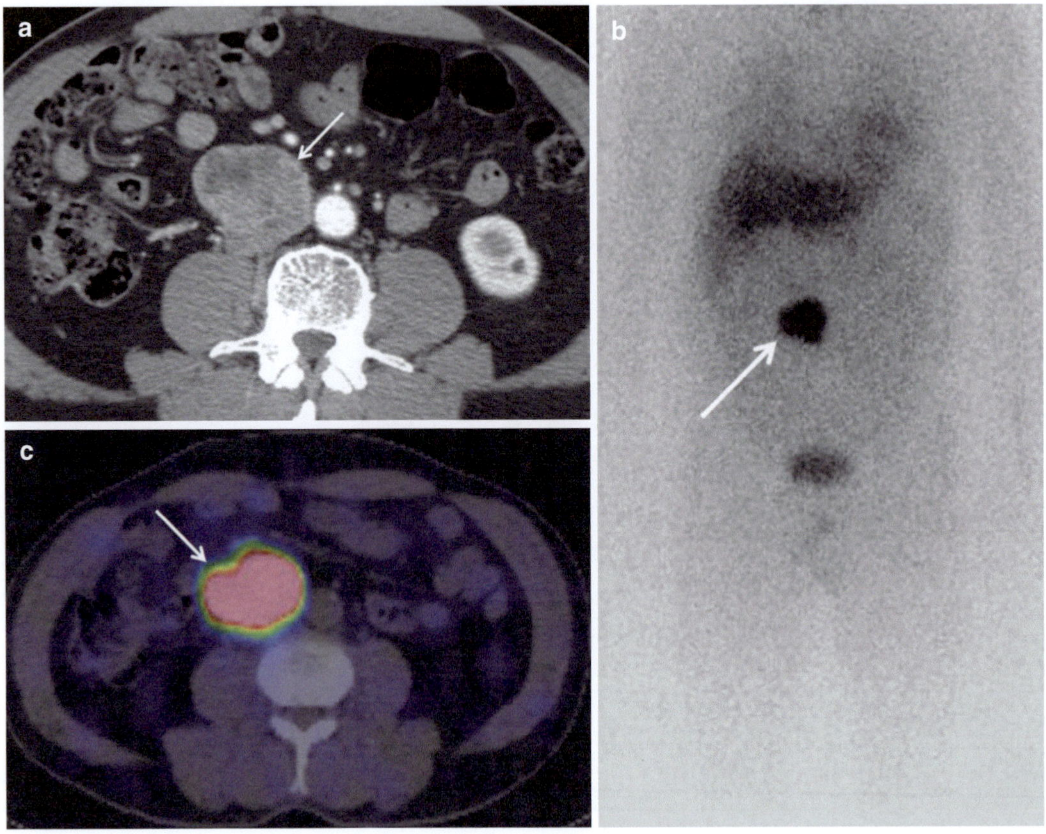

Fig. 6.16 Paraganglioma in a 69-year-old man. (**a**) Post-contrast axial CT image shows a well-defined, solid mass (*arrow*) with heterogeneous enhancement and abutting inferior vena cava. (**b**, **c**). 131I-MIBG scintigraphy (**b**) and SPECT-CT (**c**) images reveal intense 131I-MIBG uptake (*arrows*) in the mass

thecomas [46]. The imaging findings are nonspecific, and CT and MR images show heterogeneous solid tumors, with heterogeneous enhancement.

6.6 Tumors of Lymphoid Origin

Lymphoma and metastatic disease are the most common causes of abdominopelvic lymphadenopathy. Imaging differentiation between metastatic and reactive lymph nodes is based on size criteria, specifically short axis dimension. Size criteria are location based: the upper limit of normal in the retrocrural space is 6 mm, in the retroperitoneum is 10 mm, and in the pelvis is 15 mm [47–49]. Relying on size criteria alone diminishes sensitivity to metastatic normal-sized lymph nodes. Most normal lymph nodes have an oval shape with a preserved fatty hilum, whereas malignant lymph nodes are often rounded [49, 50].

6.6.1 Lymphoma

The retroperitoneum is an uncommon location for primary lymphomatous involvement. By including lymph nodes as a retroperitoneal organ, lymphoma is not considered as a primary retroperitoneal tumor by some authors. However, lymphoma is the most frequent retroperitoneal malignancy, accounting for 33 % of all of these cases [22]. Lymphoma can be broadly divided into Hodgkin lymphoma and non-Hodgkin lymphoma. Non-Hodgkin lymphoma (93.7 %) occurs in retroperitoneum more commonly than does Hodgkin lymphoma (6.3 %) [11, 51, 52].

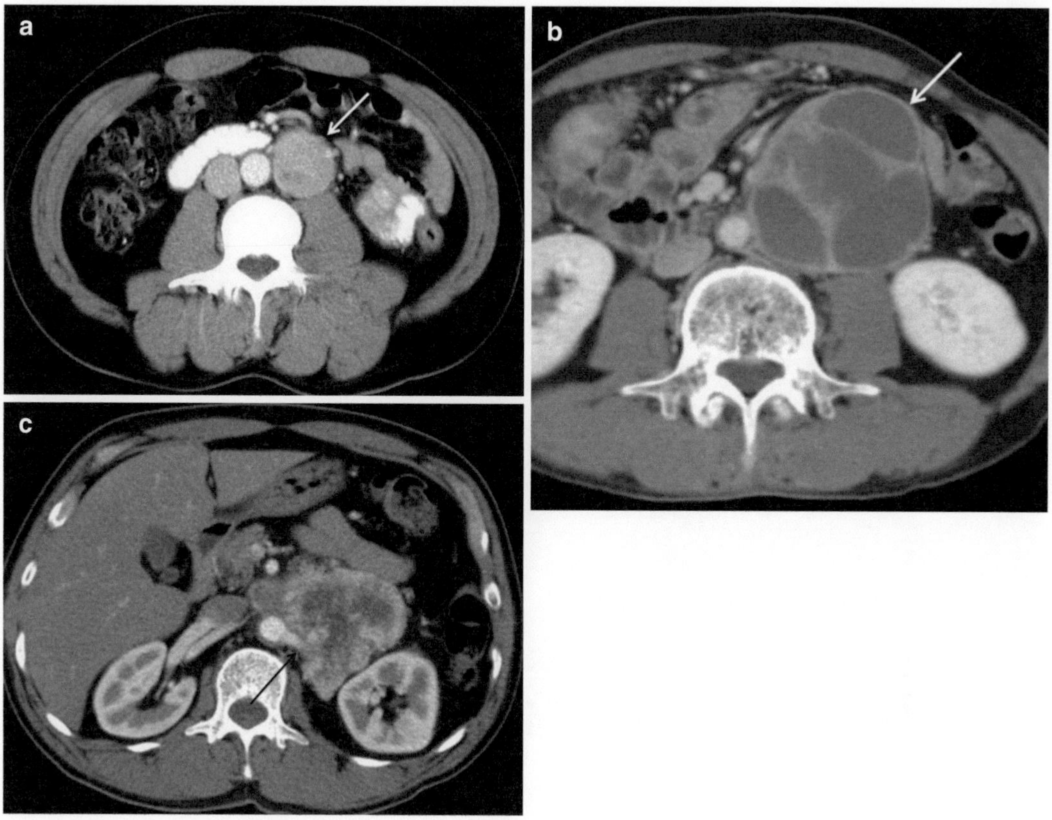

Fig. 6.17 Paraganglioma: various patterns on axial contrast-enhanced CT images. (**a**) A paraganglioma in a 50-year-old woman is seen as a homogeneously enhancing, round mass (*arrow*) at left para-aortic region. (**b**) A paraganglioma in a 55-year-old-man is seen as a multiloculated cystic mass (*arrow*) at left para-aortic region. (**c**) In a 58-year-old man, contrast-enhanced axial CT image shows a peripheral enhancing, heterogeneous mass with lobulated contour, internal necrosis, and encasement of left renal artery (*black arrow*) and vein. The histopathologic findings showed that this mass was a paraganglioma with high risk of malignancy

Para-aortic lymph nodes are involved in 25 % of the patients with Hodgkin lymphoma and 55 % of the patients with non-Hodgkin lymphoma [1].

Approximately 14 % of the patients with non-Hodgkin lymphoma present with a retroperitoneal mass [1]. Lymphoma affects mostly middle-aged and elderly persons. The neighboring retroperitoneal organs are often involved by the tumor. However, bone marrow dissemination of disease is not common. Lymphoma is seen as a well-defined homogeneous mass, with mild homogeneous contrast enhancement, that spreads between normal structures without compressing them [1]. Sometimes, the aorta and IVC are immersed in the tumor, producing the "floating aorta" sign (Fig. 6.19). This sign is characteristic of lymphoma and is generally not seen in other retroperitoneal disorders. Calcification and necrosis are uncommon before therapy (Figs. 6.19 and 6.20) [1]. At MR imaging, lymphoma is usually isointense on T1-weighted images and iso- to hyperintense on T2-weighted images, with moderate homogeneous or patchy enhancement after contrast material administration [11]. Obstruction of the ureters and IVC may be found [1].

6.6.2 Metastatic Retroperitoneal Lymphadenopathy

Retroperitoneal lymphatic spread can occur in a variety of cancers including renal cell, cervical,

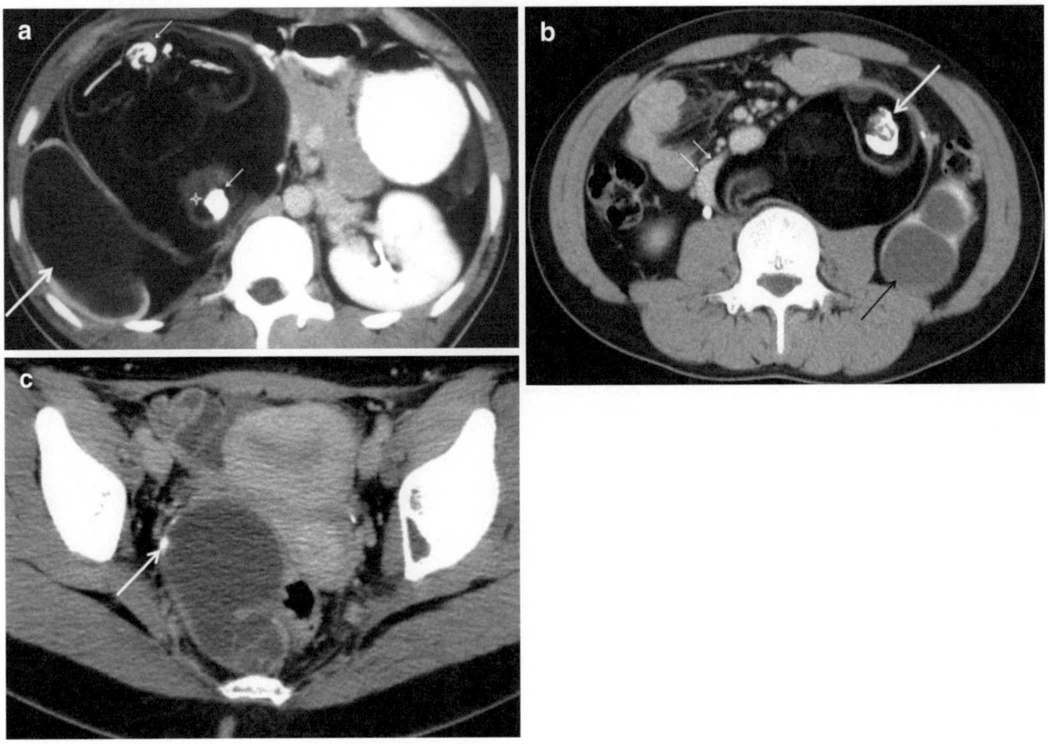

Fig. 6.18 Three cases of retroperitoneal teratoma. (**a**) Axial CT image of a 19-year-old man with a mature teratoma shows a well-defined large mass in right retroperitoneal space that contains large amount of fat (*arrow*) and several teeth (*small arrows*). (**b**) Axial CT image of a 33-year-old man with a mature teratoma shows a fatty mass that contains a nodular calcification (*arrow*) and extends into the retro-aortic space with compressing IVC (*small arrows*). Note the dilated calyces (*black arrow*) in the covered lower portion of the left kidney with severe parenchymal atrophy, which may represent the chronic obstruction of left ureter by the mass. (**c**) Axial CT image of a 31-year-old woman with a sacrococcygeal teratoma shows a cystic mass with focal wall calcifications (*arrow*) and septations in the right-side pelvis. Neither fat nor solid component is present in the mass. The histopathologic findings showed that this mass was a mature cystic teratoma

testicular, and prostatic carcinomas. Although metastatic lymphadenopathy is not strictly a primary retroperitoneal lesion, it is important to differentiate metastatic lymphadenopathy from other diseases such as lymphoma, Castleman disease, sarcoidosis, or infections. Imaging features may significantly overlap. History of primary malignancy and the presence of necrosis suggest metastatic lymphadenopathy. The imaging appearance is variable, from discrete enlarged nodes to a single conglomerate mass, which may not be recognizable as lymphadenopathy (Figs. 6.21 and 6.22) [3]. The upper limit of normal size of the lymph node at this location is 10 mm, but multiple lymph nodes smaller than 10 mm also should be viewed with suspicion.

Malignant neoplasms in pelvis tend to spread initially to the pelvic nodes. However, testicular, ovarian, and fallopian tube malignancies spread first to the retroperitoneal nodes adjacent to or near the renal hila because of spread along the gonadal vessels and may involve the pelvic nodes by retrograde spread [49]. Retroperitoneal lymph node metastasis may be difficult to differentiate from primary extragonadal tumor in a rare phenomenon known as burned-out seminoma of the testis in which spontaneous regression of a primary testicular tumor occurred after demonstration of retroperitoneal lymph node metastasis.

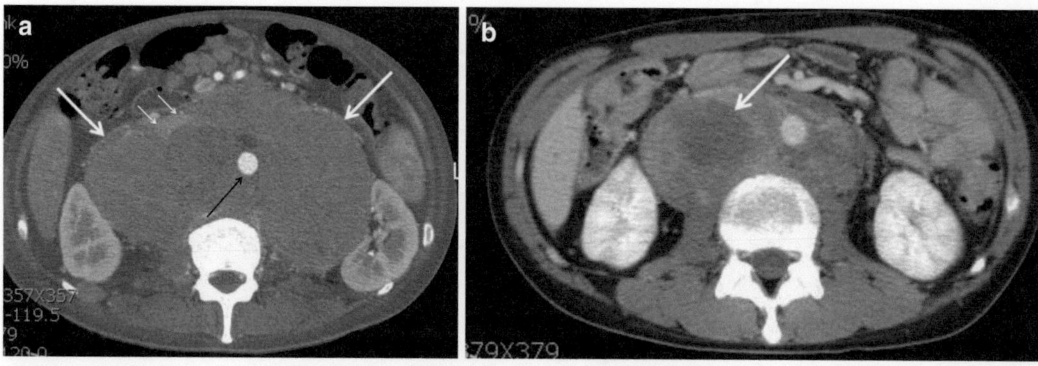

Fig. 6.19 Hodgkin lymphoma in a 28-year-old man. (**a**) Axial contrast-enhanced CT image shows a large homogeneous mass (*arrows*) that is encasing and anteriorly displacing the abdominal aorta (*black arrow*), producing the characteristic floating aorta sign. IVC (*small arrows*) is also displaced anteriorly. (**b**) Follow-up CT at 4 months after chemotherapy shows marked size reduction of the retroperitoneal mass with newly appeared nonenhancing or necrotic portion (*arrow*) in the mass

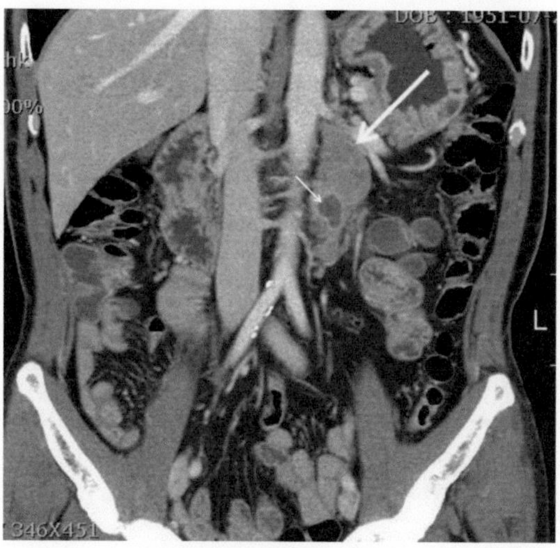

Fig. 6.20 Diffuse large B-cell lymphoma in a 61-year-old man. Coronal reformatted, contrast-enhanced CT image shows an elongated-shaped solid mass (*arrow*) with small internal cystic portion (*small arrow*) at left para-aortic region. It is very hard to differentiate from other tumor types

6.7 Miscellaneous Retroperitoneal Conditions

6.7.1 Erdheim–Chester Disease

Erdheim–Chester disease is a rare, non-inherited disease that is a rare form of non-Langerhans cell histiocytosis characterized by long bone sclerosis. Patients with Erdheim–Chester disease may present with widespread manifestations and of highly variable severity. Approximately one-half of the patients may have extraskeletal or multifocal disease. Its retroperitoneal manifestations may occur in isolation or as a component of disseminated disease [53]. Retroperitoneal involvement in Erdheim–Chester disease may produce thickened soft tissue rind of perinephric tissue and infiltration along the ureters, which can cause hydronephrosis or renal failure (Fig. 6.23). MR imaging shows low signal intensity of the thickened soft tissue rind on T1- and T2-weighted images, with minimal contrast enhancement. Distinguishing retroperitoneal infiltration in Erdheim–Chester disease from other kinds of retroperitoneal fibrosis is not easy. Occasionally, the diagnosis will require biopsy with histologic confirmation [53].

6.7.2 Castleman Disease

Castleman disease, also known as giant or angiofollicular lymph node hyperplasia, is a rare benign lymphoproliferative disorder that may be localized to a single lymph node (unicentric) or occur systemically (multicentric). Histologically, there is an abnormal overgrowth of cells of the lymph system that is similar in many ways to

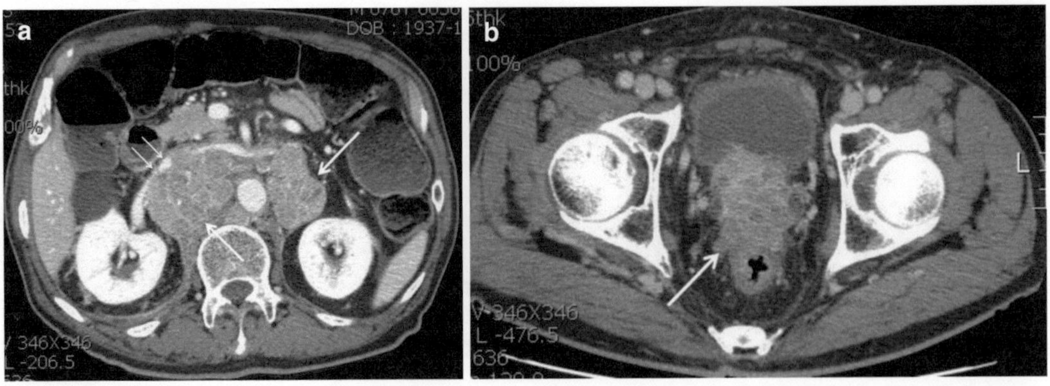

Fig. 6.21 Metastatic retroperitoneal lymphadenopathy in a 76-year-old man. (**a**) Axial contrast-enhanced CT image shows large inhomogeneous para-aortic mass (*arrows*) that is anteriorly displacing the inferior vena cava (*small arrows*). Septum-like enhancing internal structures in the mass represents conglomerate mass formed by multiple enlarged lymph nodes. (**b**) The presence of primary tumor in the same study as well as history of primary malignancy helps determine the diagnosis. CT scan reveals the presence of prostate cancer (*arrow*) with invasion of seminal vesicle and rectum

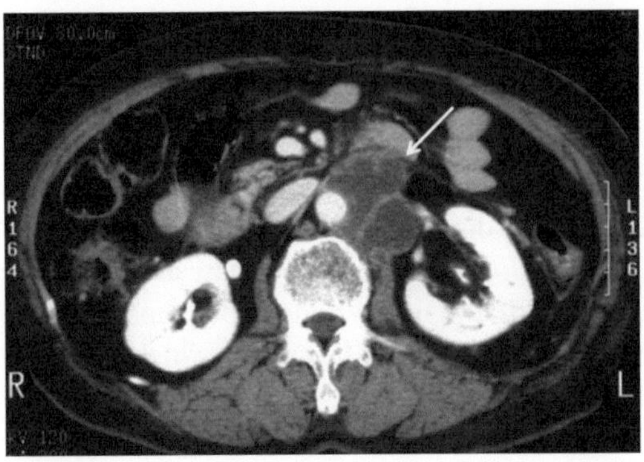

Fig. 6.22 Metastatic retroperitoneal lymphadenopathy in a 67-year-old woman with a history of endometrial carcinoma. Axial contrast-enhanced CT image shows a septate cystic mass (*arrow*) at left para-aortic region, which is difficult to differentiate from other types of primary retroperitoneal tumors. The mass was proved to be metastatic lymph nodes with necrotic changes

lymphoma. It can be classified into microscopic subtypes, mainly hyaline vascular and plasma cell types. The hyaline vascular subtype accounts for 85–90 % of cases of Castleman disease and tends to be localized (unicentric) and usually have a good prognosis. It may occur anywhere along the lymphatic chain, and about 70 % occur in the mediastinum [15].

The characteristic imaging features of localized form of Castleman disease include a well-circumscribed solitary mass or a dominant mass with small satellite nodules, showing intense enhancement [15] (Fig. 6.24). The central area of fibrosis, if seen, is one of the characteristic features and manifests as hypointense signal on both T1- and T2-weighted images [51]. Central cystic areas or necrosis is rare. The plasma cell type or multicentric form of Castleman disease may show hepatosplenomegaly, ascites, and lymphadenopathy, which generally shows lesser enhancement than in the localized form [52].

6.8 Cystic Neoplastic Masses in Retroperitoneum

The detection rate of retroperitoneal cystic masses has increased owing to the widespread use of CT and MR imaging. They are found incidentally and are usually asymptomatic but may produce symptoms that depend on the location, size, or complications. Contrast-enhanced images help in differentiating between cystic and solid renal lesions. Complex cystic and solid lesions can be characterized further. Imaging can help to support clinical management in patients with retroperitoneal cystic masses by depicting certain lesions that do not require treatment. Although many overlapped radiologic features have been shown to exist among the various retroperitoneal cystic masses, imaging can help to support clinical management for follow-up or planning specific surgical approaches. Therefore, an accurate

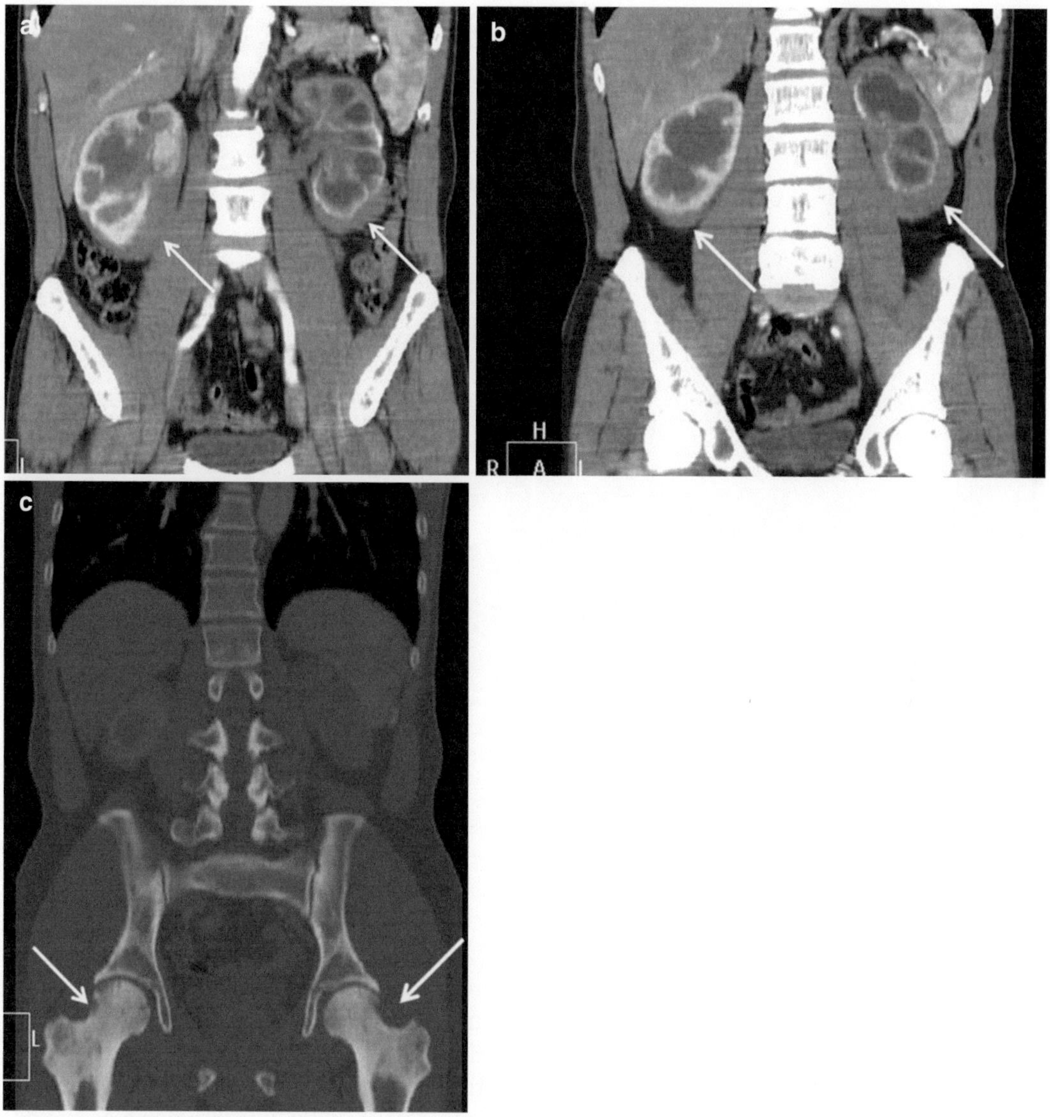

Fig. 6.23 Erdheim–Chester disease in a 45-year-old man. (**a**, **b**) Contrast-enhanced, coronal reformatted CT images demonstrate bilateral hydronephrosis with parenchymal atrophy. Note rindlike soft tissue lesions (*arrows*) surrounding both kidneys with probable compromise of ureteropelvic junction. (**c**) Coronal reformatted CT image with bone window setting demonstrates symmetric osteosclerosis (*arrows*) of the head and neck of bilateral femurs

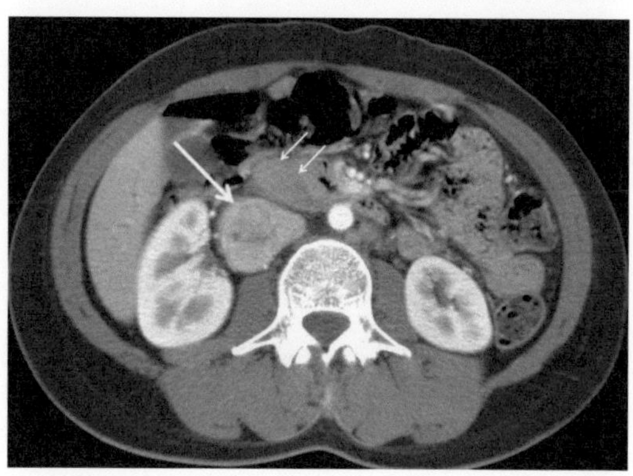

Fig. 6.24 Castleman's disease in a 35-year-old woman. Contrast-enhanced axial CT image shows a well-defined homogeneously enhancing hypervascular mass (*arrow*) at retrocaval region, separated from the right kidney. The inferior vena cava (*small arrows*) is displaced anteromedially without compression by the tumor. The histopathologic findings showed that this mass was a hyaline vascular-type Castleman's disease

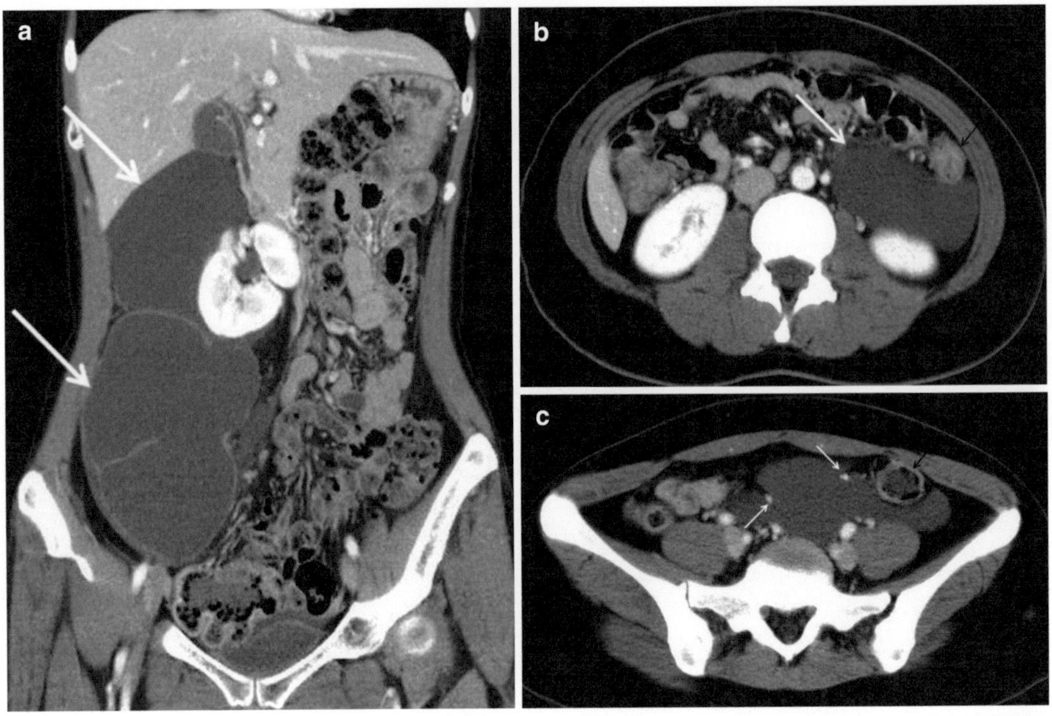

Fig. 6.25 Cystic lymphangioma. (**a**) Contrast-enhanced coronal reformatted CT image in a 35-year-old woman shows a huge lobulated–septated cystic mass (*arrows*) in the right retroperitoneum that displaces the right kidney medially. The fluid content of the mass is homogeneous with low attenuation values. (**b**, **c**) Another case of lymphangioma in a 23-year-old woman is seen as a unilocular cystic mass (*arrows*) with homogeneous fluid density and thin wall in left retroperitoneal space. The mass is indented by surrounding structures such as mesenteric vessels (*small arrows*) and descending colon (*black arrows*), which means that mass effect on the adjacent structures is only minimal

characterization of retroperitoneal cystic masses is essential to ensure appropriate management. Retroperitoneal cystic neoplasms include cystic lymphangioma, mucinous cystadenoma, cystic teratoma, cystic mesothelioma, Müllerian cyst, epidermoid cyst, tailgut cyst, bronchogenic cyst, cystic change in solid neoplasms, pseudomyxoma retroperitonei, and perianal mucinous carcinoma [54]. They should be differentiated from nonneoplastic retroperitoneal cystic lesion (pancreatic pseudocyst, nonpancreatic pseudocyst, lymphocele, urinoma, hematoma), mesenteric, and enteric duplication cysts [54].

6.8.1 Lymphangioma

Lymphangioma is a developmental malformation that occurs due to failure of communication of retroperitoneal lymphatic tissue with the main lymphatic vessels [55]. Lymphangiomas in retroperitoneum are uncommon and may occur in the perirenal, pararenal, or pelvic extraperitoneal spaces. Occasionally, lymphangioma occurs diffusely with widespread bony and soft tissue involvement, which is referred to as generalized lymphangiomatosis or cystic angiomatosis [2]. At pathologic analysis, cystic lymphangiomas are unilocular or multilocular cysts containing clear or milky fluid and lined with a single layer of flattened endothelium [1, 54]. On imaging, lymphangioma appears as large, thin-walled, unilocular, or multiseptated cystic mass, with fluid attenuation or fluid-signal intensity and no significant enhancement on post-contrast images (Fig. 6.25). It may involve more than one retroperitoneal compartment and is seen to invaginate between structures without displacing them [3]. Calcifications are rare.

6.8.2 Mucinous Cystadenoma and Cystadenocarcinoma

Mucinous cystadenomas are common ovarian or appendiceal tumors, but they are extremely rare in the retroperitoneum. The histogenesis of this rare tumor is uncertain, but a hypothesis suggested that it arises from invaginations of the multipotential coelomic epithelium with subsequent mucinous metaplasia [56]. Primary retroperitoneal mucinous cystadenomas are usually unilocular or multilocular cystic masses separated from the retroperitoneal organs. Because of their nonspecific radiologic features, it is difficult to distinguish them from other retroperotoneal cystic lesions. Complete surgical resection is recommended because of their potential for malignant transformation to cystadenocarcinoma [57].

6.8.3 Tailgut Cyst

Tailgut cysts, also known as tailgut duplication cysts or retrorectal cystic hamartomas, are rare congenital lesions that are thought to originate from embryonic hindgut remnants. They are usually asymptomatic and show strong female predilection. Tailgut cysts are most commonly seen in the retrorectal or presacral space. CT and MR imaging may show a well-marginated multilocular mass in the presacral space that demonstrates attenuation values ranging from that of water to that of soft tissue (Fig. 6.26). Calcifications may be seen in the cyst wall, and concurrent infection or malignant transformation may occur.

6.8.4 Bronchogenic Cyst

Bronchogenic cysts are developmental abnormalities of the primitive foregut that are usually found above the diaphragm. Rarely, they can occur in a subdiaphragmatic location, and a retroperitoneal position is distinctly unusual. Most retroperitoneal bronchogenic cysts are found near the left adrenal gland or the peripancreatic region. These cysts are diagnosed incidentally and are generally too small to cause symptoms. They appear as sharply defined, thin-walled, cystic lesions (Fig. 6.27). Fluid–fluid levels caused by complex internal contents, mural calcification, layering milk of calcium, and rim enhancement may be seen [5].

6.8.5 Cystic Change in Solid Neoplasms

Some types of solid retroperitoneal neoplasms such as paraganglioma and neurogenic tumor often can be cystic. These are typically seen in the paravertebral region. Leiomyosarcoma can have extensive areas of necrosis and may be predominantly cystic. Solid retroperitoneal neoplasms may show prominent cystic change resulting from secondary degenerative change caused by an inadequate blood supply to the center. Chemotherapy may reduce the bulk of the solid retroperitoneal neoplasms and induces tumor necrosis and cystic hemorrhage that may produce cystic appearance of the tumors after chemotherapy.

6.9 Pathologic Consideration of Retroperitoneal Tumors

6.9.1 Schwannoma

Schwannoma is a well-demarcated mass with yellow-whitish color and myxoid cut surface (Fig. 6.28a). Cystic change and hemorrhages can be found. Microscopically schwannoma frequently shows alternating Antoni A and B areas (Fig. 6.28b). Antoni A area is hypercellular area with spindle cells arranged in fascicles. Tumor cells frequently show nuclear palisading and often form Verocay body which is formed by palisaded nuclei with central anuclear zone composed of cell processes (Fig. 6.28c). Antoni B area is hypocellular area having loosely arranged tumor cells with myxoid stroma. Degenerative nuclear atypia, cystic change, and hyaline change can be present (Fig. 6.28d).

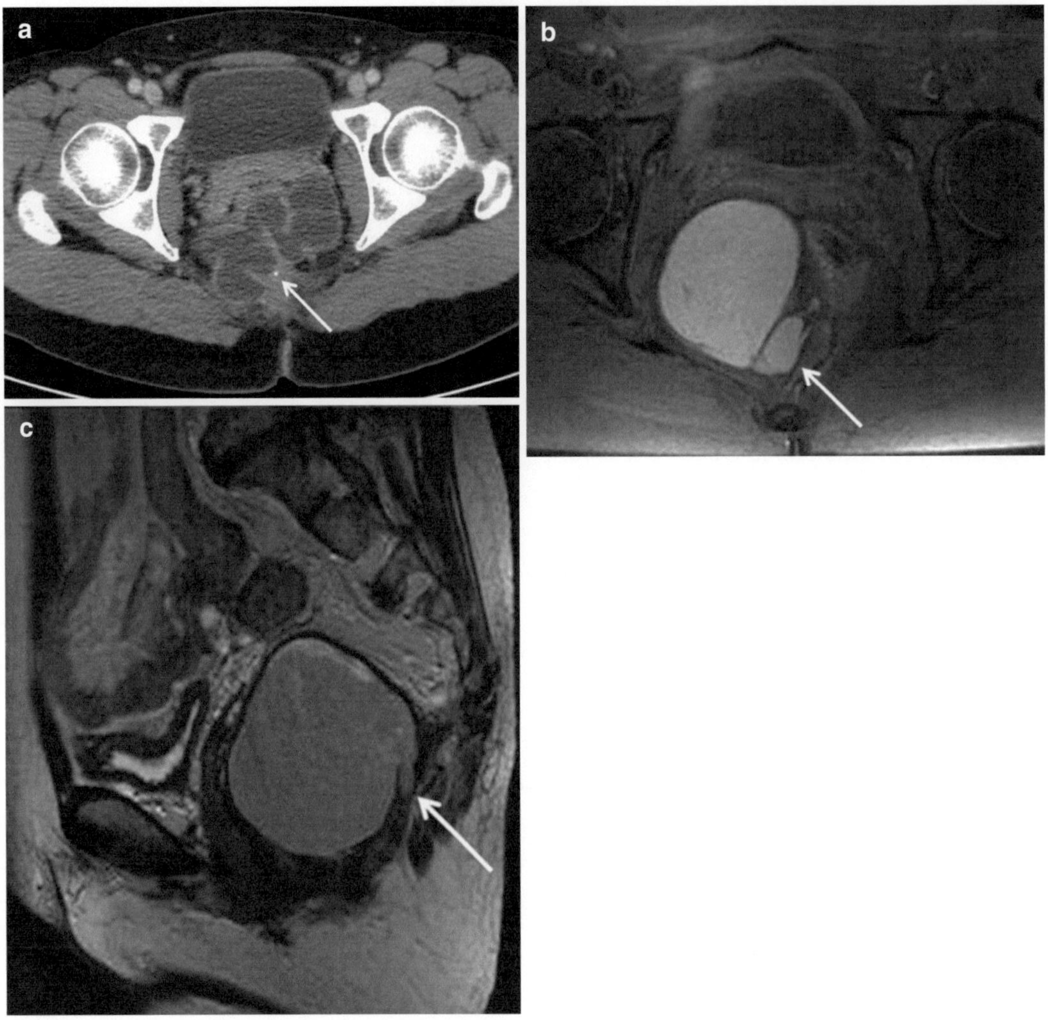

Fig. 6.26 Two cases of tailgut cyst. (**a**) Axial CT image in a 44-year-old woman with a tailgut cyst shows a multiloculated cystic mass with a tiny focal wall calcification (*arrow*) at retrorectal space. (**b**, **c**) Another case of tailgut cyst in a 53-year-old woman is seen as a well-circumscribed mass with a taillike structure (*arrows*) at retrorectal space. The mass has homogeneous high signal intensity on T1-weighted fat-suppressed axial image (**b**) and intermediate signal intensity on T2-weighted images

6.9.2 Liposarcoma

Liposarcoma can be classified into several subtypes, and most liposarcomas of retroperitoneum are well-differentiated liposarcoma and dedifferentiated liposarcoma. Retroperitoneal myxoid liposarcoma is very rare or absent [58, 59]. Grossly well-differentiated liposarcoma is a large yellowish mass resembling normal fat tissue (Fig. 6.29a). On cut surface, fibrous bands are frequently found. Dedifferentiated liposarcoma has firm, tan to gray non-adipogenic area (Fig. 6.30a). Microscopically well-differentiated liposarcoma is mainly composed of well-developed adipocytes with varying numbers of lipoblasts and atypical stromal cells in fibrous bands (Fig. 6.29b, c). Dedifferentiated liposarcoma has the area containing non-lipogenic sarcoma (Fig. 6.30b).

6.9.3 Leiomyosarcoma

Grossly leiomyosarcoma is a large white-gray mass with whirling appearance (Fig. 6.31a).

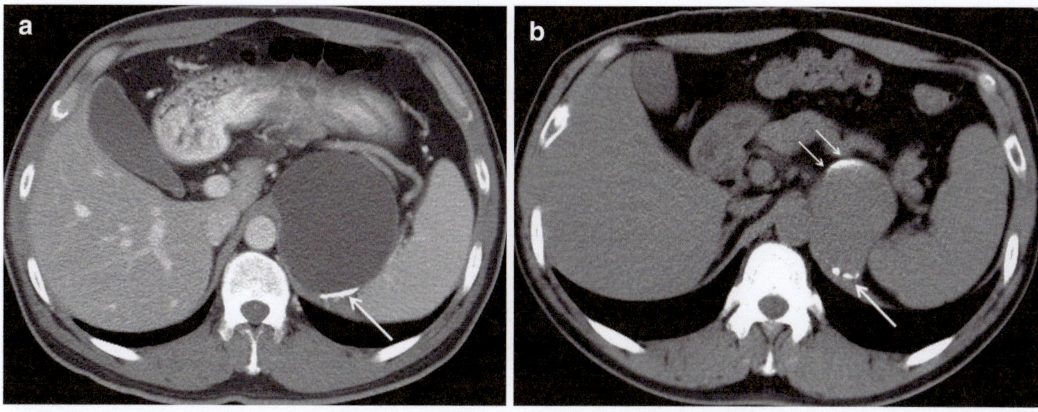

Fig. 6.27 Bronchogenic cyst in a 41-year-old man. (**a**) Axial CT image shows a well-defined unilocular cystic mass that demonstrates clear-fluid density and calcifications (*arrow*) at dependent portion of the mass. (**b**) Additional CT scan in the prone position reveals that the cyst has intraluminal milk of calcium (*small arrows*) as well as focal wall calcifications (*arrow*) at posterior wall

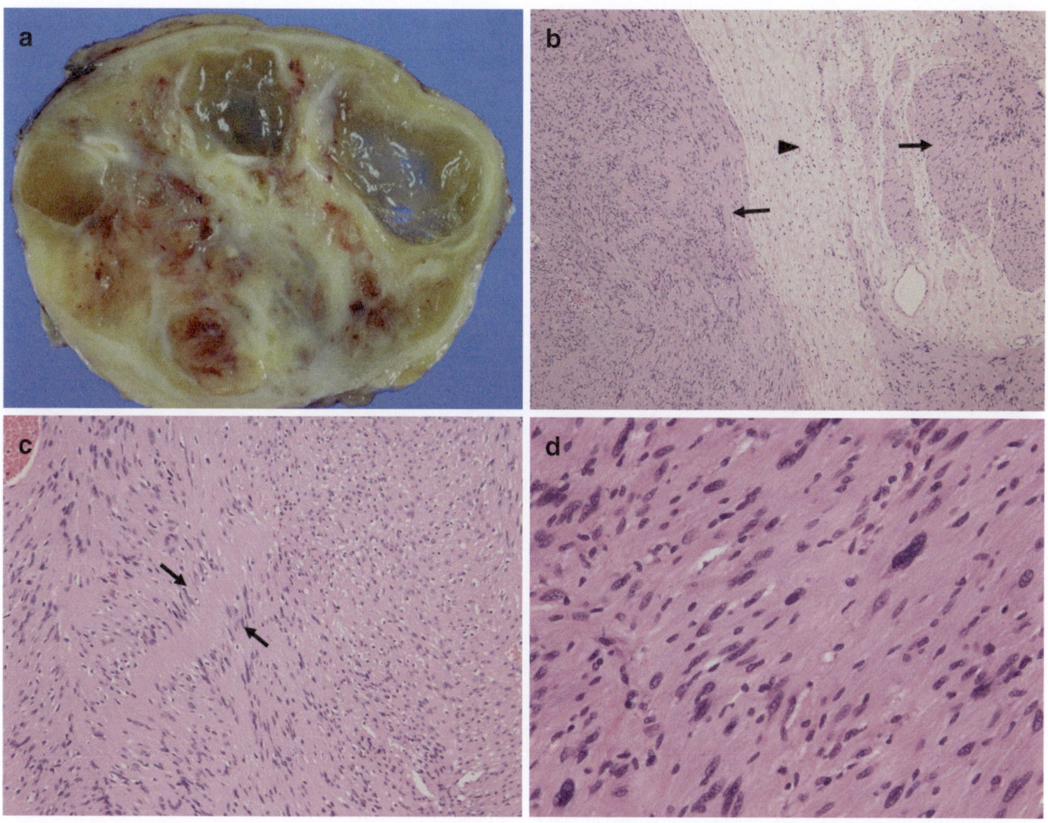

Fig. 6.28 (**a**) Grossly schwannoma shows yellowish myxoid cut surface with frequent cystic change. (**b**) Hypercellular Antoni A area (*arrows*) and hypocellular Antoni B area (*arrow head*). (**c**) Verocay body (*arrows*) by palisaded nuclei and central anuclear zone. (**d**) Degenerative nuclear atypia is common finding of old schwannoma

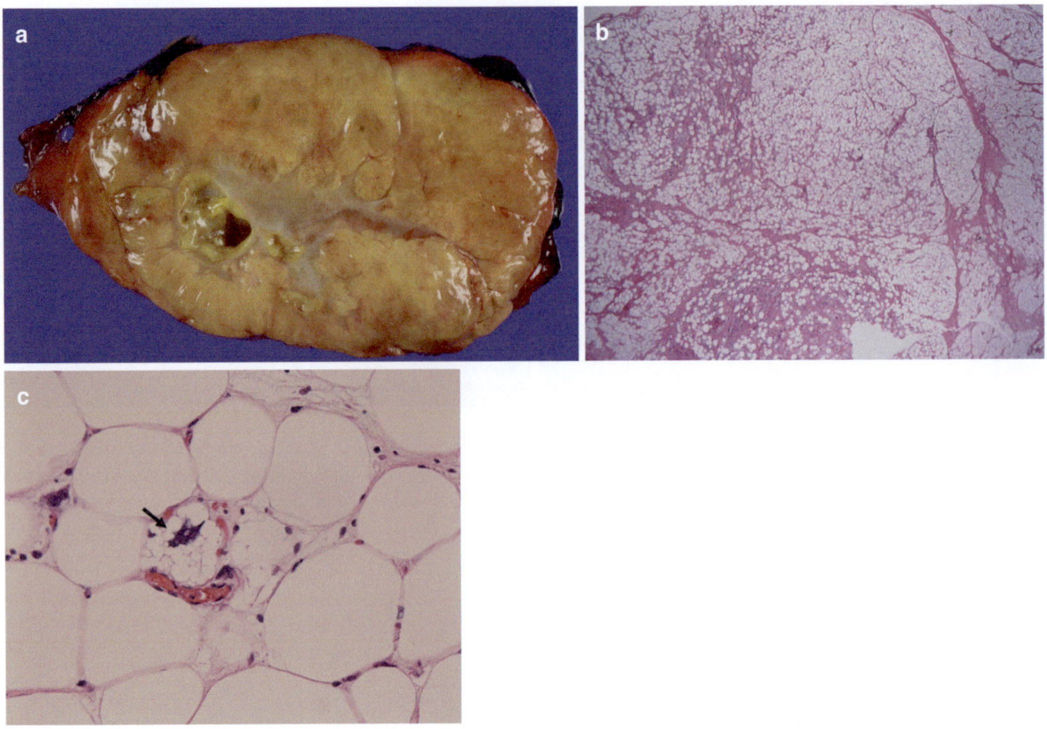

Fig. 6.29 (**a**) Microscopically well-differentiated liposarcoma contains well-developed adipocytes with thick fibrous septa. (**b**) A typical lipoblast is found (*arrow*)

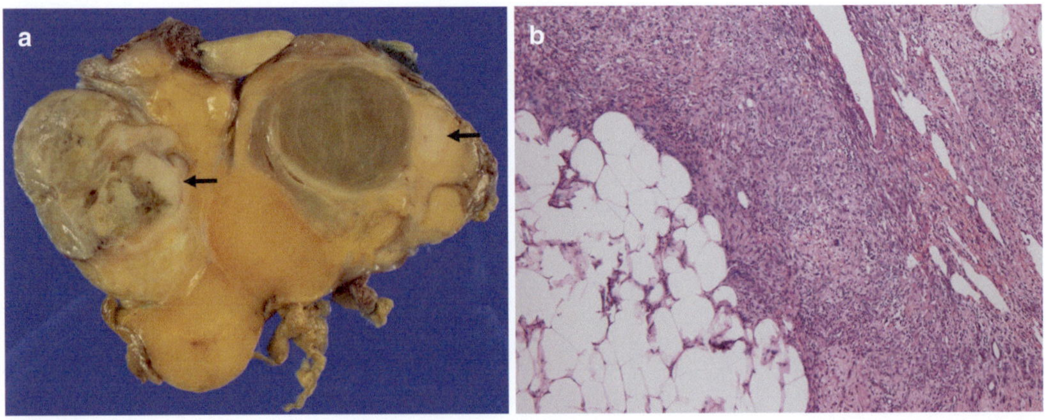

Fig. 6.30 (**a**) Dedifferentiated liposarcoma shows non-lipogenic whitish area (*arrows*) in the background of well-differentiated liposarcoma composed of yellowish fatty tissue. (**b**) Microscopically non-lipogenic spindle cell sarcoma (*right*) is present adjacent to well-differentiated liposarcoma (*left*)

Infiltration into other organs such as the kidney and pancreas is common. On cut surface, hemorrhage and necrosis can be found (Fig. 6.31b). Microscopically leiomyosarcoma is mainly composed of elongated spindle cells with cigar-shaped nuclei (Fig. 6.31c). Tumor cells frequently reveal fascicular arrangement. Less differentiated cases show more nuclear pleomorphism and high mitotic rate. Hemorrhage, necrosis, or myxoid change can be found.

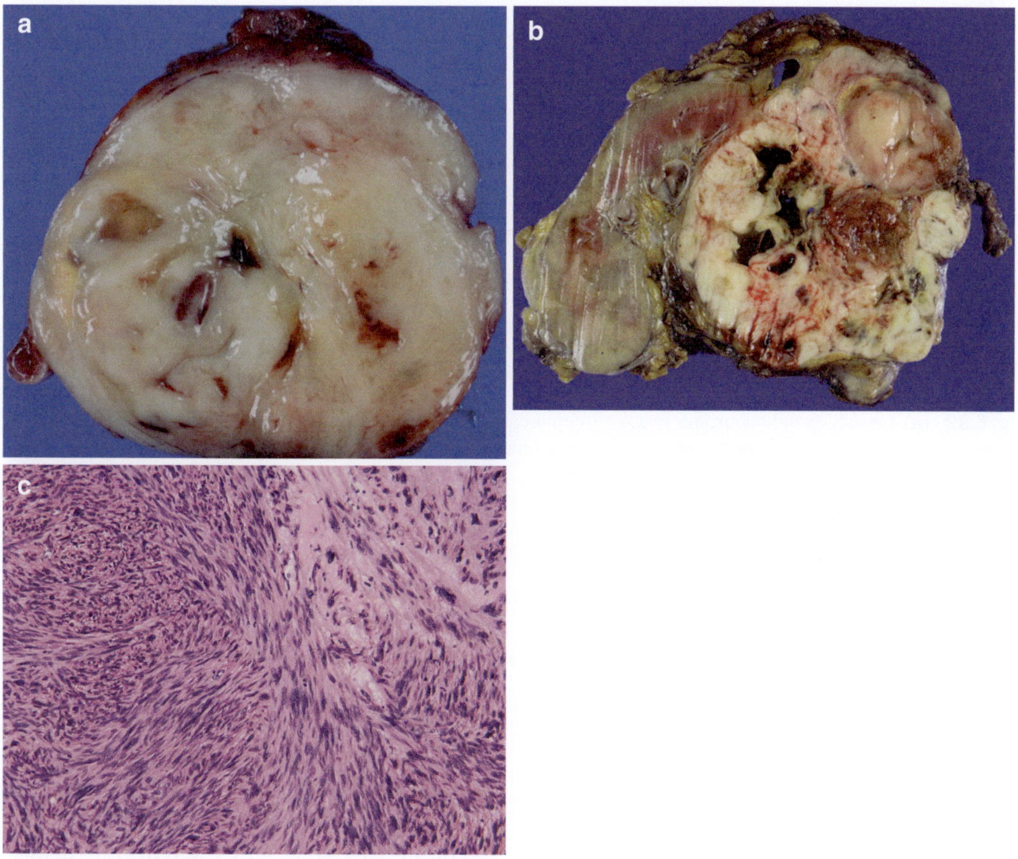

Fig. 6.31 (**a**) Gross photograph of leiomyosarcoma shows whitish cut surface. (**b**) Another leiomyosarcoma case shows hemorrhage and necrosis. (**c**) Microscopic examination reveals intersecting malignant spindle cell bundles with frequent mitosis

6.9.4 Ganglioneuroma

Gangliomeuroma can arise in adrenal medulla and more commonly in mediastinum and retroperitoneum [60]. Grossly, ganglioneuroma is a large well-demarcated and encapsulated mass showing homogeneous gray-white cut surface (Fig. 6.32a). Microscopically this tumor is fully differentiated tumor and entirely composed of ganglion cells and schwannian stroma (Fig. 6.32b).

6.10 Surgery of Retroperitoneal Tumor

6.10.1 Introduction

The retroperitoneal space is located between the peritoneum and the posterior abdominal wall and ranges from the pelvic floor to the diaphragm. Primary tumors of retroperitoneum may arise from tissues in this space. They may be originated from adipose tissue, connective tissue or fascia, muscle, vascular tissue, nervous tissue, and lymph nodes, which can be encountered in retroperitoneal space [61]. Of primary retroperitoneal tumors, over 80 % are malignant, and sarcomas are most common malignant tumor which occurs in retroperitoneal space [62]. Because retroperitoneal tumors tend to give no symptom until they grow up to substantial size, they are usually found to be large size at presentation [63].

Complete surgical resection is the treatment of choice for retroperitoneal tumors. Especially in retroperitoneal sarcoma, complete resection of the tumor only can offer the chance of cure [64]. Complete macroscopic removal has known to be the most powerful prognostic factor that has impact on survival of patients with retroperitoneal sarcoma in many studies [19, 65–68]. Also,

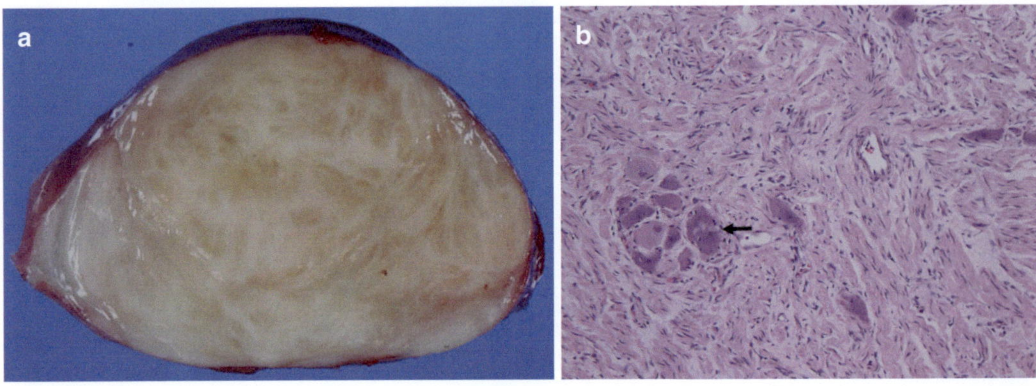

Fig. 6.32 (**a**) Grossly ganglioneuroma is a well-demarcated mass with whitish cut surface. (**b**) Ganglioneuroma is composed of ganglion cells (*arrow*) and schwannian stroma

in the management of benign lesion including lipoma or neurogenic tumors, complete resection is recommended because of the risk of malignant transformation and recurrence [69, 70]. Several large series regarding retroperitoneal sarcomas reported that the complete resection of tumor was obtained in 55–78 %, and 5-year overall survival ranges from 39 to 68 % [19, 66, 68, 71, 72].

Although complete resection with enough resection margins is the surgical principal of retroperitoneal tumors, it may be hampered by the invasion of tumors to adjacent organs. Retroperitoneal space hosts various critical organs, and retroperitoneal tumors often abut against them. Although preoperative image study enables access to adjacent involvement of retroperitoneal tumor, definite decision is made intraoperatively in many cases [73]. Large case series reported that over 80 % of surgical cases needed simultaneous resection of affected organs with tumor [19, 63]. Affected organs may be the major vessels, diaphragm, kidney, spleen, pancreas, and intestine, and the colon, kidney, pancreas, and spleen are commonly affected by retroperitoneal sarcomas and often simultaneously resected with tumor [63]. A review reported that 20 % of patients who underwent surgery for retroperitoneal sarcoma need to have nephrectomy simultaneously [74]. Often, major vessels are affected by tumor, and concomitant resection is needed. In a case series of 63 retroperitoneal tumors, concomitant resection of major blood vessel was necessitated in 5 % of all cases [73]. Inferior vena cava (IVC) is known as the most affected major blood vessel by retroperitoneal tumor. In most cases with IVC resection, synthetic graft is used to reconstruct IVC [75–77]. Occasionally, subtotal resection is needed for the relief of symptom; however, it must be decided considering benefit and risk preoperatively. Complications following retroperitoneal tumor excisions are bleeding, infection, and delayed wound healing. Perioperative mortality rate is reported as 1–3 % according to large series and recent database review [19, 63, 78].

Recently laparoscopic resection of retroperitoneal tumor has been emerging in selected cases. In benign retroperitoneal mass without affected adjacent organ, laparoscopic resection of tumor showed good perioperative outcomes [78, 79]. Also, in the case of sarcoma, a few case report of laparoscopic resection has been reported [80–83]. However, considering the principal of surgery of retroperitoneal tumor especially in malignant tumors and high probability of open conversion, the selection of cases have to be made with very strict preoperative assessment.

6.10.2 Surgical Procedure and Anatomy

Surgeon can approach in several ways including long midline, chevron, subcostal, thoracoabdominal, and flank incision to resect retroperitoneal tumors. Also, laparoscopic approaches may be

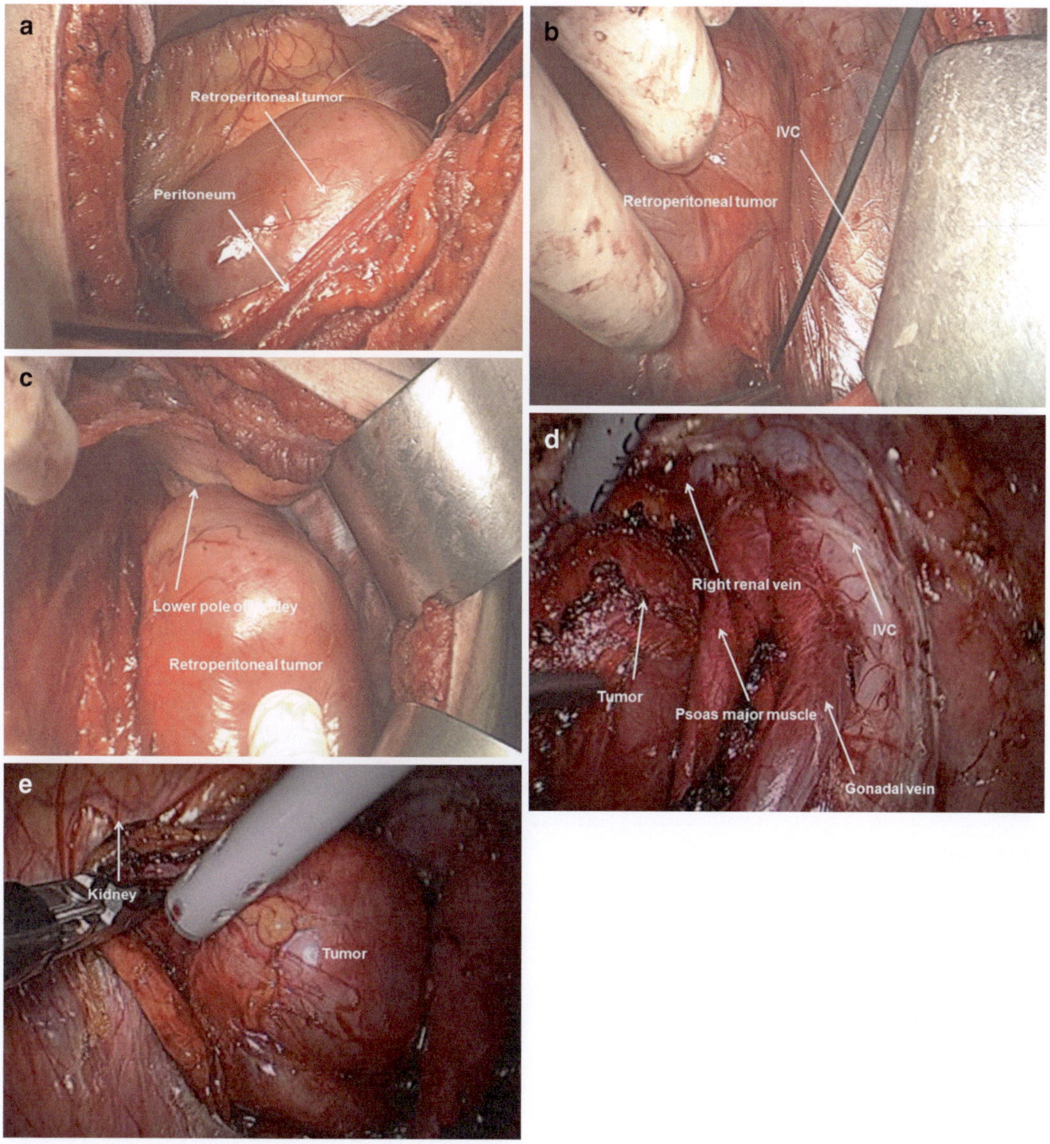

Fig. 6.33 Surgery for a retroperitoneal tumor. (**a**) Retroperitoneal tumor and peritoneum, (**b**) IVC and tumor, (**c**) kidney and tumor, (**d**) medial and superior side of tumor, and (**e**) lateral side of tumor

the option for the resection of benign retroperitoneal tumors. The location and size of tumor have to be considered preoperatively in making decision of which approaches is made. Flank incision is made at the skin of 10th intercostal space. After approaching the retroperitoneal space, the posterior layer of the tumor is dissected from the posterior abdominal wall. Genitofemoral nerve and psoas major muscle are visualized after dissection of the posterior layer. To expose the tumor, peritoneum overlying the tumor is retracted medially, and plane between tumor and peritoneum is developed with blunt and sharp dissection (Fig. 6.33a). After peritoneum is completely separated from the tumor, IVC and lower pole of the kidney are visualized at the medial side and superior side of the tumor, respectively (Fig. 6.33b, c).

Postoperative motor or sensory neurogenic disturbance is a major complication following resection of schwannoma. The dissection of the nerve fascicle along the tumor is known to be mainly responsible for postoperative neurologic deficit [84, 85]. To avoid injury to nerve fascicle, meticulous dissection between tumor and fascicle is needed. Intraoperative nerve stimulation helps surgeons to know whether the tissue planned to dissect or divide is a functional nerve fascicle or not.

In laparoscopic retroperitoneal tumor resection, port placement is made considering the location of tumor (Fig. 6.33d, e). In this case, about a 3 cm-sized benign neurogenic tumor is located between the inferior vena cava and right kidney. To expose the tumor, a peritoneal incision parallel to the lateral border of duodenum is made, and duodenum and ascending colon are mobilized medially. After medial mobilization of duodenum and colon, IVC and psoas major muscle are visualized. The tumor is abutting psoas major medially, right renal vein superiorly (Fig. 6.33d), and right kidney laterally (Fig. 6.33e). Following careful dissection of the medial, lateral, and superior planes, the vascular pedicle of the tumor is exposed and divided.

References

1. Rajiah P, Sinha R, Cuevas C, Dubinsky TJ, Bush Jr WH, Kolokythas O. Imaging of uncommon retroperitoneal masses. Radiographics. 2011;31:949–76.
2. Osman S, Lehnert BE, Elojeimy S, Cruite I, Mannelli L, Bhargava P, Moshiri M. A comprehensive review of the retroperitoneal anatomy, neoplasms, and pattern of disease spread. Curr Probl Diagn Radiol. 2013;42(5):191–208.
3. Scali EP, Chandler TM, Heffernan EJ, Coyle J, Harris AC, Chang SD. Primary retroperitoneal masses: what is the differential diagnosis? Abdom Imaging. 2015;40(6):1887–903.
4. Virseda Rodríguez JA, Donate Moreno MJ, Pastor Navarro H, Carrión López P, Martínez Ruiz J, Martínez Sanchiz C, Perán Teruel M. Primary retroperitoneal tumors: review of our 10-year case series. Arch Esp Urol. 2010;63(1):13–22.
5. Goenka AH, Shah SN, Remer EM. Imaging of the retroperitoneum. Radiol Clin North Am. 2012;50(2):333–55.
6. Heslin MJ, Lewis JJ, Nadler E, et al. Prognostic factors associated with long-term survival for retroperitoneal sarcoma: Implications for management. J Clin Oncol. 1997;15:2832–9.
7. Tambo M, Fujimoto K, Miyake M, Hoshiyama F, Matsushita C, Hirao Y. Clinicopathological review of 46 primary retroperitoneal tumors. Int J Urol. 2007;14(9):785–8.
8. Koh DM, Moskovic E. Imaging tumours of the retroperitoneum. Imaging. 2000;12:49–60.
9. Solla JA, Reed K. Primary retroperitoneal sarcomas. Am J Surg. 1986;152:496–8.
10. Storm FK, Mahvi DM. Diagnosis and management of retroperitoneal soft-tissue sarcoma. Ann Surg. 1991;214:2–10.
11. Elsayes KM, Staveteig PT, Narra VR, Chen ZM, Moustafa YL, Brown J. Retroperitoneal masses: magnetic resonance imaging findings with pathologic correlation. Curr Probl Diagn Radiol. 2007;36(3):97–106.
12. Nishino M, Hayakawa K, Minami M, et al. Primary retroperitoneal neoplasms: CT and MR imaging findings with anatomic and pathologic diagnostic clues. Radiographics. 2003;23:45–57.
13. Sanyal R, Remer EM. Radiology of the retroperitoneum: case-based review. Am J Roentgenol. 2009;192:S112–7.
14. Gustafson P, Herrlin K, Biling L, et al. Necrosis observed on CT enhancement is of prognostic value in soft tissue sarcoma. Acta Radiol. 1992;33(5):474–6.
15. Brennan C, Kajal D, Khalili K, Ghai S. Solid malignant retroperitoneal masses-a pictorial review. Insights Imaging. 2014;5(1):53–65.
16. Fletcher CDM, Bridge JA, Hogendoorn PCW, Mertens F, editors. WHO classification of tumours of soft tissue and bone. Pathology and genetics of tumours of soft tissue and bone. 4th ed. Lyon: IARC Press; 2013.
17. Jo VY, Fletcher CD. WHO classification of soft tissue tumours: an update based on the 2013 (4th) edition. Pathology. 2014;46(2):95–104.
18. Pham TH, Iqbal CW, Zarroug AE, Donohue JH, Moir C. Retroperitoneal sarcomas in children: outcomes from an institution. J Pediatr Surg. 2007;42(5):829–33.
19. Lewis JJ, Leung D, Woodruff JM, et al. Retroperitoneal soft-tissue sarcoma: analysis of 500 patients treated and followed at a single institution. Ann Surg. 1998;228(3):355–65.
20. Makela J, Kiviniemi H, Laitinen S. Prognostic factors predicting survival in the treatment of retroperitoneal sarcoma. Eur J Surg Oncol. 2000;26(6):552–5.
21. Swallow CJ, Catton CN. Local management of adult soft tissue sarcomas. Semin Oncol. 2007;34(3):256–69.
22. Neville A, Herts BR. CT characteristics of primary retroperitoneal neoplasms. Crit Rev Comput Tomogr. 2004;45(4):247–70.
23. Cormier JN, Pollock RE. Soft tissue sarcomas. CA Cancer J Clin. 2004;54:94–109.
24. Kim T, Murakami T, Oi H, et al. CT and MR imaging of abdominal liposarcoma. Am J Roentgenol. 1996;166:829–33.
25. Evans HL, Soule EH, Winkelmann RK. Atypical lipoma, atypical intramuscular lipoma, and well differentiated retroperitoneal liposarcoma: a reappraisal of 30 cases formerly classified as well differentiated liposarcoma. Cancer. 1979;43:574–84.

26. Fletcher CDM, Unni KK, Mertens F. WHO classification of tumours of soft tissue and bone. 3rd ed. Lyon: IARC Press; 2002.
27. Song T, Shen J, Liang BL, Mai WW, Li Y, Guo HC. Retroperitoneal liposarcoma: MR characteristics and pathological correlative analysis. Abdom Imaging. 2007;32:668–74.
28. Chang I-YJ, Herts BR. Retroperitoneal liposarcoma. J Urol. 2013;189:1093–4.
29. Kumarasamy NA, Gayer G. Retroperitoneal sarcomas. Semin Ultrasound CT MR. 2011;32:422–32.
30. Craig WD, Fanburg-Smith JC, Henry LR, Guerrero R, Barton JH. Fat-containing lesions of the retroperitoneum: radiologic-pathologic correlation. Radiographics. 2009;29(1):261–90.
31. Pereira JM, Sirlin CB, Pinto PS, et al. CT and MR imaging of extrahepatic fatty masses of the abdomen and pelvis: techniques, diagnosis, differential diagnosis, and pitfalls. Radiographics. 2005;25:69–85.
32. Hartman DS, Hayes WS, Choyke PL, Tibbetts GP. From the archives of the AFIP. Leiomyosarcoma of the retroperitoneum and inferior vena cava: radiologic-pathologic correlation. Radiographics. 1992;12:1203–20.
33. Fletcher CD, Gustafson P, Rydholm A, Willen H, Akerman M. Clinicopathologic re-evaluation of 100 malignant fibrous histiocytomas:prognostic relevance of subclassification. J Clin Oncol. 2001;19:3045–50.
34. O'Brien JE, Stout AP. Malignant fibrous xanthomas. Cancer. 1964;17:1445–55.
35. Coindre JM, Mariani O, Chibon F, et al. Most malignant fibrous histiocytomas developed in the retroperitoneum are dedifferentiated liposarcomas: a review of 25 cases initially diagnosed as malignant fibrous histiocytoma. Mod Pathol. 2003;16(3): 256–62.
36. Kim EE, Valenzuela RF, Kumar AJ, Raney RB, Eftekari F. Imaging and clinical spectrum of rhabdomyosarcoma in children. Clin Imaging. 2000;24:257–62.
37. Murphey MD, Walker EA, Wilson AJ, Kransdorf MJ, Temple HT, Gannon FH. From the archives of the AFIP: imaging of primary chondrosarcoma: radiologic-pathologic correlation. Radiographics. 2003;23(5): 1245–78.
38. van Rijswijk CS, Lieng JG, Kroon HM, Hogendoorn PC. Retroperitoneal extraskeletal osteosarcoma. J Clin Pathol. 2001;54(1):77–8.
39. Rha SE, Byun JY, Jung SE, Chun HJ, Lee HG, Lee JM. Neurogenic tumors in the abdomen: tumor types and imaging characteristics. Radiographics. 2003; 23(1):29–43.
40. Hughes MJ, Thomas JM, Fisher C, Moskovic EC. Imaging features of retroperitoneal and pelvic schwannomas. Clin Radiol. 2005;60:886–93.
41. Otal P, Mezghani S, Hassissene S, et al. Imaging of retroperitoneal ganglioneuroma. Eur Radiol. 2001; 11(6):940–5.
42. Lonergan GJ, Schwab CM, Suarez ES, Carlson CL. Neuroblastoma, ganglioneuroblastoma, and ganglioneuroma: radiologic-pathologic correlation. Radiographics. 2002;22(4):911–34.
43. Hruby G, Lehman M, Barton M, Peduto T. Malignant retroperitoneal paraganglioma: case report and review of treatment options. Australas Radiol. 2000;44: 478–82.
44. Feng N, Zhang W-Y, Wu X-T. Clinicopathological analysis of paraganglioma with literature review. World J Gastroenterol WJG. 2009;15(24):3003–8.
45. Scholz M, Zehender M, Thalmann GN, Borner M, Thöni H, Studer UE. Extragonadal retroperitoneal germ cell tumor: evidence of origin in the testis. Ann Oncol. 2002;13(1):121–4.
46. Keitoku M, Konishi I, Nanbu K, et al. Extraovarian sex cord-stromal tumor: case report and review of the literature. Int J Gynecol Pathol. 1997;16(2):180–5.
47. Balfe DM, Mauro MA, Koehler RE, et al. Gastrohepatic ligament: normal and pathologic CT anatomy. Radiology. 1984;150(2):485–90.
48. Dorfman RE, Alpern MB, Gross BH, et al. Upper abdominal lymph nodes: criteria for normal size determined with CT. Radiology. 1991;180(2):319–22.
49. Einstein DM, Singer AA, Chilcote WA, et al. Abdominal lymphadenopathy: spectrum of CT findings. Radiographics. 1991;11(3):457–72.
50. Coakley FV, Hricak H. Imaging of peritoneal and mesenteric disease: key concepts for the clinical radiologist. Clin Radiol. 1999;54(9):563–74.
51. Zhou LP, Zhang B, Peng WJ, Yang WT, Guan YB, Zhou KR. Imaging findings of Castleman disease of the abdomen and pelvis. Abdom Imaging. 2008;33:482–8.
52. Kim TJ, Han JK, Kim YH, Kim TK, Choi BI. Castleman disease of the abdomen: imaging spectrum and clinicopathologic correlations. J Comput Assist Tomogr. 2001;25:207–14.
53. Brian J, Douglas P. Erdheim-Chester disease of the retorperitoneum. Am J Roentgenol. 2001;176: 1130–1.
54. Yang DM, Jung DH, Kim H, Kang JH, Kim SH, Kim JH, Hwang HY. Retroperitoneal cystic masses: CT, clinical, and pathologic findings and literature review. Radiographics. 2004;24(5):1353–65.
55. Davidson AJ, Hartman DS. Lymphangioma of the retroperitoneum: CT and sonographic characteristic. Radiology. 1990;175(2):507–10.
56. Banerjee R, Gough J. Cystic mucinous tumours of the mesentery and retroperitoneum: report of three cases. Histopathology. 1988;12:527–32.
57. Lee SA, Bae SH, Ryoo HM, Jung HY, Jang SB, Kum YS. Primary retroperitoneal mucinous cystadenocarcinoma: a case report and review of the literature. Korean J Intern Med. 2007;22(4):287–91.
58. Singer S, Antonescu CR, Riedel E, et al. Histologic subtype and margin of resection predict pattern of recurrence and survival for retroperitoneal liposarcoma. Ann Surg. 2003;238(3):358–70; discussion 370–351.
59. de Vreeze RS, de Jong D, Tielen IH, et al. Primary retroperitoneal myxoid/round cell liposarcoma is a nonexisting disease: an immunohistochemical and molecular biological analysis. Mod Pathol Off J U S Can Acad Pathol Inc. 2009;22(2):223–31.

60. Geoerger B, Hero B, Harms D, et al. Metabolic activity and clinical features of primary ganglioneuromas. Cancer. 2001;91(10):1905–13.
61. Mirilas P, Skandalakis JE. Surgical anatomy of the retroperitoneal spaces, part V: surgical applications and complications. Am Surg. 2010;76(4):358–64.
62. Van Roggen JF, Hogendoorn PC. Soft tissue tumours of the retroperitoneum. Sarcoma. 2000;4(1–2):17–26.
63. Strauss DC, Hayes AJ, Thway K, Moskovic EC, Fisher C, Thomas JM. Surgical management of primary retroperitoneal sarcoma. Br J Surg. 2010; 97(5):698–706.
64. Strauss DC, Hayes AJ, Thomas JM. Retroperitoneal tumours: review of management. Ann R Coll Surg Engl. 2011;93(4):275–80.
65. Neuhaus SJ, Barry P, Clark MA, Hayes AJ, Fisher C, Thomas JM. Surgical management of primary and recurrent retroperitoneal liposarcoma. Br J Surg. 2005;92(2):246–52.
66. Bonvalot S, Rivoire M, Castaing M, Stoeckle E, Le Cesne A, Blay JY, Laplanche A. Primary retroperitoneal sarcomas: a multivariate analysis of surgical factors associated with local control. J Clin Oncol Off J Am Soc Clin Oncol. 2009;27(1):31–7.
67. Gronchi A, Lo Vullo S, Fiore M, Mussi C, Stacchiotti S, Collini P, Lozza L, Pennacchioli E, Mariani L, Casali PG. Aggressive surgical policies in a retrospectively reviewed single-institution case series of retroperitoneal soft tissue sarcoma patients. J Clin Oncol Off J Am Soc Clin Oncol. 2009;27(1):24–30.
68. Anaya DA, Lahat G, Wang X, Xiao L, Tuvin D, Pisters PW, Lev DC, Pollock RE. Establishing prognosis in retroperitoneal sarcoma: a new histology-based paradigm. Ann Surg Oncol. 2009;16(3):667–75.
69. Gubbay AD, Moschilla G, Gray BN, Thompson I. Retroperitoneal schwannoma: a case series and review. Aust N Z J Surg. 1995;65(3):197–200.
70. Cury J, Coelho RF, Srougi M. Retroperitoneal schwannoma: case series and literature review. Clinics. 2007;62(3):359–62.
71. Lehnert T, Cardona S, Hinz U, Willeke F, Mechtersheimer G, Treiber M, Herfarth C, Buechler MW, Schwarzbach MH. Primary and locally recurrent retroperitoneal soft-tissue sarcoma: local control and survival. Eur J Surg Oncol J Eur Soc Surg Oncol Br Assoc Surg Oncol. 2009;35(9):986–93.
72. Hassan I, Park SZ, Donohue JH, Nagorney DM, Kay PA, Nasciemento AG, Schleck CD, Ilstrup DM. Operative management of primary retroperitoneal sarcomas: a reappraisal of an institutional experience. Ann Surg. 2004;239(2):244–50.
73. Tseng WW, Wang SC, Eichler CM, Warren RS, Nakakura EK. Complete and safe resection of challenging retroperitoneal tumors: anticipation of multiorgan and major vascular resection and use of adjunct procedures. World J Surg Oncol. 2011;9:143.
74. Russo P, Kim Y, Ravindran S, Huang W, Brennan MF. Nephrectomy during operative management of retroperitoneal sarcoma. Ann Surg Oncol. 1997; 4(5):421–4.
75. Schwarzbach MH, Hormann Y, Hinz U, Leowardi C, Bockler D, Mechtersheimer G, Friess H, Buchler MW, Allenberg JR. Clinical results of surgery for retroperitoneal sarcoma with major blood vessel involvement. J Vasc Surg. 2006;44(1):46–55.
76. Sarkar R, Eilber FR, Gelabert HA, Quinones-Baldrich WJ. Prosthetic replacement of the inferior vena cava for malignancy. J Vasc Surg. 1998;28(1):75–81; discussion 82–73.
77. Kieffer E, Alaoui M, Piette JC, Cacoub P, Chiche L. Leiomyosarcoma of the inferior vena cava: experience in 22 cases. Ann Surg. 2006;244(2):289–95.
78. Zhang Z, Xiu D. Laparoscopic surgery for primary retroperitoneal tumors: a single institution experience of 14 cases. Surg Laparosc Endosc Percutan Tech. 2010;20(6):399–403.
79. Ahn KS, Han HS, Yoon YS, Kim HH, Lee TS, Kang SB, Cho JY. Laparoscopic re0ion of nonadrenal retroperitoneal tumors. Arch Surg. 2011;146(2):162–7.
80. Ball AJ, Siddiq FM, Garcia M, Ganjei-Azar P, Leveillee RJ. Hand-assisted laparoscopic removal of retroperitoneal liposarcoma. Urology. 2005;65(6): 1226.
81. Dalpiaz O, Gidaro S, Lipsky K, Schips L. Case report: laparoscopic removal of 10-cm retroperitoneal liposarcoma. J Endourol Endourol Soc. 2007;21(1):83–4.
82. Viani MP, Poggi RV, Pinto A, Maruotti RA. Gasless laparoscopic removal of retroperitoneal leiomyosarcoma. J Laparoendosc Surg. 1995;5(1):47–54.
83. Agresta F, De Simone P, Michelet I, Bedin N. Retroperitoneal leiomyosarcoma mimicking acute appendicitis: laparoscopic management. JSLS J Soc Laparoendosc Surg Soc Laparoendosc Surg. 2003; 7(2):177–9.
84. Park MJ, Seo KN, Kang HJ. Neurological deficit after surgical enucleation of schwannomas of the upper limb. J Bone Joint Surg. 2009;91(11):1482–6.
85. Sawada T, Sano M, Ogihara H, Omura T, Miura K, Nagano A. The relationship between pre-operative symptoms, operative findings and postoperative complications in schwannomas. J Hand Surg. 2006; 31(6):629–34.

MIX
Papier aus verantwortungsvollen Quellen
Paper from responsible sources
FSC® C105338

If you have any concerns about our products,
you can contact us on
ProductSafety@springernature.com

In case Publisher is established outside the EU,
the EU authorized representative is:
Springer Nature Customer Service Center GmbH
Europaplatz 3, 69115 Heidelberg, Germany

Printed by Libri Plureos GmbH
in Hamburg, Germany